**SECOND EDITION**

# Quality
# Improvement

## A Guide for Integration in Nursing

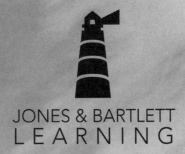

JONES & BARTLETT
LEARNING

# SECOND EDITION

# Quality
# Improvement

## A Guide for Integration in Nursing

**Anita Finkelman, MSN, RN**

Visiting Lecturer, Nursing Department
Recanati School for Community Health Professions
Faculty of Health Sciences
at Ben-Gurion University of the Negev
Beersheba, Israel
Visiting Lecturer

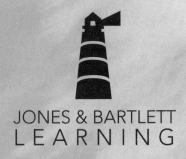

JONES & BARTLETT
LEARNING

*World Headquarters*
Jones & Bartlett Learning
5 Wall Street
Burlington, MA 01803
978-443-5000
info@jblearning.com
www.jblearning.com

Jones & Bartlett Learning books and products are available through most bookstores and online booksellers. To contact Jones & Bartlett Learning directly, call 800-832-0034, fax 978-443-8000, or visit our website, www.jblearning.com.

22505-1

**Production Credits**

VP, Product Management: Christine Emerton
Director of Product Management: Matthew Kane
Product Manager: Tina Chen
Content Strategist: Melina Leon
Project Manager: Kristen Rogers
Project Specialist: Madelene Nieman
Director of Marketing: Andrea DeFronzo
Senior Marketing Manager: Jennifer Scherzay
Production Services Manager: Colleen Lamy
VP, Manufacturing and Inventory Control: Therese Connell
Product Fulfillment Manager: Wendy Kilborn

Composition: S4Carlisle Publishing Services
Project Management: S4Carlisle Publishing Services
Cover Design: Scott Moden
Text Design: Kristin E. Parker
Senior Media Development Editor: Troy Liston
Rights & Permissions Manager: John Rusk
Rights Specialist: Maria Leon Maimone
Cover Image (Title Page, Part Opener, Chapter Opener): © Siripong Kaewla-iad/Moment/Getty Images
Printing and Binding: McNaughton & Gunn

**Library of Congress Cataloging-in-Publication Data**

Names: Finkelman, Anita Ward, author.
Title: Quality improvement : a guide for integration in nursing / Anita Finkelman.
Description: Second edition. | Burlington, Massachusetts : Jones & Bartlett Learning, [2021] | Includes bibliographical references and index.
Identifiers: LCCN 2020030736 | ISBN 9781284225051 (paperback)
Subjects: MESH: Quality Improvement | Nursing Process | Integrative Medicine | United States
Classification: LCC RT51 | NLM WY 100 AA1 | DDC 610.73—dc23
LC record available at https://lccn.loc.gov/2020030736

6048

Printed in the United States of America
24 23 22 21 20    10 9 8 7 6 5 4 3 2 1

# Brief Contents

# Contents

## SECTION II  Understanding the Healthcare Environment to Improve Care     121

## CHAPTER 5  Entering the Quality Improvement World . . . .123

## CHAPTER 6  Patient and Family Engagement in Quality Improvement . . . . . . . . . . . 151

## CHAPTER 7  Quality and Safety: Basic Understanding . . . . . . . . . . . 181

## CHAPTER 8  Setting the Stage for Quality Improvement . . . . . . . .217

**SECTION III  Ensuring the Healthcare Environment Is Focused on Quality  321**

# Acknowledgments

I thank my family, Fred, Shoshannah, and Deborah, for tolerating my long years of writing and supporting my efforts—being there when I was frustrated and also celebrating goals met. I dedicate this book to my new grandson, Matanel Yizhar, who was born as I completed this edition. The Jones & Bartlett Learning team is always a joy to work with on projects, and I appreciate the long support of Amanda Martin, as well as the team that worked on this edition: Tina Chen, Christina Freitas, and the marketing and production teams. My experiences in practice, administration, and education and all my students have given me opportunities to consider many aspects of nursing practice and education and the critical need for improvement.

# Preface

*Alice in Wonderland* provides a window into a world that is confusing, often viewed as nonsensical, where language and terminology are not clear, where characters change forms and their identities are uncertain, and where time is not always based on reality. One of the main characters, the Red Queen, makes it clear that you cannot expect to improve if you allow the status quo to continue. Alice, the main character, struggles in this world to find her way, as if in a maze, not knowing where to go or what her destination may be. Alice is full of questions as she tries to make Wonderland clearer to herself and engage others in it. She does discover that to be shown something improves her understanding. "What is the use of a book," thought Alice, "without pictures and conversation?" Alice also comments on change: "How puzzling all these changes are! I'm never sure what I'm going to be, from one minute to another."

Why have I chosen to use *Alice in Wonderland* to introduce this preface and also each section in the text? The world of healthcare and quality improvement is also confusing— language and terminology, roles and responsibilities, functions, the quality improvement process and measurement, and many other elements are not always clear. Trying to understand the system and quality improvement takes effort and comes with frustration. You need to ask questions and seek out information that changes and expands your knowledge. Quality improvement itself is based on change: data and measurement.

If we want to provide quality care, it is clear we cannot continue with the status quo. You will be entering a maze of information about quality improvement, which at times is confusing and at other times makes perfect sense. As a nurse, you must engage as Alice did in the journey to reach the goal.

As is typically the case when a nurse feels motivated to write a textbook, I was driven by the desire to provide resources for students to expand learning opportunities. This desire is influenced by my clinical and teaching experiences. Specifically, I sensed the need to help guide efforts toward quality improvement in nursing. As described in this text, the quality of healthcare in the United States has been the subject of intense scrutiny—for example, in May 2016, a study noted that if errors were considered in the listing of causes of death, they would be the third most common cause of death in the United States (Makary & Daniel, 2016). This statistic represents one example of many supporting the need for quality improvement.

In exploring the specifics of quality improvement, it is important to understand the national view of healthcare quality, which is fairly new and has been strongly influenced by the Institute of Medicine's *Quality Chasm* reports. Quality improvement is related to change, but not all change is improvement. Knowledge is very important to improvement, but not all knowledge leads to improvement. We need more than knowledge about quality improvement; we must take action and implement effective changes. The complexity of improvement is one of the difficulties we have in healthcare, and this complexity is compounded by both the complex healthcare system and the complexity of health problems and treatments for individual patients. None of these challenges, however, should be used as excuses to avoid what must be done: improve care daily, one patient at a time and throughout the system, whether that be within the healthcare delivery system, within an individual healthcare organization, or at the local, state, national, or even global level. To accomplish this goal requires a clear, effective framework that provides direction for planning and implementation of continuous quality improvement (CQI). Nurses must be prepared to engage in CQI in all settings and positions, demonstrating leadership. As Kennedy (2016) states, "A Culture of Safety begins with us. We need to follow the evidence and own up to our role" (p. 7). As this text moved to publication, globally we are challenged with COVID-19, a challenge that requires us to continue to be vigilant in maintaining an accessible, effective, quality healthcare delivery system. Nurses need to step up and help lead this effort.

This text is divided into 3 sections and 12 chapters. Section I covers Chapters 1–4, focusing on healthcare quality perspectives. The chapters consider the attributes of quality care and factors that influence it, such as ethical and legal concerns, accreditation, standards, education, professional concerns, and change. Section II includes Chapters 5–10, focusing on planning and measurement to meet CQI outcomes. The final section, Section III, includes Chapters 11–12 and covers the last phase of the quality improvement process: preventing quality problems or responding to problems based on measurement. In conclusion, Chapter 12 discusses the need for nursing engagement and effective leadership in CQI.

Each chapter begins with Chapter Objectives, a Chapter Outline, and Key Terms relevant to chapter content. Following the chapter Summary at the back of the chapter, Apply CQI includes the following resources and activities for additional student learning:

- *Chapter Highlights* identify some of the key points in the chapter.

- *Exemplars: Quality Improvement Roles and Responsibilities* for staff nurses, nurse managers, and advanced practice registered nurses are found at the conclusion of the chapter summary.
- *Critical Thinking and Clinical Reasoning and Judgment* provides opportunities for students to more deeply explore the chapter content by completing individual and team activities, including written assignments, development of presentations and visuals, and discussion in class or online.
- *Connect to Current Information* identifies web links related to some of the chapter content—for example, government sites and healthcare profession organizations.
- *Connect to Text Current Information with the Author* directs the reader to monthly updates from the author in the form of a blog, QI news, and literature review.
- *EBP, EBM, and Quality Improvement: Exemplar* provides a citation for a reference that explores evidence-based practice (EBP), evidence-based medicine (EBM), and quality improvement. Questions are posed to consider about the reference.
- *Evolving Case Study* is a case scenario focused on CQI with questions to consider.
- *References* identify sources used to develop the chapter content.

Chapters include figures, exhibits, and tables that provide additional data and information supporting chapter content. Chapters also include Stop and Consider features, which highlight important thoughts relating to the content. As students read the chapter, they should stop and consider the statement in relation to the content and their personal views.

One appendix is included at the end of the text:

- *Appendix A: Examples of Major Healthcare Organizations and Agencies, Governmental and Nongovernmental, Related to Quality Improvement*

# References

Carroll, L. (1865). *Alice's adventures in wonderland*. London, UK: Macmillan Publishing.

Carroll, L. (1872). *Through the looking-glass and what alice found there*. London, UK: Macmillan Publishing.

Kennedy, M. (2016). A culture of safety starts with us. *American Journal of Nursing, 116*(5), 7.

Makary, M., & Daniel, M. (2016, May 3). Medical error—the third leading cause of death in the US. *BMJ*. Retrieved from http://www.bmj.com/content/353/bmj.i2139/rr-40

---

**Special Note on the Affordable Care Act of 2010**

This text includes some information about the Affordable Care Act of 2010 (ACA); however, it does not cover this law in detail. The law has already undergone changes since its passage, and its long-term status is unclear. Other legislation is also discussed in the content. Students are encouraged to use the **Connect to Text Current Information with the Author** found at the end of each chapter in the **Apply CQI** section. On the accompanying **Navigate Companion Website**, the author posts monthly information in the form of a Blog, QI News, and Literature Review. ACA information will be updated there. In addition, students are encouraged to keep up to date with healthcare legislation and policy. This is rarely a static area and requires ongoing review.

# Healthcare Quality Perspectives

*"Begin at the beginning," the King said, very gravely, "and go on till you come to the end: then stop."*

Lewis Carroll, *Alice's Adventures in Wonderland* (1865)

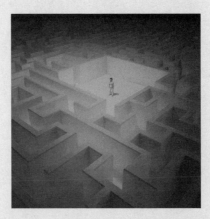

The goal of the maze is to reach a state of quality care. To find your way out of the Continuous Quality Improvement Maze you first must begin to understand quality care and improvement: What is it? What is the status of quality care? What influences quality care? Ethics, legal, accreditation, standards, education, professional concerns, and change.

# CHAPTER 1

# Healthcare Quality

## CHAPTER OBJECTIVES

At the conclusion of this chapter, the learner will be able to:

- Describe quality care and its history.
- Examine the Quality Chasm reports and their impact on healthcare delivery.
- Analyze the current status of healthcare quality in the United States.
- Synthesize the key elements of the vision of healthcare quality.
- Examine the relationship between value and costs in healthcare delivery.
- Appraise critical healthcare legislation and regulations.
- Assess the National Quality Strategy and implications for nursing.
- Appraise the status of leadership, interprofessional teamwork, and nursing responsibility for continuous quality improvement.

## OUTLINE

## KEY TERMS

Continuous quality
  improvement (CQI)
Discrimination
Disparities
Diversity
Error
Health literacy
Healthcare organizations
  (HCOs)

Learning health system
Macrosystem
Macroview
Mesosystems
Microsystems
Microview
Outcomes
Pay for performance
Process

Quality care
Quality gap
Safety
STEEEP®
Structure
Surveillance
System
System thinking
Triple Aim

# Introduction

As expressed by Nance (2008), the medical community has made great strides toward acknowledging and correcting the problem of medical injury in our society: "We know how to prevent medical injuries. The Institute of Medicine [IOM] report that received so much attention also made a clear and unambiguous observation: It's not bad people; it's bad systems. Fix those systems! More than a half-century of thought, experimentation, and hard work in cognitive psychology, human factors engineering, and several high-hazard fields, most notably aviation, underlie that recommendation. System failures cause human failures. Fix systems if you want to stop medical mistakes and injuries. The efforts to fix systems have been enormous. Since the Institute

of Medicine [IOM] report, there has been a steady crescendo of increasing development, testing, and implementation of new safe practices by hospitals throughout country" (p. vii). The emphasis on systems continues to be important in the complex area of quality care.

As we learn more about **continuous quality improvement (CQI)**, we are better able to appreciate its complexity. Many **healthcare organizations (HCOs)** are revising visions of how healthcare delivery should be viewed, initiating innovations, and developing leadership required for integration and coordination of care so that care is patient centered (Bisognano & Kenney, 2012). The publication of *To Err Is Human* (IOM, 1999) and *Crossing the Quality Chasm* (IOM, 2001a) is sometimes described as the "Big Bang" in healthcare quality. In the words of Sollecito and Johnson (2013), "Suddenly, quality improvement was acknowledged to be a professional responsibility, a quality-of-care issue rather than a managerial tactic" (p. 25).

The content in this chapter reviews the overall perspective on healthcare quality—the CQI framework—and other background information needed to begin an examination of CQI. It echoes the sentiment of a question posed by Nash, Evans, and Bowman (2006): "After decades of research and numerous press reports indicating just how poor the quality of health care is in the United States, how can we continue denying that improving the quality of care is one of the most, if not the most, pressing public health issue today?" (p. 3).

Nurses have a responsibility to participate actively in improving care in their daily practice, whether that be in care delivery, management, education, or research; in all types of settings and positions, such as staff nurse, manager, and advanced practice; and in healthcare policy making at local, state, federal, and global levels. This text supports the need for nursing engagement and leadership, but to achieve this objective requires knowledge and then application.

## Healthcare Quality in the United States

The early reports from the National Academy of Medicine (NAM) [the former Institute of Medicine (IOM) and referred to as NAM for publications from 2015 to the current year (IOM, 2015)] describe **quality care** as "providing patients with appropriate services in a technically competent manner, with good communication, shared decision-making, and cultural sensitivity" (IOM, 2001a, p. 232). This definition emphasizes an active relationship with the patient and expectation of high performance on the part of the system and its providers.

Efforts to improve care have a long history, although major initiatives toward this end were slow in arriving. Nursing was directly involved early on with the work of Florence Nightingale in the late 1800s and early 1900s. Nightingale began to examine the healthcare environment, collecting and analyzing data and recommending changes, although this was largely not noted as part of the nursing profession at the time. With greater recognition of her work, the Institute for Healthcare Improvement (IHI) has honored Nightingale by naming an IHI meeting room after her and highlighting her contributions to care improvement (McGaffigan, 2019):

- **Everyone in the healthcare system contributes to quality and safety.** Nightingale emphasized the team.

- **Using the right improvement tools and methods matter.** Nightingale used data collection, description, and analysis to make decisions.

- **Improving quality means address what matters to patients.** Nightingale recognized the need to assist patients and to make a difference in their care with dignity and respect.

- **Culture and outcomes are linked.** Nightingale advocated for the patient, recognizing the importance of individual characteristics and needs.

- **Nurses are high-impact leaders.** Nightingale led initial steps to recognize nursing as a profession that has much to offer patients and the care delivery system, including quality improvement.

- **Understanding data is essential for improvement.** Nightingale used statistics, which was a new approach to healthcare problems and assessment of change.

Others also began to address healthcare delivery problems, but systematically assessing care and then determining solutions were unknown areas. Later in this text, expansion of models and theories about CQI and their influence on the development of effective methods to measure and improve care over time are discussed. It is critical for nurses to continue to actively participate in CQI, including the development of measurement methods—monitoring, collecting and analyzing data, creating new solutions—to help prevent or respond to quality care problems. We have made progress, with acceleration in ideas, technology, and research, but from this expansion we have also learned that we do not know enough. We now look at CQI from the system perspective, but each nurse must also consider key concerns from an individual provider perspective: (1) How can I improve care for my patients? (2) How can I improve the system of care? Individuals and populations must be considered. Other industries have made great strides in addressing safety concerns, but healthcare has been much slower in developing improvement efforts in a highly complex system with complex needs. Berwick, a leading authority in healthcare quality improvement, suggested that it is time to "break the rules for better care," recommending that healthcare leaders ask this of staff and patients: If you could break or change a rule in service of a better care experience for patients and staff, what would it be? (Berwick, Loehrer, & Gunther-Murphy, 2017). Examples of issues that might be considered are visiting hours, licensure, patient access such as appointment processes, waiting times for appointments and clinical reports, engaging families, paperwork, patient sleep interruption, and so on. This is not the usual approach, but asking this question may get to important aspects of care that could be improved, may not be necessary, or could be changed.

Millenson (2006) aptly described one of the key obstacles to the quality improvement initiative: "Like the civil rights movement, the quality improvement movement cast doubts on deeply held traditional beliefs; in this case, those of the individual physician. While it might have been the individual doctor's 'duty' to pursue process improvement and outcomes measurement, it was in his 'interest,' given traditional financial incentives" (p. 15). This view of "duty" rather than "interest" did slow

down CQI efforts; however, this trend has changed with the greater emphasis on the need for improvement. One might also consider how nurses have responded, as nursing has also been slow to become more competent in CQI and assume greater leadership. Elements of CQI have been included in nursing standards for a long time, but until recently these efforts had not been enough to move CQI toward center stage in nursing. Consider, for example, the publication of *The Future of Nursing* (IOM, 2010) and its emphasis on nursing competency and leadership as a requirement for CQI, which is discussed in this text.

**STOP AND CONSIDER 1-1**

Up until 1999, we had limited in-depth knowledge of healthcare quality.

# The *Quality Chasm* Reports and the Healthcare Delivery System

As articulated by Gantz, Sorenson, and Howard (2003) two decades ago, "The movement [quality improvement] now reaches beyond the walls of health care since *quality* is a part of everyday conversation not only among providers and payers but also consumers" (p. 324). This insight remains true today, and consumers are even more involved in commenting on healthcare. To appreciate the current views and status of U.S. healthcare, it is necessary to gain a historical perspective, particularly focusing on the 1990s to today. Why is this background important? Healthcare delivery is influenced by healthcare policy, and so it is important to examine some of the policy issues—that is, how they are identified and their impact. For nurses to assume greater leadership, they need this background information. The place to begin is with President Bill Clinton's administration.

Presidents may form short-term commissions without approval of Congress to examine issues and problems. President Clinton established the President's Advisory Commission on Consumer Protection and Quality in the Health Care Industry, which published a final report, *Quality First: Better Health Care for All Americans* (1998). The report indicated that there was concern about healthcare quality and a lack of understanding about its status and how quality improvement is accomplished and maintained. The commission recommended that the Institute of Medicine (IOM/NAM) assume the responsibility for additional extensive examination. The IOM/NAM is a nonprofit agency that is located in Washington, DC. The organization is not connected to the government but, rather, serves as an advisor to government, policy makers, businesses, educators, and professionals. Since its work is highly respected, it has great influence. How does the organization provide advice? Typically, it is asked to examine a specific problem by an external party such as Congress, the president, government agencies, professional organizations, and so on, as was the case with President Clinton's Advisory Commission on Consumer Protection and Quality in the Health Care Industry. The NAM staff invites a panel of experts to examine the problem. The panel is provided with staff support. Often a panel will work for several years, examining information and data and asking for expert testimony. Then a report is published that provides information and recommendations. These recommendations may be ignored or may be used to initiate changes in policy, laws, regulations, education, and so on. The reports cover a broad range of topics, including healthcare. See the Connect to Current Information section at the end of this chapter for a link to the site, which provides free access to the reports.

Since 1999, the NAM has examined many issues and published reports related to healthcare quality and generally referred to as the *Quality Chasm* reports. Through this process of using multiple panels of experts representing a variety of professions, these reports describe the problems, define critical terms for consistency, develop aims or goals and a vision of a quality healthcare system, develop a framework for national monitoring, and address the issue of healthcare professions competencies that are needed to meet the goals and the vision. The following descriptions provide an overview of the critical reports in this series. These reports have a major impact on how the United States views its healthcare system and provide important direction for planning and implementing national and state CQI initiatives and HCO quality improvement programs (Finkelman, 2019).

## To Err Is Human (1999)

As requested by President Clinton's commission, the IOM/NAM began to examine healthcare, focusing on errors. This report (IOM, 1999) did not just become a policy report that sat on a bookshelf; it was the report that opened a "Pandora's box". The media took note of this report and ran stories on the radio and television news, in newspapers, and in other print publications. Why was this topic so interesting? The report noted that approximately 44,000 to nearly 100,000 patients died annually in the United States due to errors. This information was overwhelming to consumers who trusted the healthcare delivery system. It came at a time when healthcare consumers had found their voice, mostly due to the experience of the managed care era when consumers became angry about the growing loss of choice in healthcare. At the time of the report, there was little systematic monitoring of healthcare data, meaning the description of death rates due to errors was probably not accurate; in all likelihood, the true rate was higher. The report's concern about errors was one aspect that was discussed, but also important was the recognition of the need for systematic monitoring.

Another issue that arose from this examination was the concern about the "blame culture" in which HCOs focus on blaming individual staff for errors and ignore the impact of system issues. This critical topic is discussed in further detail in other chapters. The report provided two important definitions: **Safety** is "freedom from accidental injury (IOM, 1999, p. 4). **Error** is the "failure of a planned action to be completed as intended or the use of a wrong plan to achieve an aim" (IOM, 1999, p. 4). Safety is part of healthcare quality. It is not the only dimension of quality, but resolving errors is important in achieving a high-quality healthcare system (IOM, 2001a; Sadeghi, Barzi, Mikhail, & Shabot, 2013).

The report concluded with recommendations, particularly noting that improving patient safety requires a comprehensive approach. There is no one magic solution. The other critical conclusion was that the system must move away from the prevailing blame culture. It is important to realize that at the time of this report the United States really had no comprehensive view or model of quality care or any method for monitoring and evaluating care. We had some pieces to the puzzle, but no system. An analysis of status two decades later indicates changes have been made but not enough (Bates & Singh, 2018).

## Crossing the Quality Chasm (2001)

With the publication of *To Err Is Human*, it was recognized that we needed to know more about the healthcare delivery system and its quality. A second panel was formed to continue this examination, resulting in *Crossing the Quality Chasm* (IOM, 2001a). This report concluded that the U.S. healthcare delivery system was dysfunctional, greatly varied in performance, fragmented and poorly organized, confusing, and complex. There was treatment overuse, underuse, and misuse, all of which have a major impact on quality. This situation is often referred to as a **quality gap**. These outcomes were disturbing. In addition, other aspects of concern were noted. Chronic disease was a growing problem, crossing the

life span with many people having more than one chronic disease. The system was not prepared to deliver quality care for this population. In addition, a problem with disparities in healthcare was noted, although there was limited understanding of this problem.

The report began the process of describing a vision of the U.S. healthcare delivery system focused on quality, and this helped to develop a structure for CQI. If the only *Quality Chasm* report had been the 1999 report, we would not be where we are today, making more and more efforts to improve care. *Crossing the Quality Chasm* examined healthcare with greater depth, which was needed to fully recognize that the system had serious problems and was very weak. However, even though the first two reports indicated there were many problems, it took more reports, examination, and work to drive the need for CQI and make it a priority (Bisognano & Kenney, 2012).

## Envisioning the National Healthcare Quality Report (2001)

As was noted in the first two *Quality Chasm* reports, there was great need for systematic monitoring of healthcare quality so that we would better understand the status of quality care and then use this information to improve care. *Envisioning the National Healthcare Quality Report* (IOM, 2001b) describes an initial framework for a national healthcare quality monitoring report that would be completed annually. As expressed in this report, "*The National Healthcare Quality Report* (NHQR) should serve as a yardstick or the barometer by which to gauge progress in improving the performance of the healthcare delivery system in consistently providing high-quality care" (p. 2). The framework for the annual report is influenced by the aims and the vision as well as other recommendations from *Quality Chasm* reports. The annual report makes data and analysis available to decision makers and the public. The original description of the framework has changed, but the core elements are the same. The Agency for Healthcare Research and Quality (AHRQ), which is an agency in the U.S. Department of Health and Human Services (HHS), is responsible for the annual *report, which is now a combined report entitled National Healthcare Quality and Disparities Report (QDR)*. Current reports are accessible at the AHRQ website. A link is provided in the Connect to Current Information with the Author section at the end of this chapter.

## Priority Areas for National Action (2003)

When the direction changed from developing a framework to routinely monitoring care quality, the question of what should be monitored arose. It was clear that not all aspects of care could or should be monitored. The *Priority Areas for National Action* report discusses the issue of prioritizing and identified the focus areas used in the first annual report (IOM, 2003a). As was expected, the focus areas have changed as certain areas have improved, reducing the need for monitoring, redefinition of areas, and new areas that need to be added.

## Health Professions Education: A Bridge to Quality (2003)

After considerable time describing healthcare delivery problems and identifying aims, a vision, and setting up a system to monitor care, attention turned to the need for healthcare professionals to be prepared and competent to ensure that care is of the highest quality possible. This need impacts both staff education and healthcare professionals' academic education, as both settings prepare staff for professional roles, such as physician, nurse, pharmacist, healthcare administrator, and many others. If the healthcare system is working toward improvement but the new healthcare professionals entering the system are not prepared in core areas, then improving care will be difficult. As a consequence of this recognition, the

report's expert panel identified five healthcare professions core competencies that are necessary to reach an acceptable level of quality care (IOM, 2003b, p. 4).

1. Provide patient-centered care.
2. Work in interdisciplinary/interprofessional teams.
3. Employ evidence-based practice.
4. Apply quality improvement.
5. Utilize informatics.

The report recommended that all healthcare profession education programs adopt these core competencies. It is significant that the emphasis is not on a specific healthcare profession but rather focuses on all healthcare professions. These competencies should be common to all healthcare professions, although other specific competencies also pertain to each profession. HCO staff that are not prepared in these areas must be updated, as the competencies apply not only to students but also to staff. These competencies are directly related to healthcare problems and possible solutions. This text emphasizes these competencies for nurses because they are integral to understanding and application of CQI; however, it is also important for CQI to be a collaborative effort among all healthcare providers.

## Nursing Reports

The IOM/NAM has had a major impact on nursing, as it has published several reports on nursing. The report *Nursing and Nursing Education: Public Policy and Private Action* (IOM, 1983) recommended that nurses should have an active role in National Institutes of Health (NIH) activities, and as a result, Congress established the Center for Nursing Research at NIH in 1993, which is now called the National Institute of Nursing Research (NINR). The NINR has an impact on nursing and CQI. It provides greater nursing professional emphasis on research, which is necessary for evidence-based practice (EBP), a critical component of CQI and focus of one of the core competencies.

The second major nursing report, *Keeping Patients Safe: Transforming the Work Environment for Nurses* (IOM, 2004a), emphasizes the need to transform the work environment for nurses, focusing on the 24/7 role of nurses in acute care and how their work impacts the quality of care. The report's recommendations focus on four areas: (1) adopting transformational leadership and evidence-based management, (2) maximizing the capability of the workforce, (3) designing work and workspaces to prevent and mitigate errors, and (4) creating and sustaining cultures of safety (IOM, 2004a, pp. 7–14). This examination of acute care nursing provides important information about the status of nursing in the healthcare system and what needs to improve. The report strongly supports the need for nurses to assume more active roles in CQI but concludes that nurses are not sufficiently prepared to do this. Nursing leadership is also emphasized in this report.

In 2010, a landmark report titled *The Future of Nursing: Leading Change, Advancing Health* was published, which continued expanding on the earlier work done (IOM, 2010). This report discusses changes needed in nursing degrees, the need to increase the number of BSN-prepared nurses and doctoral-prepared nurses, barriers to scope of practice, the need for lifelong learning, workforce issues, and other relevant professional concerns. *Keeping Patients Safe* (IOM, 2004a) provides the critical groundwork for *The Future of Nursing* report. In many respects, *Keeping Patients Safe* discusses more significant information about nursing practice, such as the major roles of nurses in the healthcare delivery system, the need for nurses to be leaders in CQI (although they are often not prepared to do so), staffing and staff schedules, the blame culture, work design and its impact on quality, the need for transformational leadership, the nursing shortage, risks of working long hours, and the need for greater use of **surveillance** or ongoing monitoring of patients. Although this report's content is significant for nursing, it received less attention when published compared

to *The Future of Nursing*. The 2010 report and a progress report (NAM, 2016) are discussed in more detail in other chapters in this text.

## Public Health Reports

The *Quality Chasm* reports also examine public health. The two major public health reports are *The Future of the Public's Health in the 21st Century* (IOM, 2003c) and *Who Will Keep the Public Healthy?* (IOM, 2003d). Although we often think of the public health system as separate from the "healthcare delivery system," it should be an integral part of the entire healthcare delivery system. Today, there is much more focus given to the entire system and recognition that more needs to be done to provide care and meet health needs within the patient's community. Public/community health delivery also requires improvement and more public health services and public health professionals. The first report identifies aspects of public health that should be reviewed: the population health approach, public health infrastructure, partnerships, accountability, evidence, and communication. In addition to the five healthcare professions competencies identified in the report *Health Professions Education* (IOM, 2003b), the second public health report notes that effective public health requires that staff be competent in informatics, genomics, communication, culture, community-based participatory research, global health, policy and law, and public health ethics.

## Impact of the *Quality Chasm* Reports

The *Quality Chasm* reports have had a major impact on U.S. views of quality care, influencing innovations to improve care and healthcare legislation, such as the Patient Protection and Affordable Care Act of 2010 (ACA). Staff may wonder why it is important to pay attention to this work on quality care and its numerous reports. The answer: It represents the leading source of critical examination of the U.S. healthcare delivery system and its outcomes. Its recommendations influence the creation of new legislation and regulations and impact government departments and agencies, such as the U.S. Department of Health and Human Services (HHS), Centers for Medicare and Medicaid Services (CMS), Food and Drug Administration (FDA), Centers for Disease Control and Prevention (CDC), AHRQ, Occupational Safety and Health Administration (OSHA), National Institute for Occupational Health and Safety (NIOSH), and state and local departments and services.

The *Quality Chasm* reports have led to many changes in healthcare. The responsibility for CQI has typically been more important to higher-level healthcare administration; however, now this responsibility has been expanded to include all levels of management and healthcare providers who make decisions about healthcare quality on a daily basis. Some of the recommendations influenced changes in HCOs and CQI-related organizations' requirements, such as those of The Joint Commission, which accredits most HCOs. Healthcare professional organizations and educational institutions also consider the *Quality Chasm* reports' recommendations relevant to their goals and use them in developing initiatives to improve care and healthcare professional education, such as the following examples, many of which are discussed in other sections of this text:

- The Joint Commission designation of annual safety goals, which are monitored by organizations accredited by The Joint Commission (the goals change annually depending on the need)
- The Joint Commission and World Health Organization (WHO) initiatives focusing on reducing errors globally
- The development of the Institute for Healthcare Improvement (IHI) and resources about CQI for staff, education programs, and healthcare professions students
- Institute for Healthcare Improvement 5 Million Lives Campaign collaborating with The Joint Commission's High 5s Project

- Centers for Medicare and Medicaid Services (CMS) reimbursement changes and development of the Hospital Acquired Complications (HACs) and the Hospital Readmission Reduction initiatives
- Development of increased interest in interprofessional collaborative teams leading to the need to improve interprofessional education; publication of major reports on these topics developed jointly by an interprofessional group
- Development of web-based information and tools to improve care
- Establishment of the CMS Hospital Quality Initiative, providing comparison information on quality
- Publication of *The Future of Nursing: Leading Change, Advancing Health* (IOM, 2010), a critical report influenced by the previous *Quality Chasm* reports on CQI and related nursing reports; subsequent progress reports
- Publication of *Educating Nurses: A Call for Radical Transformation* (Benner, Sutphen, Leonard, & Day, 2010), a major report about a study that concludes there is needed to improve nursing education
- Passage and implementation of critical federal legislation focused on healthcare delivery, access to care, costs, and state legislation
- Healthy People 2030 (revisions of this initiative)
- U.S. Patient Safety Awareness Week held annually to increase awareness (HHS, AHRQ, 2019a) and also World Patient Safety Day (WHO, 2019)
- To improve the overall quality, efficiency, and value of the health care services provided by the nation's health centers, and to celebrate their recent achievements in providing care to more than 28 million patients, Health Resources & Services Administration (HRSA) provides Quality Improvement Awards (QIA). These awards recognize the highest performing health centers nationwide as well as those health centers that have made significant quality

improvement gains from the previous year. In FY 2019, the U.S. Department of Health and Human Services (HHS) announced nearly $107 million in Quality Improvement Awards to 1,273 health centers across all U.S. states, territories, and the District of Columbia. Health centers will use these one-time grant funds to expand their achievements in clinical quality improvement, care delivery efficiency, and the overall value of healthcare in the communities they serve (HHS, HRSA, 2019).

- National Steering Committee for Patient Safety established in 2018; co-led by AHRQ and the IHI along with the National Patient Safety Foundation (NPSF), which has merged with IHI (NPSF, 2017), collaborates with more than 20 organizations including the American Nurses Association to develop a national blueprint to reduce patient harm (HHS, AHRQ, 2019b).

The pressure to focus more on CQI has been influenced by the *Quality Chasm* reports, but also by initiatives that developed from these reports and other reports that followed (Draper, Felland, Liebhaber, & Melichar, 2008). Changes, such as the preceding examples, are ongoing. The Joint Commission changed its focus to requiring that its accredited HCOs report on core quality measures for accreditation rather than using a broad-based approach that tries to assess all aspects of an HCO. Since insurers typically expect HCOs such as hospitals to be accredited, there is now increased HCO motivation to meet these requirements to ensure reimbursement of services. The Magnet Recognition Program® places greater emphasis on HCO nursing service responsibilities and leadership in HCO quality improvement, supporting the recognition of nurses meeting critical CQI responsibilities and the need for this leadership. These examples and others are discussed in more detail throughout this text, but they are mentioned here to illustrate the major impact of the *Quality Chasm* reports on health policy, healthcare delivery, nursing practice, and healthcare profession education. In 2014, The U.S. Senate Committee on Health, Education, Labor, and Pensions held meetings on healthcare quality and discussed the recommendations from the *Quality Chasm* reports, their outcomes, and the current quality status, bringing this critical problem area to Congress. **Exhibit 1-1** provides excerpts of this discussion, illustrating how important this topic is in the United States and the concern about the need for improvement.

---

**Exhibit 1-1** Excerpts from Expert Testimony, U.S. Senate Committee on Health, Education, Labor, and Pensions (HELP), Subcommittee on Primary Health and Aging. Patient Safety Hearing (July 17, 2014)

**Peter Pronovost, MD, PhD, FCCM:** Medicine today has preventable harm as the third leading cause of death. We do not. Bates and I used published literature to estimate that over 220,000 preventable deaths occur from healthcare; that is over 600 deaths daily, which is far more than from mining or faulty automobiles, yet receiving far less attention. This estimate is conservative and does not include more than 120,000 deaths from teamwork failures, 80,000 deaths from misdiagnosis, or thousands of deaths from sepsis. Medicine today squanders a third of every dollar spent on therapies that do not get patients well, that result from treating preventable complications, and that result from administrative inefficiencies and fraud. This is about $9,000 per U.S. household (Fineberg, 2012), money that could be better spent on preschool education and STEM, on innovation, and on securing a better tomorrow for all Americans. Medicine today invests heavily in information technology. The federal government and healthcare organizations have spent hundreds of billions of dollars on health information technology with little to show for it. The promised improvements in safety have not been realized, and productivity has decreased rather than increased.

**Ashish Jha, MD, MPH:** So here we are, 15 years after *To Err Is Human*, and it is critical to ask a simple question: How much progress have we made? First, I want to start off with some good news. We have dramatically increased our awareness of patient safety issues and changed how we think about medical errors. In the past, medical errors were thought to be the result of individuals behaving badly. We blamed the doctor who ordered the wrong treatment, the pharmacist who dispensed the wrong dose, or the nurse who gave the medication to the wrong patient. This idea that adverse events were due to bad people led to a "deny and defend" culture among healthcare professionals and prevented progress on patient safety. Today, we know better. We know that medical errors are largely the result of bad systems of care delivery, not individual providers.

Four years ago, the *New England Journal of Medicine* published a terrific study from North Carolina hospitals which found that between 2002 and 2007, there had been little or no progress in reducing harm from unsafe medical care (Landrigan, Parry, Bones, Hackbarth, Goldman, & Sharek, 2010). A recent study led by Dr. John James found that between 200,000 and 400,000 Americans die each year from unsafe medical care, which makes it the third leading killer in the United States, behind only heart disease and cancer (James, 2013). Finally, in an eye-opening November 2011 report on adverse events in hospitals, the Office of the Inspector General (OIG) in the Department of Health and Human Services found that 13.5% of Medicare patients suffered an injury in the hospital that prolonged their stay or caused permanent harm or death. An additional 13.5% of Medicare patients suffered temporary harm, such as an allergic reaction or hypoglycemia. Together, the data suggest that more than one in four hospitalized Medicare beneficiaries suffers some sort of injury during their inpatient stay, much higher than previous rates. The OIG report also found that unsafe care contributes to 180,000 deaths of Medicare beneficiaries each year and that Medicare pays at least $4.4 billion to treat these injuries (HHS/OIG, 2010).

Despite all the focus on patient safety, it seems we have not made much progress at all. The news is not all bad, of course—and there are areas where we have made meaningful gains. The area of safety that has seen the biggest improvement is healthcare-associated infections.

While much attention in patient safety has been paid to acute hospitals, we have generally paid far less attention to what happens when patients are discharged. In a different report, the OIG at HHS found that 22% of Medicare beneficiaries in skilled nursing facilities (SNFs) suffered a medical injury that prolonged their stay or caused permanent harm or death. An additional 11% suffered temporary medical injury. All told, OIG estimates that adverse events cost Medicare roughly $2.8 billion per year, and about half of these events are preventable. The OIG report is particularly alarming given that about 20% of hospitalized Medicare patients go to a SNF after discharge (HHS/OIG, 2014). We need a renewed call to improve patient safety as a national priority.

The strategy for improvement has to focus on three main areas: metrics, accountability, and incentives. Getting the metrics right may be the most important. The fundamental problem is that most healthcare organizations don't track the safety of their care. In addition, I believe that health information technology has a critical role to play in improving patient safety. But metrics and reporting alone will not be enough. We also need to make safe care part of the business of providing healthcare. And this requires incentives.

**Tejal Gandhi, MD, MPH, CPPS:** I would like to talk to you today about ambulatory patient safety and the priorities and challenges that we currently face. Much of the effort of the patient safety movement over the past 15 years, since the Institute of Medicine report *To Err Is Human* (http://www.nap.edu/catalog.php?record_id=9728), has focused on improving patient safety in the hospital setting. However, it is important to remember that most care is given outside of hospitals, and there are numerous safety issues that exist in other health settings that are quite different from those we face in hospitals (Gandhi, 2010). The setting that we know the most about, in terms of ambulatory safety issues, is primary care. I will touch on three areas in particular: medication safety, missed and delayed diagnoses, and transitions of care. Studies have shown that medication errors are common in primary care and that adverse drug events, or injuries due to drugs, occur in up to 25% of patients within 30 days of being prescribed a drug (http://www.ncbi.nlm.nih.gov /pubmed/12700376). In addition, a key medication safety issue in ambulatory care, which is not an issue in hospitals, is nonadherence. Missed and delayed diagnosis is a key issue as well—this is the most common type of outpatient malpractice claim (usually missed and delayed diagnosis of cancer in primary care). Last, we know that patients are vulnerable during transitions in care. These transitions occur all the time in healthcare—hospital to home, nursing home to emergency department, rehabilitation center to visiting nurse. Transitions are high-risk times, when key pieces of information—for example, medication changes, pending test results, additional workups that need to happen—can be lost. One study found that after hospital discharge, within 3 to 5 days, one-third of patients were taking their medications differently than how they were prescribed at discharge (Schnipper et al., 2006). A major theme throughout ambulatory safety is patient engagement—partnering with patients to achieve safer care.

**Joanne Disch, PhD, RN, FAAN:** The estimate by James (2013) that possibly 400,000 preventable deaths (PDs) occur each year is more accurate than the previous Institute of Medicine (IOM) projection of 98,000/year (*To Err Is Human*, 1999). However, I would respectfully suggest that the title of this hearing understates the problem—and the title of the hearing should be changed to "More than 1,000 preventable deaths—and 10,000 preventable serious complications a day—is too many."

This morning, I will highlight some of the key factors influencing patient safety and make three recommendations, which I know from my 46 years as a nurse make a difference: (1) ensuring an adequate and appropriately educated supply of registered nurses at the bedside, (2) actively engaging patients and families as partners in their care, and (3) moving hospitals and other healthcare settings to embrace a safety culture and become high-reliability organizations. My comments focus on the hospital setting since that is where we have the most data, although the principles apply to other settings.

Nurses are the cornerstones of the American healthcare system. Registered nurses form the largest element (2.6 million), with more than half (58%) working in medical and surgical hospitals (Bureau of Labor Statistics [BLS], 2013). They provide care 24/7 and are on the "ground floor" of care delivery. They are the eyes and ears of patients and their families, as well as physicians and other healthcare practitioners (HCPs) who are interacting with the patient intermittently. The nurse's role is to assess the patient's condition and response to treatment, perform indicated treatments, prevent complications, assist the patient and family in adjusting to the treatment or impact of chronic illness, and create a safe environment within which health, healing, or a peaceful death can occur. It is the nurse who sees a skin breakdown that will lead to a bedsore; it is the nurse who notices the older woman's unsteady gait and puts in place strategies to prevent a fall; it is the nurse who notices that the dose of the drug ordered is not relieving the pain and who initiates a conversation with the physician to get the order changed. Individuals who have been hospitalized, or have had a family member hospitalized, understand the essential role of the nurse. Actually, nursing care is the reason for hospitalization—and it is the nurse who is the "last line of defense" against error.

**Other references noted in comments from the congressional testimony:**

Bureau of Labor Statistics (BLS). (2013). Employment projections 2012–2022. Retrieved from http://www.bls.gov/news.release/ecopro.t08.htm

Fineberg, H. (2012). Shattuck lecture. A successful and sustainable health system—how to get there from here. *New England Journal of Medicine, 366*, 1020–1027.

Gandhi, T. (2010). Patient safety beyond the hospital. *New England Journal of Medicine, 363*, 1001–1003.

Institute of Medicine (IOM). (1999). *To err is human*. Washington, DC: The National Academies Press.

Landrigan, C., Parry G., Bones C., Hackbarth A., Goldmann D., Sharek P. (2010). Temporal trends in rates of patient harm resulting from medical care. *New England Journal of Medicine, 363* (22) 2010, 2124–2134.

James, J. (2013). A new, evidence-based estimate of patient harms associated with hospital care. *Journal of Patient Safety, 9*(3): 122–128.

Schnipper, J., et al. (2006). Role of pharmacist counseling in preventing adverse drug events after hospitalization. *Archives of Internal Medicine, 166*(5), 565–571.

U.S. Department of Health and Human Services (HHS), Office of Inspector General (OIG). (November 2010) Adverse events in hospitals: National incidence among Medicare beneficiaries. Washington, DC: Author.

U.S. Department of Health and Human Services (HHS), Office of Inspector General (OIG). (2014). Adverse events in skilled nursing facilities. Washington, DC: Author.

Excerpts are taken from expert testimony provide to the U.S. Senate Committee on Health, Education, Labor, and Pensions Subcommittee on Primary Health and Retirement Security. Patient Safety Hearing. (July 17, 2014). Access meeting information at http://www.help.senate.gov/hearings /more-than-1-000-preventable-deaths-a-day-is-too-many-the-need-to-improve-patient-safety

Since the publication of the first report in the *Quality Chasm* series in 1999, there have been many other reports, in addition to reports mentioned in this chapter. These reports expand on the topic and also focus on more specific issues related to quality care and specialty care, such as emergency care, oncology, women's health, pediatrics, pain management, chronic disease, genomics, EBP, and others. See **Exhibit 1-2** for examples. All reports are available through the NAM website, listed in the Connect to Current Information section at the end of this chapter.

## Reports on Diversity and Disparities in Healthcare

With the extensive examination of the healthcare system, the early *Quality Chasm* reports noted that there was most likely a serious problem with disparities in healthcare, which is also related to efforts to improve public/ community health (IOM, 2001a). This led to additional reports on this problem and to the development of a *National Healthcare Disparities Report* that would be available annually *and later became a combined report on quality and disparities known as the QDR* and

administered by the AHRQ. In 2010, the IOM was asked to review the AHRQ monitoring system, and this led to a number of improvement recommendations. It was then recognized that quality, diversity, and disparities were interrelated, and there was greater need for benchmarking, analysis of data, and sharing of all of this information across the healthcare delivery system.

## *Guidance for the National Healthcare Disparities Report (2002)*

*Guidance for the National Healthcare Disparities Report* describes how disparities should be monitored and how to best integrate this information with quality monitoring (IOM, 2002). There are now 16 years of reports, though currently there is one combined report (HHS, AHRQ, 2019c). If healthcare disparities are to be reduced, a comprehensive review of the status and the need to monitor change over time is critical. Developing interventions to improve has become an important goal for HCOs and healthcare professions. Other content in this text elaborates on healthcare diversity and the problem of disparities.

**Exhibit 1-2** Examples of Other Reports Published by the NAM 2015–2020

- Collaboration Between Health Care and Public Health—Workshop in Brief (2015)
- Vital Signs: Core Metrics for Health and Health Care Progress (2015)
- The Future of Home Health Care: Workshop Summary (2015)
- Informed Consent and Health Literacy: Workshop Summary (2015)
- Sharing Clinical Trial Data: Maximizing Benefits, Minimizing Risks (2015)
- Health Literacy: Past, Present, and Future: Workshop Summary (2015)
- A Framework for Educating Health Professionals to Address the Social Determinants of Health (2016)
- Communicating Clearly About Medications (2017)
- Community-Based Health Literacy Interventions (2018)
- Improving Access to and Equity of Care for People with Serious Illness (2019)
- School Success: An Opportunity for Population Health: Workshop Summary (2019)
- Guiding Cancer Control (2019)
- Role of Nonpharmacological Approaches to Pain Management: Workshop Summary (2019)
- A Roadmap to Reducing Childhood Poverty (2019)
- Taking Action Against Clinician Burnout: A Systems Approach to Professional Well-Being (2019)
- Virtual Clinical Trials Challenges and Opportunities (2019)
- Guiding Cancer Control: A Path to Transformation (2019)
- Criteria for Selecting the Leading Health Indicators for Healthy People 2030 (2019)
- Integrating Social Care into the Delivery of Health Care: Moving Upstream to Improve the Nation's Health (2019)

Reports are accessible at http://www.nationalacademies.org/hmd/Reports.aspx.

In addition to reviewing these important reports, it is necessary to consider diversity in healthcare professions. In the Sullivan Commission on Diversity in the Healthcare Workforce report (Sullivan, 2004), it is noted that the United States needs greater workforce diversity to better meet the needs of a growing diverse patient population and reduce healthcare disparities. Since the publication of this report, there has been greater emphasis on increasing the number of minorities in all healthcare professions. In nursing, funding has been granted to assist in examining diversity in the profession and to support programs in nursing schools to increase faculty and student diversity; however, lack of diversity continues to be a concern despite these efforts.

### Unequal Treatment (2003)

*Unequal Treatment* (IOM, 2003e) examined healthcare disparities and noted that bias, prejudice, and stereotyping may result in disparities and that the healthcare delivery system had

a healthcare disparities problem. This problem is found consistently across a variety of healthcare settings and diagnoses. **Disparities** is defined as "racial or ethnic differences in the quality of healthcare that are not due to access-related factors or clinical needs, preferences, and appropriateness of intervention" (IOM, 2003e, pp. 3–4). Any **diversity** characteristic could be applied to this definition—for example, gender, religion, ethnicity, and so on. Among the goals of Healthy People 2030, a federal initiative and the newest revision, is to continue to address diversity. One of its overarching goals is to "eliminate disparities, achieve equity, and attain literacy to improve the health and well-being for all" (HHS, Office of Disease Prevention and Health Promotion [ODPHP], 2019). This objective relates to conclusions and recommendations in the *Quality Chasm* reports on quality and disparities. At the time there was concern that discrimination existed in the healthcare system, and there was and continues to be discrimination. The goal is to reduce **discrimination**, defined as "differences in care that result from bias, prejudices, stereotyping, and uncertainty in clinical communication and decision-making" (IOM, 2002, p. 4). Achieving health equity is a current goal to reduce disparities related to racial or ethnic group, religion, geographic location, or other characteristics associated with discrimination or exclusion (Wyatt, Laderman, Botwinick, Mate, & Whittington, 2016).

## Health Literacy (2004)

*Health Literacy* (IOM, 2004b) expanded the discussion about diversity to include **health literacy**, defined as "the degree to which individuals have the capacity to obtain, process, and understand basic information and services needed to make appropriate decisions regarding their health" (HHS, AHRQ, 2019d). Health literacy has a major impact on quality care and the health of individuals and communities. For example, if a patient or family cannot understand medication directions, then an error may occur or the patient may not take medication as prescribed, influencing health outcomes. Healthcare providers need to recognize that understanding may be more than just the ability to read. Vulnerable populations are at greater risk for health literacy problems. In 2011, the AHRQ announced that low health literacy in older Americans is linked to poorer health status and a higher risk of death, more emergency room visits, and more hospitalizations (HHS, AHRQ, 2011). Today, efforts are being made to address this problem, but much more needs to be done. Health literate organizations should meet the following criteria (HHS, AHRQ, 2019e):

1. Has leadership that makes health literacy integral to its mission, structure, and operations.
2. Integrates health literacy into planning, evaluation measures, patient safety, and quality improvement.
3. Prepares the workforce to be health literate and monitors progress.

4. Includes populations served in the design, implementation, and evaluation of health information and services.
5. Meets the needs of populations with a range of health literacy skills while avoiding stigmatization.
6. Uses health literacy strategies in interpersonal communications and confirms understanding at all points of contact.
7. Provides easy access to health information and services and navigation assistance.
8. Designs and distributes print, audiovisual, and social media content that is easy to understand and act on.
9. Addresses health literacy in high-risk situations, including care transitions and communications about medicines.
10. Communicates clearly what health plans cover and what individuals will have to pay for services.

Health literacy is discussed in other chapters, as it is highly relevant to meeting CQI outcomes and nursing care. If the healthcare system is to successfully transform into a value-based payment system, these "health systems will have to address health literacy. Health care has become so complicated that nearly everyone has difficulty understanding health information and navigating the healthcare system. Furthermore more than 1 in 3 adults have limited health literacy, which means they have difficulty with basic health-related tasks" (Brach, 2019). To reach a value-based system, four elements are identified: patients as empowered consumers, providers as accountable patient navigators, payment for outcomes, and prevention of disease—these four "Ps" provide a roadmap to better value (Brach, 2019). The NAM has continued to publish reports on health literacy that are important to understanding this complex area; examples are *Building the Case for Health Literacy* (2018a) and *Health Literacy and the Older Adult* (2018b). There is also need to continue to develop and use measurements to assess health literacy status (Brega et al., 2019).

# Healthy People 2030

The Healthy People initiative focuses on community and public health. This initiative published the fifth revision in 2030; revisions are on a 10-year cycle. The HHS Office of Disease Prevention and Health Promotion (HHS, ODPHP) (2019) describes the Healthy People initiative as follows:

> Vision: A society in which all people can achieve their full potential for health and well-being across the lifespan.

> Mission: To promote, strengthen and evaluate the Nation's efforts to improve the health and well-being of all people.

*Foundational principles explain the thinking that guides decisions about Healthy People 2030.*

- Health and well-being of all people and communities are essential to a thriving, equitable society.
- Promoting health and well-being and preventing disease are linked efforts that encompass physical, mental, and social health dimensions.
- Investing to achieve the full potential for health and well-being for all provides valuable benefits to society.
- Achieving health and well-being requires eliminating health disparities, achieving health equity, and attaining health literacy.
- Healthy physical, social, and economic environments strengthen the potential to achieve health and well-being.
- Promoting and achieving the nation's health and well-being is a shared responsibility that is distributed across the national, state, tribal, and community levels, including the public, private, and not-for-profit sectors.
- Working to attain the full potential for health and well-being of the population is a component of decision-making and policy formulation across all sectors.

Overarching Goals:

- Attain healthy, thriving lives and well-being, free of preventable disease, disability, injury, and premature death.
- Eliminate health disparities, achieve health equity, and attain health literacy to improve the health and well-being of all.
- Create social, physical, and economic environments that promote attaining full potential for health and well-being for all.
- Promote healthy development, healthy behaviors and well-being across all life stages.
- Engage leadership, key constituents, and the public across multiple sectors to take action and design policies that improve the health and well-being of all.

The goals are directly related to the work of the NAM, and there has been collaboration between the NAM and the Healthy People initiative. At the request of Healthy People, IOM/NAM participated in a review of Healthy People and provided comments about the revision of its leading indicators (IOM, 2011a; NAM, 2019). This collaboration demonstrates how the NAM is integrated throughout many aspects of healthcare policy and initiatives that address improving health and healthcare delivery. It also developed criteria to assist in the identification of leading health indicators or objectives for the 2030 revision, which included public health burden, magnitude of the health disparity, and the degree to which health equity would be achieved; the degree to which the objective would serve as a warning of problems; and actionability of the objective (NAM, 2019). Further information can be accessed through the Healthy People website, listed in the Connect to Current Information with the Author section at the end of this chapter.

**STOP AND CONSIDER 1-2**

Since 1999 many reports focusing on a variety of issues related to quality improvement have been published, and these reports guide the development of quality improvement.

# Status of Healthcare Quality

As we get into a more detailed examination of CQI and how nurses can be involved in the effort, it is important to review the current status of healthcare quality and disparities. We now know we have annual reports on quality and disparities to help us monitor and analyze the status, and the current reports are accessible through the AHRQ website. Where do we stand, and what should concern us? Since the publication of the 1999 *Quality Chasm* report, additional concerns have been identified and discussed, such as missed care, over- and under-treatment, problems with diagnosis, need for more patient engagement in CQI, development and utilization of measurement tools, greater sharing of information, disparities, and so on, as discussed throughout this text. "Health disparities have persisted, despite extensive research and a decades-long mandate to eliminate them" (NIH, 2019a). Due to this result the National Institute on Minority Health and Health Disparities (NIMHD) led a two-year science visioning process to provide guidance for research to improve minority health and reduce disparities. This is an example of how learning about quality can lead to initiatives and strategies to improve care.

Based on comments like this and others, much work still must be done. Despite reports, initiatives, and work done by the government, HCOs, and healthcare providers, the United States continues to have quality care problems. In 2016, a study noted that if healthcare errors were considered a disease, errors would be the third leading cause of death in the United States (Makary & Daniel, 2016). This is a significant statement, particularly if this study is considered alongside the 1999 report *To Err Is Human* (IOM, 1999), which identified a high rate of errors many years ago. The continuing problems are expected to result in 115 safety events for every 1,000 hospitalizations in the United States, costing $6,000 to $20,000 per event (Khanna, 2019a).

In 2016, it was revealed that the National Institutes of Health Clinical Center had major quality problems (Bernstein & McGinley, 2016). The Clinical Center serves as a hospital for clinical trials and is the largest hospital of its kind in the world. It has a long history of providing care that is needed and exemplary; however, an independent review board "concluded that patient safety had become "subservient to research demands" (Sun, 2016). The review also noted that, compared to other hospitals, the center had no adequate systems for staff to anonymously report problems, such as near misses and errors, and supervisors did not address problems. This conclusion demonstrated grave problems and indicated that even with all the discussion about CQI, and in a well-known hospital, there are HCOs providing care in an environment in which CQI is not a priority. There have been changes in this system with actions taken to improve the environment, and current data indicate that identifying problems and responding to and ideally preventing them are important, but sometimes this is not recognized in a timely manner (NIH, 2019b).

Since 1999, the healthcare community has recognized some elements of CQI that are important determinants of whether quality care is provided. Examples include movement toward a patient-centered system, greater engagement of patients and families, health informatics that continues to develop and provide tools that can be used while providing care, monitoring care, measuring CQI, and more. As a result of the *Quality Chasm* reports, there is now greater recognition for more national approaches; many of the current initiatives are discussed in this text. We know we need leadership that guides CQI and staff engaged in the process, but despite all of these insights, much more needs to be learned about CQI and how to achieve it. CQI is not something that has an end point, which is why quality improvement is referred to as *continuous* quality improvement.

## Quality Care

As noted in *To Err Is Human*, an organized process was begun to examine the U.S. healthcare system (IOM, 1999). After several expert panels and published reports, it was clear that the system had major problems; however, efforts have been made to improve since 2004 by more effective implementation of CQI (IOM, 2001a). There has also been some effort to include CQI content in academic nursing programs, although more is required. Monitoring is now done on an annual basis, with some of the resulting information available to the public and healthcare providers on the Internet.

In addition, the federal government has assumed a major role in monitoring and developing solutions to improve care as well as funding initiatives to improve care. The HHS is the major federal agency responsible for protecting the health of all Americans and providing essential health services. The department has a number of agencies that assist in meeting HHS goals, particularly to better ensure quality care, for example (HHS, 2019):

- *Centers for Medicare and Medicaid Services (CMS)*. Manages all aspects of the Medicare program and the Medicaid program. Medicaid is a shared program, functioning at both the federal and the state levels, and Medicare is a federal program.
- *Agency for Healthcare Research and Quality (AHRQ)*. Focuses on improving the quality, safety, efficiency, and effectiveness of healthcare for all Americans. As one of the agencies within the HHS, the AHRQ supports research and programs that help consumers, healthcare professionals, and

HCOs to make more informed decisions and that improve the quality of healthcare services and outcomes.

- *Centers for Disease Control and Prevention (CDC)*. Collaborates to create the expertise, information, and tools that people and communities need to protect their health through health promotion, prevention of disease, injury and disability, and preparedness for new health threats; also offers information and resources about workplace safety, although the primary responsibility for this charge rests with the U.S. Department of Labor.
- *Food and Drug Administration (FDA)*. Ensures safe use of food, drugs, and medical devices and equipment.
- *Indian Health Service (IHS)*. Focuses on providing quality care to Native Americans and Alaska Native populations.
- *Substance Abuse and Mental Health Services Administration (SAMHSA)*. Focuses on quality care for substance abuse and mental health needs.
- *Health Resources and Services Administration (HRSA)*. Serves as the primary federal agency for improving access to healthcare services for people who are uninsured, isolated, or medically vulnerable, including people living with HIV/AIDS, pregnant women, and mothers and children. The HRSA provides leadership and financial support to healthcare providers in every state and U.S. territory. The agency trains health professionals and improves systems of care in rural communities. It also oversees organ, bone marrow, and cord blood donation and supports programs that prepare against bioterrorism, compensates individuals harmed by vaccination, and maintains databases that protect against healthcare malpractice and healthcare waste, fraud, and abuse.
- *National Institutes of Health (NIH)*. Seeks fundamental knowledge about the nature and behavior of living systems and the application of that knowledge to enhance

health, lengthen life, and reduce the burdens of illness and disability. The NIH includes the National Institute of Nursing Research (NINR).

These federal government agencies are not new, but today they have been influenced by the *Quality Chasm* reports and recommendations, leading to an increase in their CQI activities. Appendix A identifies examples of major healthcare organizations and agencies, governmental and nongovernmental, related to quality improvement.

The National Quality Forum (NQF), a public–private partnership established in 1999, is now an important organization leading healthcare performance improvement and advising policy makers. Its mission is to "enhance healthcare value, make patient care safer, and achieve better outcomes" (NQF, 2019). The NQF is particularly recognized for establishing NQF-endorsed measures, now considered by many to be the gold standard in measurement, providing advice about CQI measurement to government agencies and others (Burstin, Leatherman, & Goldmann, 2016). Additional information about its measures is found in this text's content about measurement and on the NQF website.

A major source of data about the status of healthcare is the *National Healthcare Quality and Disparities Report* (HHS, AHRQ, 2019c). As mentioned earlier, the *Quality Chasm* reports recommended annual monitoring of quality care and of disparities. It is a reporting system that is congressionally mandated and has provided reports since 2003. The new version combines both quality and disparities data and also includes data from the National Quality Strategy (NQS) priorities. Examples of results noted in the QDR for 2018 include these, among others: More than half of the measures focused on improved access; one-third did not improve; and 14% worsened (HHS, AHRQ, 2019c). The data should be reviewed by healthcare organizations and healthcare professionals to better understand the current status of healthcare quality and provide direction for further improvement. These reports are typically not focused on the current year because it takes time to collect the data and complete analysis. More detailed, comprehensive, and current *QDR* data are available at the AHRQ website, which is identified in the Connect to Current Information section at the end of this chapter. The CQI work is not completed; it is ongoing to ensure that there is a health system that meets the NQS to provide better, more affordable care for the individual and the community (HHS, AHRQ, 2017).

## Disparities

Healthcare disparities, a component of healthcare quality, continue to be of concern throughout the United States, supported by data from the QDR (*HHS, AHRQ, 2018a*). As of the date of this report, the Affordable Care Act of 2010 (federal legislation) reduced the number of uninsured. However, as noted in the introductory material for this text, this law is at risk for continued changes and may even be cancelled. Affordable care, including access to health insurance, does have an impact on healthcare disparities—it may limit access to care and impact the quality of care and health outcomes for individuals and populations. Social determinants of health (economic stability, neighborhood and physical environment, education, food, community and social context, healthcare system) are interrelated and have an impact on healthcare disparities (HHS, CDC, 2014).

## Global Healthcare Quality

Quality healthcare is not just a concern in the United States. There is global interest in quality care and initiatives to improve health in many countries. The World Health Organization (WHO) has long worked to improve health and healthcare delivery, particularly in developing countries, although its work applies to all countries, noting "the centrality of patient safety in health services delivery for a strengthened health care system, and the importance of governments and policy makers to prioritize patient safety in their policies and programs. Patient safety was identified crucial for countries to progress towards universal health coverage as extending heath care should mean extending safe care" (WHO, 2019). The WHO website devotes space to patient safety, access through the link in the Connect to Current Information section at the end of this chapter. There are several critical types of resources for the global community, such as a multi-professional patient safety curriculum guide, safe childbirth checklist, surgical safety checklist, medication without harm, and patient engagement. Many of its resources are offered in multiple languages.

The NAM published a report entitled *Crossing the Global Quality Chasm: Improving Health Care Worldwide*. This report recognizes that the effort to improve care is not just a national issue but also a global one (NAM, 2018c). There are gaps and uneven progress in healthcare improvement; of particular concern are low- and middle-income countries. Access and quality are the critical elements to improve care and health.

The nursing profession is also involved in initiatives to improve global health. In 2015, the Global Advisory Panel on the Future of Nursing and Midwifery (GAPFON) met for the first time (Wallis, 2016). This organization, which was established by Sigma Theta Tau International (STT), works with the International Council of Nurses (ICN). The GAPFON is concerned with nursing, but it also sees the value in collaborating globally with leaders in other areas, such as economics, government, education, and regulatory agencies.

Supporting further global concern about patient safety and efforts to improve healthcare, a global seminar was held in 2019. This initiative identified eight global principles for the measurement of patient safety. These are identified in **Exhibit 1-3**. They represent a call to action for all healthcare stakeholders, crossing all types of healthcare settings.

Interconnection is a key characteristic of the world today. Informatics allows greater communication and sharing of information, which can improve the quality of care. For example, healthcare providers and researchers can easily share information and collaborate. Problems such as natural (e.g., hurricanes, volcanic eruptions, floods, fires) or human-caused disasters, epidemics, refugee health and social concerns, poor nutrition, impact of war and injuries to civilians and military, terrorism, and other problems require that countries work together to ensure greater health and safety for all. Medical technology and healthcare informatics are developed in many countries and then used globally, improving care in more than one country and thereby demonstrating greater collaboration. While modern transportation allows people to travel anywhere, it should be noted that travel does present some risks, such as transmitting infectious diseases, which is a particular problem in areas of the world that do not have effective control of diseases, such as the COVID-19 pandemic.

---

**STOP AND CONSIDER 1-3**

Healthcare disparities are interrelated with quality care.

---

# The Vision of Healthcare Quality

In the words of Cosgrove (2013), "Quality is elusive. Not only achieving it. But defining it. Measuring it. Planning it and improving it" (p. ix). The healthcare system has focused sporadically on different aspects of quality improvement but has now moved to a major emphasis on CQI (Hall, Moore, & Barnsteiner, 2008). From the mid-1970s to today, The Joint Commission and regulatory agencies have agreed that quality care is an important issue.

**Exhibit 1-3** Global Principles for Measuring Patient Safety

1. The purpose of measurement is to collect and disseminate knowledge that results in action and improvement. Measures must feed into a learning health system focused on improvement. Selected measures must be evidence-based, balanced between assessing downstream harm and informing upstream risk, and incorporate measures that matter to patients and all staff.

2. Effective measurement requires the full involvement of patients, families, and communities within and across the health system. Patients and families must be involved in the co-design of measures and processes, meaningful patient reported outcome measures, and feedback loops. Patients should also directly contribute data on outcomes, system structures, processes, and degree of patient-centeredness. Safety measures must be transparent and readily accessible to patients and their families.

3. Safety measurement must advance equity. Equity, the absence of avoidable, unfair, or remediable differences among groups of people, must be considered in the development and collection of new and existing measures. All safety and quality data should be stratified and analyzed by key demographic characteristics that reflect the community served.

4. Selected measures must illuminate an integrated view of the health system across the continuum of care and the entire trajectory of the patient's health journey. Measures should be applicable across the continuum of care and focus safety of care as it matters through the eyes of the patient. Selected sets of measures should be relevant across the entire trajectory of each patient's care rather than at single disconnected points in time.

5. Data should be collected and analyzed in real time to proactively identify and prevent harm as often as possible. New and existing technologies should be harnessed to shorten the life cycle between data collection, analysis, and action. New predictive technologies can help understand and intervene in high-risk situations before harm occurs and measurement should focus on identifying these risky situations to allow for real-time response.

6. Measurement systems, evidence, and practices must continuously evolve and adapt. New technology and best practices should be adopted to make measurement simple, modern, and consistently relevant within changing systems of care. Measures and methods should be selected to include both quantitative and qualitative data that is applicable to the specific context in which care is provided.

7. The burden of measures collected and analyzed must be reduced. Organizations and regulatory bodies must optimize systems to reduce collection burden, facilitate analysis and data sharing, and eliminate the collection of ineffective measures that result in fruitless actions and impede care. The creation and implementation of new measures should be driven by multiple relevant stakeholders, with resource- and cost-effectiveness as a key consideration.

8. Stakeholders must intentionally foster a culture that is safe and just to fully optimize the value of measurement. All leaders must invest in and commit to eliminating cultures of fear and blame and replacing them with cultures that are just, welcoming, and nurturing of curiosity and innovation. Culture should be measured consistently and in a way that is transparent and promotes action and improvement.

Managed care concerns, with its emphasis on reimbursement and some quality improvement elements, were the focus from 1980 to 2000. Quality assurance programs were focused on from 1980 through 2008; however, this term is not used today. EBP and health informatics became important in 1990 and continue to expand in all types of HCOs. Quality improvement moved into focus in the mid-1990s, with changes in terminology from quality assurance to quality assessment, quality improvement, and also CQI. Around 2000, patient safety became more of a concern and is considered to be a dimension of quality care.

Before this text focuses into the specifics of quality improvement, it is important to describe the national view of healthcare quality, which is fairly new and has been strongly influenced by the *Quality Chasm* reports and the extensive work done to develop these reports. Quality improvement is related to change, but not all change is improvement. Knowledge is very important to improvement, but not all knowledge leads to improvement. We need more than knowledge about quality improvement; we must take action and implement effective changes. The complexity of improvement is one of the difficulties we have in healthcare, and this complexity is compounded by both the complex healthcare system and the complexity of health problems and treatment for individual patients and population health. None of these challenges, however, should be used as excuses to avoid what must be done: improve care daily, one patient at a time and throughout the system, whether the focus is at the level of the collective HCO system, the individual HCO level, or the local, state, national, or even global level. To accomplish this goal requires a clear, effective framework that provides direction for planning, implementing, and evaluating CQI.

## Vision

*Crossing the Quality Chasm* (IOM, 2001a) extended the examination of the healthcare delivery quality problem, but it also supported steps toward developing a more systematic view of quality care and improvement strategies. Included in this vision is the comparison of the current vision with a future vision, which is referred to as "new" rules for redesigning the system and improving care that are intended as improvements to current rules, which continue to apply today (IOM, 2001a, pp. 61–62):

1. *Care based on continuous health relationships.* Patients should receive care whenever they need it and in many forms, not just face-to-face visits, and should have opportunity to access consistent healthcare providers whenever possible. For example, access to care may also be provided over the Internet, telephone, telehealth, and by other means.

2. *Customization based on patient needs and values.* The system of care should be designed to meet the most common types of needs, but it should also respond to individual patient choices and preferences.

3. *The patient as the source of control.* Patients should be given the necessary information and opportunity to exercise the degree of control they choose over healthcare decisions that affect them. The health system should be able to accommodate differences in patient preferences and encourage decision-making.

4. *Shared knowledge and the free flow of information.* Patients should have easy access to their own medical information and clinical knowledge. Clinicians and patients should communicate effectively and share information, with privacy and confidentiality maintained.

5. *Evidence-based decision-making.* Patients should receive care based on the best available scientific knowledge. Based on evidence-based practice care should not vary illogically from clinician to clinician or from place to place.

6. *Safety as a system property.* Patients should be safe from injury caused by the care system. Reducing risk and ensuring safety require greater attention to systems that help prevent and mitigate errors.

7. *The need for transparency.* The healthcare system should make information available to patients and their families so that they can make informed decisions when selecting a health plan, hospital, or clinical practice or when choosing among alternative treatments. This information should include a description of the system's performance in achieving measures relating to quality, EBP, and patient satisfaction.

8. *Anticipation of needs.* The health system should anticipate patient needs rather than simply react to events.
9. *Continuous decrease in waste.* The health system should not waste resources or patient time.
10. *Cooperation among clinicians.* Clinicians and healthcare organizations should actively collaborate and communicate to ensure an appropriate exchange of information and coordination of care.

These rules should not be viewed as a list of choices but rather a package that is needed to improve care (IOM, 2001a). This perspective crosses all types of healthcare settings and applies to all healthcare professions. Since the publication of these rules, much has been done to address them, but much more is still required. Content in this text relates to all of these rules, and CQI models include many, if not all, of these rules in their approaches. One can also see how they are related to the six aims or goals identified in the following section and can then compare them with the five healthcare professions core competencies. The work done in the *Quality Chasm* reports connects the elements discussed so that in the end there should be a complete picture.

## Aims

*Crossing the Quality Chasm* also identified six aims or goals. Clear direction and leadership are needed to improve healthcare, and these aims provide that direction. The following six aims or goals guide this process (IOM, 2001a, pp. 39–40):

1. *Safe.* Avoiding injuries to patients from the care that is intended to help them
2. *Timely.* Reducing waits and sometimes harmful delays for both patients who receive and those who give care
3. *Effective.* Providing services based on scientific knowledge to all patients who could benefit from those services and refraining from providing services not likely to benefit the patient

4. *Efficient.* Avoiding waste of equipment, supplies, ideas, and energy
5. *Equitable.* Providing care that does not vary in quality because of personal characteristics, such as gender, ethnicity, geographic location, and socioeconomic status
6. *Patient-centered.* Providing care that is respectful of and responsive to individual patient preferences, needs, and values, ensuring that patient values guide all clinical decisions

Some organizations refer to the aims as **STEEEP®**. Each aim is now important in healthcare delivery and in CQI and emphasized in this text. They should be integrated into nursing education and nursing practice.

## Framework for Monitoring Quality

As mentioned earlier, monitoring care is required to effectively improve care, and the AHRQ now monitors care annually. Federal legislation mandates this monitoring. In 2014, substantial changes were made in this monitoring and annual reporting. The rules and aims mentioned earlier are now part of monitoring and help to provide a framework for this process.

## System Approach

A **system** is a group of parts that work together as a whole. With greater interest in viewing healthcare as a system comes greater emphasis on understanding the healthcare system in order to improve it. In addition, with efforts to establish a patient-centered approach to care, understanding how the patient views the healthcare system is also important.

There are two important approaches to viewing the overall picture of healthcare quality—the macroview and the microview. The **macroview** of healthcare quality focuses on the broader issues from a local, state, federal, or even global perspective. At this broad level, there is much interaction not only between people and healthcare providers but also between services and funding. Funding may be provided by local, state, or federal sources, with federal sources providing a lot of the funding for healthcare services and research. The national reports on healthcare quality and disparities are examples of a CQI macroview focus. The **microview** of healthcare quality focuses on the healthcare provider, which can be an HCO or individual healthcare provider, such as a physician, nurse, or pharmacist. The macroview provides many of the standards that are used to assess care as well as regulate care, whereas the microview implements and ensures that these standards are met and, if not, makes changes to improve care at the patient care level.

Healthcare today is complex, and so it is not always easy to separate these perspectives. For example, when people travel they interact with healthcare delivery systems nationally or globally. Both views must use the same terminology and measurement, share information, apply a similar understanding of the roles of all providers, collaborate, and provide patient-centered care. Such a system, however, has not yet been fully realized.

One can also apply the system approach to an individual HCO. In this case the **macrosystem** applies to an HCO (e.g., a hospital or a medical corporation with multiple hospitals). Within the macrosystem are mesosystems and microsystems (Nelson et al., 2008). If the macrosystem is a large multistate corporation, then the mesosystem might be individual HCOs within the system, such as a hospital or a home health agency that is part of the healthcare system. Within one HCO, the **mesosystems** are departments, clinical centers, or services. Regardless of the type of organizational structure, drilling down to the microsystem level is critical in improving care. It is at this level that most nurses practice, and they have the most to offer in improving care. **Microsystems** are the clinical units, the smallest unit of the system, and it is here that the patient has the most influence.

Nurses work within all of these systems and need to understand them and how they impact nurses and nursing practice—structures, processes, and outcomes. Healthcare systems are neither simple nor stagnant; they change, requiring adaptation. **System thinking**—seeing the whole, how its parts interrelate, and how these parts all impact workflow—is important for success. This type of thinking is an integral part of effective CQI, allowing us to prevent, identify, and lessen the harm of errors; use problem solving and critical thinking along with clinical reasoning and judgment to make sound decisions based on best evidence; plan and use effective timelines; use interprofessional teams; and evaluate to determine outcomes. As stated by Fallon, Begun, and Riley (2013), "systems thinking encourages consideration of unintended consequences of an intervention. Unintended consequences are results that are different from the outcomes expected as a result of a purposeful action" (p. 220). When nurses focus only on what they are doing each day, their views and options are limited, and improved care will not occur.

## Need for Definitions

Definitions are important in CQI. If the CQI process is undertaken with unclear definitions or if staff involved in any step of the process use different definitions, then data and outcomes will be negatively impacted. For example, if two people are measuring the length of the same room and each person is using a different definition for a foot, then it will not be possible to compare the results. While this logic may seem rather obvious, in healthcare quality there has been limited consensus on definitions of critical terms. The *Quality Chasm* reports build on one another, defining terms and then using them consistently across the reports. Defining key terms, such as quality, safety, and error, was a critical part of developing a clear framework; the effort to standardize terminology remains crucial to the CQI process; and that approach is embraced by this text.

The definition of quality care used in the *Quality Chasm* reports and mentioned earlier in this chapter (IOM, 2001a) supports earlier work by Donabedian (1980). Donabedian described quality care as having three elements: structure, processes, and outcomes. As the topic of CQI is examined in this text, it is important to keep this definition. When **structure** is examined, the focus is on how the organization's elements are put together and how this coming together of parts impacts quality. This view recognizes that an organization is a system that has parts, and a thorough understanding of an organization considers both the whole and the parts. When **process** is reviewed, the focus is on how the parts of the system function independently and interact. **Outcomes** are critical; considering them turns the focus to results. Historically, healthcare professionals had problems agreeing on a universally accepted definition of quality care. The definition in the *Quality Chasm* reports, noted in this chapter, was used as the guide in developing a vision, goals, framework to monitor care, and recommendations. It has been used by many of the major CQI initiatives that followed.

CQI is defined as "a structured organizational process for involving personnel in planning and executing a continuous flow of improvements to provide quality healthcare that meets or exceeds expectations and usually involves a common set of characteristics," such as staff education, CQI teams, inclusion of CQI in HCO planning, and commitment and engagement to CQI (Sollecito & Johnson, 2013, pp. 4–5). Quality improvement has also been influenced by approaches and methods found in other businesses—for example, safety in the aviation industry. Key strategies to achieve improved quality include the following (Draper et al., 2008, p. 3):

- Having supportive hospital leadership and keeping them actively engaged in the work
- Setting expectations for all staff—not just nurses—that quality is a shared responsibility
- Holding staff accountable for individual roles

- Inspiring and using physicians and nurses to champion efforts
- Providing ongoing, visible, and useful feedback to engage staff effectively
- Applying the most current and rigorous techniques of the scientific method and statistical process control

Today, CQI is the most common approach used to improve care that supports the definition of quality care found in this chapter. As the topic of CQI is further examined in this text, there will be continued discussion of what it means and how it is implemented to achieve positive outcomes.

> **STOP AND CONSIDER 1-4**
>
> The most accepted view of healthcare quality is the application of STEEEP®.

# Value and Cost

Although some may find this claim difficult to accept, cost and quality are connected, but maybe not in the direction expected. The U.S. healthcare system is the most expensive healthcare system in the world, and yet it does not have the best quality. In one study that examined costs associated with harm while hospitalized, results noted that there were increased total costs, variable costs, and length of stay, and these factors had a negative impact on long-term hospital finances. This problem will increase as healthcare delivery focuses more on value and performance rather than focusing just on volume (Adler et al., 2015). However, increasing cost does not necessarily mean better care. We must get much better at providing efficient *and* effective care. The report *Best Care at Lower Cost: The Path to Continuously Learning Health Care in America* (IOM, 2012) presents "a vision of what is possible if the nation applies the resources and tools at hand by marshaling science, information technology, incentives, and care culture to transform the effectiveness and efficiency of care—to produce high-quality health care that continuously learns

# Healthy People 2020

## *A society in which all people live long, healthy lives*

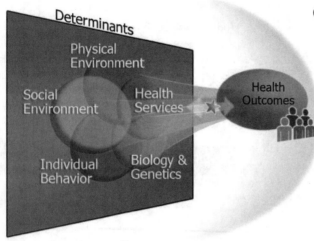

**Overarching Goals:**

- Attain high quality, longer lives free of preventable disease, disability, injury, and premature death.
- Achieve health equity, eliminate disparities, and improve the health of all groups
- Create social and physical environments that promote good health for all.
- Promote quality of life, healthy development and healthy behaviors across all life stages.

**Figure 1-1**  Schematic of the Healthcare System

Reproduced from Institute of Medicine. (2012). Best care at lower cost: The path to continuously learning health care in America. Washington, DC: The National Academies Press. Courtesy of the National Academies Press, Washington, DC.

to be better" (p. ix). The report recognizes that there is a connection between cost and quality, and it needs to be addressed. **Figure 1-1** describes missed opportunities in reducing waste and harm. Missed opportunities act as barriers to best care at lower cost and are discussed throughout this text.

To achieve the goal of best care at lower cost, the healthcare system needs to manage ever-increasing complexity and reduce ever-increasing costs (IOM, 2012). Discussed in this text, other reports emphasize the complexity and rapidly expanding knowledge (science and research) within the healthcare system; such reports focus on EBP, clinical guidelines, and comparative research (IOM, 2011b, 2011c, 2011d). In general, the U.S. healthcare system needs to improve care while reducing expenses and waste; consider the cost of care and determine if the cost is reasonable, such as the extremely high costs of some medications and treatments (Rockoff & Silverman, 2015).

Addressing the key concerns found in Figure 1-1, *Best Care at Lower Cost,* concludes with the overall recommendation of achieving a learning health system. What is meant by the **learning health system** discussed in this critical report and emphasized by HHS (HHS, AHRQ, 2019f)? The AHRQ defines a learning health system as "a health system in which internal data and experience are systematically integrated with external evidence, and that knowledge is put into practice." As a result, patients get higher quality, safer, more efficient care, and healthcare delivery organizations become better places to work. Learning health systems are characterized as follows:

- Have leaders who are committed to a culture of continuous learning and improvement.

- Systematically gather and apply evidence in real time to guide care.
- Employ IT methods to share new evidence with clinicians to improve decision making.
- Promote the inclusion of patients as vital members of the learning team.
- Capture and analyze data and care experiences to improve care.
- Continually assess outcomes, refine processes and training to create a feedback cycle for learning and improvement.

The CDC tracks and publishes data about healthcare expenditures, although the results are typically published several years behind the current year. Examples of some of the CDC data on U.S. healthcare expenditures include the following (HHS, CDC, 2017): National health expenditures were $3.3 trillion for 2017 compared to $3.0 trillion for 2014. The percentage of health expenditures for hospital care was 32.4% (2016); nursing home and continuing care retirement 4.9%; physician and clinical services 19.9%; and prescriptions 9.8%. Current CDC data are found at the CDC website.

Data comparing the United States with other countries indicate that the United States spends more on healthcare. According to the Organization for Economic Co-operation and Development (OECD, 2019), "Health spending measures the final consumption of health care goods and services (i.e., current health expenditure) including personal health care (curative care, rehabilitative care, long-term care, ancillary services and medical goods) and collective services (prevention and public health services as well as health administration), but excluding spending on investments. Health care is financed through a mix of financing arrangements including government spending and compulsory health insurance ('Government/compulsory') as well as voluntary health insurance and private funds such as households' out-of-pocket payments, NGOs and private corporations ('Voluntary')." The OECD rates for the United States are higher than rates for other major countries such as France, Germany, and the United Kingdom. The key question remains, if the United States spends more money on healthcare, is its care better? We know there are major quality care issues in the United States, as there are in other countries. We cannot rely on improving care by increasing costs. This may or may not make a difference.

The U.S. has consistently not done well when compared to other countries—quality and cost of care. It has been hoped that the U.S. will improve access and care and reduce costs in the years to come. Access to care is a critical element in ensuring health and care quality—impacting length of life and quality of life. However, current data indicate that the United States has much work to do to improve, as noted below. It is also important to recognize that many of the countries in the ranking have universal healthcare coverage, which the United States does not have. Examples of findings about the U.S. healthcare rankings include the following (Kaiser Family Foundation [KFF], 2019):

- Mortality amenable to healthcare is a measure of the rates of death considered preventable by timely and effective care, measured by the Healthcare Access and Quality (HAQ) Index. The U.S. ranks last among comparable countries on the HAQ index with a score of 88.7.
- Premature deaths are measured in Years of Life Lost (YLL), which is an alternative to overall mortality rate. The U.S. and comparable OECD countries have improved in this rating, but the U.S. continues to trail comparable countries by a significant margin (12,282 v. 7,764 YLLs in 2017).
- Disability adjusted life years are a measure of disease burden and the rate per 100,000, the total number of years lost to disability and premature death. The U.S. continues to have higher age-adjusted rates than those of comparable countries (2017, the U.S. 31% higher than the comparable country average).

- Hospital admission rates in the United States are higher than in comparable countries for congestive heart failure, asthma, and complications due to diabetes. However, the United States has lower rates for hypertension on average than comparably wealthy countries do: In total across these four disease categories, the United States has a 37% higher rate of hospital admissions than the average of other countries.
- Mortality within 30 days of being admitted to a hospital is not entirely preventable, but can be reduced for certain diagnoses and services. Improvement in this area is often linked to improved quality of care. The 30-day mortality rate for ischemic strokes (caused by blood clots) is 4.2 deaths per 100 patients in the United States, compared to an average of 6.9 deaths per 100 patients in similar countries. The 30-day mortality rates after hospital discharge for heart attacks (acute myocardial infarction) and hemorrhagic stroke (caused by bleeding) are similar in the United States and comparable countries.
- According to a recent survey by the Commonwealth Fund, patients in the United States are more likely than those in comparable countries to experience a medical error at some point during their care. In this case, medical errors include being given the wrong medication or dose, or experiencing delays or errors in laboratory test results. In 2016, 19% of patients in the United States experienced a medical error compared to 12% of patients in similar countries.
- With the exception of Canada and Sweden, patients in the United States have a harder time making a same-day appointment when in need of care. In 2016, 51% of patients in the United States were able to make a same-day appointment with a provider, compared to 57% of patients in similar countries.
- According to a recent survey by the Commonwealth Fund, patients in the United States visit the emergency department for conditions that could have been treated by a regular doctor or place of care nearly twice as often as in comparable countries. In similar countries, 9% of patients visited an ER for nonemergency care, compared to 16% of patients in the United States.

Data have improved since 1999 when the IOM/NAM began to examine care and published the first *Quality Chasm* report, *To Err Is Human*; however, current data does not demonstrate enough improvement.

The reason for providing examples in this chapter is to present a better picture of how cost and quality are connected. An important change related to the cost of care and its relationship to quality is the demonstrated by greater emphasis on **pay for performance**. This emphasis can be positive, as it may stimulate improvement, but it can also be problematic if providers are focused on "how they appear" rather than actually providing quality care. For example, an opinion column published in the *New York Times*, written by a surgeon, noted that there are problems with using quality report cards when reported information may be used to penalize physicians, and this may then influence physicians to be too cautious (Jauhar, 2015; McCabe, Joynt, Welt, & Resnic, 2013). As stated by Jauhar (2015), "Surgical report cards are a classic example of how a well-meaning program in medicine can have unintended consequences . . . . It would appear that doctors, not patients, are the ones focused on doctors' grades—and their focus is distorted and blurry at best" (p. A27).

One of the NQS six priorities is to "make quality care more affordable for individuals, families, employers, and governments by developing and spreading new healthcare delivery models, and the goal is associated with its two long-term goals related to care affordability:

1. Ensure affordable and accessible high-quality healthcare for people, families, employers, and governments.

2. Support and enable communities to ensure accessible, high-quality care while reducing waste and fraud.

The strategy recognizes that while this will be a challenge, the goal of reducing healthcare costs is important to everyone because of the impact of rising costs on families, employers, and state and federal governments. Reducing costs must be considered hand in hand with the aims of better care, healthier people and communities, and affordable care" (HHS, AHRQ, 2018a).

This priority is associated with paying, rewarding, and incentivizing providers to deliver high-quality, patient-centered care. The focus needs to move from volume to value in the purchase of healthcare or quality. In trying to meet this priority, there are challenges to measurement that must be considered—for example, measures must be accurate and reliable and should not set up a scenario where the provider and others view the measures as the end point, thus limiting the understanding of quality care. Effective, efficient healthcare measurement is weak, and it is an important topic discussed in this text.

# Critical Healthcare Legislation and Regulation

Both federal and state legislation has an impact on healthcare delivery. At the state level the emphasis is on an individual state; however, states cannot ignore federal legislation that may supersede state laws or may influence how a state healthcare system functions. Federal healthcare law and regulations have a major impact on healthcare. State–federal system legislation is more complex, and this influences both the content and process of

health policy. The following content discusses some examples and content related to critical healthcare legislation and regulation.

# Healthcare Reform and Quality Improvement

The United States is unusual in that most developing countries have universal healthcare coverage; however, to date, there has been insufficient political support in the United States for this type of coverage. The Affordable Care Act of 2010 (ACA) does not support universal healthcare coverage, and as discussed in the introduction to this text, it is a law that is changing.

This text does not focus on the ACA but rather discusses how it and other healthcare legislation impact, or might impact, quality improvement. The law has been changed and may likely be changed further.

In addition to the Affordable Care Act of 2010, which has had an impact on healthcare coverage, costs, and quality care issues, CQI has been greatly affected by recent national legislation, such as the Health Insurance Portability and Accountability Act (HIPAA) of 1996, the American Recovery and Reinvestment Act (ARRA) of 2009, and the Health Information Technology for Economic and Clinical Health (HITECH) Act of 2008, which requires the establishment of a National Coordinator for Health Information Technology in HHS (Fallon et al., 2013). The ARRA provides funding to assist physicians in adopting electronic records. As of 2015, to avoid Medicare payment penalties, physicians who care for Medicare patients must use electronic records. The HITECH also requires that physicians document clinical quality measures. There is also mandated reporting of measures to ensure quality and federally mandated establishment of the NQS. States have also moved to more direct monitoring of healthcare quality by requiring reporting of serious adverse events. Examples of some of the ACA impact follow; however, since this law has changed and more change is predicted, some of these examples may be affected in the future:

- Funding: grants and loans for students and faculty
- Education and training funds focused on geriatrics
- Primary care: advanced practice traineeships
- Funding for nurse-managed clinics
- Health prevention and public health
- Increased workforce diversity
- Community-based transition programs
- Establishment of the Patient-Centered Outcomes Research Institute
- Efforts toward nondiscrimination in healthcare
- Continued support for the Preventive Services Task Force
- Creation of the National Health Care Workforce Commission

As discussed in this chapter, the *Quality Chasm* reports brought the problem of healthcare disparities to the forefront (IOM, 2001a, 2001b, 2002, 2003a). It is now recognized that it is difficult to resolve issues of reimbursement, cost, access, and quality without consideration of disparities. For example, health literacy is discussed in the ACA as a provision "to communicate health and healthcare information clearly; promote prevention; be patient-centered and create medical or health homes; assure equity and cultural competence; and deliver high-quality care" (Somers & Mahadevan, 2010, p. 4).

## Current Status

Since 1999, we have been able to get a better picture of the healthcare delivery system with the annual QDR. In 2014, the journal *Patient Safety and Quality Healthcare*, which began publishing in 2004, devoted its August issue to the future, asking patient safety experts to look 5 years into the future and predict the status of healthcare quality. Generally, the comments predicted modest improvement

focused on continuing progress with current changes in the CQI process. Carr (2014) reports the following expert opinion from a former hospital CEO, Paul Levy, predicting that healthcare will continue to be "'islands of excellence surrounded by a sea of mediocrity" because medical education is largely unchanged and hospital leaders are focused more on market concentration and the bottom line than on safety and quality. Other experts share this view, as Carr (2014) further elucidates: "Jim Conway, adjunct lecturer at the Harvard School of Public Health. . . reminds us that there is no end to that journey and expects that 'sustainability' will be a new challenge, especially for organizations that engage in isolated, limited improvement projects. Sustainability comes from system-wide commitment to continual improvement. Organizations that work to embody the principles of high reliability know that sustaining the gains they have made means never taking those gains for granted or believing that past or even performance offers protection from future hazards."

Why do problems persist despite some improvement? The work described in the *Quality Chasm* reports clarified many of the problems, but Fineberg (2012), who led the IOM in its early years, identified some of the critical inefficiencies that also continue to cause current problems in the healthcare system (p. 1023):

- Less emphasis on patient outcomes in the payment system
- Reward for inefficiency such as complications and readmissions
- Indifference of providers to reduce costs; lack of personal and professional concern about this problem
- Failure to take full advantage of professional skills of nurses
- Lack of uniform systems and processes to ensure safe and high-quality care
- Problems with patient flow, use of services, overcrowding (such as in emergency

departments delaying treatment and admissions)

- Insufficient involvement of patients in decision making
- Insufficient attention to prevention, disparities, primary care, health literacy, population health, and long-term results
- Fragmented and uncoordinated delivery, without continuity of care
- Lack of information on resource costs, performance, comparative effectiveness, quality of care, and health outcomes
- Scientific uncertainty about effectiveness and cost
- Cultural predisposition to believe that more care is better
- Administrative complexity related to multiple insurers
- Fraud and a problematic malpractice system

There are other issues, but the issues listed here summarize some of the key healthcare quality concerns.

The Trump administration developed a blueprint to lower drug prices and out-of-pocket costs, American Patients First (HHS, 2018). There are many drugs in the United States available for treatment, but if one cannot afford them, then access is limited to valuable treatment. The United States faces challenges related to drugs, including high list prices for drugs; seniors and government programs overpaying for drugs due to inadequate negotiation for prices; high and rising out-of-pocket consumer costs; and foreign governments free-riding off American investment in innovation. The major strategies in the blueprint are to improve competition, offer better negotiation, provide incentives for lower list prices for drugs, and lower out-of-pocket costs. The United States has the highest drug prices in the world, and this proposed blueprint addresses this issue; however, as of 2019, the results are not yet clear (Dabbous, Francois, Chachoua, & Tourni, 2019). It will take more time to determine results, and this type of change is also related to the status of the ACA and any changes that might be made in future healthcare coverage legislation.

**STOP AND CONSIDER 1-6**

State and federal legislation makes healthcare policy, laws, and regulations complex.

# An Important Step Toward Improvement: National Quality Strategy

As discussed throughout this chapter, the *Quality Chasm* reports and similar initiatives focused the U.S. healthcare system on CQI. There was a great need to identify the problems and examine approaches to address them. Laying the groundwork and then recommending annual monitoring of healthcare quality and disparities were major steps toward a healthcare environment that commits to quality at its core. There was, however, still a need to have a clearer overall national perspective of CQI. The *Quality Chasm* reports and other sources, such as the Institute for Healthcare Improvement, provided initial ideas for a framework.

One of the ACA provisions related to quality improvement was the establishment of the National Quality Strategy (NQS), which addresses the need for a national quality improvement framework and adds an additional focus on population health and reduction in healthcare disparities (Burstin et al., 2016; HHS, AHRQ, 2017). After the publication of the first *Quality Chasm* report in 1999, it took 12 years for the federal government to develop this national framework for healthcare quality. A variety of theories and models supporting improvement had an impact on the NQS. There is additional information about quality improvement theories and models in other chapters of this text. It is important in this chapter, which focuses on the introduction of CQI, to recognize the importance of the NQS and understand its framework and implications of its use.

# Development and Purpose of the National Quality Strategy

The NQS is now an important part of the national initiative to improve care. The development of the NQS framework was led by the AHRQ, and it continues to lead its implementation. To ensure a collaborative effort, the AHRQ included feedback from over 300 stakeholders representing the federal government, especially the HHS, the states, the private sector, and multi-stakeholder groups, such as healthcare professional organizations, and recommendations found in the *Quality Chasm* series. An evidence-based approach was used to develop the NQS.

In a 2011 press release, the HHS commented that the NQS was a groundbreaking initiative supporting an approach that quality care can be measured and improved at multiple levels—namely at the level of the community, practice settings, and individual physicians (HHS, 2011). A critical problem noted was that there were too many measures and no control or evaluation of them. This problem has led to redundancies and some overlap in measurement, which impacts the value of results. More systematic methods are needed to measure care quality and maintain the CQI process. Patient-centered care needs to be at the core of the NQS, as it is now considered the core concern in care delivery. The major purpose of the NQS is to provide a national approach to measure quality and ensure higher-quality care for all.

# National Quality Strategy Design

The NQS consists of three aims, six priority strategies for improvement, and levers.

The NQS is also working toward a greater measure of alignment across the HHS to establish core sets of measures that would be useful and meaningful for different groups of stakeholders. This effort is motivated by the concern about the proliferation of measures.

## Aims

The three NQS aims are based on the **Triple Aim** framework and incorporate elements of STEEEP®. It is recommended that HCOs adopt all of the aims. The Triple Aim is discussed in other sections of this text, but it is important to introduce it at the beginning of the discussion about quality improvement due to its influence on the NQS (HHS, AHRQ, 2017):

1. *Better Care.* Improve overall quality by making healthcare more patient-centered, reliable, accessible, and safe.
2. *Healthy People in Healthy Communities.* Improve the health of the U.S. population by supporting proven interventions to address behavioral, social, and environmental determinants of health in addition to delivering higher-quality care (HHS, CDC, 2015).
3. *Affordable Care.* Reduce the cost of quality healthcare for individuals, families, employers, and government.

The second aim is important because it illustrates how various initiatives are connected to the NQS. An effective national view of quality requires collaborative initiatives and a consistent framework. With development of the NQS, these long-standing programs are brought into the overall national strategy.

## Prioritizing Strategies

The aims connect to the NQS six priorities and strategies, examining the most common health concerns. It is recommended that HCOs use these priorities to guide efforts to improve health and healthcare quality. The six priorities are as follows and are highlighted in **Figure 1-2** (HHS, AHRQ, 2017):

- Making care safer by reducing harm caused in the delivery of care
- Ensuring that each person and family is engaged as a partner in care
- Promoting effective communication and coordination of care
- Promoting the most effective prevention and treatment practices for leading causes of mortality
- Working with communities to promote wide use of best practices to enable healthy living
- Making quality care more affordable for individuals, families, employers, and government by developing and spreading new healthcare delivery models

## Levers

Nine levers are identified for the strategies. Each lever "represents a core business function, resource, and/or action that stakeholders can use to align to the strategy. In many cases, stakeholders may already be using these levers but have not connected these activities to NQS

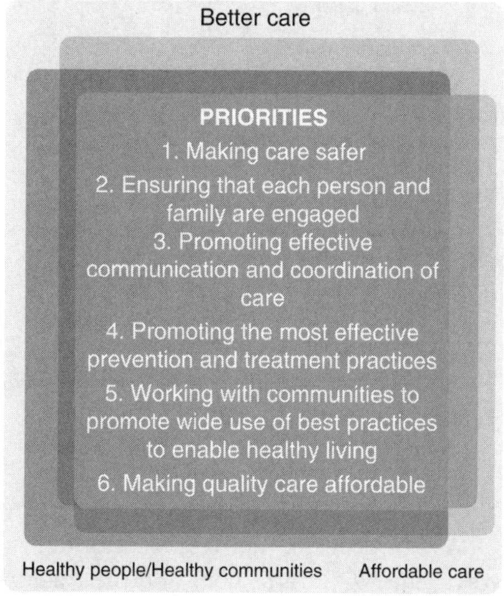

**Figure 1-2** National Quality Strategy—Three Aims and Six Priorities

Reproduced from Centers for Medicare and Medicaid Services, Center for Clinical Standards and Quality. (2018). 2018 national impact assessment of the Centers for Medicare & Medicaid Services (CMS) quality measures report. Retrieved from https://www.cms.gov/Medicare/Quality-Initiatives -Patient-Assessment-Instruments/QualityMeasures/National-Impact-Assessment-of-the-Centers -for-Medicare-and-Medicaid-Services-CMS-Quality-Measures-Reports

alignment" (HHS, AHRQ, 2017). In addition to developing a national framework, the NQS also addresses the problem of too many measures and the negative impact that this has on CQI and healthcare providers. It results in confusion, lack of consistency, and disorganization. Given that the healthcare system is described as dysfunctional, this has an impact on the CQI approach. The levers are identified in **Figure 1-3**. The relationship between the aims and the levers is found in **Figure 1-4**. It is recommended that HCOs focus on at least one of the levers.

Federal healthcare programs now apply the NQS. It is recommended that other healthcare programs—both private and public— adopt the NQS; however, it is not required. The AHRQ provides tools and resources to support implementation of the NQS (HHS, AHRQ, 2016). The NQS must provide an annual report to Congress, and the reports are posted on the AHRQ website. Key findings from the 2015 report (reports are typically several years behind the publication date) include the following (HHS, AHRQ, 2018b):

- Access to healthcare has improved dramatically, led by sustained reductions in the number of Americans without health insurance and increases in the number of Americans with a usual source of medical care.
- Quality of healthcare continues to improve, but wide variation exists across the National Quality Strategy priorities.
  - Effective Treatment measures indicate success at both improving overall performance and reducing disparities.
  - Care Coordination measures have lagged behind other priorities in overall performance.
  - Patient Safety, Person-Centered Care, and Healthy Living measures have improved overall but few disparities have been reduced.
  - Care Affordability measures are limited for summarizing performance and disparities.
- Disparities related to race and socioeconomic status persist among measures of

| National Quality Strategy Levers | | | |
|---|---|---|---|
| **Lever** | **Icon** | **Definition** | **Example** |
| Payment | | Reward and incentivize providers to deliver high-quality, patient-centered care. | Join a regional coalition of purchasers that are pursuing value-based purchasing. |
| Public Reporting | | Compare treatment results, costs, and patient experience for consumers. | A regional collaborative may ask member hospitals and medical practices to align public reports to the National Quality Strategy aims or priorities. |
| Learning and Technical Assistance | | Foster learning environments that offer training, resources, tools, and guidance to help organizations achieve quality improvement goals. | A Quality Improvement Organization may disseminate evidence-based best practices in quality improvement with physicians, hospitals, nursing homes, and home health agencies. |
| Certification, Accreditation, and Regulation | | Adopt or adhere to approaches to meet safety and quality standards. | The National Quality Strategy aims and priorities may be incorporated into continuing education requirements or certification maintenance. |
| Consumer Incentives and Benefit Designs | | Help consumers adopt healthy behaviors and make informed decisions. | Employers may implement workforce wellness programs that promote prevention and provide incentives for employees to improve their health. |
| Measurement and Feedback | | Provide performance feedback to plans and providers to improve care. | A long-term care provider may implement a strategy that includes the use of Quality Assurance and Performance Improvement data to populate measurement dashboards for purposes of identifying and addressing areas requiring quality improvement. |
| Health Information Technology | | Improve communication, transparency, and efficiency for better coordinated health and health care. | A hospital or medical practice may adopt an electronic health record system to improve communication and care coordination. |
| Workforce Development | | Investing in people to prepare the next generation of health care professionals and support lifelong learning for providers. | A medical leadership institution may incorporate quality improvement principles in their training. |
| Innovation and Diffusion | | Foster innovation in health care quality improvement, and facilitate rapid adoption within and across organizations and communities. | Center for Medicare & Medicaid Innovation tests various payment and service delivery models and shares successful models across the Nation. |

**Figure 1-3** National Quality Strategy Levers

Reproduced from U.S. Department of Health and Human Services. (2014). National Quality Strategy: Using levers to achieve improved health and healthcare. Retrieved from https://www.ahrq.gov/workingforquality/about/nqs-fact-sheets/nqs-fact-sheet-using-levers.html

access and all National Quality Strategy priorities, but progress is being made in some areas. Disparities in quality of care and disparities in access to care typically follow the same pattern, although disparities in access tend to be more common than disparities in quality.

As healthcare delivery continues to evolve, the NQS framework and the tracking data found in the *National Healthcare Quality and Disparities Report* can help identify system successes that should be celebrated, as well as aspects of the system that require attention.

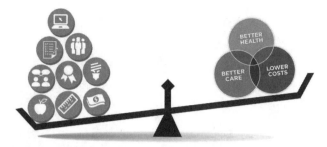

**Figure 1-4** Relationship of the National Quality Strategy Aims and Levers

Reproduced from U.S. Department of Health and Human Services. (2016). National Quality Strategy: Overview [PowerPoint presentation]. Retrieved from http://www.ahrq.gov/workingforquality/nqs/overview2016.pptx

How should the healthcare delivery system implement the NQS (HHS, AHRQ, 2017)? It is hoped that HCOs are knowledgeable about the NQS and adopt its elements as recommended. Adopters should also include healthcare profession education programs such as all nursing academic programs including this content and ensuring that nursing students at all levels know about NQS and can apply it to their practice. The overall goal is an effective healthcare delivery system that is consistent and emphasizes CQI from the same perspective. The NQS website offers resources such as tools and reports for healthcare providers, policy makers, and healthcare educators. The Connect to Current Information section at the end of this chapter provides a link to this site.

## Current Status of the National Quality Strategy

The NQS priorities are patient safety, person-centered care, care coordination, effective treatment, healthy living, and care affordability. As noted previously, they are also monitored as part of the annual *QDR*. This information is then included in the annual NQS report to Congress. Multiple healthcare organizations and government agencies participate in providing data for the report. **Figure 1-5** provides an overview of how the NQS works.

# Introduction to Leadership, Interprofessional Teamwork, and Nursing Responsibility for Continuous Quality Improvement

Leadership, including nursing leadership, is required in all phases of CQI. HCO leaders ensure that CQI is part of all aspects of the organization, including the mission, goals and objectives, organization structure, processes, policies and procedures, position descriptions and performance appraisal, and all aspects of clinical practice. They must work to integrate standards, accreditation requirements, staff education, ethics, and legal requirements into the organization. Teamwork is critical to successful CQI, and leaders in the HCO must provide support to teams with resources, guidance, and staff education about teams. As articulated by Gantz and colleagues

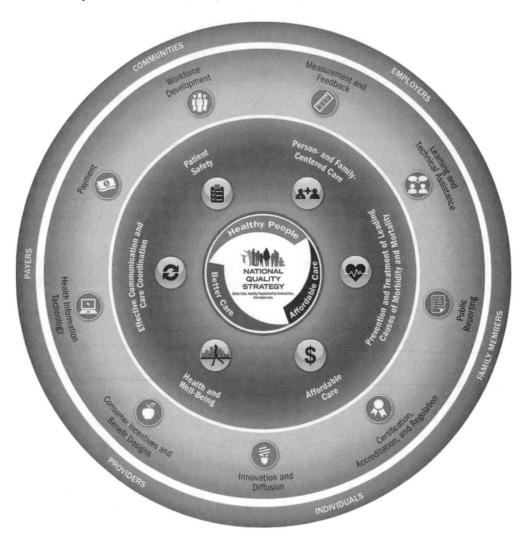

**Figure 1-5** National Quality Strategy: How It Works

(2003), "Quality improvement and performance should be a way of life for best practices and high performers who seek to understand, change, improve, and enhance patient care outcomes" (p. 329).

Nurses usually think of nursing leaders as being in management or administration positions; however, every nurse needs to be a leader and develop leadership competencies—staff nurses, advanced practice registered nurses (APRNs), nurses with a doctorate of nursing practice (DNPs) in all types of settings and positions (Finkelman, 2020). These competencies are needed as nurses provide care working with teams, advocating for patients, and engaging in CQI in direct care. Nurses also need these competencies when they participate in organizational activities such as committees, task forces, and other situations where professional issues are considered, and nurses need to share the nursing perspective. *The Future of Nursing* report includes the following recommendation: "expand opportunities for nurses to lead and diffuse collaborative improvement efforts" (IOM, 2010, p. S-9).

Responsibility for CQI is the core issue in this text. Every healthcare profession has the responsibility to (1) ensure that its educational programs prepare graduates who can apply quality improvement in their individual practice and participate in CQI programs within HCOs and (2) actively commit to improving care in all types of healthcare settings. These objectives are not simple to accomplish. CQI has not always been an important content topic in healthcare professions education, including nursing. It is mentioned, of course, but there is typically limited in-depth examination of quality care and methods to improve care—although this situation is slowly improving. One of the five healthcare professions core competencies is to apply quality improvement, and this core competency is tied to the other four core competencies, and all are needed to effectively continuously improve care.

The *Quality Chasm* series has had an impact on the entire healthcare system. Not only has the recognition of CQI as a professional responsibility influenced how HCOs view quality care and how the government at local, state, and federal levels works toward improving care but also now there is much more emphasis on the role of individual healthcare providers—and in this text, the focus is on nurses. CQI is not something that is just done by a single department in an HCO with staff occasionally hearing about it. It must be part of daily work and the provision of care, and it must impact all staff, both professional and nonprofessional. Each staff member must ask: How can I improve what I do?

## STOP AND CONSIDER 1-8

Nursing must develop more leadership in quality improvement.

# Summary

This chapter sets the stage for an in-depth examination of the healthcare system from the perspective of quality care and the roles and responsibilities of nurses in CQI. Two decades ago the road to change that focused on CQI began in earnest with the initiation of the *Quality Chasm* reports. The AHRQ assumed a more major role in the nation's initiatives to improve healthcare; as the third decade approaches, the AHRQ notes "But, like other organizations in healthcare, we recognize that the agency is at a crossroads. The healthcare landscape is changing—the way it's delivered, paid for, and regulated. The population is aging. Mergers, acquisitions, and consolidations are accelerating. Networked medical devices are proliferating. And we are witnesses to a digital revolution that is upending the volume, variety, and velocity of healthcare data" (Khanna, 2019b). What does the future hold, and how might the AHRQ continue to contribute? It has identified three focus areas: (1) improving care for Americans living with multiple chronic conditions, (2) providing data and analytics to policymakers to empower informed decision making, and (3) reducing diagnostic errors (Khanna, 2019b). This is not to say that these are the only issues that need to be addressed, but they are important and reflect some of the current problems in healthcare quality. Others will be discussed in this text.

Healthcare quality improvement is a complex area, involving many viewpoints and methods. Nurses should assume more CQI responsibilities at the point of care and within HCOs. This chapter provides background information and an overview of our current knowledge of CQI so that nurses will be well informed as they begin their journey toward competence in quality improvement. Fineberg (2012) frames this journey in the following manner: "To achieve a successful and sustainable health system, we must be able and willing to try many different things. But therein lies a unifying idea: Do many things.

No single stroke will solve this problem. A successful and sustainable health system will not be achieved by supporting prevention, it will not be achieved by championing competition, it will not be achieved by comparing the effectiveness of different practices, it will not be achieved by striking commercial influence from professional decision making, it will not be achieved by changing the way we pay doctors, and it will not be achieved by just reengineering the system. It requires all these changes and more. We need the cleverness of the fox and the persistence of the hedgehog. We must be willing to adopt many strategies and use them to reach one big goal" (p. 1026). Exemplars of quality improvement roles and responsibilities for staff nurses, nurse managers, and APRNs are found in **Exhibit 1-4**.

---

**Exhibit 1-4** **Exemplars: Quality Improvement Roles and Responsibilities**

---

**Staff Nurse**

The staff nurse who works in a clinical unit in a hospital can consider how the STEEEP® can be applied to the nurse's practice. An example is the nurse admitting a patient to the surgical unit. The plan for the patient should include consideration of safe, timely, effective, efficient, equitable, patient-centered care: ensure the patient's medications prior to surgery are administered as ordered and when needed; ensure the assessment is complete and all surgical permissions are signed and patient states the information was discussed; supplies used for intravenous medication used in manner and amount required; nurse treats patient with respect and shares same information would share with all patients who are preparing for surgery; patient asked questions/ asked to give feedback/asked to engage in CQI and how might do this/patient asked who he/she wants staff to share information with, such as wife, daughter, and so on.

**Nurse Manager**

The nurse manager of a medical unit reviews the hospital's CQI plan, which is based on the NQS. The manager then ensures that the plan is implemented on the unit with staff knowledge and engagement. Data are shared with staff routinely in staff meetings.

**Advanced Practice Registered Nurse (APRN)\***

Four APRNs work in the ambulatory care setting for a 300-bed hospital. In their positions in a variety of clinics (pediatrics, maternity, medicine, surgical) they work with the CQI Program staff in collecting data and analysis of data. For example, to ensure STEEEP® they assist CQI staff by reviewing and analyzing data collected related to these elements: safe, timely, effective, efficient, equitable, patient-centered. They are also involved in developing strategies when problems are identified—for example, to better engage patients in their care, education about their care, and get patient feedback on a routine basis. The APRNs work with other staff to ensure that the strategies are implemented and evaluated.

---

\* Advanced Practice Registered Nurse includes Clinical Nurse Specialist, Clinical Nurse Leader, APRN, and nurses with DNP.

# APPLY CQI

## Chapter Highlights

- Healthcare quality improvement is complex and continues to develop.
- Concern about the quality of healthcare in the United States has been particularly high since 1999 when a report *To Err Is Human* was published, followed by a number of other critical reports referred to as the *Quality Chasm* reports.
- The Institute of Medicine (IOM), whose name has been changed to the National Academy of Medicine (NAM), has a major role in examining healthcare quality through its review panels and published reports with recommendations.
- Five healthcare professions core competencies were identified by one of the major reports, *Health Professions Education* (2003), and apply to all healthcare professions.
- The *Quality Chasm* reports identified the need for national annual reports on healthcare quality and disparities administered by the Agency for Healthcare Research and Quality (AHRQ) and provided in a combined report focused on quality and disparities.
- Continuous quality improvement (CQI) is now a major concern of all healthcare organizations (HCOs) and professions, with emphasis on STEEEP® (safe, timely, effective, efficient, equitable, patient-centered).

- Based on data and reports that indicate certain populations do not receive equitable care, leading to healthcare disparities; diversity and disparities in healthcare are now integrated as a part of CQI.
- Healthy People 2030 is a national health initiative that guides perspectives on healthy individuals and communities (2019).
- U.S. healthcare does not rate as high as it should when compared to other countries' healthcare systems.
- The *Quality Chasm* reports provide a vision of U.S. healthcare that is now incorporated into many quality improvement initiatives.
- Macro- and microviews of healthcare quality are integrated into CQI. The macrosystem, mesosystem, and microsystem should be understood for each HCO.
- Value and cost are related and have to be considered in CQI.
- State and federal legislation is interrelated and complex; influencing healthcare policy.
- The National Quality Strategy (NQS) is a significant national initiative assisting in developing and maintaining quality care within the healthcare delivery system.
- Every nurse needs to be a leader and assume an active role in CQI.

## Critical Thinking and Clinical Reasoning and Judgment: Questions and Learning Activities

1. Select one of the *Quality Chasm* reports described in this chapter. Go to the National Academies/Science, Engineering, Medicine website (https://www.nap.edu) and find the report. Read the executive summary, and then in your own words describe why the report is important to healthcare delivery and to nursing.

2. Review this chapter's discussion of the NQS, and visit the AHRQ's website to further research the NQS. How is the

NQS directly related to nursing care and the nursing profession? Identify the NQS elements that are based on important CQI elements discussed in this chapter. Discuss your views with your student team.

3. Discuss the relationship and relevance to the NQS of the Triple Aim, STEEEP®, and structure/process/outcomes.

4. Compare and contrast value and cost in healthcare delivery and quality improvement. Why is this important for nurses? Provide examples.

5. Why do you need to be actively engaged in CQI as a student and then as a practicing nurse?

## Connect to Current Information

- National Academy of Medicine
  https://nam.edu
- U.S. Department of Health and Human Services
  http://www.hhs.gov
- Agency for Healthcare Research and Quality
  http://www.ahrq.gov
- Healthy People 2030
  http://www.healthypeople.gov

- National Healthcare Quality and Disparities Reports (current annual reports)
  http://nhqrnet.ahrq.gov/inhqrdr
- National Quality Strategy
  http://www.ahrq.gov/workingforquality
- World Health Organization
  http://www.who.int/en
- National Quality Forum
  http://www.qualityforum.org/Home.aspx

### Connect to Text Current Information with the Author

Go to the update for this text to review the Blog, QI News, and Literature Review. Access this regular update at: http://nursing.jbpub.com/Finkelman/QualityImprovement/2e.

## EBP, EBM, and Quality Improvement: Exemplar

Ryan, C. et al. (2017). Nurses' perceptions of quality care. *Journal of Nursing Care Quality*, 32(2), 180–185.

This article describes a study that examines the perceptions of quality care of nurses in practice. There is not always consensus on the definition of quality care, and how one perceives quality care may impact the response to engagement in quality improvement. This study identifies some key themes related to these perceptions, which may apply

more broadly, though with this study they reflect a specific sample.

### Some Questions to Consider

1. Is this study quantitative or qualitative? How do you support your answer?
2. What method was used to collect data? What do you think of this method?
3. What is your opinion of the results?

# EVOLVING CASE STUDY

Your hospital has recently revised its CQI vision and aims based on work done in the *Quality Chasm* series and the NQS recommendations. As nurse manager for an emergency department (ED), you need to take this information and make it "real" for staff in the ED. You and the medical director will present this information to the staff, but you need to figure out how it applies to daily work and how to engage staff. You both agree that the staff will not appreciate the "words" on the paper unless you can attach their meaning to their daily work in the ED.

## Case Questions

**1.** What information would you use as your base to discuss the vision and the aims?
**2.** How would you then apply this information to the ED and daily work done by staff?
**3.** What are several questions you might expect, and how might you answer them to better ensure that staff understand and get engaged?

## References

Adler, L., Yi, D., Li, M., McBroom, B., Hauck, L., Sammer, C., . . . Classen, D. (2015). Impact of inpatient harms on hospital finances and patient clinical outcomes. *Journal of Patient Safety.* doi:10.1097/PTS.0000000000000171

Bates, D., & Singh, H. (2018). Two decades since *To Err Is Human*: An assessment of progress and emerging priorities in patient safety. *Health Affairs, 37*(11), 1736–1743.

Benner, P., Sutphen, M., Leonard, V., & Day, L. (2010). *Educating nurses: A call for radical transformation.* San Francisco, CA: Jossey-Bass.

Bernstein, L., & McGinley, L. (2016, April 21). NIH hospital needs sweeping reform to better protect patient safety, panel says. *Washington Post.* Retrieved from https://www.washingtonpost.com/national/health-science/nih-hospital-needs-sweeping-reform-to-better-protect-patient-safety-panel-says/2016/04/21/52c1cb00-080d-11e6-b283-e79d81c63c1b_story.html?tid=a_inl

Berwick, D., Loehrer, S., & Gunther-Murphy, C. (2017). Breaking the rules for better care. *JAMA, 317*(21), 2161–2162.

Bisognano, M., & Kenney, C. (2012). *Pursuing the triple aim.* San Francisco, CA: Jossey-Bass.

Brach, C. (2019). Achieving value in health care through health literacy. Retrieved from https://health.gov/news/blog/2019/10/achieving-value-in-health-care-through-health-literacy

Brega, A.G., Hamer, M. K., Albright, K., Brach, C., Saliba, D., Abbey, D., & Gritz, R. M. (2019). Organizational health literacy: Quality improvement measures with expert consensus. *Health Literacy Research and Practice, 3*(2), e127–e146.

Burstin, H., Leatherman, S., & Goldmann, D. (2016). The evolution of healthcare quality measurement in the United States. *Journal of Internal Medicine, 279,* 154–159.

Carr, S. (2014). Looking to the future of patient safety. *Patient Safety and Healthcare Quality.* Retrieved from http://www.psqh.com/july-august-2014/looking-to-the-future-of-patient-safety

Cosgrove, D. (2013). Foreword. In S. Sadeghi, A. Barzi, O. Mikhail, & M. Shabot (Eds.), *Integrating quality and strategy in health care organizations.* Burlington, MA: Jones & Bartlett Learning.

Dabbous, M., Francois, C., Chachoua, L., & Tourni, M. (2019). President Trump's prescription to reduce drug prices: From the campaign trail to American Patients First. *Journal of Market Access & Health Policy, 7*(1), 1579597.

Donabedian, A. (1980). *Explorations in quality assessment and monitoring, volume 1: The definitions of quality and approaches to its assessment.* Ann Arbor, MI: Health Administration Press.

Draper, D., Felland, L., Liebhaber, A., & Melichar, L. (2008). The role of nurses in hospital quality improvement. Center for Studying Health System Change. *Research Brief, March*(3), 1–8.

Fallon, L., Begun, J., & Riley, W. (2013). *Managing health organizations for quality performance.* Burlington, MA: Jones & Bartlett Learning.

Fineberg, H. (2012). A successful and sustainable health system—How to get there from here. *New England Journal of Medicine, 366*(11), 1020–1027.

Finkelman, A. (2019). *Professional nursing concepts. Competencies for quality leadership* (4th ed.). Burlington, MA: Jones & Bartlett Learning.

Finkelman, A. (2020). *Leadership and management for nurses. Core competencies for quality care* (4th ed.). Upper Saddle River, NJ: Pearson Education.

Gantz, N., Sorenson, L., & Howard, R. (2003). A collaborative perspective on nursing leadership in quality improvement. *Nursing Administrative Quarterly, 27*(4), 324–329.

Hall, L., Moore, S., & Barnsteiner, J. (2008). Quality and nursing: Moving from a concept to a core competency. *Urological Nursing, 28*(6), 417–425.

Healthy People. (2019). Healthy people 2030. Retrieved from http://www.healthypeople.gov

Institute of Medicine (IOM). (1983). *Nursing and nursing education: Public policy and private action.* Washington, DC: The National Academies Press.

Institute of Medicine (IOM). (1999). *To err is human.* Washington, DC: The National Academies Press.

Institute of Medicine (IOM). (2001a). *Crossing the quality chasm.* Washington, DC: The National Academies Press.

Institute of Medicine (IOM). (2001b). *Envisioning the national healthcare quality report.* Washington, DC: The National Academies Press.

Institute of Medicine (IOM). (2002). *Guidance for the national health care disparities report.* Washington, DC: The National Academies Press.

Institute of Medicine (IOM). (2003a). *Priority areas for national action.* Washington, DC: The National Academies Press.

Institute of Medicine (IOM). (2003b). *Health professions education: A bridge to quality.* Washington, DC: The National Academies Press.

Institute of Medicine (IOM). (2003c). *The future of the public's health in the 21st century.* Washington, DC: The National Academies Press

Institute of Medicine (IOM). (2003d). *Who will keep the public healthy?* Washington, DC: The National Academies Press.

Institute of Medicine (IOM). (2003e). *Unequal treatment.* Washington, DC: The National Academies Press.

Institute of Medicine (IOM). (2004a). *Keeping patients safe. Transforming the work environment of nurses.* Washington, DC: The National Academies Press.

Institute of Medicine (IOM). (2004b). *Health literacy: A prescription to end confusion.* Washington, DC: The National Academies Press.

Institute of Medicine (IOM). (2010). *The future of nursing: Leading change, advancing health.* Washington, DC: The National Academies Press.

Institute of Medicine (IOM). (2011a). *Leading health indicators for Healthy People 2020: Letter report.* Washington, DC: The National Academies Press.

Institute of Medicine (IOM). (2011b). *Learning what works: Infrastructure required for effectiveness research: Workshop summary.* Washington, DC: The National Academies Press.

Institute of Medicine (IOM). (2011c). *Finding what works in health care: Standards for systematic reviews.* Washington, DC: The National Academies Press.

Institute of Medicine (IOM). (2011d). *Clinical practice guidelines we can trust.* Washington, DC: The National Academies Press.

Institute of Medicine (IOM). (2012). *Best care at lower cost: The path to continuously learning health care in America.* Washington, DC: The National Academies Press.

Institute of Medicine (IOM). (2015). Press release: Institute of Medicine to become National Academy of Medicine. Retrieved from http://www.iom.edu/Global/News%20Announcements/IOM-to-become-NAM-Press-Release.aspx

Jauhar, S. (2015, July 22). Giving doctors grades. *New York Times*, p. A27.

Kaiser Family Foundation (KFF). (2019). Peterson-Kaiser health system tracker: How does the quality of the U.S. healthcare system compare to other countries? Retrieved from https://www.healthsystemtracker.org/chart-collection/quality-u-s-healthcare-system-compare-countries/#item-start

Khanna, G. (2019a). AHRQ's commitment to meeting unmet needs in the healthcare system. Retrieved from https://www.ahrq.gov/news/blog/ahrqviews/ahrqs-commitment-to-meeting-unmet-needs.html

Khanna, G. (2019b). After 20 years of improving America's healthcare, AHRQ makes bold plans for future successes. Retrieved from https://www.ahrq.gov/news/blog/ahrqviews/bold-plans-future-successes.html

Makary, M., & Daniel, M. (2016). Medical error: The third leading cause of death in the U.S. *BMJ*, May 3. Retrieved from http://www.bmj.com/content/353/bmj.i2139/rr-40

McCabe, J., Joynt, K., Welt, F., & Resnic, F. (2013). Impact of public reporting and outlier status identification on percutaneous coronary intervention case selection in Massachusetts. *JACC Cardiovascular Interventions, 6*(6), 625–630.

McGaffigan, P. (2019). Why Florence Nightingale's lessons matter today. Retrieved from http://www.ihi.org/communities/blogs/why-florence-nightingales-improvement-lessons-still-matter-today

Millenson, M. (2006). Duty versus interest. The history of quality health care. In D. Nash & N. Goldfarb (Eds.), *Closing the quality chasm* (pp. 15–29). Sudbury, MA: Jones & Bartlett Publishers.

Nance, J. (2008). *Why hospitals should fly? The ultimate flight plan to patient safety and quality care.* Bozeman, MT: Second River Healthcare Press.

Nash, D., Evans, A., & Bowman, K. (2006). An overview of quality in the healthcare system. In D. Nash & N. Goldfarb (Eds.), *The quality solution: The stakeholder's guide to improving health care* (pp. 3–14). Sudbury, MA: Jones & Bartlett Publishers.

National Academy of Medicine (NAM). (2016). *Assessing progress on the IOM report The Future of Nursing*. Washington, DC: The National Academies Press

National Academy of Medicine (NAM). (2018a). *Building the case for health literacy*. Washington, DC: The National Academies Press.

National Academy of Medicine (NAM). (2018b). *Health literacy and the older adult*. Washington, DC: The National Academies Press.

National Academy of Medicine (NAM). (2018c). *Crossing the global quality chasm: Improving health care worldwide*. Washington, DC: The National Academies Press.

National Academy of Medicine (NAM). (2019). *Criteria for selecting the leading health indicators for healthy people 2030*. Washington, DC: The National Academies Press.

National Institute of Health (NIH). (2019a). The future of minority health and health disparities research is here. Retrieved from https://www.nih.gov/news-events/news-releases/future-minority-health-health-disparities-research-here

National Institute of Health (NIH). (2019b). NIH Clinical Center patient safety and clinical quality improvements. Retrieved from https://clinicalcenter.nih.gov/about/safety/improvements.html

National Patient Safety Foundation (NPSF). (2017). The Institute for Healthcare Improvement and the National Patient Safety Foundation merge. Retrieved from http://www.npsf.org/news/333839/Institute-for-Healthcare-Improvement-and-NPSF-Agree-to-Merge.htm

National Quality Forum (NQF). (2019). About us. Retrieved from http://www.qualityforum.org/About_NQF

Nelson, E. C., Godfrey, M. M., Batalden, P. B., Berry, S. A., Bothe, A. E., Jr., McKinley, K. E.,. . . Nolan, T. (2008). Clinical microsystems: Part 1. The building blocks of health systems. *The Joint Commission Journal of Quality and Patient Care, 34*(7), 367–378.

Organization for Economic Co-Operation and Development (OECD). (2019). Health spending (Indicators). Retrieved from https://data.oecd.org/healthres/health-spending.htm

President's Advisory Commission on Consumer Protection and Quality in the Health Care Industry. (1998). *Quality first: Better health care for all Americans*. Retrieved from https://govinfo.library.unt.edu/hcquality

Rockoff, J., & Silverman, E. (2015, April 26). Pharmaceutical companies buy rivals' drugs and then jack up the prices. *Wall Street Journal*. Retrieved from http://www.wsj.com/articles/pharmaceutical-companies-buy-rivals-drugs-then-jack-up-the-prices-1430096431#:HilJLi6HwyKdqA

Sadeghi, S., Barzi, A., Mikhail, O., & Shabot, M. (2013). *Integrating quality and strategy in health care organizations*. Burlington, MA: Jones & Bartlett Learning.

Sollecito, W., & Johnson, J. (2013). The global evolution of continuous quality improvement: From Japanese manufacturing to global health services. In W. Sollecito & J. Johnson (Eds.), *McLaughlin and Kaluzny's continuous quality improvement in healthcare* (4th ed., pp. 1–48). Burlington, MA: Jones & Bartlett Learning.

Somers, S., & Mahadevan, R. (2010). *Health literacy implications of the Affordable Care Act*. Hamilton, NJ: Center for Health Care Strategies.

Sullivan, L. (2004). *Missing persons. Minorities in health professions*. Washington, DC: Sullivan Commission on Diversity in the Healthcare Workforce. Retrieved from https://drum.lib.umd.edu/bitstream/handle/1903/22267/Sullivan_Final_Report_000.pdf?sequence=1&isAllowed=y

Sun, L. (2016, May 10). Exclusive: Patient safety issues prompt leadership shake-up at NIH hospital. *Washington Post*. Retrieved from https://www.washingtonpost.com/national/health-science/exclusive-patient-safety-issues-prompt-leadership-shake-up-at-nih-hospital/2016/05/10/ad1f71f6-0ffb-11e6-8967-7ac733c56f12_story.html

U.S. Department of Health and Human Services (HHS). (2011). Press release: National quality strategy will promote better health, quality care for Americans. Retrieved from http://www.businesswire.com/news/home/20110321006087/en/National-Quality-Strategy-Promote-Health-Quality-Care

U.S. Department of Health and Human Services (HHS). (2018). American patients first. Retrieved from https://www.hhs.gov/sites/default/files/AmericanPatientsFirst.pdf

U.S. Department of Health and Human Services (HHS). (2019). About HHS. Retrieved from https://www.hhs.gov/about/index.html

U.S. Department of Health and Human Services (HHS), Agency for Healthcare Research and Quality (AHRQ). (2011). Low health literacy linked to higher risk of death and more emergency room visits and hospitalizations. Retrieved from http://archive.ahrq.gov/news/newsroom/press-releases/2011/lowhlit.html

U.S. Department of Health and Human Services (HHS), Agency for Healthcare Research and Quality (AHRQ). (2016). The National Quality Strategy: Fact sheet. Retrieved from https://www.ahrq.gov/workingforquality/about/nqs-fact-sheets/fact-sheet.html

U.S. Department of Health and Human Services (HHS), Agency for Healthcare Quality and Research (AHRQ). (2017). About the National Quality Strategy. Retrieved from https://www.ahrq.gov/workingforquality/about/index.html

U.S. Department of Health and Human Services (HHS), Agency for Healthcare Quality and Research (AHRQ). (2018a). 2015 National Healthcare Quality and Disparities Report and 5th anniversary update on the National Quality Strategy. Retrieved from https://www.ahrq.gov/research/findings/nhqrdr/nhqdr15/executive-summary.html

U.S. Department of Health and Human Services (HHS), Agency for Healthcare Research and Quality (AHRQ). (2018b). Chartbook on care affordability. Retrieved from https://www.ahrq.gov/research/findings/nhqrdr/chartbooks/careaffordability/careaffordability.html

U.S. Department of Health and Human Services (HHS), Agency for Healthcare Research and Quality (AHRQ). (2019a). Patient Safety Awareness Week. Retrieved from https://www.ahrq.gov/patient-safety/psaw-2019/index.html

U.S. Department of Health and Human Services (HHS), Agency for Healthcare Research and Quality (AHRQ). (2019b). National steering committee for patient safety. Retrieved from https://www.ahrq.gov/patient-safety/about/national-steering-committee.html

U.S. Department of Health and Human Services (HHS), Agency for Healthcare Research and Quality (AHRQ). (2019c). National healthcare quality and disparities reports. Retrieved from https://www.ahrq.gov/research/findings/nhqrdr/index.html

U.S. Department of Health and Human Services (HHS), Agency for Healthcare Research and Quality (AHRQ). (2019d). Health literacy online. Retrieved from https://health.gov/communication/literacy/quickguide/factsbasic.htm

U.S. Department of Health and Human Services (HHS), Agency for Healthcare Research and Quality (AHRQ). (2019e). Ten attributes of health literate health care organizations. Retrieved from https://www.ahrq.gov/professionals/quality-patient-safety/quality-resources/tools/literacy/ten-attributes.html

U.S. Department of Health and Human Services (HHS), Agency for Healthcare Research and Quality (AHRQ).

U.S. Department of Health and Human Services (HHS), Centers for Disease Control and Prevention (CDC). (2014). Social determinants of health: Definitions. Retrieved from http://www.cdc.gov/socialdeterminants/Definitions.html

U.S. Department of Health and Human Services (HHS), Centers for Disease Control and Prevention (CDC). (2015). Healthy communities program. Retrieved from https://www.cdc.gov/nccdphp/dch/programs/healthycommunitiesprogram

U.S. Department of Health and Human Services (HHS), Centers for Disease Control and Prevention (CDC). (2017). Health expenditures. Retrieved from https://www.cdc.gov/nchs/fastats/health-expenditures.htm

U.S. Department of Health and Human Services (HHS), Health Resources & Services Administration (HRSA). (2019). Quality improvement awards (QIA). Retrieved from https://bphc.hrsa.gov/program-opportunities/funding-opportunities/quality

U.S. Department of Health and Human Services (HHS), Office of Disease Prevention and Health Promotion (ODPHP). (2019). *Healthy people 2030 framework*. Retrieved from https://www.healthypeople.gov/2020/About-Healthy-People/Development-Healthy-People-2030/Framework

Wallis, L. (2016). Global advisory panel on the future of nursing. *American Journal of Nursing, 116*(4), 18–19.

World Health Organization. (WHO). (2019). World patient safety day. Retrieved from https://www.who.int/campaigns/world-patient-safety-day/2019

Wyatt, R., Laderman, M., Botwinick, L., Mate, K., & Whittingon, J. (2016). Achieving health equity: A guide for health care organizations. IHI white paper. Cambridge, Massachusetts: Institute for Healthcare Improvement. Retrieved from http://www.ihi.org/resources/Pages/IHIWhitePapers/Achieving-Health-Equity.aspx

U.S. Department of Health and Human Services (HHS). (2019f). About learning health systems. Retrieved from https://www.ahrq.gov/learning-health-systems/about.html

# Quality Improvement: Ethics, Standards, Regulatory, Accreditation, and Legal Issues

## CHAPTER OBJECTIVES

At the conclusion of this chapter, the learner will be able to:

- Analyze ethical issues in healthcare delivery and nursing implications.
- Apply standards to the continuous quality improvement process.
- Illustrate the implications of government standards, legislation, and regulations to continuous quality improvement.
- Examine accreditation and its importance to quality healthcare.
- Examine legal issues that relate to quality healthcare.

## OUTLINE

## KEY TERMS

| | | |
|---|---|---|
| Accreditation | Ethics | Scope of practice |
| Autonomy | Fraud | Self-determination |
| Beneficence | Justice | Self-regulation |
| Certification | Malpractice | Standard |
| Code of ethics | Negligence | Veracity |
| Collaboration | Nursing regulation | Whistleblower |
| Ethical dilemma | Reasonably prudent nurse | |

# Introduction

Moving beyond the previous content—an overview of the history, key players, and current initiatives of the continuous quality improvement (CQI) movement—this chapter considers ethics, standards, legislation, regulations, accreditation, and legal issues related to CQI. These issues apply to all healthcare settings and all healthcare professionals and staff and can affect CQI by acting as barriers and also as support for positive CQI outcomes. "Research in patient safety and medical liability in recent years has widened our definition of these terms. Patient safety improvement is no longer a preventive strategy to protect medical facilities from lawsuits—it is a serious and wide-reaching effort to measurably improve the safety culture among staff in medical institutions, to find lasting and systemic prevention strategies for adverse events, and to work with patients—and with their families and caregivers—as equals to both address their care needs and to earnestly reconcile when their care does not go as planned. Working with patients as partners has become increasingly important in our rapidly changing medical landscape. Patients are experts in their own care and their own needs. Too often, we medical professionals ignore their expertise and opinion. In addition, caregivers and family members have knowledge and perspectives about the patient and his or her condition that can contribute to better care and improved patient safety" (Battles, Azam, Grady, & Reback, 2017). Transparency and ethics are critical elements that healthcare organizations (HCOs) and healthcare professionals need to consider in quality improvement. Ethical and legal concerns are often related.

# Ethical Concerns

Finkelman (2019) frames the discussion of **ethics** by comparing ethics to a related concept, *morals*: "Ethics refers to a standardized code or guide to behaviors. Morals are learned through growth and development, whereas ethics typically is learned through a more organized system, such as standardized ethics code developed by a professional group" (p. 170). Ethical standards, often presented as a **code of ethics**, guide professional behaviors. These standards are part of quality care and should not be ignored. Since there is greater concern today about ethical behavior, or the rightness and wrongness of the behavior of organizations and individual staff, healthcare organizations (HCOs) emphasize ethics more. For example, the American Nurses Association (ANA) designated 2015 as the year of ethics, recognizing its importance to the profession. The following are four major principles of ethics (**Figure 2-1**). The principles are part of nursing professional ethics (ANA, 2015a; Finkelman, 2019, pp. 171–172; Koloroutis & Thorstenson, 1999).

1. **Autonomy.** *Patients have the right to determine their own rights.* This principle applies to CQI when you consider issues such as patient-centered care, patient decision making, and privacy and confidentiality.
2. **Beneficence.** *Nurses should not inflict harm and should safeguard the patient.* This principle applies to CQI when you consider prevention of errors, quality monitoring, analysis of quality care concerns, such as errors and failure to meet outcomes, and development and evaluation of solutions to problems.

3. **Justice.** *Patients should be treated fairly.* This principle applies to CQI when you consider patient equality, health literacy, and methods to reduce healthcare disparities.
4. **Veracity.** *Patients should be told the truth.* This principle applies to CQI when staff communicate clear information about patient care, obtain patient consent, report concerns about care delivery, and disclose errors to patients.

# Nursing's Social Policy Statement: The Essence of the Profession

*Nursing's Social Policy Statement* (ANA, 2016) describes the scope of nursing practice and how the nursing profession relates to the public for whom it is accountable. Nursing practice is directly related to a number of social concerns, one of which specifically addresses the need for quality healthcare delivery and outcomes. Social responsibility requires nurses to assist with social concerns, providing nurses with the authority to do

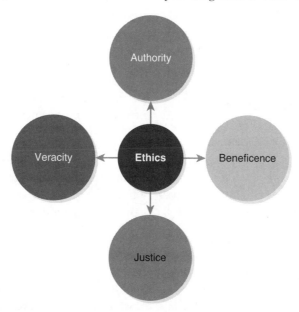

**Figure 2-1** Critical Ethical Principles

this; however, nurses need to be competent and follow a code of ethics. They are accountable for the care they provide based on their scope of practice. Professional **collaboration**, which is directly related to the need for teamwork, is required to meet the goal of effective nursing practice, working together with other nurses and healthcare professionals to meet agreed-upon outcomes, recognizing the contributions of collaborators.

## Guide to the Code of Ethics for Nurses: Interpretation and Application

The primary source for a code of ethics for nurses was developed by the ANA "as a guide for carrying out nursing responsibilities in a manner consistent with quality in nursing and the ethical obligations of the profession" (Fowler, 2015, p. xix). Provision 3 in the ANA Code focuses on issues related to CQI: "Protection of the rights of privacy and confidentiality, protection of human participants in research, performance standards and review mechanisms, professional responsibility in promoting a culture of safety, protection of patient health and safety by acting on questionable practice, and patient protection and impaired practice" (ANA, 2015a, p. 9). Many of the code's other provisions are indirectly related to CQI.

## Fraud and Healthcare Quality

When fraud occurs there are both ethical and legal issues. Fraud and abuse in healthcare are not rare. **Fraud** is intentional deception for one's own gain, and it is a criminal act. Abuse and fraud are similar acts, but with abuse it is often difficult to prove intention. Healthcare fraud and abuse have increased over the years. In some instances, HCOs and individuals that work for HCOs have committed fraud or deliberately deceived another person or organization for personal gain. In other instances, patients, such as those undergoing

mental health treatment, have been abused, as described in this section. Nurses have been involved in these problems. Healthcare is a business, a very large industry, and it provides many opportunities for fraud, particularly related to reimbursement. Healthcare fraud and abuse impact healthcare quality and also loss of funds that could be used to provide and improve care.

The most common fraud example is deceiving reimbursement sources such as the federal government, particularly the Medicare and Medicaid programs, although fraud also occurs with other types of reimbursement/insurers. During 2018 the federal government won or negotiated over $2.3 billion that was returned to the federal government or to private persons; Medicare received $1.2 billion and Medicaid $232 million. During this year the U.S. Department of Justice (DOJ) opened 1,139 criminal actions against individuals or entities for fraud-related crimes and 918 new civil healthcare fraud investigations. The U.S. Department of Health and Human Services (HHS) opened 679 criminal actions against individuals or entities for fraud-related crimes and 795 new civil healthcare fraud investigations (HHS, DOJ, OIG, 2019). This provides some perspective on the size of this problem.

It is important that this money was recovered; even though this instance does not represent all of the money that is lost, it represents a poor statement about ethics and legal concerns. For example, this fraud was related to common methods used to commit healthcare fraud such as billing for "phantom patients" (patients who did not exist), billing for medical goods or services that were not provided, billing for more hours than there are in a day, and double-billing for healthcare goods and services provided (HHS, CMS, 2014). In 2015, more than 240 individuals (doctors, nurses, and other licensed professionals) were arrested in one week for alleged participation in Medicare fraud involving $712 million in false billings (DOJ, FBI, 2015).

These major fraud issues involving Medicare led the Centers for Medicare and Medicaid (CMS) to create a website focused on fraud called Stop Medicare Fraud. Because Medicare fraud exhausts healthcare resources and thereby contributes to rising healthcare expenses, it impacts all Americans as well as patient outcomes and quality care. Identifying and preventing such corruption can improve the quality of healthcare and help make it more affordable for families, businesses, and the federal government (HHS, 2015). The CMS identifies the following examples of healthcare fraud, which continue to be committed (HHS, 2015):

- A healthcare provider bills Medicare for services patients never received.
- A supplier bills Medicare for equipment patients never received.
- Someone uses another person's Medicare card to get medical care, supplies, or equipment.
- Someone bills Medicare for home medical equipment after it has been returned.
- A company offers a Medicare drug plan that has not been approved by Medicare.
- A company uses false information to mislead potential Medicare beneficiaries into joining a Medicare plan.

It is important for consumers to be more aware of this fraud. They should ask questions when they are concerned or not clear of actions or requests and should report concerns to the CMS or other insurer and, when needed, to the healthcare provider. For example, the CMS website encourages Medicare beneficiaries to report problems and ask questions they may have about billing and other issues so that potential problems can be investigated; the website provides information about the problems and a reporting link. The Connect to Current Information section at the end of this chapter provides a link to this site.

Nurses may assume that nurses are not involved in healthcare fraud cases, but this is not a correct assumption. An example is a major HHS healthcare fraud effort in 2017 that involved 1,000 law enforcement staff. The investigation concluded by serving 295 individuals with exclusion notices, which means they can no longer submit claims for payment to any federal healthcare programs, including Medicare and Medicaid. In this group were 57 doctors, 162 nurses, and 36 pharmacists. The number of nurses might be thought to be questionable because "nurses do not prescribe medication," but now advanced practice registered nurses (APRNs) may have prescription authority. Many of the cases dealt with overprescription of narcotics (HHS, CMS, 2017). All healthcare professionals including nurses must follow their professional ethics code along with laws, as ethics and legal concerns are related.

Healthcare fraud does not just happen through Medicare and Medicaid claims and may be associated with CQI if staff members use a cover-up to limit knowledge about fraud. An example occurred in 2016 at an academic medical center (Beckers Hospital Review, 2016). What is notable about this case is that a nurse served as a **whistleblower**: a person who reports to authorities about fraud committed by an employer. The whistleblower laws protect the whistleblower from retaliation when such lawsuits are initiated (Westrick, 2019). In this 2016 case, the nurse filed a whistleblower civil lawsuit that led to an investigation of the number of patients, estimated at 100, who experienced infections after bronchoscopy. The medical center decided the best way to deal with the increase in infections was to just stop checking the bronchoscopes routinely. In doing this, they of course did not identify any problems. The nurse asked that this not be done and recommended that the hospital use an external agency to investigate this quality care problem, but this was not done. This case is significant as it includes a cover-up to make CQI look better and includes a healthcare professional who asks for help outside the organization and then files a lawsuit. It takes great personal strength to make this type of stand against inadequate care or, in some cases, fraud. Nurses and others encounter such situations in their workplaces and must decide how to address it.

Another example of major fraud and patient abuse episodes occurred in the 1980s and 1990s. During this period there were many large national psychiatric healthcare corporations, which were investor owned or for profit. Many new hospitals of this type were built, and there was a great deal of merging of corporations and competition. The following types of fraud and abuse are now known to have occurred in this patient care specialty (U.S. House of Representatives, 1992, 1994; U.S. Senate, 1992):

- HCOs documented admissions when the patients were never actually admitted.
- Parents were told that their children were seriously ill and needed admission when this was not the case.
- Patients were given medications they did not need, or there was documentation indicating patients received large amounts of medications that were never actually given; in either case, the hospitals billed for the medications.
- Patients were charged for treatment they never received.
- Patients were restrained unnecessarily and for long periods without appropriate care.
- Patients were denied their rights.
- Patients were subjected to verbal abuse.
- Staff did not follow expected healthcare standards.

When these problems were finally identified on a national level, there were extensive U.S. congressional reviews that detailed a lack of professional and business ethics in healthcare delivery (U.S. House of Representatives, 1992, 1994; U.S. Senate, 1992). Some states, such as Texas, had worse problems than others. Senator Mike Moncrief commented in Congress that "in Texas, we have uncovered some of the most elaborate, aggressive, creative, deceptive, immoral, and illegal schemes being used to fill empty hospital beds with insured and paying patients" (U.S. House of Representatives, 1992, p. 7). Hospital administration, physicians, nurses, and others were involved in these activities, although some physicians and nurses did report the activities to the authorities, such as to their state board of nursing (Mohr, 1996, 1997). However, some of them experienced negative results for stepping up to report unethical and illegal activities. For example, some of these employees reported being blacklisted so that it was difficult to get a new job, being victims of false claims to licensing boards about use of drugs, being subjected to verbal abuse, and receiving other threats.

An example of this type of complexity related to CQI occurred in 2014, when a major healthcare fraud concern was identified in Veterans Health Administration (VA) hospitals and their services. This healthcare system identified measures/indicators to determine quality status outcomes and in many cases to assess performance of providers and administrators. Some of these measures/indicators were connected to wait times for initial appointments. Some of the hospitals were involved in elaborate schemes to demonstrate that they met the measures/indicators; these schemes included changing or falsifying documentation. All of this fraud had a direct impact on the quality of care received; access was delayed, and in some cases care was never received. This is a clear example of the relationship between ethics and legal issues and quality care. In this case, the focus on CQI outcomes incentivized staff to do the wrong thing, to make the wrong decisions to meet the outcomes. Even in 2016, problems continued in some VA medical centers—for example, care and misconduct allegations at a Cincinnati, Ohio, VA hospital prompted an Inspector General investigation and in a Long Island, New York, VA hospital (Krause, 2016; Rebelo & Santora, 2016).

Such behavior is always a risk when outcomes are set and then used to assess performance of individuals and organizations. With the increasing use of this method in CQI, it has become even more important for health-care professionals to understand ethics and apply ethical principles, recognizing the need to maintain ethics in decisions and practice.

Fraud persists and is a major problem. Because this problem has increased and drains resources, it is addressed in the Affordable Care Act of 2010 (ACA) by increased penalties, expanded screening for fraud, and improved coordination of information across states. The U.S. Department of Health and Human Services (HHS) Healthcare Fraud Prevention and Enforcement Action Team (HEAT) is an example of the government's efforts to decrease healthcare fraud. HEAT brings together multiple stakeholders to prevent waste, fraud, and abuse in Medicare and Medicaid (HHS, OIG, 2017). Its mission statement includes the importance of preventing fraud, as it impacts quality care. The HHS works closely with the DOJ in this initiative. The federal government has increased monitoring and enforcement of laws to prevent fraud. Who has been involved in the fraud? Physicians, nurses, pharmacists, healthcare administrators, and other healthcare providers have been involved in fraud cases as have a variety of types of healthcare organizations such as hospitals, home healthcare agencies, long-term-care facilities, medical supply companies, pharmacies, and so on. Every staff member has an obligation to follow the four ethical principles and to report concerns to an organization's administration or, if necessary, to legal authorities.

## Organizational Ethics

With the increased number of ethical and legal concerns in healthcare, such as the healthcare fraud examples discussed in this chapter, HCOs have become more interested in organizational ethics. This is now a problem in many industries, but what does *organizational ethics* mean?

Organizations develop organization compliance committees with the goal of ensuring ethical business practices. These committees establish standards; provide staff education on ethics; develop systems for staff to report ethical and legal concerns, including policies, procedures, and staff education; and develop audits and monitor outcomes. Staff members need to understand how the organization's mission, vision, and goals relate to a code of conduct and its relationship to the HCO's compliance program.

When the program is developed, a critical element is implementation of a method for staff to anonymously report ethical concerns. Staff must feel that their identity will be protected and that reporting concerns will not lead to any personal negative result. In the preceding psychiatric care fraud and abuse examples, nurses had limited confidential methods to report their concerns, and those who stepped forward met with negative consequences. This type of culture does not lead to an effective compliance program. The need for healthcare organization monitoring of ethical concerns has become so important that in 1996 the Health Care Compliance Association (HCCA) was established, and it has expanded over the years as need increased (HCCA, 2019). Staff can now complete certification requirements in healthcare compliance to more effectively assist HCOs in their compliance efforts.

## Ethical Leadership

Leaders need to apply ethical principles in their decision making and ensure that the staff applies these principles in their work settings. All types of healthcare providers and HCOs need to ensure that there is a process for measuring quality and that strategies are used to improve care (Baily, Bottrell, Lynn, & Jennings, 2006; Jennings, Baily, Bottrell, & Lynn, 2007; White & O'Sullivan, 2012). There is greater emphasis today on pushing CQI activities down to the bedside level or the direct care level. This means that CQI is no longer just the responsibility of management and CQI programs/departments within HCOs; it is also the responsibility of each staff member. Healthcare leaders need to communicate to staff that attending to CQI efforts are an expectation and directly connected to the organization's ethics.

Ethical decision making is connected to decisions nurses make about CQI. Typically, this process occurs when there is an ethical dilemma. When **ethical dilemmas** occur, significant emotions are often involved, making it even more difficult to resolve them. Using facts is an important part of describing and understanding an ethical dilemma. HCO leaders need to actively support an ethical environment and work processes. The ethical environment should also include patient, family, and staff perspectives. In the end, choices must be made, and typically none of the options are ideal, creating an ethical dilemma. There is no "magic" answer to an ethical dilemma.

### STOP AND CONSIDER 2-1

Nurses have been involved in healthcare fraud.

# Standards and Quality Improvement

Standards impact practice, management, and CQI in healthcare and relate to individual professions, HCOs, and the government (local, state, and national). A **standard** is an "authoritative statement defined and promoted by a profession by which the quality of practice, service, or education can be evaluated" (ANA, 2015b, p. 146). Standards are viewed as the minimum, not maximum, expectation. They should be met, but they are not the end point in improvement. These nursing standards of practice include both standards of care that guide the provision of care and standards of professional performance describing the competent level of professional practice. Standards are an important part of CQI in that individual healthcare professions have standards that guide practice (e.g., nursing, medicine, pharmacy). States and the federal government

have standards, often incorporated in laws and regulations, and HCOs and healthcare professionals must commit to apply them—for example, state scope of practice and licensure requirements. Scope of practice is an area that changes, and with the growth in APRNs states are reviewing this issue—for example, in 2019 six states passed legislation related to prescribing ability and signage authority (Scope of Practice Policy, 2019). Accrediting organizations establish standards required for accreditation of HCOs and healthcare profession academic programs. Individual HCOs also have standards that must be followed.

## Professional Standards

**Self-regulation** is an important aspect of a profession. Nurses are expected to maintain their competence, often through required continuing education for licensure and/or certification. Even if this is not required, it is expected as part of self-regulation. If HCOs use peer review, nurses need to participate in this process. ANA's *Nursing: Scope and Standards of Practice* emphasizes the "essential role of the nurse in care coordination, promoting wellness, providing individualized care in nurse-managed health centers, and participation in medical homes. It identifies these and other nursing services as vital to the effort—to alleviate the financial and social costs of treating preventable and chronic diseases" (ANA, 2015b, p. 26).

Healthcare professional organizations develop standards for their members. For example, the ANA standards *Nursing: Scope and Standards of Practice* (ANA, 2015b) are the major nursing standards. The ANA also has developed standards focused on specific practice areas, such as nursing administration, staff education, gerontology, informatics, and other areas. Other healthcare professions, such as medicine, respiratory therapy, pharmacy, social work, laboratory services, radiology, and so on, have similar types of standards. The main goal for these standards is to ensure quality care and provide a description of professional responsibility required to reach the profession's goals.

Typically, specialty groups within a profession also have standards. Examples of nursing specialty organizations include the American Organization for Nursing Leadership, formerly known as the American Organization of Nurse Executives; Association of Occupational Health Nurses; American Association of Nurse Anesthetists; Association of Perioperative Registered Nurses; National Association of Neonatal Nurses; Infusion Nurses Society; and others. Nurses who work in these specialty areas are also expected to follow specialty standards. Standards change periodically due to changes in healthcare knowledge, research, and delivery needs, as well as changes within the health professions. Nurses and HCOs need to be aware of changes. Ideally, nurses will actively participate in the development of changes in standards and apply them. The *Quality Chasm* five healthcare professions core competencies are now integrated into some healthcare professions education requirements, including nursing, although more needs to be done to implement this recommendation. Over time, other important standards have been developed, such as Quality and Safety Education for Nurses (QSEN) standards associated with nursing education and the American Nurses Association Credentialing Center Magnet® standards. In addition, all of the standards must relate to The Joint Commission standards. Having so many standards can be confusing and also limits their value (Lyle-Edrosola & Waxman, 2016). Using methods such as a crosswalk description to compare standards is helpful in reducing confusion.

## Healthcare Organization Standards

HCOs also establish standards that apply to their staff and work processes within the organization. It is important that HCOs remain aware of other standards—those of government and other healthcare organizations such as ANA and other specialty organizations—to avoid conflicts. For example, is the HCO requiring staff to practice in a certain way that is not in accord with the staff members' professional standards or other relevant standards such as the state board of nursing? If so, this has a negative impact on quality care.

**STOP AND CONSIDER 2-2**

Standards are described as minimum standards.

# Government Standards, Legislation, and Regulations

Government at the local, state, and federal levels has many standards that are integrated into laws and regulations. These standards should be based on best evidence but also consider expert advice and other sources of information. HCOs and healthcare professionals are required to follow all relevant standards.

## Government Standards

The HHS is particularly tasked with development of healthcare policy and ensuring effective healthcare delivery on the federal level. It has many agencies that do this work for the department, as described in other chapters. The National Academy of Medicine (NAM), formerly known as the Institute of Medicine (IOM), and its *Quality Series* reports and subsequent reports have an impact on the HHS. The HHS often turns to this source to request in-depth examination of problems and provide external advice. State and federal governments establish standards in laws and related regulations that must be met. Many of these government standards are more than a guide; they are legal requirements. An example is the Emergency Medical Treatment and Active Labor Act of 1986 (EMATALA), which establishes the standard that all patients who require emergency treatment or who are in labor must be provided care regardless of ability to pay. This act establishes a level of care that is enforced under penalty of law. An emergency department must monitor this activity in its CQI program. Now, in some situations it is difficult to determine what is an emergency, but emergency departments have no choice but to make every effort to meet this standard.

## Legislation and Regulation

State laws and regulations also have a major impact on how nursing is practiced within a state, which in turn impacts the status of healthcare delivery. The American Nurses Association describes the Model of Professional Nursing Practice Regulation as a guide for the profession. Nursing practice integrates scope of practice, standards, ethics, specialty certification, nurse practice acts, rules and regulations, healthcare organization policies and procedures, and individual self-determination in care delivery. Quality, safety, and evidence are critical supporting elements of this practice (ANA, 2015b; Styles, Schuman, Bickford, & White, 2008). The guiding principles of nursing regulation are protection of the public, competence of all practitioners regulated by the board of nursing, due process and ethical decision making, shared accountability, strategic collaboration, evidence-based regulation, response to the marketplace and healthcare environment, and globalization of nursing (National Council State Boards of Nursing [NCSBN], 2007).

**Self-determination** is a very important part of the ANA practice model. During practice, each nurse must determine if there is a match with the scope of practice; clinical setting in which care is provided and the patient; individual skills and competencies; and the healthcare team's competencies. Individual

judgment is part of this process. **Scope of practice** is "the description of the *who, what, where, when,* and *how* of nursing practice that addresses the range of nursing practice activities common to all registered nurses" (ANA, 2015b, p. 67). The ANA *Standards of Practice* and the *Code of Ethics* influence the scope of practice that is designated by each state's nurse practice act. All of these impact evidence-based practice and quality.

## State Boards of Nursing and Nurse Practice Acts

**Nursing regulation**, as defined by the NCSBN (2007), "exists to protect the health, safety, and welfare of the public in their receipt of nursing services—and much more." This sets state-specific regulatory nursing standards. State boards of nursing are responsible for ensuring that each state's nurse practice act is followed in order to demonstrate effective practice and quality care for patients, the state's citizens. Each state has its own practice act, which is a law with regulations. The state boards also evaluate schools of nursing within the state to ensure that they meet the requirements established by the state board, and these requirements are influenced by standards. The NCSBN is an independent, nonprofit organization that provides counsel to all state boards of nursing but cannot tell individual state boards what they must do. The NCSBN is also responsible for the nursing licensure exams (NCSBN, 2020a). The purpose of the state boards and the NCSBN is to address issues related to public health, safety, and welfare. For example, the NCSBN description of effective transition to practice and its relationship to CQI are discussed in this text. It is not only important to the nursing profession but also to healthcare delivery.

The NCSBN is also involved in health policy—providing information, lobbying, and so on—with all levels of government. For example, the NCSBN assists in developing policies related to interstate practice and tele-health, both of which have implications for CQI. In 2015, the NCSBN held a conference, Leadership and Public Policy, to examine these issues and their relationship to nursing. Other activities related to CQI are improving simulation education for nurses and research about workforce needs. The NCSBN publishes the *Journal of Nursing Regulation* to provide a discussion forum about regulation and the profession. It also develops reports and books, such as *Nursing Pathways for Patient Safety* (Benner, Malloch, & Sheets, 2010).

The NCSBN is also involved in helping state boards of nursing with their professional discipline activities. It is not possible to eliminate risk in nursing practice, and state boards of nursing know this but are mandated by their state nurse practice act to protect the public. The NCSBN (2020b) summarizes its role in nursing discipline as follows: "While the vast majority of nurses are competent and caring individuals who provide care according to the standard, violations of the Nurse Practice Act do happen. When violations occur, the board of nursing takes formal action if it finds sufficient basis that the nurse violated the act or regulations. Currently, the rate of discipline on a license is less than 1 percent."

The NCSBN is engaged in patient safety by offering a national web-based network for anonymous reporting of student errors and near misses (2019a). The Safe Student Report (SSR) was developed in 2013. There is no similar program for other health professions inside or outside the United States. Data are compared among multiple prelicensure academic nursing programs, providing nurse educators with valuable data that can be used to improve nursing education.

## Professional Licensure

Professional licensure is administered at the state level through each state's board of nursing, but the licensure exam is offered on a national basis and administered through the NCSBN. The purpose of professional licensure is to ensure that all registered nurses and licensed practical nurses meet required standards to enter nursing practice at the *minimum* level of competence. The overall goal is to better ensure that patients receive quality care. Renewal of licensure is required for practice, but no testing is done. However, states may have different requirements—for example, completion of a certain number of continuing education credits. Despite the requirement for continuing education in some states, there is no current method to determine if this requirement makes any difference in practice and quality of care. For example, if a nurse completes a continuing education program on infections, how do the nurse and employer determine knowledge and application? Typically, the employer does not know what programs the nurse has completed, and if it is known, there is no way to determine outcomes. Continuing education programs require testing, but this testing is not rigorous, and it is easy to get passing scores. One can go back and look at content to answer questions and so on.

## Certification

**Certification** is available for many nursing specialties. Through standardized examination, nurses are able to demonstrate expertise in a specialty area and validate knowledge for certification as determined by the ANCC, although this is not the only provider of certification (ANCC, 2019). The goal is the same as for licensure: to ensure excellence in practice and thus impact the quality of care. To apply for certification, all eligibility requirements must be met, which may include practice requirements. Exams, portfolios, and continuing education are methods used to establish certification. The same problems encountered with continuing education for licensure are found in certification; thus, it is difficult to determine if this makes a difference in practice.

# Accreditation

Thus far, this chapter has presented individual professional responsibilities and methods to ensure that individual healthcare providers meet certain standards. Attention to the individual provider, however, is not enough, as HCOs have critical responsibilities in working to improve care. **Accreditation** is a method used to assess organizations and determine if they meet *minimum* established standards.

## The Joint Commission: Purpose and Description of Accreditation Process

The Joint Commission is an independent, not-for-profit organization that accredits and certifies HCOs and healthcare programs. The Joint Commission (2019a) vision is "all people always experience the safest, highest quality, best value health care across all settings." This vision correlates with the NAM work, the Triple Aim (better care, healthy people/healthy communities, affordable care), and the National Quality Strategy. Most hospitals are accredited by this organization. Although it is a voluntary process, accreditation has implications for marketing, receipt of federal funds such as Medicare payment, and insurers. Healthcare profession student clinical experiences must be offered in accredited HCOs. Accreditation focuses on hospitals, ambulatory healthcare, behavioral healthcare, critical access hospitals, home care, laboratory services, and nursing care centers. Although accreditation is typically associated with HCOs in the United States, The Joint Commission also accredits HCOs in other countries.

As is the case with other types of accreditation organizations, The Joint Commission has established *minimum* standards, which it periodically reviews and updates. HCOs that apply for accreditation or renewal of accreditation use these standards as guidelines as they prepare to ensure that they can gain accreditation during the official process. Standards vary depending on the type of HCO. Examples of standard topics for one type of HCO—hospitals—include the following: the environment of care, human resources, infection prevention and control, information management, leadership, life safety, medical staff, and medication management. The Joint Commission identifies annual National Patient Safety Goals, which for hospitals in 2020 were to identify patients correctly, improve staff communication, use medicines safely, use alarms safely, identify patient safety risks, and prevent mistakes in surgery (The Joint Commission, 2019b). These goals typically relate to the common areas of concern to better ensure quality improvement and are reviewed and changed annually.

The Joint Commission has developed a measurement system with measure sets focused on specific medical problems—for example, acute myocardial infarction, pneumonia, heart failure, and so on. This measurement system includes a review of medical records documentation. This approach provides an assessment of quality; however, it does not require a review of all HCO activities. The Joint Commission provides resources to both healthcare providers and the consumer/patient. From The Joint Commission website, consumers/patients can link to Quality Check to search for information about specific HCOs—information on measures that best indicate the status of quality care in a Joint Commission–accredited HCO. These measures are based solely on the perspective of The Joint Commission (2018). Consumers/patients can also report a safety or other type of concern about an HCO accredited by The Joint Commission to the website link for this purpose.

Additional information about The Joint Commission and its CQI activities and resources is found in other chapters. The Joint Commission website includes information about important content for healthcare providers, particularly focused on quality care, such as the listing of the current National Patient Safety Goals, sentinel event alerts, staff training, and so on. The Connect to Current Information section at the end of this chapter provides a link to its site.

## Nursing and The Joint Commission Accreditation

Nurses in all types of HCOs accredited by The Joint Commission are involved in all phases of the accreditation process. Nurses in leadership and management positions must be actively engaged in all steps within the HCO—planning, implementation, and evaluating the process at its conclusion. Clinical nursing staff is also involved, and now, compared to the past, all staff members, clinical and nonclinical, are more involved in the actual survey visit. This should also include nursing students who are assigned to clinical sites that may be undergoing accreditation. Surveyors speak with staff and engage them in the on-site process. Nurses need to also participate in CQI, which is part of accreditation; however, CQI should not be dependent on accreditation. CQI does not end when accreditation is received, nor is it ignored until the accreditation period concludes and a renewal is needed.

The Joint Commission accreditation process and its standards provide an objective process for HCOs to assess, measure, and improve performance (2019c). The objectives of the survey are not only to evaluate the organization but also to provide education and "good practice" guidance that will help staff continually improve the HCO's performance. Preparing for accreditation and the survey visit is part of the process. All levels of staff participate in the preparation and the survey on site. HCOs conduct self-assessments to prepare for an accreditation survey visit. The preparation includes the following:

1. Planning, which requires time and input from relevant stakeholders
2. Offering effective staff education about accreditation
3. Implementing an effective plan for the accreditation process
4. Providing ongoing evaluation of the implemented plan

The danger is always that the HCO does all the work for accreditation and then takes a long break until accreditation time comes around again. This is not the intent of accreditation and in the end harms the HCO. These activities should be ongoing.

## Examples of Other Accrediting Organizations

The following examples illustrate that accreditation is relevant to a variety of HCOs and associated organizations and processes, including nursing academic programs. Other healthcare profession programs, such as medicine, pharmacy, and physical therapy, also participate in the accreditation process for their specific professional academic programs based on their professional standards.

### Community Health Accreditation Partner

The Community Health Accreditation Partner (CHAP) has existed for more than 50 years (CHAP, 2019). It provides accreditation to community-based HCOs and related businesses. These HCOs include hospice, private duty agencies, home medical equipment businesses, home health, infusion therapy nursing, pharmacy, and public health. As is typical for most accreditation processes, the CHAP process includes a self-study and site visit. The review includes all aspects of the organization and its services.

### Accreditation Commission for Health Care

The Accreditation Commission for Health Care (ACHC) is an accreditation program that focuses on accreditation of hospice; home health; durable medical equipment, prosthetics, orthotics, and supplies (DMEPOS); pharmacy; private duty services; sleep lab/center; and behavioral health. Quality improvement is an important component of ACHC accreditation (ACHC, 2019). The CMS recognizes this accreditation for home health, hospice, and DMEPOS. This accreditation applies a process similar to the process used for other accrediting organizations.

### Utilization Review Accreditation Commission

The Utilization Review Accreditation Commission (URAC) is an independent, nonprofit organization that provides accreditation for health insurance plans (URAC, 2019). The goal is to promote CQI through its accreditation education and measurement programs—for example, by using benchmarking to compare insurance plan outcomes.

### Accreditation of Nursing Academic Programs

Nursing academic programs also undergo an accreditation process. There are two organizations that accredit schools of nursing: the American Association of Colleges of Nursing's accreditation Commission on Collegiate Nursing Education (CCNE) and the Accreditation Commission for Education in Nursing (ACEN) associated with the National League for Nursing. Both accreditation programs use similar processes based on their own required standards, self-study, and survey or site visit.

Nursing academic programs choose which accreditation they wish to obtain; however, the types of degree programs offered by schools of nursing may impact their choice of accreditation organization. The CCNE accredits collegiate professional education (baccalaureate and graduate nursing programs, including the doctor of nursing practice [DNP] degree but excluding PhD programs) and post-baccalaureate nurse residency programs (AACN, 2019). Programs that may be accredited by CNEA are practical (vocational), diploma, associate degree, baccalaureate, master's, and DNP programs that prepare advanced practice nurses, nurse executives, and nurse educators (CNEA, 2019).

The purpose of academic accreditation is to ensure that the nursing programs meet standards related to students, organization, curriculum, faculty, and program assessment to ensure that students get effective education and meet requirements to practice as designated by the school's state nurse practice act and its scope of nursing practice and other role requirements. The process recognizes the need to focus on self-assessment and growth and improvement.

### STOP AND CONSIDER 2-4

Healthcare organization accreditation is not required but is common.

## Legal Issues

Legal issues are connected with ethics, standards, and regulation. HCOs retain attorneys to assist with legal concerns and risk factors related to potential legal problems. These attorneys work with HCO staff on risk management and quality care to prevent legal problems and to resolve them when they occur. All nurses need to understand negligence and malpractice and how their practice can be at risk. Disclosure of errors is an important topic and part of patient-centered care today. This topic is discussed further in other chapters of this text.

# Negligence and Malpractice

Standards serve another function, which is also related to quality care. They are used by state boards of nursing and by the legal system to address nursing actions in licensure concerns and in legal cases, such as determining nursing negligence and malpractice. The nurse is expected to practice as a **reasonably prudent nurse**. *Reasonably prudent* means a nurse who has similar education and experience and average intelligence, judgment, foresight, and skill would respond like other similar nurses to the same situation, case, facts, or emergency using the standard of care and particularly should follow professional standards (Westrick, 2019). Standards are used as a guide for expected care, although other sources are also used in legal cases, such as clinical guidelines, expert testimony, and other documents that might clarify practice expectations. **Negligence** is "failure to exercise reasonable care, or the degree of care that a reasonably prudent person would exercise under the same or similar circumstances" (Westrick, 2019, p. 369). Negligence may be intentional or unintentional. **Malpractice** is similar to negligence but more specific. It is "professional negligence committed by a person in his or her professionally licensed capacity" (Westrick, 2019, p. 369). Specific legal requirements must be met for negligence: (1) duty to the patient, (2) proximate cause, and (3) damages or injury.

Nurses can be sued, and when this occurs it is important to consider the nurse's practice and whether or not expected standards were followed. Nurses in the employ of an HCO may also be sued as individual healthcare providers in lawsuits against that HCO. In these cases, it is recommended that the nurse consult an attorney that represents the nurse, not the HCO. Many nurses carry professional insurance, and when the nurse is involved in a potential lawsuit of this type, the insurer may require that the nurse take certain steps and use an attorney recommended by the insurer.

Negligence and malpractice and situations in which nurses are identified as having practice problems by their board of nursing are directly related to quality care. Something may have been done or not done that impacted practice and patient outcomes, and standards may not have been met.

# Guide to Nurses' Responses to Legal Problems Related to Errors

Nurses need to know the legal requirements within their state and federal requirements. They must follow the state nurse practice act and report practice that does not meet the standards. This is part of professional responsibility. Complaints to a board of nursing typically focus on nursing practice that is unsafe; incompetent; unethical; affected by alcohol, drugs, or other chemicals or by a physical or mental condition; and/or in violation of a nursing or nursing-related law or rule (NCSBN, 2019b). Each board of nursing describes its procedure for reporting concerns to the board. The NCSBN (2019b) states the following: "A nurse's practice and behavior is [sic] expected to be safe, competent, ethical, and in compliance with applicable laws and rules. Any person who has knowledge of conduct by a licensed nurse that may violate a nursing law or rule or related state or federal law may report the alleged violation to the state board of nursing where the situation occurred."

---

**STOP AND CONSIDER 2-5**

Nurses are sued for malpractice.

---

# Summary

CQI does not stand alone. It is influenced by critical aspects of healthcare delivery, particularly ethics, standards, legislation and regulation, accreditation, and legal concerns. Nurses are expected to understand all of these aspects

**Exhibit 2-1** Exemplars: Quality Improvement Roles and Responsibilities

**Staff Nurse**

Staff nurses in a medical unit are meeting with their nurse manager to discuss plans for the coming year, which includes preparation for an accreditation renewal survey culminating in an on-site survey at the end of the year. Each nurse is responsible for understanding the process and participating. At the time of the on-site survey, surveyors stop a staff nurse who is walking down the hall in the unit. They ask her to explain the importance of accreditation to her, the unit, the hospital, and the patients. This nurse has to be prepared for this type of question and engage when asked.

**Nurse Manager**

A nurse manager in the pediatric unit is meeting with the chief nurse executive and one of the hospital's attorneys. A patient (parents of a patient in the name of the 5-year-old) who had major complications that might have been due to a medication error has filed a lawsuit. Some of the questions the attorneys ask focus on the role of the nurse manager in supervising and quality improvement. The nurse knows he must be involved but also that he needs legal counsel separate from hospital counsel. After hearing about the case and realizing that this will be ongoing as it has not been resolved, he calls the representative for his professional insurance, who gives him a name of an attorney to call. The representative emphasizes that the nurse needs to contact and work with this attorney to ensure professional coverage. The nurse calls the attorney.

**Advanced Practice Registered Nurse***

The manager of the emergency department informs the department's APRN that she must prescribe certain medications when appropriate and does not need to be supervised by a physician. The APRN reviews the list of medications and wonders about several of them and the need for physician approval. The APRN contacts the state board of nursing to review scope of practice and other issues around prescriptive authority.

* Advanced Practice Registered Nurse includes APRN, Clinical Nurse Specialist, Clinical Nurse Leader, and nurses with DNP

as members of a profession, and they need to participate actively in following requirements to improve care. The profession uses specific methods and organizations, such as professional organizations and state boards of nursing, which focus on all of these concerns.

All of these methods relate to CQI—ensuring quality care for patients. Exemplars of quality improvement roles and responsibilities for staff nurses, nurse managers, and APRNs are found in **Exhibit 2-1**.

# APPLY CQI

## Chapter Highlights

- Ethical concerns are present every day in all healthcare settings and relate to all healthcare professionals.
- Professional codes of ethics are related to CQI.

- Healthcare fraud causes the nation to lose money that could have been used on healthcare delivery, and it impacts quality; the problem is increasing.

- Ethical leadership should be part of each HCO, but achievement requires effort.
- Individual professional standards, HCO standards, and government standards all have an impact on how we practice and on CQI.
- Regulations and legislation may indirectly or directly impact CQI.
- Accreditation of HCOs and health profession academic programs are important parts of ensuring CQI. Practice is based on standards. Academic programs follow standards to meet consistent education requirements, and both HCOs and educational programs include CQI in their ongoing activities.
- Negligence and malpractice are related to the quality of practice and related outcomes.

## Critical Thinking and Clinical Reasoning and Judgment: Discussion Questions and Learning Activities

1. Why is professional ethics part of a discussion about quality improvement? Provide three examples to support your answer.
2. You are part of a standards committee at your HCO. The committee is working on its annual review of standards. What internal and external information should be reviewed?
3. Review your state's nurse practice act and visit your state board of nursing website. Summarize key points you want to remember. Discuss what you find with your student team.
4. You and several classmates plan to ask about accreditation at the HCOs where the students are performing clinical rotations. Before interviewing HCO staff, work together to prepare a list of key questions. After the interview, summarize the interview information and discuss how it relates to quality improvement. Compare the data you obtained.
5. Scope of practice continues to be an issue that requires nurses to be aware of changes within their states and also national trends. Visit the following website and search for information related to your state, then discuss your findings with your student team: https://campaignforaction.org/

## Connect to Current Information

- Help Fight Medicare Fraud
  https://www.medicare.gov/forms-help
  -resources/help-fight-medicare-fraud
- The Joint Commission
  http://www.jointcommission.org
- American Association of Colleges of Nursing
  https://www.aacnnursing.org/CCNE
- National League for Nursing
  http://www.acenursing.org
- American Nurses Credentialing Center
  https://www.nursingworld.org/our
  -certifications
- Scope of Practice Policy/Legislation by State
  http://scopeofpracticepolicy.org/legislative
  -search
- ANA's *Code of Ethics for Nurses with Interpretive Statements*
  https://pdfs.semanticscholar.org/5e53
  /bafd3cb3d02efa0ef20fbcd71fbcf5001c54
  .pdf

**Connect to Text Current Information with the Author**

Go to the update for this text to review the Blog, QI News, and Literature Review. Access this regular update at: http://nursing.jbpub.com/Finkelman/QualityImprovement/2e.

## EBP, EBM, and Quality Improvement: Exemplar

Millikin, A. (2018). Ethical awareness: What it is and why it matters. *The Online Journal of Nursing, 23*(1). Retrieved from http://ojin.nursingworld.org/MainMenuCategories/ANAMarketplace/ANAPeriodicals/OJIN/TableofContents/Vol-23-2018/No1-Jan-2018/Ethical-Awareness.html

### Questions to Consider

1. What is ethical awareness?
2. Discuss the examples provided and their implications.
3. How might you use the information found in this article?

# EVOLVING CASE STUDY

As a member of the staff development department, you and others in the department are beginning preparations for an upcoming Joint Commission survey—a process that takes many months. Five staff members, including the director, are involved; however, two of you have not been through an accreditation survey as a staff educator. Since the last survey, the hospital has added 40 beds; there is a shortage of registered nurses in two medical units and one surgical unit; and there has been an increase in CQI activities and an increase in CQI program staff. There are still concerns about quality care problems that have not improved, such as medication errors.

### Case Questions

1. What should your staff development group include in the plan to prepare for The Joint Commission process? Your plan should identify a timeline.
2. What are the differences in the accreditation role of staff educators, administration/management, clinical staff (staff nurses, APRNs), and nonclinical staff? How should you collaborate?
3. As part of your preparation of staff and expansion of accreditation content in staff orientation, how would you include accreditation, standards, regulation, and ethical and legal issues in the orientation discussion? What teaching–learning methods might you use?

# References

Accreditation Commission for Health Care (ACHC). (2019). ACHC: For providers. By providers. Retrieved from https://www.achc.org

American Association of Colleges of Nursing. (AACN) (2019). Vizient/AAN Nurse Residency Program. Retrieved from https://www.aacnnursing.org/Nurse-Residency-Program

American Nurses Association (ANA). (2015a). *Code of ethics with interpretive statements* (3rd ed.). Silver Spring, MD: Author.

American Nurses Association (ANA). (2015b). *Nursing: Scope and standards of practice.* Silver Spring, MD: Author.

American Nurses Association (ANA). (2016). *Guide to nursing's social policy statement: Understanding the profession from social contract to social covenant.* Silver Spring, MD: Author.

American Nurses Credentialing Center (ANCC). (2019). Our certifications. Retrieved from https://www.nursing world.org/our-certifications

Baily, M., Bottrell, M., Lynn, J., & Jennings, B. (2006). *The ethics of using QI methods to improve healthcare quality and safety.* New York, NY: The Hastings Center.

Battles, J., Azam, I., Grady, M., & Reback, K. (Eds.) (2017). Advances in Patient Safety and Medical Liability. AHRQ Publication No. 17-0017. Rockville, MD: Agency for Healthcare Research and Quality.

Beckers Hospital Review. (2016). UC health nurse sues health system for covering up scope-related outbreak. Retrieved from http://www.beckershospitalreview .com/quality/uc-health-nurse-sues-health-system-for -covering-up-scope-related-outbreak.html

Benner, P., Malloch, K., & Sheets, V. (Eds.). (2010). *Nursing pathways for patient safety.* St. Louis, MO: Mosby.

Community Health Accreditation Partner (CHAP). (2019). Accreditation. Retrieved from https://chapinc.org /accreditation-process

Commission for Nursing Education Accreditation (CNEA). (2019). Overview: National League for Nursing Commission for Nursing Education Accreditation (CNEA). Retrieved from http://www.nln.org /accreditation-services/overview

Finkelman, A. (2019). *Professional nursing concepts: Competencies for quality leadership* (4th ed.). Burlington, MA: Jones & Bartlett Learning.

Fowler, M. (2015). *Guide to the code of ethics for nurses with interpretive statements. Development, interpretation, and application* (2nd ed.). Silver Spring, MD: American Nurses Association.

Health Care Compliance Association (HCCA). (2019). About CCB. Retrieved from https://www.hcca-info .org/certification

Jennings, B., Baily, M., Bottrell, M., & Lynn, J. (2007). *Healthcare quality improvement: Ethical and regulatory issues.* Garrison, NY: The Hastings Center.

Koloroutis, M., & Thorstenson, T. (1999). An ethics framework for organizational change. *Nursing Administrative Quarterly, 23*(2), 9–18.

Krause, B. (2016, February 15). Cincinnati VA at center of misconduct investigation. Retrieved from http:// www.disabledveterans.org/2016/02/15/cincinnati -va-at-center-of-misconduct-investigation

Lyle-Edrosola, G., & Waxman, K. (2016). Aligning healthcare safety and quality competencies: Quality and Safety Education for Nurses (QSEN), The Joint Commission, and American Nurses Association Credentialing Center (ANCC) Magnet® standards crosswalk. *Nurse Leader, 14*(1), 70–75.

Mohr, K. (1996). Dirty hands: The underside of marketplace healthcare. *Advances in Nursing Science, 19*(1), 28–37.

Mohr, K. (1997). Outcomes of corporate greed. *Image: Journal of Nursing Scholarship, 29*(1), 39–45.

National Council State Boards of Nursing (NCSBN). (2007). *Guiding principles.* Retrieved from https:// www.ncsbn.org/1325.htm

National Council State Boards of Nursing (NCSBN). (2019a). Safe student reports (SSR) research study. Retrieved from https://www.ncsbn.org/safe-student -reports.htm

National Council State Boards of Nursing (NCSBN). (2019b). Filing a complaint. Retrieved from https://ncsbn.org /What_Every_Nurse_Needs_to_Know.pdf

National Council State Boards of Nursing (NCSBN). (2020a). Index. Retrieved from https://www.ncsbn .org/index.htm

National Council State Boards of Nursing (NCSBN). (2020b). Discipline. Retrieved from https://www .ncsbn.org/discipline.htm

Rebelo, K., & Santora, M. (2016, September 19). Deaths, fraud allegations, and an inquiry into a Long Island V.A. hospital. Retrieved from http://www.nytimes .com/2016/09/20/nyregion/inquiry-into-northport -va-hospital-long-island.html?_r=

Scope of Practice Policy. (2019). Legislative search. Retrieved from http://scopeofpracticepolicy.org/legislative-search

Styles, M., Schuman, M., Bickford, C., & White, K. (2008). Specialization and credentialing in nursing revisited: Understand the issues, advancing the profession. Retrieved from https://www.ovid.com/product -details.8282.html

The Joint Commission. (2018). About Quality Check. Retrieved from http://qualitycheck.org/help_qc_facts .aspx

The Joint Commission. (2019a). Facts about The Joint Commission. Retrieved from https://www.jointcommission .org/about-us/

The Joint Commission. (2019b). 2020 Hospital National Patient Safety Goals. Retrieved from https://www .jointcommission.org/assets/1/6/2020_HAP_NPSG _goals_final.pdf

The Joint Commission. (2019c). Fact sheets. Retrieved from https://www.jointcommission.org/resources/news -and-multimedia/fact-sheets

U.S. Department of Health and Human Services (HHS), Centers for Medicare and Medicaid Services (CMS). (2014). Common Medicaid rip-offs and tips to prevent fraud. Retrieved from http://www.cms.gov /Medicare-Medicaid-Coordination/Fraud-Prevention /FraudAbuseforConsumers/Ripoffs_and_Tips.html

U.S. Department of Health and Human Services (HHS). (2015). Stop Medicare Fraud. About fraud. Retrieved from https://www.justice.gov/archives/opa/blog/stop -medicare-fraud

U.S. Department of Health and Human Services (HHS), Centers for Medicare and Medicaid Services (CMS). (2017). Healthcare fraud and abuse control program protects consumers and taxpayers by combating healthcare fraud. Retrieved from https://www.cms .gov/newsroom/fact-sheets/health-care-fraud-and -abuse-control-program-protects-consumers-and -taxpayers-combating-health-care-0

U.S. Department of Health and Human Services (HHS) and the Department of Justice (DOJ). Office of the Inspector General (OIG). (2019). The Department of Health and Human Services and the Department of Justice Health Care Fraud and Abuse Control Program, annual report for fiscal year 2018. Retrieved from https://oig.hhs.gov/publications/docs/hcfac/FY2018 -hcfac.pdf

U.S. Department of Health and Human Services (HHS), Office of Inspector General (OIG). (2017). 2017 national healthcare fraud takedown. Retrieved from https://oig.hhs.gov/newsroom/media-materials /2017/2017HealthCareTakedown_FactSheet.pdf

U.S. Department of Justice (DOJ), Federal Bureau of Investigation (FBI). (2015). Healthcare fraud takedown. Retrieved from https://www.fbi.gov/news/stories/2015 /june/health-care-fraud-takedown/health-care -fraud-takedown

U.S. House of Representatives. (1992, April 28). The profits of misery: How inpatient psychiatric treatment bilks the system and betrays our trust. Hearing before the Select Committee on Children, Youth and Families, One Hundred Second Congress, Second Session. Washington, DC: U.S. Government Printing Office.

U.S. House of Representatives. (1994, July 19). Deceit that sickens America: Health care fraud and its innocent victims. Hearings before the Subcommittee on Crime and Criminal Justice of the Committee on the Judiciary House of Representatives, One Hundred and Third Congress, One Hundred Congress, Second Session. Washington, DC: U.S. Government Printing Office.

U.S. Senate. (1992, July 28). Hearing before the Committee on the Judiciary United States Senate, Senate Bill 2652, One Hundred Second Congress, Second Session. Washington, DC: U.S. Government Printing Office.

Utilization Review Accreditation Commission (URAC). (2019). URAC. Retrieved from https://www.urac.org

Westrick, S. (2019). *Essentials of nursing law and ethics* (3rd ed.). Burlington, MA: Jones & Bartlett Learning.

White, K., & O'Sullivan, A. (Eds.). (2012). *The essential guide to nursing practice: Applying ANA's scope and standards in practice and education.* Silver Spring, MD: American Nurses Association.

## CHAPTER 3

# Healthcare Professions Core Competencies to Improve Care

## CHAPTER OBJECTIVES

At the conclusion of this chapter, the learner will be able to:

- Analyze the five healthcare professions core competencies and implications for continuous quality improvement (CQI) and nursing identified in *Health Professions: A Bridge to Quality*.
- Discuss critical nursing education documents and initiatives and their implications to healthcare CQI.

## OUTLINE

## KEY TERMS

Attitudes
Comparative effectiveness
   research
Competency
Continuing education (CE)
Evidence-based management
   (EBM)

Evidence-based practice (EBP)
Interprofessional education
Knowledge
Learning health system
Lifelong learning
Point-of-care learning
Skills

Systematic review
Workplace learning

## Introduction

Today, it is clearly recognized that in order for healthcare to improve in the United States, there must be improvement and ongoing changes in healthcare education in academic healthcare professional programs, staff education in the workplace, and professional continuing education. This chapter offers a description of relevant competencies that are important to improving practice and care outcomes, along with a discussion of important strategies needed to improve care through more competent staff practice that are supported by accreditation of education programs, education standards, innovative education approaches such as simulation, staff education, interprofessional education, and improvement in continuing education for healthcare professionals. The goal is to establish a learning healthcare system that, in the words of the Institute of Medicine (IOM, 2007), is "designed to generate and apply the best evidence for the collaborative healthcare choices of each patient and provider; to drive the process of discovery as a natural outgrowth of patient care; and to ensure innovation, quality, safety and value in healthcare. Advances in computing, information science, and connectivity can improve patient–clinician communication, point-of-care guidance, the capture of experience, population surveillance, planning and evaluation, and the generation of real-time knowledge—features of a continuously learning health care system" (p. 37).

## Health Professions: A Bridge to Quality

The publication of *Health Professions: A Bridge to Quality* (IOM, 2003a), one of the early *Quality Chasm* reports, was an important step in the development of the reports on quality care. The *Quality Chasm* reports published prior to this report primarily focused on understanding the status of care and healthcare delivery problems; describing a vision, aims, and framework for quality care; and offering recommendations for measuring and tracking progress. The piece that was missing in the process is greater understanding of the implications of the competency of the healthcare professionals and others who are associated with care delivery on continuous quality improvement (CQI) process (Finkelman, 2020).

The *Health Professions* report discussed this concern, as well as the connection of this report to previous reports: *To Err Is Human* leading to additional quality reports.

One can spend a lot of effort trying to improve care during the care process and within healthcare organizations (HCOs), but something was missing from this effort. Are healthcare professions ready to provide quality care and work to ensure that there is CQI? This CQI agenda is really the critical topic of this text. If HCOs work to improve but staff and new graduates from the various healthcare professions are not prepared in understanding and applying CQI every day in care settings, can we really ever reach the aims of safe, effective, timely, efficient, equitable, and patient-centered (STEEEP®) care (IOM, 2001)?

The first step was to identify the core competencies, and the approach taken was highly significant. Rather than identify core competencies for specific healthcare professions, the decision was made to identify core competencies for all healthcare professions— the same competencies to ensure a base of functioning in the healthcare delivery system. This approach had never been tried before. A **competency** is "an expected and measurable level of nursing performance that integrates knowledge, skills, abilities, and judgment

based on established scientific knowledge and expectations for nursing practice" (American Nurses Association [ANA], 2015, p. 64). The five competencies are based on this definition. These core competencies are highlighted in **Figure 3-1** and discussed in the following sections. Healthcare professions meeting these competencies then act as a bridge to quality.

## Provide Patient-Centered Care: Application to Nursing and CQI

The core competency to provide patient-centered care is described by the IOM (2003a) as follows: "Identify, respect, and care about patients' differences, values, preferences, and expressed needs; relieve pain and suffering; coordinate continuous care; listen to, clearly inform, communicate with, and educate patients; share decision making and management; and continuously advocate disease prevention, wellness, and promotion of healthy lifestyles, including a focus on population health" (p. 4). **Figure 3-2** highlights key elements of this competency.

Focusing on the patient in healthcare has had a fluctuating history. Some healthcare professions, such as nursing, have historically put patients at the center of care.

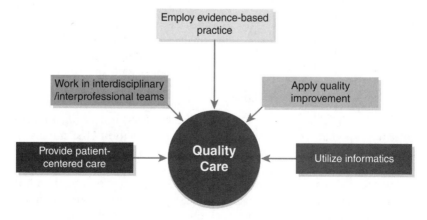

**Figure 3-1** The Five Healthcare Professions Core Competencies

Data from Institute of Medicine. (2003). *Health professions education: A bridge to quality.* Washington, DC: National Academies Press.

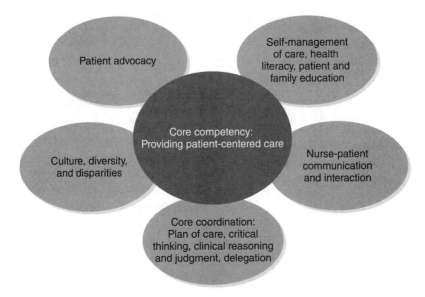

**Figure 3-2** Providing Patient-Centered Care: Key Elements

With the increasing concern about the quality of care and the work done by the National Academy of Medicine (NAM), this focus has increased. Now, the term "patient-centered" applied to care is commonly used, and when appropriate this concept has been expanded to "family-centered" care.

As discussed in this text, this competency supports greater patient participation in CQI—for example, patients are encouraged to comment on care concerns (e.g., ask questions about their medications, request information about diagnosis and treatment, note if staff are washing their hands, and so on) and are asked to complete evaluation surveys, and then HCOs use the data to improve. The focus of care is the patient, and this approach should improve care when nurses do the following:

- Recognize the importance of patient- and family-centered care and encourage patients to actively participate in decisions.
- Understand the patient's and the family's journey—that is, their experiences with the healthcare system, both current and past.
- Incorporate patient rights and preferences in care.

- Incorporate elements of patient- and family-centered care in their daily work.
- Consider how they can improve the implementation of effective patient- and family-centered care.

Cosgrove (2012) explains the ideal approach to patient-centered care as follows: "Patient-centered care requires shared decisions and open communication with patients. This type of decision making requires listening to the patient and assists staff when they need to discuss benefits and risks with patients about their care so that the patient is prepared to participate actively in decision making. The discussion should be based on evidence of best practice" (p. 18).

Healthy People 2030, as discussed in other chapters, is a national initiative to improve the health of U.S. citizens. This initiative also has an impact on quality of care for individuals and populations, and it is also patient centered, connecting it with the *Quality Chasm* recommendations. Its vision supports a society in which all people live long, healthy lives by focusing on four goals: healthcare quality, equity of healthcare, a healthy social and physical environment, and healthy development and behaviors across the life span (Healthy People, 2020). The patient is the center of each of the goals. Additional content about patient-centered care is found throughout this text.

## Work on Interdisciplinary/ Interprofessional Teams: Application to Nursing and CQI

The core competency of interdisciplinary or interprofessional teams is described as "cooperate, collaborate, communicate, and integrate care in teams to ensure that care is continuous and reliable" (IOM, 2003a, p. 4). **Figure 3-3** highlights key elements of this competency.

Teams are used in all HCOs. Some teams are composed of the same type of staff (intraprofessional), such as a nursing team, and some teams are interprofessional, representing multiple professions. All staff need to understand how teams are structured and function in order to participate effectively in the team environment. Organizations have their own cultures, and this culture impacts how the organization

is structured and functions. The team approach to CQI is a key topic of this text.

## Employ Evidence-Based Practice: Application to Nursing and CQI

The core competency of employ evidence-based practice (EBP) is described as "integrate best research with clinical expertise and patient values for optimum care, and participate in learning and research activities to the extent feasible" (IOM, 2003a, p. 4). **Figure 3-4** highlights key elements of this competency. Given the emphasis in this text on quality improvement, it is important to address the issue of similarities and differences in EBP, quality improvement, and research (Carter, Mastro, Vose, Rivera, and Larson, 2017). How might these be compared? Here's an example: A hospital wants to introduce a checklist for care of patients with diabetes. With an EBP emphasis, a nurse-led team reviews and assesses literature on diabetes and use of checklists with the goal of developing a checklist, policy, and procedure. From a QI perspective the hospital tracks data on patient knowledge of diabetes care and notes that patients lack critical information,

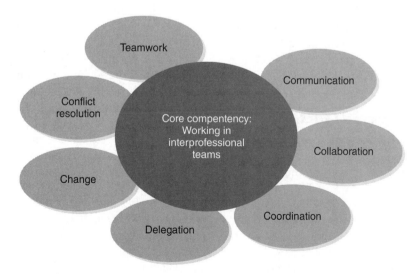

**Figure 3-3** Working Interprofessional Teams: Key Elements

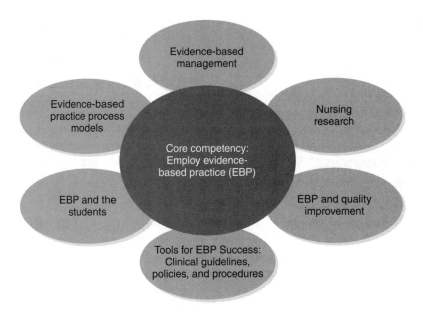

**Figure 3-4** Employ Evidence-Based Practice: Key Elements

this is not routinely documented, and change in care occurs using the new checklist. A nurse from the local school of nursing approaches the chief nurse executive to suggest a research study that would compare use of two different diabetes checklists over time. EBP provides opportunities to bridge the knowledge gap leading to new solutions. "Improvement comes from the application of knowledge, the more complete the appropriate knowledge, the better the improvement will be when this knowledge is applied to making change" (Leming-Lee & Watters, 2018, p. 1).

## Evidence-Based Practice

What is **evidence-based practice (EBP)**? EBP is making clinical decisions using the best evidence possible. There are four types of evidence used in EBP (Melnyk & Fineout-Overholt, 2010): "(1) evidence from research, (2) evidence from the patient's history and assessment, (3) clinical expertise, and (4) patient values and preferences. It is accepted that EBP has a positive impact on "constraining health costs, reducing geographic

variation in the use of healthcare services, improving quality, supporting consumer-directed healthcare, and improving health coverage decisions" (IOM, 2008, p. 3).

EBP is now an integral part of undergraduate and graduate nursing education. It took time for this to happen and pressure from HCOs, as they needed new graduates with at least baseline EBP knowledge. The process of recognizing and determining how to add this content so that this competency could be met varied. Some nursing academic programs dealt with this new need by eliminating research courses, adding EBP courses, combining research and EBP into one course, and/or adding EBP student projects, and eventually academic programs developed content and approaches for preparing students. Most academic nursing programs did not consider EBM content, but it too is important to include in leadership and management content, as is CQI content (Kovner & Rundall, 2010). The IOM (2008) describes the need for continued efforts toward EBP as follows: "The nation's capacity has fallen far short of its need for producing reliable and practical information about the care that works best. Medical-care decision making is now strained, at both the level of the individual patient and the level of the population as a whole, by the growing number of diagnostic and therapeutic options for which there is insufficient evidence to make a clear choice" (p. 17).

Even though EBP is now integrated in most HCOs, particularly hospitals, we still have much to do to ensure that best evidence is used in all healthcare organizations and all healthcare professionals, as articulated by the IOM (2011a): "The demand for better evidence to guide healthcare decision making is increasing rapidly for a variety of reasons, including the adverse consequences of care administered without adequate evidence, emerging insights into the proportion of healthcare interventions that are unnecessary, recognition of the frequency of medical errors, heightened public awareness and concern about the very high costs of medical care, the burden on employers and employees, and the growing proportion of health costs coming from out of pocket" (p. 1). To support EBP improvement, more nursing research is needed to answer questions about best practice, staff understanding of EBP and EBM, and effective methods to implement and maintain EBP and EBM.

### *Evidence-Based Management*

Evidence should not just be associated with clinical care. It is very important to use evidence to support other decisions in healthcare, decisions typically made by managers. This is something that is usually not thought of in nursing curricula or by managers themselves. **Evidence-based management** is the "systematic application of the best available evidence to the evaluation of managerial strategies for improving the performance of health services organizations" (Kovner & Rundall, 2010, p. 56). **Figure 3-5** provides an overview of the EBM steps.

HCO managers and leaders must be concerned with two aspects of the organization:

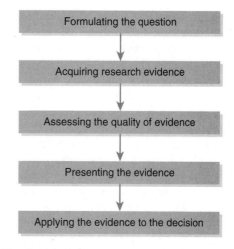

**Figure 3-5** The Evidence-Based Management Process

Data from Kovner, A., Fine, D., & D'Aquila, R. (2010). *Evidence-based management in healthcare.* Chicago, IL: Health Administration Press.

its functioning and its services (products). They are interconnected, although the latter focuses more on clinical care and EBP. EBM is concerned more with organization functioning. How does the use of best evidence relate to management? For example, managers consider the effect of staffing levels on patient outcomes or evaluate a change in services that would impact CQI. An EBM approach provides evidence for making management decisions about these issues or problems, which in turn may impact EBP. Decision making is complex and requires a thoughtful process supported by best evidence, as described by the IOM (2008): "The era of physician as sole healthcare decision maker is long past. In today's world, multiple people make healthcare decisions, individually or in collaboration, in multiple contexts for multiple purposes. The decision maker is likely to be the consumer choosing among health plans, patients or patients' caregivers making treatment choices, payers or employers making health coverage and reimbursement decisions, professional medical societies developing practice guidelines or clinical recommendations, regulatory agencies assessing new drugs or devices, or public programs developing population-based health interventions. Every decision maker needs credible, unbiased, and understandable evidence on the effectiveness of health interventions and services" (pp. 2–3).

Is manager and team leader decision making the same as decision making for clinicians? There are some differences. Clinicians may make more decisions than managers, but the decisions that managers make often involve and impact more people and costs and may require major changes in a unit, department, or HCO. Management decision making often takes more time—for example, it can take weeks, months, or years to develop a plan and make long-range decisions, implement them, identify and monitor outcomes, and complete evaluation of outcomes. While clinical decisions tend to be more focused or specialized, management decisions are more heterogeneous.

There is great variety in management problems and approaches. Intuition is frequently used, with managers saying they had a gut feeling that some type of decision should be made. This approach is not EBM, although experience does help in making decisions, and sometimes gut feelings are based on past experiences and may be effective—but managers should seek other evidence when possible. Management decisions should involve multiple levels of staff, even though the manager may make the final decision. Reality has to be considered, such as the organizational hierarchy and its impact on decisions, but the manager should role model the importance of EBM and share information about factors that may impact decisions so that staff better understand the process and final decisions. Examples of HCO factors that might be considered are budget, changes in services or community health needs, staffing, staff and management changes, systemwide issues, policies and procedures, accreditation and government requirements, standards, and so on. EBM may be used to get needed support for changes from higher levels of management

and also when needed from healthcare providers—supporting decisions with objective evidence. While clinical decision making has been influenced more and more by EBP and staff are more prepared today to use EBP, managers still tend to follow trends or fads in management or use consultants to help them make decisions, but effective quality improvement also requires more active use of EBM. Despite the common decision-making practices of managers, effective decisions should be based on solid evidence. HCOs are complex and demand clear decision making. Patient care is the focus, and this means that use of careful decision making is even more important. As Walshe and Rundall (2001) explain, "Research evidence is more likely to be used in organizations that have a culture that values and encourages innovation, experimentation, data collection and analysis and the development of critical appraisal skills among managers. Organizations must cultivate what has been called a culture of learning through research" (p. 431).

Evidence that exists is often not shared even within the same system. It must be noted that there is minimum evidence available related to best management practices, making it difficult for most managers to actively use EBM. This, however, should not be viewed as a barrier for using EBM. There also are potential barriers that make it difficult to effectively implement EBM, and understanding them helps managers as they make decisions and involve staff. Examples of the barriers are workload and deadlines and access to information.

EBM is fairly new from the perspective of a structured approach to decision making to ensure use of evidence. It would be incorrect to say that management decisions have not been based on evidence, as many decisions are. The difference in using EBM is that it is a specific process that consciously recognizes the importance of research evidence as well as other forms of evidence for best management practice. Managers may know what would be the best approach to take, but there are factors within the organization that make it difficult to make decisions and implement them (Pearlman, 2006). More needs to be done to limit this problem and use EBM in as many management decisions as possible, particularly CQI decisions. Examples of strategies to improve use of EBM include the following (Rundall, Martelli, McCurdy, Graetz, & Arroyo, 2010, p. 15):

- Ask what evidence supports decisions.
- Brief managers routinely on recent management research related to the organization's operational and strategic concerns.
- Incorporate research assessments into due diligence reports.
- Train management team members in the steps of evidence-based decision making—about the process and its application.
- Establish ties with academic institutions and research centers.

It is also important that staff (clinical and management) be informed about EBM in the same manner that they are informed about EBP. Information is key when making any decision, and HCOs need to make sure information is available when needed, which typically today includes use of electronic communication methods. Effective HCOs recognize the need to develop a questioning culture, one that encourages and supports staff to ask questions and seek answers. The following are strategies that an organization might use to develop this type of culture (Kovner & Rundall, 2010, p. 69):

- Organize research rounds (e.g., presentations by experts, updates on research, management research journal clubs, and research seminars).
- Analyze the results of past operational and strategic decisions, including comparing the system's performance with findings from research about other organizations.
- Conduct staff development programs to enhance managers' abilities to find, assess, and apply research findings.
- Link compensation to metrics related to obtaining and using relevant evidence in decision making and sharing evidence with key stakeholders.
- Develop guidelines for decision making that require an assessment of research evidence.

## Learning Health System

Other reports, such as *Learning What Works: Infrastructure Required for Effectiveness Research: Workshop Summary* (IOM, 2011a), provide further examination of EBP and application to the EBP competency for all healthcare professions. The goal is to develop a **learning health system**. This is a system that applies evidence to the care process. A learning health system focuses on the organization culture and the system, which supports engagement and patients and families at its core focused on psychological safety, accountability, teamwork and communication, negotiation, continuous learning, improvement and measurement, reliability, transparency, and leadership, representing the learning health system framework (Federico, 2017). For example, if a healthcare organization (HCO) needs to improve medication administration, this framework should be applied to the process of improvement.

Along with the use of EBP and EBM, there is need for greater **comparative effectiveness research** to provide healthcare professionals with state-of-the-science information to make the best quality and cost decisions for patients. Comparing evidence should be an active part of this process. The federal government provides resources for this through various agency websites, such as the Agency for Healthcare Research and Quality (AHRQ) and the Centers for Medicare and Medicaid Services (CMS). Another report, *Finding What Works in Health Care: Standards for Systematic Reviews* (IOM, 2011b), adds to this expanding examination of what is needed to apply EBP and, in doing so, relates to the EBP competency. A **systematic review** is a summary of evidence focused on a specific clinical question and provides critical appraisal of the evidence to determine if bias exists. Experts who understand the systematic review appraisal process should be the source of these reviews. Ideally, when EBP decisions are made in practice, they are based on these reviews, although in nursing there are not yet sufficient reviews, mostly due to the need for more research to use as evidence. Research is the highest level of evidence; however, other types of evidence are also important. *Finding What Works* focuses on setting standards for the expanding development of systematic reviews to better ensure that these reviews provide effective information for clinical application.

Accelerating Change and Transformation in Organizations and Networks (ACTION) is an initiative led by the AHRQ (U.S. Department of Health and Human Services [HHS], AHRQ, 2018). This initiative supports delivery system research in clinical sites by partnering with the clinical sites and supporting their efforts to test interventions to improve care. The focus is on real-world concerns in healthcare delivery. ACTION is associated with the mission of AHRQ, which is "to produce evidence to make health care safer, higher quality, more accessible, equitable, and affordable, and to work with HHS and other partners to make sure that the evidence is understood and used" (HHS, AHRQ, 2018). Accelerating means pushing forward, and this effort is needed in all aspects of healthcare delivery and CQI. Effective change requires evidence.

## Apply Quality Improvement: Application to Nursing and CQI

The core competency of apply quality improvement is described (IOM, 2003a) as follows: "Identify errors and hazards in care; understand and implement basic safety design principles, such as standardization and simplification; continually understand and measure quality of care in terms of structure, process, and outcomes in relation to patient and community needs; and design and test interventions to change processes and systems of care, with objective of improving care" (p. 4). **Figure 3-6** highlights the key elements.

Performance accountability is a critical factor in healthcare today. As more has been learned about the quality of U.S. healthcare, there has been greater need to evaluate performance: individual provider performance, team performance, and healthcare organization performance. This need is connected to CQI, which requires aggregation of state and national performance. Many external organizations make demands on HCOs for performance data. Some of the organizations are The Joint Commission, which accredits most of the HCOs in the United States; the CMS, the federal agency that administers both Medicare and Medicaid and funds these services

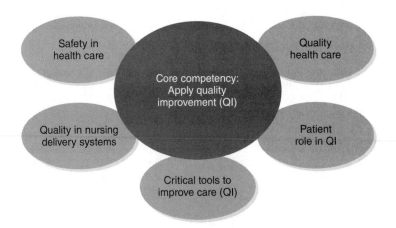

**Figure 3-6** Apply Quality Improvement: Key Elements

(although Medicaid is jointly funded by the states and the federal government); and other organizations and government agencies as discussed in other chapters.

Nursing practice has long been involved in CQI; however, as noted in many sources, including *Keeping Patients Safe: Transforming the Work Environment for Nurses* (IOM, 2003b) and *The Future of Nursing: Leading Change, Advancing Health* (IOM, 2010), nursing is a critical component of healthcare, with nurses providing care that is integral to patient outcomes. Both reports, however, comment on the need for greater nursing leadership in CQI. To accomplish this goal, nurses must know more about CQI and then apply this information. This text provides information to help nurses as they practice and improve care and meet this core competency. Other content in this text discusses the current status of this report's recommendations.

## Utilize Informatics: Application to Nursing and CQI

The core competency of utilize informatics is described as "communicate, manage knowledge, mitigate error, and support decision making using information technology" (IOM, 2003a, p. 4). **Figure 3-7** highlights key elements of this competency.

Since the publication of *Health Professions Education* (IOM, 2003a), much more has been done to expand health informatics technology (HIT) and develop resources for healthcare professions and HCOs, along with expanding medical technology used in care delivery. In a report on HIT, the issue of preparing staff to better utilize informatics is addressed. Staff who are not knowledgeable about HIT and do not apply their knowledge will not effectively use HIT and meet this core competency (IOM, 2012). It is a complex task to engage nursing staff in CQI, and to make this task easier nurse managers need to depend on hiring new graduates who have a basic understanding of the CQI process and use of HIT in the process (Odell, 2011). HIT is discussed in more detail in other chapters in

**STOP AND CONSIDER 3-1**

The Institute of Medicine decided it is important for all healthcare professions to meet five core competencies.

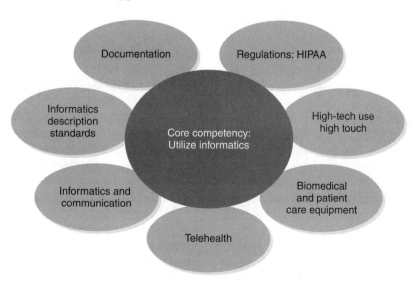

**Figure 3-7** Utilize Informatics: Key Elements

this text, notably its relationship to measurement and solutions to resolve problems and improve care.

# Education to Improve Quality of Care

The *Health Professions* report (IOM, 2003a) concludes that ensuring a competent healthcare staff is critical to healthcare improvement, but this requires healthcare profession education that supports inclusion of CQI in the curriculum and use of outcome-based education. There has been movement to increase content and learning experiences focused on CQI, although much more is needed. The ANA practice and professional standards, *Nursing: Scope and Standards of Practice,* also support the need for staff education to improve care (ANA, 2015). In addition to the traditional teaching practices, such as lectures, exams, and written assignments and clinical experiences, other teaching–learning practices should be used—for example, grand rounds, root cause analysis assignments, use of structured communication methods in simulation and clinical settings, greater use of simulation that integrates CQI, interprofessional workshops on CQI, cases, web-based activities such as discussion, and team projects—emphasizing the use of critical thinking and clinical reasoning and judgment (Benner, Sutphen, Leonard, & Day, 2010). Multiple methods should be used in academic nursing programs and in staff education. In a recent study, baccalaureate degree and associate degree graduates compared their quality improvement preparation (Djukic, Stempfel, & Kovner, 2018). The study's conclusion was that baccalaureate degree graduates were better prepared; however, it is important to ask why there should be a difference in two prelicensure nursing degrees when all registered nurses need to actively engage in quality improvement, which requires knowledge of QI.

# Critical Nursing Documents and Initiatives Emphasizing CQI Through Education

Nursing professional organizations have long developed and published information about nursing practice and the healthcare delivery system. It is important to consider examples of some of these publications and initiatives that impact nursing practice and nursing education and their relationship to the five healthcare professions core competencies to improve practice.

## *The American Association of Colleges of Nursing and the National League for Nursing: Nursing Education Standards*

The American Association of Colleges of Nursing (AACN) nursing education standard publications are *The Essentials of Baccalaureate Education for Professional Nursing Practice* (2008), *The Essentials of Master's Education in Nursing* (2011), and *The Essentials of Doctoral Education for Advanced Nursing Practice* (2006). All three of these publications comment on and/or integrate the healthcare professions core competencies. Nursing programs that follow AACN standards apply the relevant *Essentials* to their programs and are accredited by the AACN accrediting body, which impacts an education program's curriculum and expected competencies of graduates. The baccalaureate *Essentials* document specifically mentions many of the core competency concerns, such as patient-centered care and quality care. One of the major goals for master's education is to lead change to improve quality outcomes, and the doctor of nursing practice (DNP) *Essentials* emphasize leadership, change, and quality. The *Essentials* are periodically reviewed and revised, and this is currently in process. See the AACN link in Connect to Current Links to obtain current information on this lengthy process.

A National League for Nursing (NLN) objective is "to promote the preparation of a diverse workforce that contributes to healthcare quality and safety" (NLN, 2019). The NLN supports nursing education and improvement in nursing education to ensure that graduates provide care which meets the healthcare professions core competencies and support the NLN's core values of caring, diversity, integrity, and excellence by providing educator resources and training and nursing education accreditation standards.

## Educating Nurses: A Call for Radical Transformation

*Educating Nurses* is a landmark report of a study that examined the status of nursing education (Benner et al., 2010). The sample for this qualitative study includes several nursing programs and provides extensive data and analysis with recommendations for nursing education. The results call for change and improvement in nursing education in order to ensure that education is in sync with practice needs and healthcare delivery. As Benner and colleagues (2010) state, "New nurses need to be prepared to practice safely, accurately, and compassionately, in varied settings, where knowledge and innovation increase at an astonishing rate. They must enter practice ready to continue learning" (p. 1). The researchers note that nurses practice in a *dysfunctional* environment (a descriptor also used in the *Quality Chasm* reports). This nursing education report supports the common messages from the *Quality Chasm* reports emphasizing the need for healthcare quality, but to accomplish this we need competent healthcare providers, nurses, and others. To meet this demand means nursing education must also change and improve.

## The Future of Nursing: Leading Change, Advancing Health

This report has had a significant impact on the nursing profession and consequently healthcare delivery (IOM, 2010). Its content was influenced by the *Quality Chasm* reports emphasizing that to maintain safe, patient-centered care across settings, nursing education also needs to improve. Along with the need for improvement in education, nurses need to be full partners in the healthcare delivery system and in CQI—assuming responsibility for identifying problems, participating in measurement and analysis of care problems, and developing interventions/strategies to prevent errors and care-quality problems or to resolve them. The competencies discussed in *The Future of Nursing* report relate to the healthcare professions core competencies. Additional discussion of this report is found in several chapters in this text.

## American Nurses Association Practice Standards

The ANA includes standards of practice for generalist and advanced practice nurses and also for a number of specialties. Some nursing specialty organizations offer standards that pertain to their specialty focus. All of these standards emphasize the need for CQI and the role and responsibilities of nurses to practice in a manner to ensure quality care, supporting the healthcare professions core competencies. These standards are reviewed and revised as needed. Nurses need to be aware of the standards that pertain to them and apply them in their practice. HCO administrators and managers need to ensure that their staff follows them. Standards are discussed in more detail in other sections of this text; however, in this chapter it is important to note that standards relate not only to practice but also to education.

## National Council of State Boards of Nursing Simulation Study

In 2009, the National Council of State Boards of Nursing (NCSBN) began a national, multisite, longitudinal study to better understand simulation outcomes in prelicensure nursing programs (NCSBN, 2015). Use of simulation increased and continues to do so today, but we need to know more about it. In addition, this study began after the publication of significant reports about healthcare professions education and the need for quality improvement.

This study was conducted in three phases. Phase I focused on a survey of prelicensure programs to provide more information on the use of simulation. Phase II was a randomized controlled trial examining the outcomes of using different levels and amounts of simulation in place of clinical site competencies. Data from 10 schools of nursing (5 associate degree and 5 baccalaureate programs) included student perceptions of meeting their learning needs in clinical and in simulation experiences and compared their licensure (National Council Licensure Examination [NCLEX]) pass rates. This study collected and analyzed data from assessment of nursing knowledge and clinical experience. Phase III followed new graduates through the first 6 months of their first clinical positions as registered nurses, focusing on their competency in practice (clinical competency, critical thinking, readiness for practice). This part of the study included data from the new graduates' nurse managers, adding an important factor: the healthcare delivery perspective of management. Data collection for Phase III concluded in June 2014.

The results provide strong evidence that when up to 50% of traditional clinical experiences in prelicensure programs were replaced by simulation, there was no significant difference in educational outcomes (Hayden, Smiley, Alexander, Kardong-Edgren, & Jeffries, 2014). The researchers note that best practices for high-quality simulation should be incorporated by nursing education, including use of consistent terminology; clear participant objectives; inclusion of professional integrity applied to participants/students; and use of active facilitation with a facilitator, debriefing process, and participant assessment and facilitator evaluation (International Association for Clinical Simulation & Learning, Board of Directors [IACSL], 2013). When changes are made in nursing education, it is important to support the changes with evidence to ensure that students will get the learning experiences they need.

The AHRQ also supports the use of simulation and provides resources about simulation, noting the following: "When applied properly, simulation-based training allows the opportunity to learn new skills, engage in deliberate practice, and receive focused and real-time feedback. The goal of simulation-based training is to enable the accelerated development of expertise, both in individual and team skills, by bridging the gap between classroom training and real-world clinical experiences in a relatively risk-free environment" (HHS, AHRQ, Patient Safety Network [PSNET], 2019). It may be used not only for task training but also for teamwork, communication, planning, quality improvement, and so on. Not all of this requires expensive equipment. Simulation can be used to train all types of healthcare professionals (Perry, 2019).

Simulation was first used in education programs for specific training, such as procedures for healthcare professions students, but now it is also found to be useful in developing teamwork, particularly for interprofessional teams; applying human factors engineering to patient safety in simulated experiences; and testing new equipment and technology in real-world situations. Systematic reviews of simulation provide evidence that it is an effective educational method (HHS, AHRQ, PSNET, 2019). Simulation is also used in part of the medical licensure exams and for specialty anesthesiology exams. At this time, it is not yet used for registered nurse licensure exams.

## National League for Nursing Simulation Innovation Resource Center

The NLN's Simulation Innovation Resource Center (SIRC) provides resources for nurse educators (NLN, SIRC, 2015). It is described as an interactive global simulation community, launched in 2008. The SIRC is also involved in offering courses and conferences and supporting simulation-focused research. Both this initiative and the extensive study done by NCSBN mentioned in this chapter indicate the importance of simulation to nursing education, and it is also expanding for other healthcare professions. Simulation is an education experience that can effectively integrate CQI and also teamwork—both included in the healthcare professions core competencies. To accomplish this goal, schools of nursing need to plan and implement initiatives to actively increase content and simulation experiences related to CQI and teamwork.

### American Organization for Nursing Leadership Competencies and Guiding Principles

The American Organization for Nursing Leadership (AONL) is the major organization for nurse leaders and managers in HCOs. It strongly supports active nursing involvement in CQI and the need to develop nursing competencies that are discussed in this chapter. The AONL identifies the need for nursing leadership, teamwork, improved care, effective use of informatics, and patient-centered care. The organization provides standards and a framework for nursing leadership that focus on effective leadership and management, improving practice and care, resources, training opportunities, and conferences. Additional content about the AONL, CQI, and leadership content is be found in other chapters in this text.

# Quality and Safety Education for Nurses

The Quality and Safety Education for Nurses (QSEN) Institute provides a variety of competency-based resources for nurse educators (QSEN, 2019a). This initiative began in 2005 with a national study funded by the Robert Wood Johnson Foundation, focused on examining education on quality and safety for nursing students. The funding was initially provided to researchers at the University of North Carolina. The QSEN is now situated at the Frances Payne Bolton School of Nursing–Case Western Reserve University. The QSEN seeks "to prepare nurses with the knowledge, skills, and attitudes necessary to continuously improve the quality and safety of the healthcare systems within which they work, based on the six quality and safety competencies" (QSEN, 2019b).

The multiphase project identified core knowledge, skills, and attitudes for prelicensure students and then examined key content areas. In 2007, Phase II turned the focus to graduate education and also initiated pilots in 15 schools of nursing (QSEN, 2019b). In the first two phases of the project, QSEN faculty—experts from institutions across the nation—focused on defining the comprehensive set of quality and safety competencies for nursing and training (QSEN, 2019b). In Phase III, which began in 2009, the project joined with the AACN to increase faculty expertise and apply the QSEN competencies. Phase IV coincided with the publication of *The Future of Nursing* (IOM, 2010). The project continues with its work to prepare nurses to ensure high-quality, patient-centered care, supporting the recommendations found in *The Future of Nursing* report.

The QSEN competencies are focused on knowledge, skills, and attitudes (KSAs) (QSEN, 2019c). **Knowledge** is the understanding of content required to meet the competencies—facts, concepts, and information and their relationships. **Skills** focus on psychomotor requirements or how something should be done to meet the competencies. **Attitudes** concern the affective, or emotions, responses, motivation, and perceptions. The QSEN competencies are based on the five healthcare professions core competencies, but they were adapted for this nursing initiative (IOM, 2003a). The QSEN competencies are the same for prelicensure and graduate levels, but KSAs vary per competency.

In regard to integration of the QSEN into systemwide nursing education, Dolansky and Moore (2013) note the following: "Many nurse educators report that the QSEN competencies are already integrated into their curriculum, but in our practice, we have noted that often this integration is at the individual level of care, rather than at the level of the system of care. The full effect of the QSEN competencies to improve the quality and safety of care can only be realized when nurses apply them at both the individual and system levels of care." The following list provides a description of the QSEN competencies (QSEN, 2019c):

- *Patient-centered care KSAs.* Recognize the patient or designee as the source of control and full partner in providing compassionate and coordinated care based on respect for the patient's preferences, values, and needs.
- *Teamwork and collaboration KSAs.* Function effectively within nursing and interprofessional teams, fostering open communication, mutual respect, and shared decision making to achieve quality patient care.
- *Evidence-based practice KSAs.* Integrate best current evidence with clinical expertise and patient/family preferences and values for delivery of optimal healthcare.
- *Quality improvement KSAs.* Use data to monitor the outcomes of care processes and use improvement methods to design and test changes to continuously improve quality and safety of healthcare systems.
- *Safety KSAs.* Minimize risk of harm to patients and providers through both system effectiveness and individual performance.
- *Informatics KSAs.* Use information and technology to communicate, manage information, mitigate error, and support decision making.

The core KSAs for the competencies are found on the QSEN website. A link to this site is found in the Connect to Current Information section at the end of this chapter. **Table 3-1** provides a brief comparison of the five interprofessional core healthcare professions competencies and the QSEN competencies for nurses.

**Table 3-1** Comparing the Five Healthcare Professions Core Competencies and the QSEN Competencies for Nurses

| Healthcare Professions Core Competencies* | QSEN Competencies for Nurses** |
| --- | --- |
| Provide patient-centered care | Patient-centered care knowledge, skills, attitudes (KSAs) |
| Work on interdisciplinary (interprofessional) teams | Teamwork and collaboration KSAs |
| Employ evidence-based practice | Evidence-based practice KSAs |
| Apply quality improvement | Quality improvement KSAs |
| — | Safety KSAs |
| Utilize informatics | Informatics KSAs |

Data from *Institute of Medicine (IOM). (2003). *Health professions education: A bridge to quality*. Washington, DC: The National Academies Press; **QSEN Institute. (2019). Definitions and prelicensure KSAs. Retrieved from http://qsen.org/competencies/pre-licensure-ksas/QSENInstitute; QSEN Institute. (2020). Graduate KSN competencies. Retrieved from http://qsen.org/competencies/graduate-ksas

## Nursing Education and CQI

As discussed previously, nursing education standards include the need for students to gain competency in CQI. However, more needs to be done to integrate effective learning experiences throughout prelicensure education and also in graduate programs. This text provides information that supports the development of CQI competency. As nurses practice, they then build on this knowledge and competency to practice with an emphasis on CQI. As noted in this chapter, there have been a number of initiatives to improve nursing education; however, this must be a continuous process as we adjust to a rapidly changing healthcare environment and expansion of knowledge.

## Staff Education and CQI

The ANA standards, *Nursing Professional Development: Scope and Standards of Practice* (Harper & Maloney, 2016), are important standards that are used to guide nursing staff education in HCOs. The goal is to orient staff and support ongoing learning so that the staff are competent to provide quality care. As is true for all of the standards, the central point of the standards is the protection of the public and provision of quality care. HCOs invest a lot of their budget in staff orientation and education. Some HCOs also include support for staff to attend conferences and in, some cases, continue academic education, such as to obtain a baccalaureate or a graduate degree, thus supporting the recommendations found in *The Future of Nursing* report (IOM, 2010).

Along with education provided by HCOs for their staff, there is also need for a more effective model of **continuing education (CE)** for nurses and other healthcare professions. *Redesigning Continuing Education in the Health Professions* (IOM, 2009) is a report that examines CE from an interprofessional perspective. Currently, typical methods used for CE include attending a conference or presentation, completing an evaluation form, and then getting the CE credit. In some states, academic credits may also be used for nursing CE credit. A third method is to complete an online course, which is often short and may require completion of a brief quiz, which often can be repeated to improve scores. A question that is often asked is, how do we know that the healthcare professional applies what is learned and there is an impact on care outcomes? The report states the following: CE "is the process by which health professionals keep up to date with the latest knowledge and advances in health care. However, the CE 'system'... is so deeply flawed that it cannot properly support the development of health professionals. CE has become structured around health professional participation instead of performance improvement. This has left health professionals unprepared to perform at the highest levels consistently, putting into question whether the public is receiving care of the highest possible quality and safety" (IOM, 2009, p. ix).

Following this 2009 report, the AACN and the American Association of Colleges of Medicine (AACM) held a conference on lifelong learning for nursing and medicine. The vision statement from the two organizations noted the following: "We envision a continuum of health professional education from admission into a health professional program to retirement that values, exemplifies, and assesses lifelong learning skills; emphasizes interprofessional and team-based education and practice; employs tested, outcomes-based continuing education methods; and links health professional education and delivery of care within the workplace" (AAMC & AACN, 2010, p. 3). This all sounds familiar, as it is another example of support for the healthcare professions core competencies; however, in this case the vision statement emphasizes the competencies not only in academic programs but also in lifelong learning for the healthcare professions. This report describes the problems and issues but does not recommend specific strategies to improve lifelong learning. More work is needed to address regulation, accreditation, education, and certification for all healthcare professions and develop and improve strategies. The content of this report focuses on the following (AAMC & AACN, 2010, pp. 6, 7, 19, 20, 22, 27):

- **Lifelong learning** is voluntary and self-motivated pursuit of knowledge for either personal or professional reasons. The report notes the need to meet the following key competencies: an understanding of evidence-based healthcare and critical appraisal, familiarity with informatics and literature search and retrieval strategies, practice-based learning and improvement methods, self-reflection and assessment, and other skill sets related to knowledge management,
- **Continuing education** has long acted as a major support to lifelong learning through CE offerings. CE is formal transmission of a predetermined body of knowledge. These activities are frequently provided with designated accreditation and generate "credits" for practitioners, necessary for most state licensure and other credentialing processes.
- **Interprofessional education** is education for individuals from different professions offered together during all or part of the professional training and in practice—in order to promote collaborative teamwork in their professional practice.
- **Workplace learning** is a way in which individuals or groups acquire, interpret, reorganize, change, or assimilate a related cluster of information, skills, and feelings, and a means by which individuals construct meaning in their personal and shared organizational lives. The report notes that workplace learning has an impact on prevention of errors, staff self-reflection on performance, and improvement of individual and organization performance outcomes.

- **Point-of-care learning** is a subset of workplace learning that occurs at the time and place (whether virtual such as simulation or actual) of a health professional–patient encounter.

The report connects the various types of education for healthcare professions and illustrates the incorporation of patient-centered care, as described in **Figure 3-8**.

## Interprofessional Education and CQI

Several years after the *Health Education Professions* report was published, there was more examination of interprofessional education (IPE). This work flowed from the identification of healthcare professions core competencies (IOM, 2003a). In 2011, a report was published about IPE that was developed by a collaborative of healthcare professions organizations: American Association of Colleges of Nursing, American Association of Colleges of Osteopathic Medicine, American Association of Colleges of Pharmacy, American Dental Education, Association of American Medical Colleges, and Association of Schools and Programs of Public Health (Interprofessional Professional Education Collaborative Expert Panel [IPECEP], 2016). This collaboration indicates the importance of this topic to healthcare and the preparation of different healthcare professions. The report identifies four competency domains:

1. Values/ethics for interprofessional practice (patient-centered, community/population orientation; shared purpose and commitment)
2. Roles/responsibilities (understanding of different roles and responsibilities and how they complement each other)
3. Interprofessional communication (support collaborative practice and teams)
4. Teams and teamwork (team player, cooperation, coordination, shared decision making)

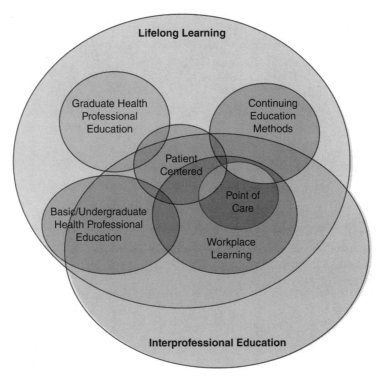

**Figure 3-8** Finalized Key Constructs for Lifelong Learning

Reproduced from American Association of Colleges of Nursing and Association of American Medical Colleges. (2010). *Lifelong learning in medicine and nursing: Final conference report.* Retrieved from https://www.policymed.com/2010/06/aamc-aacn-report-lifelong-learning-in-medicine-and-nursing.html

We have basic competencies for all, but we also now need to determine how to apply more IPE to develop and improve interprofessional competencies and teamwork within healthcare professions education and staff education. It is easy to view IPE as a course in which different healthcare professions students are enrolled, and they sit next to each other in the classroom. This is not IPE. Students need to engage in the learning process together, participating in learning activities that require them to interact and work together. The World Health Organization has published a number of reports on the need for IPE that describe it in the following manner: "[IPE] occurs when two or more professionals learn about, from, and with each other to enable effective collaboration and improve health outcomes" (World Health Organization

[WHO], 2010, p. 13). This collaborative approach is not simple to accomplish. Schools of nursing that are not near other healthcare professions programs have major problems providing IPE. Simulation is also effective in bringing together different students for teamwork and can also be used in interprofessional staff education. Understanding of roles and responsibilities—differences and similarities—is a critical part of IPE. It is best achieved when students or staff interact with one another and collaborate on their learning. The core competency of working in interprofessional teams is difficult to accomplish if students cannot experience interprofessional interactions before they enter practice.

The report notes that there needs to be greater connection between changes in the redesign of practice and healthcare professions

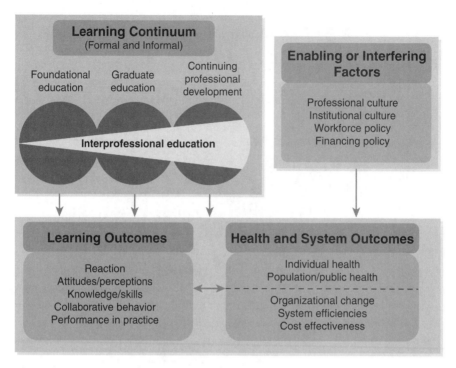

**Figure 3-9** The Interprofessional Learning Continuum (IPLC) Model

Reproduced with permission from Institute of Medicine and Committee on Patient Safety and Health Information Technology Board on Health Care Services. (2012). Health IT and patient safety: Building safer systems for better care. Washington, DC: National Academies Press. Courtesy of the National Academies Press, Washington, DC.

education. A change in one impacts the other. There is also greater need for widespread adoption of IPE. There is need for a framework to measure IPE interventions and their outcomes; collaborative behavior is critical (IOM, 2015). The components of healthcare professions education (prelicensure and graduate), workplace education, and continuing education need to be linked and improved to include IPE. **Figure 3-9** provides a model for the interprofessional-learning continuum. These components should be directed at learning outcomes that address reaction, attitudes/perceptions, knowledge/skills, collaborative behavior, and performance in practice. The learning outcomes are influenced by and also influence health and system outcomes associated with individual health, population/public health, organizational change, system efficiencies, and cost-effectiveness. Enabling

or interfering factors that impact the health and system outcomes are professional culture, institutional (organizational) culture, workforce policy, and financing policy.

**STOP AND CONSIDER 3-2**

Nursing education must be an active participant in continuous quality improvement, at all levels of nursing education and practice.

## Summary

Since the publication of the *Quality Chasm* landmark reports on health professions education, recognizing that to reach the goal of improving care we must consider the competency of the staff providing care, there is now more concern about healthcare professions education and staff competency. As discussed in this chapter, the five core competencies have been adapted by nursing in the QSEN initiative (Cronenwett et al., 2007, 2009); however, this does not negate the need to follow the recommended core competencies that focus on interprofessional needs (IOM, 2003a). In meeting the five core competencies, healthcare professionals practice from the same core base of competencies, even though there are differences in practice per profession. With the growing need to improve care and practice, healthcare professions education and continuing education have also been examined and require improvement. This text is about quality improvement, and education is a critical strategy for improving care. Exemplars of quality improvement roles and responsibilities for staff nurses, nurse managers, and APRNs are found in **Exhibit 3-1**.

---

**Exhibit 3-1** Exemplars: Quality Improvement Roles and Responsibilities

### Staff Nurse

As a staff nurse, you are working on the policy and procedure committee. The committee is reviewing the current policy and procedure on medication administration. As part of the process you are asked to work with a small group to review current QI data on medication administration. The group also decides that more evidence is needed to support changes in the policy and procedure. You ask the hospital librarian to obtain systematic reviews on the question, and this is then used to apply EBP to the process.

### Nurse Manager

At the weekly nurse manager meeting in a rural hospital, the managers discuss HIT. The hospital has an electronic medical record system that is fairly new. The managers ask that data about its use and problems be presented monthly by HIT staff and quality improvement staff. The managers also discuss this topic with their staff on their units and bring this information to the nurse manager meeting.

### Advanced Practice Registered Nurse*

An APRN in an ambulatory care clinic prepares staff education. The focus of the program is patient-centered care when providing care in a variety of clinics. The APRN asks several questions to organize the presentation, such as these: What is patient-centered care? How does it apply to ambulatory care (identifying specific examples)? How can each staff member (clinical and nonclinical) better ensure patient-centered care? After the APRN presents the staff education program, he monitors responses—such as staff feedback to the content, asking staff how they are applying the contact, monitoring patient surveys, monitoring QI data pertaining to patient-centered care (such as timeliness for appointments, wait times upon arrival for appointments, implementation and evaluation of patient education, and so on).

\* Advanced Practice Registered Nurse includes APRN, Clinical Nurse Specialist, Clinical Nurse Leader, and nurses with DNP.

# APPLY CQI

## Chapter Highlights

- The IOM/NAM has been very active in the CQI movement by examining problems and providing recommendations. One of its major recommendations is the need for a consistent base of core competencies for all healthcare professions. In this approach, competencies are not identified for a specific profession; rather, they apply to all healthcare professions.

- Quality and Safety Education for Nurses (QSEN), a nursing initiative, focuses on improvement. It adapted the IOM/NAM core competencies to nursing, emphasizing knowledge, skills, and attitudes (KSAs). QSEN provides resources, training, and research for nursing education.

- Nursing education programs must integrate the competencies, CQI content, and new approaches to learning, such as simulation.

- Professional continuing education (CE) is also more important today than ever before. Evaluation of outcomes indicates that CE needs to be improved, although accomplishing this is not easy. Attendance is the major evaluation criterion and, in some cases, completion of a brief quiz. In addition, more CE should be interprofessional to support effective use of interprofessional teams.

- There is greater emphasis today on interprofessional education within healthcare profession degree programs, although it is a challenge to accomplish.

## Critical Thinking and Clinical Reasoning and Judgment: Discussion Questions and Learning Activities

1. What impact do you think the healthcare professions core competencies have on healthcare delivery? Discuss the pros and cons of the same competencies for all healthcare professions.

2. Compare and contrast the five IOM/NAM core healthcare competencies with the QSEN competencies. Provide examples for each competency and how it relates to your practice.

3. Attend a continuing education offering. Critique the experience and what you observe. If the offering was interprofessional, what impact might this approach have had on the content and attendees? If it was not interprofessional, how could it have been changed to an interprofessional focus? Identify how greater emphasis on IPE might impact practice. Review *Core Competencies for Interprofessional Collaborative Practice* (IPECEP, 2016) and relate this content to your experience.

4. Access *The Future of Nursing* (IOM, 2010) report and review the sections on education and competence. Summarize the key points in a list of items you want to remember. Identify why the items are important. Review the progress data and outcomes. Discuss relevance of results with your student team.

## Connect to Current Information

- American Association of Colleges of Nursing (AACN)
  https://www.aacnnursing.org
- National League for Nursing (NLN)
  http://www.nln.org
- Quality and Safety Education for Nurses (QSEN)
  http://qsen.org
- American Organization of Nursing Leadership (AONL)
  http://www.aonl.org
- *Core Competencies for Interprofessional Collaborative Practice* (2011)

  https://www.aacom.org/docs/default
  -source/insideome/ccrpt05-10-11.pdf?
  sfvrsn=77937f97_2
- *Redesigning Continuing Education in the Health Professions* (2009)
  http://www.nap.edu/catalog/12704
  /redesigning-continuing-education-in
  -the-health-professions
- Accelerating Change and Transformation in Organizations and Networks (ACTION) (2015)
  http://www.ahrq.gov/research/findings
  /factsheets/translating/action/index.html

## Connect to Text Current information with the Author

Go to the update for this text to review the Blog, QI News, and Literature Review. Access this regular update at: http://nursing.jbpub.com/Finkelman/QualityImprovement/2e.

## EBP, EBM, and Quality Improvement: Exemplar

Melnyk, B. et al. (2018). The first U.S. study on nurses' evidence-based practice competencies indicates major deficits that threaten healthcare quality, safety, and patient outcomes. *Worldviews on Evidence-Based Nursing, 15*(1), 16–25.

This extensive study focuses on the critical issue of evidence-based practice and impact on healthcare quality. It applies nursing EBP competencies that were developed in 2014.

### *Questions to Consider*

1. What is the design used for this study, including research question(s), sample, interventions, data collection, and analysis?
2. What are the results of this study?
3. How might these results be applied to nursing education, practice, and management?

# EVOLVING CASE STUDY

You are one of the staff education instructors in a 500-bed acute care hospital. The department staff includes the director and four instructors. Each clinical unit has a designated staff member who assists with staff education and collaborates with the staff education department. With the increased concern about quality of care in the hospital and an error rate that does not meet the desired standard, it has been a stressful time. Sometimes you feel like "the dump department." If there is a problem, staff education will fix it. However, not all problems can be fixed with education alone, and for some problems this is not even a realistic strategy. During your weekly meeting with the director and other instructors, you are all having a difficult discussion as again the department is asked to fix it.

## Case Questions A

*The following questions relate to the staff meeting.*

1. One of the instructors says, "I don't understand why they think we are the ones to fix the error rate." Why do you think this might be a common response from the hospital administration?
2. How might you engage the staff on the units who offer unit education in this discussion?
3. How does the core competency focused on quality improvement relate to your conversation and interprofessional teams and education?

## Case Questions B

*You have moved past the venting, and you are trying to understand the problem so that you can move to action.*

1. The department decides to prepare a brief summary of issues that the hospital should consider related to staff education and CQI. How would you design this document, and what content would you include?
2. Describe specific strategies the department will use to ensure that CQI is integrated in staff education.
3. Describe how the department will assess outcomes. What measures will it use?
4. When issues and problems are outside its domain, how will the department communicate this to administration?

# References

American Association of Colleges of Nursing (AACN). (2006). *The essentials of doctoral education for advanced nursing practice.* Washington, DC: Author.

American Association of Colleges of Nursing (AACN). (2008). *The essentials of baccalaureate education for professional nursing practice.* Washington, DC: Author.

American Association of Colleges of Nursing (AACN). (2011). *The essentials of master's education in nursing.* Washington, DC: Author.

American Nurses Association (ANA). (2015). *Nursing: Scope and standards of practice* (3rd ed.). Silver Spring, MD: Author.

Association of American Medical Colleges (AAMC) & American Association of Colleges of Nursing (AACN). (2010). *Lifelong learning in medicine and nursing: Final conference report.* Retrieved from https://www.policymed.com/2010/06/aamc-aacn-report-lifelong-learning-in-medicine-and-nursing.html

Benner, P., Sutphen, M., Leonard, V., & Day, L. (2010). *Educating nurses: A call for radical transformation.* San Francisco, CA: Jossey-Bass.

Carter, E., Mastro, K., Vose, C., Rivera, R., & Larson, E. (2017). Clarifying the conundrum: Evidence-based practice, quality improvement, or research? *JONA, 47*(5), 266–270.

Cosgrove, D. (2012). Appendix B: A CEO checklist for high-value health care. Washington, DC: The Institute of Medicine. Retrieved from http://www.ncbi.nlm.nih.gov/books/NBK207215

Cronenwett, L., Sherwood, G., Barnsteiner, J., Disch, J., Johnson, J., Mitchell P.,... Warren, J. (2007). Quality and safety education for nurses. *Nursing Outlook, 55*(3), 122–131.

Cronenwett, L., Sherwood, G., Pohl, J., Barnsteiner, J., Pohl, J., Barnsteiner, J.,... Warren, J. (2009). Quality and safety education for advanced nursing practice. *Nursing Outlook, 57*(6), 338–348.

Dolansky, M., & Moore, S. (2013). Culture of safety. *OJIN: The Online Journal of Issues in Nursing, 18*(3). Retrieved from http://www.nursingworld.org/Quality-and-Safety-Education-for-Nurses.html

Djukic, M., Stempfel, A., & Kovner, C. (2018). Bachelor's degree nurse graduates report better quality and safety educational preparation than associate degree graduates. *Joint Commission Journal of Quality and Safety, 45*(3), 180–186.

Federico, F. (2017). Who has time for the big (patient safety) picture? Retrieved from http://www.ihi.org/communities/blogs/who-has-time-for-the-big-patient-safety-picture?utm_campaign=tw&utm_source=hs_email&utm_medium=email&utm_content=77385244&_hsenc=p2ANqtz-8sum8EM-dC4HJQ_cAaxmtcYmcvrqF37dT5Au-uztMrr9Bs2adjKoEZE0kbXvOYwsVaVSm6RabOfUL6t9lRdM4ZYW08rA&_hsmi=77432990

Finkelman, A. (2020). *Leadership and management for nurses* (4th ed.). Upper Saddle River, NJ: Pearson.

Harper M., & Maloney P. (2016). *Nursing professional development: Scope and standards of practice* (3rd ed.). Chicago, IL: Association for Nursing Professional Development.

Hayden, J., Smiley, R., Alexander, M., Kardong-Edgren, S., & Jeffries, P. (2014). The NCSBN national simulation study: A longitudinal, randomized, controlled study replacing clinical hours with simulation in pre-licensure nursing education. *Journal of Nursing Regulation, 5*(2), Supplement. Retrieved from https://www.ncsbn.org/JNR_Simulation_Supplement.pdf

Healthy People. (2020). About healthy people. Retrieved from https://www.healthypeople.gov/2020/About-Healthy-People

Institute of Medicine (IOM). (2001). *Crossing the quality chasm*. Washington, DC: The National Academies Press.

Institute of Medicine (IOM). (2003a). *Health professions education: A bridge to quality*. Washington, DC: The National Academies Press.

Institute of Medicine (IOM). (2003b). *Keeping patients safe: Transforming the work environment for nurses*. Washington, DC: The National Academies Press.

Institute of Medicine (IOM). (2007). *The learning healthcare system: Workshop summary*. Washington, DC: The National Academies Press.

Institute of Medicine (IOM). (2008). *Knowing what works in health care: A roadmap for the nation*. Washington, DC: The National Academies Press.

Institute of Medicine (IOM). (2009). *Redesigning continuing education in the health professions*. Washington, DC: The National Academies Press.

Institute of Medicine (IOM). (2010). *The future of nursing: Leading change, advancing health*. Washington, DC: The National Academies Press.

Institute of Medicine (IOM). (2011a). *Learning what works: Infrastructure required for effectiveness research. Workshop summary*. Washington, DC: The National Academies Press.

Institute of Medicine (IOM). (2011b). *Finding what works in health care: Standards for systematic reviews*. Washington, DC: The National Academies Press.

Institute of Medicine (IOM). (2012). *Health IT and patient safety: Building safer systems for better care*. Washington, DC: The National Academies Press.

Institute of Medicine (IOM). (2015). *Measuring the impact of interprofessional education on collaborative practice and patient outcomes*. Washington, DC: The National Academies Press.

International Association for Clinical Simulation & Learning, Board of Directors (IACSL). (2013). Standards of best practice: Simulation. *Clinical Simulation in Nursing, 9*(6), S1–S32.

Interprofessional Professional Education Collaborative Expert Panel (IPECEP). (2016). *Core competencies for interprofessional collaborative practice: 2016 Update*. Retrieved from https://www.asha.org/uploadedFiles/Interprofessional-Collaboration-Core-Competency.pdf

Kovner, A., & Rundall, T. (2010). Evidence-based management reconsidered. In A. Kovner, D. Fine, & R. D'Aquila (Eds.), *Evidence-based management in healthcare* (pp. 53–78). Chicago, IL: Health Administration Press.

Harper M., & Maloney P. (2016). *Nursing professional development: Scope and standards of practice* (3rd ed.). Chicago, IL: Association for Nursing Professional Development

Leming-Lee, S., & Watters, R. (2018). Translation of evidence-based practice. Quality improvement and patient safety. *Nursing Clinics of North America, 54l*, 1–20.

Melnyk, B., & Fineout-Overholt, E. (2010). *Evidence-based practice in nursing and healthcare* (2nd ed.). Philadelphia, PA: Lippincott Williams & Wilkins.

National Council State Boards of Nursing (NCSBN). (2015). Simulation study. Retrieved from https://www.ncsbn.org/685.htm

National League for Nursing (NLN). (2019). Mission and strategic plan. Retrieved from http://www.nln.org/about/mission-goals

National League for Nursing (NLN), Simulation Innovation Resource Center (SIRC). (2015). About SIRC. Retrieved from http://www.nln.org/sirc/about-sirc

Odell, E. (2011). Teaching quality improvement to the next generation of nurses: What nurse managers can do to help. *Journal of Nursing Administration, 41*(12), 553–557.

Pearlman, E. (2006). Robert I. Sutton: Making a case for evidence-based management. Retrieved from http://www.cioinsight.com/c/a/Expert-Voices/Robert-I-Sutton-Making-a-Case-for-EvidenceBased-Management

Perry, A. (2019). 3 myths about healthcare simulation. Retrieved from http://www.ihi.org/communities/blogs/3-myths-about-health-care-simulation

Quality and Safety Education for Nurses (QSEN). (2019a). QSEN: About. Retrieved from http://qsen.org/about-qsen

Quality and Safety Education for Nurses (QSEN). (2019b). Project overview (November 2005). Retrieved from http://qsen.org/about-qsen/project-overview

Quality and Safety Education for Nurses (QSEN). (2019c). QSEN competencies. Retrieved from http://qsen.org/competencies/pre-licensure-ksas

Rundall, T., Martelli, P. F., McCurdy, R., Graetz, I., & Arroyo, L. (2010). Using research evidence when making decisions: Views of health service managers and policymakers. In A. Kovner, D. Fine, & R. D'Aquila (Eds.), *Evidence-based management in healthcare* (pp. 3–16). Chicago, IL: Health Administration Press.

U.S. Department of Health and Human Services (HHS), Agency for Healthcare Research and Quality (AHRQ). (2018). Accelerating change and transformation in organizations and networks III. Retrieved from https://www.ahrq.gov/research/findings/factsheets/translating/action3/index.html

U.S. Department of Health and Human Services (HHS), Agency for Healthcare Research and Quality (AHRQ) & Patient Safety Network (PSNET). (2019). Simulation training. Retrieved from https://psnet.ahrq.gov/primer/simulation-training

Walshe, K., & Rundall, T. (2001). Evidence-based management: From theory to practice in healthcare. *The Milbank Quarterly, 79*(3), 429–457.

World Health Organization (WHO). (2010). Health workforce: Framework for action on interprofessional education and collaborative practice. Retrieved from https://www.who.int/hrh/resources/framework_action/en

# Change and Healthcare Delivery

## CHAPTER OBJECTIVES

At the conclusion of this chapter, the learner will be able to:

- Examine change as a process and understand its relationship to continuous quality improvement.
- Discuss the role of stakeholders in the change process.
- Examine the change process.
- Analyze the barriers to change and strategies to prevent or overcome the barriers.
- Apply methods to assess and describe the need for change and develop solutions.

## OUTLINE

## KEY TERMS

| | | |
|---|---|---|
| Brainstorming | Gap analysis | Proactive change |
| Change | Groupthink | Reactive change |
| Change agents | Nominal group | Six hat method |
| Decision tree | Pass the problem | Solution analysis |
| Delphi technique | Plan-do-study-act (PDSA) | Stakeholder |
| GANTT chart | PERT chart | |

## Introduction

Change is discussed in the first section of this text because it is a critical element of healthcare delivery and continuous quality improvement (CQI). The healthcare system is not a static system and undergoes changes daily as care is provided. As noted in previous chapters, the system is in need of improvement in all sectors and among all healthcare practitioners. Achieving this improvement requires change, and change is not something most people like to experience. This also applies to healthcare organizations (HCOs), where effective change is often resisted. "Effective" is a key term here, as not all change effects positive outcomes. Another view is that, even though improvement requires change, change does not necessarily represent improvement. Negative responses to change are often due to past negative experiences with the change process and/or results. However, when healthcare practitioners come to understand the vital role of change in the CQI process, they will be more apt to buy into change. All managers and staff should be engaged in change—looking for opportunities to change, participating actively to integrate changes, and evaluating changes that are made and then using these insights to effect further change. The overall goal should be to adapt the common perspective of change from a dreaded experience to an opportunity. **Change agents**, or those who work to bring about change, are important to success. Effective change must consider and include individuals, interpersonal relationships (staff acting together), and the system (Hilton & Anderson, 2018).

## Change: An Ongoing Experience in Healthcare Delivery and Quality Improvement

Maureen Bisognano, president and CEO of the Institute for Healthcare Improvement, identified the first factor in influencing improvement as that of "building will." She explains this idea as follows: "When someone is tired, when they implemented change and they haven't seen dramatic results, or when they find resistance in their peers or they find problems in the supply chain—when they come up against those walls, I believe it's our obligation to help them to see the end result. And that is to tell the story of the patient. Often I think when we have a team that's demoralized or tired or overloaded by too many projects, the sense making that can come from telling a story and combining that with data is very powerful" (U.S. Department of Health and Human Services [HHS], Agency for Healthcare Research and Quality [AHRQ], 2015).

As noted in the previous comments, patient-centered care is emphasized throughout the CQI decision process and changes within the healthcare system. To **change** is to do something to cause something to be different—for the patient, system, healthcare services, and so on. This concept seems simple enough to accomplish, but it is not. Bringing about change is a complex process. Every human being experiences changes. HCOs also change daily. There is change that just happens, and there is change that is planned, implemented, and evaluated, which may or may not be connected to quality improvement. As staff work, they have to make decisions, and the outcome of these decisions may lead to small or major changes. This chapter primarily focuses on the process of change as a basis for further understanding and application in CQI and CQI planning. "The healthcare landscape is facing dramatic changes. Transformation is being driven by unprecedented mergers and acquisitions, new technologies in the marketplace, and the volume, variety, and velocity of available data. Change is occurring with phenomenal speed across the healthcare ecosystem. We must harness this change to address the serious health challenges we continue to face" (HHS, AHRQ, 2019).

There is no doubt that whether change just occurs or it is planned, equilibrium (individual and organizational) is disturbed. Change may involve eliminating something (e.g., process, procedure, program service); improving or enhancing current activities,

which may include adding new approaches; or it may involve a combination of these approaches. Change can be negative or positive, and while HCOs and healthcare providers can learn from both types of change, CQI supports positive change. The vision of the healthcare system and the aims for improvement, as identified by major quality initiatives, all involve changes. With the rapidly changing healthcare delivery system and health knowledge, along with the expansion of health informatics and technology (HIT), *change* is an everyday experience for those who work in healthcare.

A common term used today in organizations is "transformation." Some believe that change and transformation are the same, but they are not (Feeley, 2019). A key difference between the two is that transformation engenders uncomfortable feelings, whereas change does not. Transformation requires major adaptations; requires a plan to reach future goals; requires taking control proactively; is led by more than a few people and impacts more than a few; and requires a clear, shared purpose. Transformation is profound change.

## Factors Influencing Change

With change being such a natural occurrence in healthcare, one might wonder, where does it come from? Change occurs daily in the healthcare delivery system, both on the macrolevel (national, state, local) and on the microlevel (HCOs of all types). Examples of influences that have a major impact on healthcare delivery include the following:

- Patient needs (individuals and populations)
- Demographic changes
- Diversity and disparities
- Expansion and change in medical knowledge, including influence of research
- Changes in treatment (e.g., pharmaceuticals, procedures)
- Healthcare reform
- Healthcare reimbursement

- Health policy and legislation
- Government programs, such as Medicare and Medicaid
- Healthcare profession education
- Use of multiple CQI methods leading to identification of change needs based on gaps
- Greater emphasis on primary care
- Population health
- Local, state, and national economics (e.g., fluctuating economy that impacts HCO reimbursement and budgets)
- Increase in aging population
- Health promotion and prevention
- Changing healthcare roles and new degrees, as in nursing
- Greater use of interprofessional collaborative teams
- Increase in chronic disease across the life span
- Increased emphasis on patient-centered care
- Increase in errors and decreased quality of care
- Expansion of health information technology (HIT)
- Expansion of medical technology
- Greater emphasis on performance outcomes requiring better monitoring of care
- Staffing concerns (e.g., level, mix, shortage, expertise and competence, retention of staff, burnout and stress)
- The uninsured and underinsured
- Patient confidentiality and rights
- Healthcare legal and ethical issues
- Access to care
- Government initiatives to improve care
- Changing vulnerable populations
- Healthcare profession changes
- Healthcare industry changes (e.g., mergers, hospital closures, development of national healthcare corporations, shortage of services, financial issues)
- Need for improvement in healthcare professions education
- Global health concerns (e.g., Ebola virus and other infectious diseases)

This list is not exhaustive, but it provides a view of how many influences may impact the healthcare delivery system and healthcare professionals. For each of the examples, there are multiple possible changes that might occur.

Sometimes trying to cope and adjust can be very tiring, but there is no avoiding it. Change can lead to positive experiences and outcomes, and it can lead to difficult and even negative experiences and outcomes. A key factor supporting successful experiences with change is to understand change and how it works. In addition, it is important to use self-reflection and understand how you personally respond to change and how you might improve your coping with change. Within an HCO, each staff member impacts the organization change process; thus, how each staff member responds to the change process can also have an impact. For example, if the staff member is in a leadership position and is hesitant to engage in change, this makes a difference. If some staff members do not engage in the process and try to block change, the power of the group may alter the change process and outcomes. Later in this chapter, stakeholders are described. Stakeholders have power to influence change either positively or negatively.

Why is change important? Consider what people, organizations, and situations would be like if there were no change. There would be no way to improve, thereby limiting recognition of new ideas, adding new people and positions, and providing different services and meeting new needs. History is all about change. Individuals and families experience change across the life span, which impacts all aspects of their lives. Communities experience change in demographics, economic status, safety, health services, and so on. Government changes to meet new needs and discard old approaches. People often question how or when the government should make these changes, but if there were no changes, government would no longer meet the many needs of citizens. As changes are made in an organization, the organization's vision, mission, and objectives must be considered. Changes should align with the current view of the organization, unless one of the changes is actually to alter the organization's vision, mission, or objectives.

Understanding the potential land mines of change is important to success, but there are also many benefits to change. It can invigorate us. We do not know all of the answers, and we often confront new issues and problems, but this should not stop us from valuing change. Complacency and isolationism lead us to becoming stale and reduce ability to respond to situations in an effective and timely manner. Isolationism—doing our work and trying to just maintain it with no interferences—can become comfortable for us. When we avoid isolationism, however, we are provided with more opportunities to develop innovative responses. Isolationism often brings rigidity, which only diminishes creativity. Then when a critical need for change occurs, as it will, we will not be ready to deal with it. The idea of change may elicit an emotional reaction, such as the following:

- A person may laugh and say "Not again—another change!"
- A person may express frustration and not know where to begin.
- A person may fear the change will blow up in his or her face.
- A person may complain about more paperwork, confusion, and poor communication.
- A person may become depressed and less productive.
- A person may become angry with management personnel who "don't know what they're doing."

None of these responses are helpful, but within the organization's culture they may become more common than embracing change. It is important to recognize that change is personal; everyone has an experience with it and a personal view of it. Leaders of change need to understand these personal reactions to better prevent barriers to change. Even leaders of change have their own personal experiences and reactions to change that need to be recognized and may influence how they lead change.

# Change Theories and Models

A successful change begins as an idea that is shaped and molded through the change process and, ideally, should be preplanned. Leadership needs to consider the process carefully. The outcome(s) should be clearly identified so that outcomes can guide the evaluation of the change. There are many theories and models that address change and the change process. Many were developed several decades ago but are still applied today. The following represent some of these theories and models.

## *Lewin's Force Field Theory*

The force field model of change focuses on the change team identifying, analyzing, and then adjusting as needed based on the driving and restraining forces (Lewin, 1947). This model applies one of three strategies to determine feasibility. The team can increase the number or strength of the driving forces, decrease the number or strength of the restraining forces, or combine these two strategies. The model includes three stages. In the *unfreezing stage*, the major issue is increasing knowledge and awareness of the problem and then identifying and decreasing any forces that do not allow change or, if required, maintaining the current situation. The *moving stage* ensures that the problem is clearly described and the team can identify change outcomes based on the problem. As the name of the stage implies, this is an active stage of implementing interventions/strategies to reach the identified outcomes. The final stage is *refreezing,* when the change is "hardwired" or becomes part of the HCO and the culture. For many changes, refreezing is not easy to accomplish as there is risk of a return to the way things were or some back and forth for a time until the change is truly integrated into the system. A criticism of this model is that it does not emphasize feelings and attitudes enough, but it is still commonly used and can be combined with other models of change that would consider more of these elements. Lewin's model emphasizes the impact of the group over individuals. With today's increasing emphasis on interprofessional collaborative teams, this focus on the group is critical. **Figure 4-1** describes this model.

This model also assumes a more episodic approach. Episodic changes are mostly infrequent, discontinuous, and intentional. In this situation, the HCO is not adapting to its needs, and the result is ineffectiveness and pressure to change. This type of change takes more time, and often staff do not feel the change process is really completed before another change begins. The organization experiences disequilibrium, and then the change moves on to a new equilibrium. Avoiding disequilibrium requires planned change. Lewin's model is one of the most commonly applied models used to make deliberate changes.

Weick and Quinn (1999) also identify the importance of continuous change or a series of fast mini-episodes of change. Change is brought about by the need to adapt, but in reality change never starts or stops. This view is helpful for appreciating how change is part of everything and ongoing; however, as will be discussed here, one can still look at specific change efforts, the process, and results that lead to decisions. As Weick and Quinn explain, "When change is continuous, the problem is not one of unfreezing [as is described by Lewin]. The problem is one of redirecting what is already under way" (p. 379). Quinn has also described "slow death" and "deep change." These terms are quite visual. If your HCO does not make needed changes, then the organization accepts "what is" as the best it can be. In these organizations, the staff often experiences this as a status quo approach, and this can limit staff enthusiasm and drive, impacting performance and productivity. Deep change often leads to significant readjustment within the HCO.

Human factors cannot be ignored in the process, whether it is episodic change or continuous change. Although presented here, the process of change may seem to be a single process or episodic, but in reality HCOs have multiple, organized, ongoing change processes occurring all the time. Waiting for one change process to complete before beginning another change is a luxury few have today in thriving HCOs and in the changing environments in which healthcare is delivered. In the background, change is always continuous.

### Havelock's Theory

Many theories and models build on one another. Havelock's theory expands Lewin's theory by focusing more on the management of change—planning and monitoring change. This theory includes the following steps (Havelock, 1973):

1. Building relationships
2. Diagnosing the need for change
3. Getting the resources needed for change
4. Selecting the best option to respond to the change and implementing it
5. Establishing and accepting change
6. Maintaining and stabilizing

The steps must be clear and include typical steps attributed to planning. When comparing

**Greater chance of positive change**

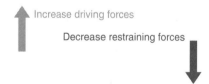

Increase driving forces

Decrease restraining forces

**Greater chance of poor outcomes**

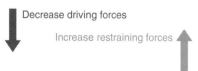

Decrease driving forces

Increase restraining forces

**Figure 4-1** Force Field Analysis

this theory/model with other theories/models, the steps or stages are different. For example, the stages in Lewin's model focus on increasing and decreasing forces that influence the problem and change, which is incorporated in this model.

### Kotter's Change Model

Kotter's model focuses on a culture of change, with emphasis on vision and leadership and greater emphasis on the implementation stage rather than the entire process. A change needs to become part of the HCO culture. The stages in this model begin with an important consideration: It is easy to become complacent—we like the way it is; we have time to make adjustments—but this response is not helpful. Kotter's model involves eight stages (Kotter, 1996):

1. Establish a sense of urgency.
2. Create a guiding coalition.
3. Develop a vision and strategy.
4. Communicate the change vision.
5. Empower broad-based action.
6. Generate short-term wins.
7. Consolidate gains and produce more change.
8. Anchor new approaches in the culture.

This model is similar to Havelock's theory, but it describes more than just planning steps, as it includes process, leadership elements, attitudes, and responses.

### Juran's Trilogy Model

Juran's model focuses on the customer—that is, the product must meet the customer's needs. In the case of healthcare, the most important customer is the patient. There are, however, other customers. For example, the HCO also views insurers as customers; or when a laboratory provides services for a nurse or physician, the laboratory views a nurse or physician as a customer in addition to the patient. The laboratory would be concerned with satisfaction in their services for both the patient and

providers. The Juran trilogy includes the following elements (Juran & Defeo, 2010):

1. *Quality planning.* Identify the customers, determine customer needs, and develop a product/service that addresses the needs.
2. *Quality improvement.* Develop a process to produce the product/service and optimize the process.
3. *Quality control.* Prove that the process will result in the product/service with minimal oversight, and transfer the change process to HCO operations.

This model emphasizes first identifying major concerns about change and then deciding what should be done to address the concerns.

## Proactive Versus Reactive Change

The discussions in this chapter and in other chapters support the use of **proactive change**, change that is planned based on assessment of need. This approach to change is much more effective than is **reactive change**. When we wait for something to happen that might require change, we often miss the opportunity to be effective. Looking ahead—projecting needs and then planning—is better than trying to handle a problem that was not foreseen, which often leads to a response that is insufficiently planned and lacks clear objectives to evaluate outcomes. The change theories and models discussed in this chapter are based on proactive change.

---

**STOP AND CONSIDER 4-1**

CQI cannot occur without change.

---

## Stakeholders

A **stakeholder** is any party that has a strong enough interest in an issue to want to give input and engage in actions relating to the issue. Such parties can be an individual (e.g., patient, staff member), a patient's family or significant others, groups/teams, staff, management, communities, government agencies, professional organizations, nonprofit organizations, insurers, or businesses.

## Identification of Stakeholders

Many possible stakeholders might be involved in the change process. Stakeholders may be internal and external to the HCO or a combination. The identification of specific stakeholders depends on the change issue and the healthcare setting. If stakeholders are not identified, then they may act as barriers to success, as they feel left out of the process. This may also reduce understanding and development of best approaches.

## Engaging Stakeholders

The change process requires that stakeholders be convinced the change is needed, and when a solution is selected, stakeholders need to be committed to it. Often, approaches used to convince stakeholders to participate are political, requiring use of influence, but it is critical to have all key players on board with the change. When talking to others and getting their support, the information collected in earlier steps may help later in the process. For some, the support may be just that they are not going to block the change. Others may provide support by doing something specific to help implement the change. Stakeholders may provide different views of a problem, assessments of solutions, evaluation of actions taken, and new information and may identify potential barriers that need to be considered during the change process. It can also be useful to include staff who are negative about a planned change on the planning team. If the team hears only positive comments, then they may be missing important factors necessary to understand the "real-world" view of the

problem. In addition, listening is very important as change proponents engage stakeholders, even if they disagree with the stakeholder's view.

One approach to increasing engagement of stakeholders is a transformation model that incorporates engagement, empowerment, and professional development, moving away from a focus on a "top down" approach (Scanlon & Woolforde, 2016). This requires that frontline leaders be change agents. This change to engagement improves care and effectiveness. Some organizations refer to these change agents as champions. This empowerment increases staff confidence. Structural empowerment means staff have "access to work conditions that make it possible to accomplish work goals in a meaningful way" (p. 39). Professional development is incorporated in order to prepare and maintain staff to assume these responsibilities related to change in the system and improve care.

### STOP AND CONSIDER 4-2

Nurses are stakeholders in the CQI change process.

## The Change Process

The process of change is a living process in that it is not exactly the same every time a change is planned. It requires careful balancing with the many factors that are involved, even with a simple change. It is important to remember that not all change is planned, and in fact most change is not planned. It happens. Unplanned change can get organizations into trouble because the change process may not be controlled and then staff usually feel more frustration and stress. "Healthcare improvers worldwide still struggle with the adaptive side of change, which relates to unleashing the power of people ("who") and their motivations ("why") to advance and sustain improvement—two commonly cited reasons for the failure of improvement initiatives"

(Hilton & Anderson, 2018, p. 4). This relates to the human side of change, which cannot be ignored if it is to be successful.

The change process includes multiple steps that influence each other. Steps may merge into future steps, particularly if all the tasks related to a step in the process are not completed. It is easy to underestimate the amount of training and time it will take. In addition, it is important to know when more help is needed, either to guide the planning or to implement the change. Data may change what might be needed to understand a problem, requiring flexibility rather than rigidity to a change approach. Rigidity is a barrier to effective CQI projects.

The focus in this chapter is on understanding change as an important process within healthcare delivery and making response to change as effective as possible. As discussed in other chapters, systems and processes are very important in improving care and in developing CQI plans. System-level factors that need to be kept in mind during the change process are identified in **Figure 4-2**.

# Identification of the Need for Change

It is key that the issue, problem, or need for change is understood in order to develop the best response. Resources are always tight (budget, staff, time, and so on); thus it is important not to waste energy and resources; this should be incorporated in planning, implementation, and evaluation. The first step is to identify the issue or problem, but often more information is needed to fully describe it, which leads to step 2. It is during the first step that change leaders decide if the effort should continue, and in steps 2 and 3 the final decision is made to complete the entire process or to stop the process if it is not needed. This type of approach may also be called proactive planning, particularly if the goal is to avert a problem. The objectives are clarified, which should be in line with the overall goals or outcomes. Other chapters expand on CQI approaches and planning used in the improvement process, as well as application of the change process.

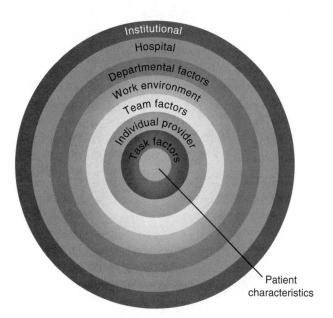

**Figure 4-2** System-Level Factors that Impact Safety

Reproduced from Agency for Healthcare Research and Quality (AHRQ). (2015). Collaborative Unit-Based Safety Program (CUSP) toolkit: Learn about CUSP. Retrieved from https://www.ahrq.gov/hai/cusp/modules/learn/index.html

# The Team: Leadership and Followership

Today, teams, both intraprofessional and interprofessional, are important in healthcare. Nurses have long worked on nursing teams, but they now must become more involved in interprofessional teams, too. Other chapters in this text discuss teamwork in greater detail; however, teamwork must be recognized as part of an effective change process. Change within an HCO does not happen with one leader or manager or with one staff member. Using a team with an effective leader and team members (followers) is the best approach for an effective change process. TeamSTEPPS® is discussed in other chapters as an effective approach to improving teamwork. **Figure 4-3** provides a description of the steps in the process to ensure effective team functioning, leadership, and followership.

# Analysis and Description of the Problem

Gap analysis is one method for better understanding a problem and describing its elements. Project teams can use this method as

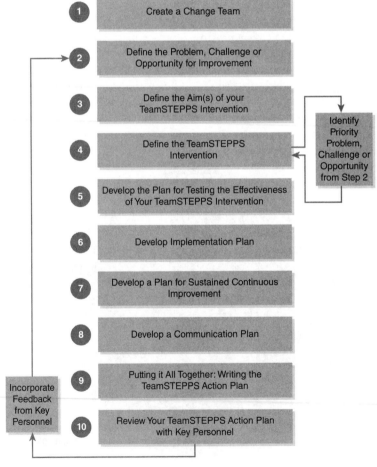

**Figure 4-3** TeamSTEPPS®: Action Planning At-A-Glance

Reproduced from Agency for Healthcare Research and Quality. (2018). The quick reference guide to TeamSTEPPS® action planning. Retrieved from https://www.ahrq.gov/teamstepps/instructor/essentials/implguide3.html

they prepare a plan. It is a written analysis that assists the team in "understanding of the differences between current practices and best practice and an assessment of the barriers that need to be addressed before successful implementation of best practices" (HHS, AHRQ, 2016). **Table 4-1** describes the AHRQ Gap Analysis Toolkit.

The amount of information or data needed to fully describe a problem or issue can vary a great deal, depending on the problem or issue. For example, if a hospital is instituting use of an electronic medical record (EMR) or electronic health record (EHR), the amount of information needed is greater, such as information about software choices, customization

of possible software, advantages and disadvantages of software options, and type of information required for the EMR/EHR to ensure that all documentation needs are met. In addition, consideration must be given to the HCO's typical CQI problems and how the EMR/EHR might help to improve care, software cost, maintenance requirements, staff education to implement the change, and so on. A smaller project that might require less information to fully describe the problem or issue might be to extend clinic hours by 1 hour. In this case, the HCO would need to understand what could be done in the extra hour that is different from the current schedule, as well as the impact the change might have on staffing,

**Table 4-1** AHRQ Gap Analysis Toolkit

Project:                                      Quality Indicator:

Individual Completing This Form:

| Best Practice Strategies | How Your Practices Differ From Best Practice | Barriers to Best Practice Implementation | Will Implement Best Practice (Yes/No; why not?) |
|---|---|---|---|
| Best Practice #1: [insert description of best practice here] | | | |
| | | | |
| | | | |
| | | | |
| Best Practice #2: [insert description of best practice here] | | | |
| | | | |
| | | | |
| | | | |
| Best Practice #3: [insert description of best practice here] | | | |
| | | | |
| | | | |
| | | | |

U.S. Department of Health and Human Services (HHS), Agency for Healthcare Research and Quality (AHRQ). (2016). Gap analysis. Retrieved from https://www.ahrq.gov/sites/default/files/wysiwyg/professionals/systems/hospital/qitoolkit/combined/d5_combo_gapanalysis.pdfv budget, space, parking needs, and issues such as better lighting for night hours, security, response of stakeholders (healthcare providers, nonclinical staff, and patients), and so on. Other decisions might have greater impact on the HCO, such as a decision to develop a home healthcare service. This type of service requires extensive marketing information, budget analysis, consideration of the impact on other HCO services and on reimbursement, input from community stakeholders, and so on. All of these examples are changes. Some may be directly related to CQI as when CQI data indicate that a problem in quality exists; others may be responding to changing trends and community needs. All represent change.

The description of data should allow decision makers to review the information and better understand the problem or issue. The result should include a clear description of the issue or problem and should connect to the predicted expected outcomes. Failure to present this information clearly can be one of the biggest barriers to effective change. Decisions must be based on the description of the issue or problem. Jumping to conclusions or selecting the most obvious description, which may seem like the easier route, may lead to problems later. Often we tend to consider the initial information or data we hear as the most important, when it may not be. More in-depth discussion of measurement and data is provided in other chapters.

## Readiness Assessment

Readiness for change is also an important factor to describe. It is critical that management and the change team understand the current status of the HCO and its staff and how this impacts their ability to handle change. This readiness is not necessarily focused on a specific change but rather on the ability to engage in the change process. Some staff are more ready to handle change than others. How is the HCO functioning? Effective

planning to respond to change is more difficult for dysfunctional organizations. Does the organization have the resources available, such as financial resources, physical space, equipment, supplies, informatics technology, and staffing levels and expertise? Have there been other recent changes, and what are their status and staff response? Is there effective leadership within the HCO to guide the change process? What is the history of changes in the HCO? Past experiences with change also have a direct impact on current change—for example, if the HCO has had a difficult experience with a change, then staff may be reluctant to get involved in another change.

It could be that it is just not the right time to make a particular change. One can never be sure that change will be successful; it is risky (Finkelman, 2019). Knowing how much the organizational culture can handle at one time can make a difference in how difficult it will be to even get the change process moving. How critical the problem or issue becomes is a major factor in determining if this change must be made now. For example, more than 10 years ago, instituting use of EMR/EHRs was not so important, although many hospitals did begin to use them. Today, there is more evidence supporting the need for EMR/EHRs and their impact on reducing errors. The federal government is pushing for use across the country in all types of healthcare settings. In the case of this issue, an HCO would not spend a lot of time debating the readiness for this change.

Budget is also an important factor in readiness for change. If an organization does not have the money to cover the expenses, then change should not happen. Budget issues are not just organization focused. State and national economic issues impact HCO budgets, as does reimbursement for healthcare services. All of these considerations must be figured into a discussion about readiness. What will be the costs? Will monies be shifted to accommodate change, and what will be the impact on current and future services—for example, on staffing or staff education?

Another readiness factor is leadership. If an organization has undergone major changes in critical leadership positions, these changes will impact the types of changes the organization is able to handle. Changes in leadership positions are major concerns in any HCO and need to settle some before other major changes are started. New leadership, however, often means that the leaders themselves recommend changes, often to demonstrate their own leadership to staff and to higher-level leadership within the HCO. Many staff members have experience working with new leaders who are eager to make changes, often with limited understanding of the new organization and staff or use of effective planning. Staff may then feel like every time they turn around there is a new change. This scenario is not effective planning for change or effective leadership. Leaders who use evidence-based management (EBM) tend to make more effective decisions about change, as they review and apply best evidence to problems to determine best possible solutions.

Assessment of readiness for change should lead to a change process plan. The plan describes how a change will occur and is critical for success of the change process. This plan of action should be written and clear to all who may be involved. Guidelines to creating a change process plan include the following:

- Clearly describe the issue or problem (the focus of the change process).
- Identify specific goals and objectives, and describe the major intervention(s) or solution(s) (the change), with rationale to support the change.
- Identify the policies and procedures needed to apply the recommendations.
- Describe the implementation phases.
- Specify the timeline in sufficient detail so that all concerned understand the due dates.

- Designate responsibilities, including specific names.
- Develop the budget.
- Describe the evaluation methods; create a timeline that includes both short-term and long-term evaluation markers.

The goals and outcomes should be measurable and achievable. The timeline is important, and it should be reasonable. Can the goals and outcomes be met in the time frame described? Moving too fast or even too slowly can interfere with meeting outcomes. The timeline may need adjustment as the change process occurs; however, frequent adjustments indicate a weak timeline and plan.

## Selection and Development of the Solution(s): Using Best Evidence

When plans are developed, EBM—and when necessary evidence-based practice (EBP)—should be used to select and develop solution options. The following are typical steps used to identify solution options and apply the best solutions:

1. *Prepare staff for the change.* Education about the need for change and the process of change is important for all staff that will be affected by the change. It is best that this effort is planned so that all information is covered and all those concerned are included. Leaving people out leads to resistance and impacts effective implementation and outcomes.

2. *Test the solution(s).* Ideally, the change process includes pilot tests to implement a change before it is used in a broader way in the HCO. Some changes are not implemented throughout the HCO, as the change is too specific—for example, the HCO may change the procedure for admitting newborns to the neonatal unit to improve the patient assessment process, although there may still be a testing time

designated to identify potential problems, get staff and parent feedback, and so on. For other changes, a rollout plan is more effective (e.g., the implementation of the EMR/EHR in a hospital). The hospital may choose to begin use of the EMR/EHR in certain departments, divisions, or units first and then expand to other areas. This approach allows for corrections before the entire hospital is moved to the new system. The difficulty with this approach is that initially the hospital would be using two documentation systems. For some changes, this approach may not be useful (e.g., the development of home care services). The hospital must weigh the pros and cons of the best method to use. Testing can be very important to work out the kinks and create more effective change. Pilot tests must be time limited and carefully evaluated by those who best understand the change and its need and by stakeholders.

3. *Implement the change (solution).* Implementing the change means all the steps necessary to start the change solution are begun as planned. Timing is important; it is particularly important to determine the best start time and the timeline for major steps in the process. During the implementation of the solution(s), change leaders should pay attention to feedback, which may be important in preventing problems. Perceiving staff feedback as resistance or mere complaining may lead to serious mistakes. In fact, it is important to incorporate feedback options as part of the implementation step, including active listening to feedback. This engages staff in the process and increases commitment. Staff, however, also have the responsibility of communicating concerns in a clear and timely manner.

4. *Spread improvement.* Supporting the integration of change within the organization is a critical part of the process. The goal is to make the change a part of the system.

Many factors can impact the success of a change, such as staff attitude and preparation, staffing levels, staff issues such as morale and frequent turnover, changes in leadership/management, work environment and the culture of safety, communication, diversity issues, collaborative approach, empowerment, commitment, budget, standards and regulations, equipment and supplies, and other changes that may be ongoing. Timing is critical, and making several major changes at one time should be avoided when possible. Staff members get tired of constantly coping with changes. It is stressful, and strain impacts work productivity and quality. Even as changes are implemented, work continues, and it is important to avoid decreasing productivity and quality whenever possible. Evaluation must be integrated through the implementation phase and at the conclusion. The evaluation data should be used to make needed adjustments and to learn about the change process for the next time change is needed.

Best practices to improve the change process, especially during major change projects, include the following (Robinson-Walker, 2011, p. 11):

- Encourage self-care by helping staff be reasonable about what needs to be done and not get overwhelmed.
- Recognize that change can lead to staff unhappiness when staff experience lack of understanding, lack of information, and/or fear about the future.
- Communicate. Even when one thinks something has been communicated, repeat it if needed. Use emails, newsletters, meetings, and so on to share. Provide opportunities for dialogue (two-way discussion). Promote trust and respect of others.
- Avoid asking specific staff or managers to keep secrets. This leads to distrust and rumors. Rumors are very destructive to the process.

- Be visible—leaders should be engaged.
- Consider how changes in titles and positions cause stress.
- Accept that change is inevitable.
- Understand how you respond to change, how you might block change, and how you can improve your response to change.
- Planned change is best, but you have to learn to cope with unplanned change.
- Lead change when needed, but also be an effective follower in the change process.
- Recognize that some change efforts are not effective.
- Learn how to effectively work to make change a positive experience rather than just blocking it.
- Communicate and collaborate with your team and organization.
- Use critical thinking effectively.
- Be willing to recognize a poor decision, admit it, and learn from it.
- Work collaboratively with others.

McCannon, Schall, and Perla (2008) pose some useful questions to consider when developing and implementing change projects: "How will your system for spreading change foster learning and create value for participants every single day? How will you collect and quickly redistribute insight from the front lines?" (p. 11). Here are some other useful questions to consider: Will you need to collect new data for the project? How can you generate information that is useful to front-line teams? Each HCO, leader, and team must continually develop change expertise.

## Roles and Responsibilities

The change agent, who may be an individual or a team, focuses on the problem or change issue and possible approaches to take. Change agents may have no formal position or may be in formal leadership positions, such as a nurse manager, the chair of a task force leading a CQI project, or the administrator responsible for development of a new service. Even if the change agent is not in a formal leadership position, the change agent needs to use leadership to accomplish tasks. The change agent is the driver of change; however, do not assume that this person or team is the only relevant party in the change process. All staff and managers are involved in change, ideally working together and not against one another. Consider the following questions when you think about the organization in which you work and the role of the change agent.

- What happens when the staff makes suggestions?
- Are staff suggestions used and, if so, are their contributions acknowledged?
- When new staff are oriented, is the value of staff involvement and creativity in the organization discussed and, if so, in what manner?
- During orientation, are new staff members given examples of how the staff participates in organization changes? Are potential staff members asked about their typical responses to change?
- How are critical thinking and clinical reasoning and clinical reasoning and judgment used in your organization? When and by whom?
- How is the change process applied in your organization?

## Evaluation and Follow-up

Evaluation is often the weakest part of the change process. It may be because change leaders and staff are tired and do not actively pursue evaluation, or it could be that no one wants to listen to outcomes. However, evaluation is critical. First, it is important to know if the change solution is working. Are the outcomes met? If not, what went wrong? Feedback from the staff who is involved in the solution is an important element of the evaluation plan. It is common to think that if evaluation is performed at the end of implementation, then the requirement for evaluation has been satisfied. The best approach, however, is to use continuous evaluation throughout implementation and then at the end. For example, evaluation points might be at month 1, month 3, and so on, and then at the conclusion of implementation with a clearly identified date.

It is important to determine any adjustments needed and implement them as needed during implementation and evaluation. With the example of implementation of changes in EMR/EHR systems, it is more than likely that many adjustments will be required, and the need for adjustments will span a long period. Due to the critical nature of documentation for patient care, quality care, and reimbursement, as well as in general communication, waiting to make some adjustments might be highly risky.

---

**STOP AND CONSIDER 4-3**

Given that change is inevitable in the work environment and a critical part of CQI, consider how you respond to change, your experience with it, and how you can improve your response.

---

# Barriers to Change and Strategies to Prevent or Overcome Barriers

As planning is begun, it is important to identify barriers to and support for change. As barriers and support may change, adjustments should continue throughout the planning and implementation of a change.

## Barriers

As noted, restraining forces are important (Figure 4-1). Sometimes the staff who are involved in a change process are reluctant to explore the barriers that may be blocking the change process, but understanding them can prevent problems later when change is planned and strategies implemented.

## Resistance

Using empathy or putting yourself in the shoes of others will help to better understand staff reactions, such as staff feeling threatened by change (Hilton & Anderson, 2018). Staff (clinical and nonclinical) resistance to change is common. Change disturbs people and the environment in which they work. For many changes, the disturbance may be minor or last only a short time, but it can last longer for other changes. Feeling comfortable with the way things are does not typically move an organization forward.

It must be understood why staff might resist a specific change. It could be just general resistance to all change, but it may also be something about the specific change. Staff may not understand why the change is necessary, may feel concerned about its effect on work processes, may fear that it will result in a loss (e.g., job, responsibility and authority, ranking or status, pay, working with a specific team, work schedule, friends within the work setting, job enjoyment and satisfaction), or they may consider the change to be a personal criticism of job performance.

How change has been experienced in the past is also important—either in the same organization or in another—can lead staff to be highly resistant, particularly if the change process was poorly planned and implemented and no one listened to the staff. Another issue related to resistance is the amount and level of change. An HCO can handle only a certain amount and level of change at one time before the change begins to negatively impact operations. Change leaders need to recognize this risk and consider it carefully. This can be a major barrier to effectively implementing a change. Typically, barriers can be classified as (1) emotional reactions, (2) perceptual issues, or view of the situation, (3) economic threat or loss, and (4) social threat or loss. Better understanding of the barriers can lead to a plan to address them up front rather than waiting for additional problems to occur. The AHRQ suggests some steps to consider when planning change, which may reduce resistance (HHS, AHRQ, 2014):

- It is important to ensure that staff understand the new roles and have the knowledge and tools to carry them out.
- Help reduce resistance to change by ensuring that staff understand the reasons for change and agree that change is needed.
- To help staff fully accept the new bundle of practices, ensure that they understand that those practices offer promising strategies for providing high-quality care for patients.
- Identify and minimize practical barriers to using the new practices, such as inadequate access to supplies.
- At all levels, engage staff to gain their support and buy-in to the improvement effort and help tailor the practices.

Not only may staff be resistant to change but also HCOs as organizations can be resistant to change. HCOs that are bureaucratic, highly structured, and heavily dependent on following policies and procedures may be less likely to change easily. Khator (2014) identified four attitudes that often get in the way of coping with and effectively managing change:

- *Ignorance.* "When did that happen?" This reaction may indicate that staff feels as though things are moving too fast and are too complicated to manage.
- *Arrogance.* "We have been doing this our way a long time and we know best." Staff often do not know what is best for the HCO as a whole and may not have the insights needed to anticipate disruption until faced directly with it. Everything seems fine to them, so why rock the boat?
- *Victimization.* "Why are they doing this to us?" Disruptions are a real part of business; they are not personal.
- *Panic.* "We have to do something! Anything! And quickly!" Panic creates a fragmented, inefficient work environment; effecting positive change requires a supportive, unified work environment. (pp. 4.2–4.3)

Support for change is also important to understand. Change leaders need to identify stakeholders who will support the change process because they believe in it. Stakeholders can help to identify barriers and ways to resolve barriers through effective strategies. For example, a staff member who fears suffering a professional setback due to a proposed change might actually get a promotion, more pay, a better work team, a better work environment, or a better work schedule. Change leaders may help stakeholders recognize, and consequently rectify, misunderstandings when stakeholders lack such insight.

The work environment should facilitate productivity and ensure patient and staff safety. Many changes can improve the work environment, though some can make it more difficult. Change leaders need to consider the impact of the planned change on the work environment. They must identify solutions in order to solve or improve the problem. In this step, planning moves from collecting data and information to putting the information together so that solutions can be identified. For most problems or issues, there are multiple options. The more that is known about problems, the more likely it is that the best change approach will be selected to resolve the problems.

### Inadequate Leadership

Leaders need to think ahead and engage in planning. This includes developing effective infrastructure, staff training, information systems, policies and procedures, and performance appraisal that includes rewards. Quinn's work on change and leaders emphasizes that often the major issue with organizational change is the leaders' fears about what might happen to them due to the change (Quinn, 1996, 2000). Effective change requires leaders who are challenged by change and do not pull away from it, as noted by Quinn, recognizing the need to engage in the heroic journey. Change is best viewed as an opportunity.

## *Groupthink*

**Groupthink** occurs when group members go along with a proposed idea as a group. There often is, however, at least one member who may disagree with the idea, but when this member sees that no one is sharing negative views, this member then keeps quiet and goes along with the group. This type of response is not that unusual and acts as a major barrier to creativity and shared ideas. It blocks an open communication environment. If members speak up and present minority views, they may fear criticism, retaliation, or be concerned that they will not be viewed as a member of the group. This dynamic is not part of a functional organizational culture, nor is it effective teamwork. Teamwork does not mean everyone must agree but rather that everyone must work together to arrive at best solutions while considering multiple viewpoints. Team members need to understand that compromise may be required.

## *Inadequate Planning*

Not all change is successful. We know change is disruptive and causes stress for staff, but why does change sometimes fail? Understanding why makes a difference in successfully managing change in the future (Ponti, 2011, p. 43). The following are possible reasons failure is associated with planning for change:

- *Lack of urgency.* Urgency is a critical change driver. Leadership and staff need to feel it is really important that a change is made. If this is not felt, moving change forward is difficult. Another problem is when the leader thinks there is urgency, but there is none. A third problem is when the leader does not take the time to work through the need for change and lead others to understand the need for change (the urgency).
- *Lack of coalition.* Who are the key people who need to be driving the change and forming a coalition? Sometimes the wrong people are chosen or someone critical is left out.

- *Lack of vision.* A plan for change requires a clear vision. It provides the goal(s) and the meaning of the change.
- *Ineffective communication.* Limited information and understanding about urgency, vision, limits a plan's effectiveness. Communication must be clear, timely, and consistent and needs to support the sharing of information.
- *Vision obstacles.* Obstacles to change are inevitable. When possible, they need to be prevented. If they cannot be prevented, then they need to be dealt with or adjusted to ensure that change occurs as planned.
- *Lack of short-term wins.* Often the focus is on the end point; however, most change takes time. It is important to also celebrate and recognize the accomplishment of interim short-term goals, allowing time for reassessment.
- *Declaring victory too soon.* Leaders have to be careful about prematurely pronouncing the change a success. Determining the status requires careful analysis.
- *Not anchoring changes.* It is critical to make sure change is part of the culture and "the way things are done." It is easy to assume this has occurred when it has not, and this can then result in losing momentum in ensuring that the change is part of the organization.

# Strategies to Prevent or Overcome Barriers

Empowering staff to make decisions is a sign of an effective, healthy organization. If all decision-making power is only focused in the top or middle level of management, this impacts how the organization functions. Staff members need some power to make decisions where decisions count and, when needed, at the direct site of work. For healthcare providers, this may mean at the bedside or on the unit. Teams are critical, and teams make decisions. If they cannot make decisions, then there is not much reason to have teams.

Trust is also an issue. During change, predictability and capability have an impact on trust. Staff feel most comfortable, as do many managers, when work expectations, schedules, processes, and so on are clear and predictable. Often during change, this predictability is lost. Capability relates to whether or not the HCO can do what needs to be done, and this also then impacts roles and responsibilities. During the change process, the HCO's capability may not be clear all the time. As a consequence, if predictability and/or capability are in flux, staff and managers may have reduced trust. This atmosphere of distrust impacts empowerment, both in managers "trusting" staff with power to make decisions or follow through and with staff "trusting" managers.

The following is a checklist of some strategies to consider when responding to resistance.

- *View resistance as a friend.* This makes you pay attention in case you are headed in the wrong direction.
- *Allow others to tell their stories.* Listen, as you may learn something important.
- *Look at resistance as a "cue."* It is difficult to listen to negative feedback, but these comments may reveal issues that may be important to further understand an issue or problem.
- *Use "no" as a connecting point.* Stop and find out why someone disagrees.
- *Stop doing what is not working.* It could be that this approach needs revision.
- *Include staff in the change process.* To provide different views, particularly include some staff who are not 100% in support of the change.
- *Identify the driving and restraining forces in language that can easily be understood.* Use the method suggested in Lewin's theory to decrease restraining forces and/or increase driving forces. First, however, you need to identify the restraining and driving forces.
- *Establish a safe environment where staff feel comfortable expressing their concerns.* Avoid letting negativity become the main theme, and avoid groupthink.

The American Organization for Nursing Leadership (AONL) [formerly the American Organization of Nurse Executives, AONE] believes that a healthful practice/work environment—an environment that is able to cope with change—is supported by the presence of the following elements (AONL, 2019):

1. *Collaborative practice culture.* The culture is marked by respectful collegial communication and behavior, team orientation, presence of trust, and respect for diversity.
2. *Communication-rich culture.* Communication is clear and respectful, open and trusting.
3. *A culture of accountability.* Role expectations are clearly defined; everyone is accountable.
4. *The presence of adequate numbers of qualified nurses.* Nurses are able to provide quality care to meet patients' needs; work–home life is balanced.
5. *The presence of expert, competent, credible, visible leadership.* Leaders serve as an advocate for nursing practice, support shared decision making, and allocate resources to support nursing.
6. *Shared decision making at all levels.* Nurses participate in system, organizational, and process decisions; formal structure exists to support shared decision making; nurses have control over their practice.
7. *The encouragement of professional practice and continued growth/development.* Continuing education/certification is supported/encouraged; participation in a professional association is encouraged; an information-rich environment is supported.
8. *Recognition of the value of nursing's contribution.* Nurses are rewarded and paid for performance; they are afforded career mobility and expansion.
9. *Recognition by nurses for their meaningful contribution to practice.* Nurses need to understand how they can make a difference and to use their position and competencies effectively.

These elements represent an important part of change within nursing. Much work needs to be done to ensure that nursing staff and leadership are able to respond to delivery and organizational issues, supporting the type of environment described in this list. Inevitably, this involves change.

> ### STOP AND CONSIDER 4-4
>
> Barriers to change can be turned into positive factors.

# Examples of Methods to Assess and Describe the Need for Change and Develop Solutions

Data have become very important in healthcare, having a direct impact on healthcare delivery, change, and CQI. Medical education has begun to address this issue, noting the need for physicians to use "health data to not only improve community-wide health but also to make a difference for their individual patients" (Frieden, 2015). Frieden interviewed Marc Triola, director of the Institute for Innovations in Medical Education, who had the following to say: "We're at this amazing time where federal and local governments are releasing health data through initiatives like data.gov, and medical schools have access to data about the health care delivered by doctors in the community. . . . With the changes happening in health care and the changing role of technology and data, teaching these [data analysis] skills seems more important than ever" (Friden, 2015). Nurses also need this same improvement. HCOs use a variety of methods to better understand problems and changes that organizations need to make, such as questionnaires or surveys, observation, and interviews, which are discussed in content about measurement. Examples of other methods that

are often used are described below. The Connect to Current Information section at the end of this chapter provides links to sites that describe figures for some of these methods.

## Solution Analysis

Deciding on the best solution requires a structured approach. The **solution analysis** method considers each of the possible solutions and then ranks them according to how effective the solution might be in meeting the objective, cost, time, and feasibility. It is often referred to as SWOT analysis, with SWOT representing the four key elements of solution analysis: **s**trengths, **w**eaknesses, **o**pportunities, and **t**hreats of a situation. This approach may be used to analyze each possible solution. During this process, all involved need to check their assumptions carefully, think through the process, and continue to increase knowledge about the issue or problem. Sometimes it is important to use intuition when appropriate and step away from rigidity. It is best not to overemphasize that decisions are final, as most are not.

## Plan-Do-Study-Act

**Plan-do-study-act (PDSA)** is an example of a rapid-cycle change method. PDSA—also referred to as the Deming cycle after its creator—is a common method used by HCOs today to assist in responding to change and in planning. The PDSA cycle can be used to help with the following (Value Based Management. net, 2019):

- Daily routine management, for the individual and/or the team
- Problem-solving process
- Project management
- Continuous development
- Human resources development
- New product or service development
- Process trials

A few key questions are first asked when applying this cycle: (1) What are we trying to accomplish? (2) How will we know that a change is an improvement? (3) What changes can we make that will result in improvement? After this analysis, the cycle is applied (Institute for Healthcare Improvement [IHI], 2012; Langley et al., 2009):

1. *Plan.* In step 1, the team describes a plan for the change. Objectives are clarified, and predictions of what will happen are identified. The team plans for the test of change. Planning should consider the five Ws: (1) who, (2) what, (3) when, (4) where, and (5) why data.
2. *Do.* In step 2, the change is pilot tested using a smaller perspective—for example, on one unit.
3. *Study.* In step 3, the focus is on collecting and analyzing data in order to better understand outcomes. Compare the data with the predictions made in step 1. If the prediction was that there would be a certain percentage of staff complaints or errors, was this met? Was it lower or higher, and why? The data are summarized so that the data can be understood and communicated. Note that some who use PDSA have changed the "S" to a "C," or check impact of the change (Sollecito & Johnson, 2013, p. 37).
4. *Act.* In step 4, the change may be adjusted based on what has been learned in the pilot test or trial. Then the next pilot test is planned, or the decision is made to apply the change to the larger system based on the specific purpose of the change initiative.

# Brainstorming

**Brainstorming** is a method used to identify as many ideas as possible so that the ideas can then be assessed to determine if they can be used or should be eliminated. In the beginning of the process, all ideas are considered relevant; they are "put on the table" for consideration and there is no "right" or "wrong" answer but rather an open forum to explore ideas and options. This approach requires input from a variety of people. It is a quick way to identify new ideas. Brainstorming might focus on identifying what change needs to be considered factors impacting the change, and solutions. Brainstorming may be unstructured or structured. Unstructured brainstorming methods use open discussion, and anyone can add ideas at any time, as there is no specific order or process. Brainstorming does not really require any preparation and may be used at any point during meetings to get ideas from the team.

Typically, the risk with asking the team for ideas is that some members may participate more than others do. Structured brainstorming methods use a specific process to elicit ideas and increase participation, reducing the chance of staff not participating. This type of process uses a leader or facilitator who guides the process. The following are some methods used in structured brainstorming.

## Delphi Technique

The **Delphi technique** is easy to use when it is difficult for staff to meet or when anonymity may be needed, such as if staff are concerned that speaking out might have a negative impact on them. Staff are provided with a questionnaire that focuses on a particular problem, and they are asked to identify possible solutions. After the results are compiled, staff that participated in the first round are given a copy of the results. This can be done on the computer; however, if anonymity is a concern and respondents can be identified, another method may need to be used. The respondents are then asked to comment on results from round 1, and these new comments are added to the round 1 results. This activity can continue for many rounds, and the information changes according to discussion results and the deletion or addition of new ideas. This method is time consuming, and participants do not get immediate feedback. Since this is a structured method, it allows time for thought and further examination of the issue or problem.

## Nominal Group

The **nominal group** is another method that may be included in brainstorming. It requires participation from all group or team members, avoiding the problem of several members controlling the brainstorming (Fallon, Begun, & Riley, 2013). The process works as follows: All members are informed of the process, and the facilitator shares information about the issue to be discussed. Then each member thinks about his or her own ideas related to the issue with no sharing of this information. After this phase, members write down their ideas and submit them to the facilitator. All of the ideas are then documented, numbered, and shared with the entire group or team, leading to a discussion about the proposed ideas and a vote on them. Items with the largest number of votes are considered to be the most important ideas. In some cases, there may be additional rounds and voting. The goal is to ensure that all relevant staff contribute to the change process to reach the most effective decision possible.

## Pass the Problem

**Pass the problem** is a method used after a problem has been described and possible causes identified. The steps are as follows:

1. Staff are divided into groups or work teams.
2. The leader creates a folder for each identified problem and potential root causes and gives one folder to each group.
3. Each group generates as many strategies as possible to address the problem in 10 minutes (time frame may vary but should not be long). The strategies are written and added to the folder.
4. Then each group passes its folder to the group on its right. This means each group has a new problem with some potential strategies to examine.
5. The new group then adds to and refines the existing list of strategies. (Steps 4 and 5 are done several times based on the number of small groups.)
6. After all groups have responded, the last round concludes by having the groups set up the list on a PowerPoint slide(s).
7. PowerPoint slides per problem are then shared.
8. As each problem and its lists of strategies are presented to the entire group, the group discusses each problem and its associated possible strategies one.

## Six Hat Method

The **six hat method** is a brainstorming method used by teams to better understand proposals for change (Fallon et al., 2013). During the process, team members assume one of the roles (hats) and discuss the proposal from that perspective. One role/hat is the facilitator. Using this method helps team members step away from their usual perspectives and better understand all aspects of the proposal as they assume different hats representing different roles.

# Examples of Methods Used to Describe Planning for Change

The following are a few examples of methods used in planning to describe actions needed, decision processes, and timelines. Additional information is found in other chapters. The Connect to Current Information section at the end of this chapter provides links to sites with examples of some of these methods.

## GANTT and PERT Charts

Effective change requires a clear implementation plan with a timeline. A **Gantt chart** may be used to display progress in a project over time. This type of chart is an important part of the plan for change. Sometimes this type of chart is referred to as a **PERT chart**, where PERT is an acronym for **p**rogram **e**valuation **r**eview **t**echnique. The PERT chart is a visual or graphic representation describing a project or a process using boxes and arrows to illustrate the sequence of tasks. It is particularly useful for viewing sequential relationships of project tasks (Langley et al., 2009).

## Decision Tree

The **decision tree** is a method that helps to identify alternatives. After a problem is identified, solutions and their potential positive and negative outcomes are identified. The goal is to identify the best solution that will yield the most positive outcomes and the least negative outcomes. The process should include staff involved in the issue or problem.

---

**STOP AND CONSIDER 4-5**

Consider how you were involved in change today, in the past week, and in the past month, and reflect on methods that were used to assess and describe the change.

---

## Summary

Now, you may still be thinking, why bother with the topic of change? The truth is you have no choice. Change is a fact of life, and certainly it is a fact of life for an HCO and its staff. Consider these quotes and note their wide range of dates and the variety of people who have been intrigued by this subject:

- *Nothing is permanent but change.* (Heraclitus, 535–475 BCE, pre-Socratic Ionian philosopher)
- *Chaos often breeds life, when order breeds habit.* (Henry Brooks Adams, 1838–1919, American writer and historian)
- *It's been a long time coming. But I know a change is gonna come.* (Sam Cooke, 1931–1964, American musician)
- *People don't resist change. They resist being changed!* (Peter Senge, 1947–, writer focused on management and famous for identifying the concept of the learning organization)
- *I am personally convinced that one person can be a change catalyst, a "transformer" in any situation, any organization. Such an individual is yeast that can leaven an entire loaf. It requires vision, initiative, patience, respect, persistence, courage, and faith to be a transforming leader.* (Stephen R. Covey, 1932–2012, business consultant focused on leadership; his book *Seven Habits of Highly Effective People* was listed in 2011 as one of the 25 most influential management books)

Exemplars of quality improvement roles and responsibilities for staff nurses, nurse managers, and APRNs are found in **Exhibit 4-1**.

---

**Exhibit 4-1** Exemplars: Quality Improvement Roles and Responsibilities

**Staff Nurse**

The staff nurses in a small hospital have asked the chief nursing officer to have more staff nurse representation in planning changes for the hospital. They expressed concern that their input is ignored and they feel they have valuable information that could improve some of the changes—for example, when changes are made in the admission process. The chief nurse executive agreed.

**Nurse Manager**

In the example above, the staff nurses first went to the nurse manager group to discuss this issue. They also told the managers that the managers should consult staff nurses more to improve policies and procedures.

**Advanced Practice Registered Nurse***

An ambulatory care center uses APRNs. The director of the center expects all APRNs to also participate in planning for the center. They are provided time for this work.

* Advanced Practice Registered Nurse includes APRN, Clinical Nurse Specialist, Clinical Nurse Leader, and nurses with DNP

# APPLY CQI

## Chapter Highlights

- Effective CQI requires use of the change process.
- Not all changes are improvements.
- Change is an ongoing experience in HCOs.
- Critical change theories and models include Lewin's force field theory, Havelock's theory, Kotter's change model, and Juran's trilogy model.
- Many factors—both internal and external to an HCO—influence the need for change.
- Stakeholders need to be identified and engaged in the change process.
- The change process includes the following steps: identification of need, development and engagement of the team requiring leadership and followership, analysis and description of the problem, readiness assessment, selection and development of the solution(s) based on best evidence,

testing and implementation of the solution(s), spreading improvement, identification of roles and responsibilities, and evaluation and follow-up.

- Barriers to change must be identified and addressed.
- Typical barriers to change are lack of readiness, inadequate leadership, groupthink, and inadequate planning.
- The planning for change must include interventions/strategies to address current and potential barriers.
- Examples of methods to assess and describe the need for change are solution analysis (SWOT), the plan-do-study-act (PDSA) approach, and brainstorming, such as the Delphi, nominal group, and pass the problem techniques.
- Examples of methods used to describe planning are GANTT and PERT charts and decision trees.

## Critical Thinking and Clinical Reasoning and Judgment: Discussion Questions and Learning Activities

1. Develop a visual that includes a minimum of three of the change theories and models discussed in this chapter. The visual (poster, PowerPoint slides, or other methods) should include the key points in each of the theories/models.

2. After reviewing the change process, apply the information to a change you think should be made in a clinical situation. This can be for a problem you have identified in your clinical experience or based on a new idea you

have read about that you think should be applied. Describe what would need to be done for each step of the change process.

3. Based on your response to exercise #2, identify the key stakeholders and why they would be considered stakeholders.

4. Assess how you respond to change. Provide several examples in your assessment. What might you do to improve your response to change?

## Connect to Current Information

- Examples of SWOT
  https://www.google.com/search?sxs-rf=ALeKk00SjknEpu79B11bMAzpyU-DOKJ-aSw:1591788212468&source=univ&tbm=isch&q=SWOT+images&client=firefox-b-d&sa=X&ved=2a-hUKEwjXu9iXkffpAhWVnVwKHefgC3Y-QsAR6BAgIEAE&biw=1867&bih=955

- Examples of decision trees
  https://www.google.com/search?sxs-rf=ALeKk03q34QWGe7DeYmp2auk_zrsEkZAcQ:1591788299136&source=univ&tbm=isch&q=images+decision+trees&client=firefox-b-d&sa=X&ved=2ahUKEwipkoLBkffpAhVLQEEAHTzADH8QsAR6BAgKEAE&biw=1867&bih=955

- Examples of GANTT charts
  https://www.google.com/search?sxsrf=ALeKk00VAFkvXncqekbXCzLoHdnUXEpaXw:1591788341315&source=univ&tbm=isch&q=images+GANTT&client=firefox-b-d&sa=X&ved=2ahUKEwi84ZDVkffpAhUaQUEAHTtFDX8QsAR6BAgKEAE&biw=1867&bih=955

- Examples of PERT charts
  https://images.search.yahoo.com/yhs/search?p=Pert+Chart

- Selecting Changes
  http://www.ihi.org/resources/Pages/HowtoImprove/ScienceofImprovementSelectingChanges.aspx

## Connect to Text Current Information with the Author

Go to the update for this text to review the Blog, QI News, and Literature Review. Access this regular update at: http://nursing.jbpub.com/Finkelman/QualityImprovement/2e.

## EBP, EBM and Quality Improvement: Exemplar

Sloane, D., Smith, H., McHugh, M, & Aiken, L. (2018). Effect of changes in hospital nursing resources on improvements in patient safety and quality of care: a panel study. *Medical Care, 56*(120), 1001–1008.

This article examines change, change management, and quality improvement.

### Questions to Consider

1. What is the study design and sample?
2. What measures were used?
3. What were the results?
4. How does the information in the article apply to nursing and change?

# EVOLVING CASE STUDY

As a staff member who serves on the Quality Improvement Planning Committee, you are at a meeting to discuss the best way to share information about recent CQI data so that staff in the hospital can appreciate the value of the data. You need to identify pros and cons of methods the committee might use to assess and describe data for planning purposes.

The committee is mostly new; some members have limited experience. You and two other members have the most experience, so you three volunteer to help the others get up to speed as quickly as possible so that decisions can be made about steps to take with the data, and you can get to decisions about strategies. You make clear to the other committee members that (1) this is a team effort and (2) the team must engage hospital staff at all levels. You comment, "We have tried to keep this to ourselves, thinking only we knew the best approaches, and we failed." Staff do not feel engaged in CQI and complain about the extra work for which they see no value.

## Case Questions A

*The following questions relate to the committee's discussion.*

1. What are some of the barriers that could be influencing limited staff engagement?
2. What strategies might be used to overcome these barriers?

## Case Questions B

*Now the committee must move to the work they must do.*

1. What are pros and cons of the methods used to assess and describe the need for change (discussed in this chapter)?
2. What are the common reasons staff members resist change?
3. How might the committee use GANTT and PERT charts and/or decision trees?

# References

American Organization for Nursing Leadership (AONL). (2019). Elements of a healthy practice environment. Retrieved from https://www.aonl.org/system/files/media/file/2019/10/healthful-practice-work.pdf

Fallon, L., Begun, J., & Riley, W. (2013). *Managing health organizations for quality performance*. Burlington, MA: Jones & Bartlett Learning.

Feeley, D. (2019). The five Ps of Triple Aim transformation. Retrieved from http://www.ihi.org/communities/blogs/the-five-ps-of-triple-aim-transformation

Finkelman, A. (2019). *Professional nursing concepts: Competencies for quality leadership* (4th ed.). Burlington, MA: Jones & Bartlett Learning.

Frieden, J. (2015). The changing face of medical education: Big data, self-paced learning. Retrieved from https://www.healthleadersmedia.com/strategy/changing-face-medical-education-big-data-self-paced-learning

Havelock, E. (1973). *The change agent's guide to innovation in education*. Englewood Cliffs, NJ: Educational Technology Publications.

Hilton, K., & Anderson, A. (2018). *IHI psychology of change framework to advance and sustain improvement*. Boston, MA: Institute for Health Improvement. Retrieved from ihi.org

Institute for Healthcare Improvement (IHI). (2012). How to improve. Retrieved from http://www.ihi.org/knowledge/Pages/HowtoImprove/default.aspx

Juran, J., & Defeo, J. (Eds.). (2010). *Juran's quality handbook* (6th ed.). Columbus, OH: McGraw-Hill Companies.

Khator, R. (2014). Innovate or perish: The future is here. In M. Fennell & S. Miller (Eds.), *Presidential perspectives, 2014–2015 series: Inspirational innovation* (pp. 4.1–4.4). Philadelphia, PA: Aramark.

Kotter, J. (1996). *Leading change*. Boston, MA: Harvard Business School Press.

Langley, G., Moen, R., Nolan, K., Nolan, T., Norman, C., & Provost, L. (2009). *The improvement guide: A practical approach to enhancing organizational performance* (2nd ed.). San Francisco, CA: Jossey-Bass Publishers.

Lewin, K. (1947). Group and social change. In T. Newcomb & E. Hartely (Eds.), *Readings in social psychology*. New York, NY: Holt, Rinehart, and Winston.

McCannon, C., Schall, M., & Perla, R. (2008). *Planning for scale: A guide for designing large-scale improvement initiatives*. IHI Innovation Series white paper. Cambridge, MA. Retrieved from http://www.ihi.org/resources/pages/ihiwhitepapers/planningforscalewhitepaper.aspx

Ponti, M. (2011). Why change fails. *Nurse Leader, 9*(8), 41–43.

Quinn, R. (1996). *Deep change: Discovering the leader within*. San Francisco, CA: Jossey-Bass.

Quinn, R. (2000). *Change the world: How ordinary people can accomplish extraordinary results*. San Francisco, CA: Jossey-Bass.

Robinson-Walker, C. (2011). Managing an onslaught of change. *Nurse Leader, 9*(7), 10–11.

Scanlon, K., & Woolforde, L. (2016). A unique improvement approach centered on staff engagement, empowerment, and professional development. *Nurse Leader, 14* (1), 38–45.

Sollecito, W., & Johnson, J. (2013). The global evolution of continuous quality improvement: From Japanese manufacturing to global health services. In W. Sollecito &

J. Johnson, (Eds.), *McLaughlin and Kaluzny's continuous quality improvement in healthcare* (4th ed., pp. 1–48). Burlington, MA: Jones & Bartlett Learning.

U.S. Department of Health and Human Services (HHS), Agency for Healthcare Research and Quality (AHRQ). (2014). How do we implement best practices in our hospital? Retrieved from https://www.ahrq.gov/patient-safety/settings/hospital/resource/pressureulcer/tool/pu4a.html

U.S. Department of Health and Human Services (HHS), Agency for Healthcare Research and Quality (AHRQ). (2015). In conversation with... Maureen Bisognano. Retrieved from https://psnet.ahrq.gov/perspective/conversation-maureen-bisognano

U.S. Department of Health and Human Services (HHS), Agency for Healthcare Research and Quality (AHRQ). (2016). Gap analysis. Retrieved from https://www.ahrq.gov/sites/default/files/wysiwyg/professionals/systems/hospital/qitoolkit/combined/d5_combo_gapanalysis.pdf

U.S. Department of Health and Human Services (HHS), Agency for Healthcare Research and Quality (AHRQ). (2019). AHRQ's commitment to meeting unmet needs in the healthcare system. Retrieved from https://www.ahrq.gov/news/blog/ahrqviews/ahrqs-commitment-to-meeting-unmet-needs.html

Value Based Management.net. (2019) The Deming cycle. Retrieved from https://www.valuebasedmanagement.net/methods_demingcycle.html

Weick, K., & Quinn, R. (1999). Organization change and development. *Annual Review of Psychology, 50,* 361–386.

# Understanding the Healthcare Environment to Improve Care

*"No, no! The adventures first, explanations take such a dreadful time."*

Lewis Carroll, *Alice's Adventures in Wonderland* (1865)

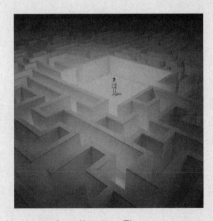

The goal of the maze is to reach a state of quality care. The maze may not be clear enough for you to fully appreciate quality improvement. To do this you must engage in continuous quality improvement planning and the measurement process within the healthcare environment. Neither is easy to understand and both take time. This is where the patient enters and is the center of all activities. How do you find the information you need to understand all of this, and where does the information take you? Answer: To an effective continuous quality improvement plan and measurement that meets required outcomes.

## CHAPTER 5

# Entering the Quality Improvement World

## CHAPTER OBJECTIVES

At the conclusion of this chapter, the learner will be able to:

- Compare and contrast examples of quality care theories, models, and approaches.
- Analyze the impact of the blame culture.
- Examine the impact of a culture of safety on the continuous quality improvement process and how to implement and maintain this culture.

## OUTLINE

## KEY TERMS

Accountability
Blame culture
Code of silence
Consonant culture
Cultural competence
Culture
Culture of safety
Dissonant culture

Healthcare disparity
Healthcare equity
Healthcare inequality
High-reliability organizations
  (HROs)
Just culture
Lean approach
Linguistic competence

Organizational culture
Rapid cycle model
Reliability
Science of improvement
Six Sigma
Social determinants of health
STEEEP®
Triple aim

## Introduction

In 2015, Dr. Gandhi, Chief Executive of the National Patient Safety Foundation (NPSF), looked back over the development of patient safety and quality since the publication of *To Err Is Human* (Institute of Medicine [IOM], 1999; Institute for Healthcare Improvement [IHI], 2015a). This review has relevance to this chapter as we begin to examine the continuous quality improvement (CQI) world—what it is and approaches that might be taken to provide a framework for the CQI work that is done by individual healthcare providers and healthcare organizations (HCOs). Dr. Gandhi notes that the first approach to quality improvement was to convince us we had a problem: we lacked the level of quality care we should have. This effort is ongoing, but the focus now is more on answering two questions: How do we improve, and what type of **culture** and leadership are needed to accomplish improvement? Since 1999, the culture has changed, engaging staff, including frontline workers, and incorporating health informatics technology (HIT). Change has been discussed and will continue to be a theme throughout this text. Engaging staff begins with knowledge; a major goal of this text is to provide more information and resources for nurses, and, as noted earlier, healthcare professions education must also include more content about CQI and its relationship to HIT. This is an expanding area,

providing us with more data, better analysis methods, and more timely communication. This chapter discusses issues related to the current focus.

## Creating a Vision of Quality Care: Theories, Models, and Approaches

There are many references that could be used to introduce this section about the vision of quality care. Since this text focuses on nurses and their engagement in CQI, we will turn to the *Quality Chasm* report *Keeping Patients Safe: Transforming the Work Environment of Nurses* (IOM, 2004a). Looking at the title of the report, there are two critical messages: (1) The patient is mentioned first, and (2) the term "transforming" is used. These choices communicate a message of positive in-depth change focused on patients. The nurse's work environment is also included in the title, and this consideration is critical if we are to meet required patient outcomes. The 2004 report makes five recommendations that nurses must consider that are still relevant today:

- Implementing evidence-based management
- Balancing tension between efficiency and reliability
- Creating and sustaining trust

- Actively managing the change process through communication, training, feedback, sustained effort and attention, and worker involvement
- Creating a learning organization

As noted in the discussion about the healthcare professions core competencies in other sections of this text, these competencies do not separate safety from quality. Quality care is "the degree to which healthcare services for individuals and populations increase the likelihood of desired health outcomes and are consistent with current professional knowledge" and safety "relates to actual or potential bodily harm" (HHS, Agency for Healthcare Research and Quality [AHRQ], 2018a). Typically, HCOs have a structural component, such as an organizational unit (e.g., department, service), focused on quality improvement, and this work includes safety for staff and patients. In the end, quality must become a systemwide attribute—so much a part of the system that it is never thought of as a separate aspect of an organization.

Current quality improvement frameworks/models tend to emphasize the six dimensions of quality care noted in the earlier *Quality Chasm* reports (IOM, 1999, 2001). The dimensions are safety, timeliness, effectiveness, efficiency, equity, and patient-centeredness (STEEEP®). With the dynamic (changing) nature of healthcare there is need for a variety of models of quality improvement. There are key similarities but also some differences in these models. Some of the models were developed specifically for healthcare, and others are borrowed from other industries and then adapted as needed and applied to healthcare. Quality improvement is also viewed as a journey, implying movement and change; data are collected, and changes are initiated when needed (Storme, 2013). According to the Health Resources and Services Administration (HRSA), an agency in the U.S. Department of Health and Human Services (HHS), "An organization that implements a quality improvement program experiences a range of benefits" (HHS, HRSA, 2011, p. 6), including the following:

- *Improved patient health (clinical) outcomes that involve both process outcomes (e.g., provide recommended screenings) and health outcomes (e.g., decreased morbidity and mortality).*
- *Improved efficiency of managerial and clinical processes.* By improving processes and outcomes relevant to high-priority health needs, an organization reduces waste and costs associated with system failures and redundancy. Often quality improvement processes are budget-neutral, where the costs to make the changes are offset by the cost savings incurred.
- *Avoided costs associated with process failures, errors, and poor outcomes.* Costs are incurred when nonstandard and inefficient systems increase errors and cause rework. Streamlined and reliable processes are less expensive to maintain.
- *Proactive processes that recognize and solve problems before they occur ensure that systems of care are reliable and predictable.* A culture of improvement frequently develops in an organization that is committed to quality because errors are reported and addressed.
- *Improved communication with resources that are internal and external to an organization, such as funders and civic and community organizations.* A commitment to quality shines a positive light on an organization, which may result in an increase of partnership and funding opportunities. When successfully implemented, quality improvement infrastructure often enhances communication and resolves critical issues. (p. 6)

Dailey (2013) offers a useful description of quality: "Quality is a concept. It expresses people's perceptions of what makes something seem better or worse in some way that can only be measured by proxy, comparison, or using some abstract metric." The following are principles on which quality is based (Galt, Paschal, & Gleason, 2011):

1. Healthcare professionals are intrinsically motivated to improve patient safety because of the ethical foundation, professional norms, and expectations of our respective disciplines.
2. Organizational leaders are responsible for setting the standards for achieving safety at the highest level and in response to societal expectations.
3. Consumers are becoming increasingly aware of healthcare safety problems and are not accepting of it.
4. There is substantial room for improvement of healthcare systems and practices that will result in a reduction in both error potential and harm. (p. 8)

A variety of models and theories apply to quality improvement. HCOs typically use one of them, a combination, or adapt one or two to serve as a guide for their quality improvement program. The following discussion describes some of the common models and theories.

## Science of Improvement

According to the Institute for Healthcare Improvement (IHI, 2015b): "The **science of improvement** is an applied science that emphasizes innovation, rapid-cycle testing in the field, and spread in order to generate learning about what changes, in which contexts, produce improvements. It is characterized by the combination of expert subject knowledge with improvement methods and tools. It is multidisciplinary—drawing on clinical science, systems theory, psychology, statistics, and other fields." It requires clear goals, which implies a plan and measurement.

The science of improvement focuses on three questions that the HCO should ask (IHI, 2015c):

1. *What are we trying to accomplish?* This question focuses on assessment, description of issues, and development of goals and a plan.

2. *How will we know that a change is an improvement?* This question is based on using the plan as a guide to identify outcomes and measurements required.
3. *What changes can we make that will result in improvement?* This question considers changes/interventions/strategies that will lead to improvement.

The **rapid cycle model** is associated with the science of improvement and related to these three key questions. The approach is used to pilot test small changes recommended by frontline staff and to actively engage staff in the CQI process, recognizing that small changes can impact the HCO with positive outcomes. The plan-do-study-act (PDSA) model is used to respond to needs and move toward improvement. PDSA is discussed in other sections of this text. Using this approach emphasizes frontline staff identification of needs for change and actively engages staff. There is then less need to "force" changes on staff. This approach is supported by government initiatives to improve healthcare (HHS, Office of the National Coordinator for Health Information Technology [ONC], 2019).

Improvement capability must be considered to ensure that the science of improvement focuses on CQI to reach improvement outcomes. Efforts include the following (IHI, 2015b):

- Building science-based improvement capability at individual, organizational, and system levels
- Arming future doctors and nurses and others preparing for careers in healthcare with quality improvement knowledge and skills before they enter the workforce
- Expanding the capability of middle managers and other operational leaders to use advanced improvement methods to guide and support frontline improvement
- Developing learning networks to accelerate implementation, spread, and scale-up of innovative approaches to improve health outcomes

- Providing a clear road map for how organizations applying the lean approach and Six Sigma (both discussed later in this chapter) can use the science of improvement to accelerate results
- Providing individuals, professional groups, organizations, and whole systems with the right "dose" of improvement capability to drive results

## The Triple Aim

In 2008, the IHI proposed a framework for CQI, which is called the **Triple Aim** (Stiefel & Nolan, 2012). Since its development, it is now used globally, and it has had an impact on the Affordable Care Act of 2010 (ACA). It is also a critical part of the National Quality Strategy (NQS), which is discussed in this text (Whittington, Nolan, Lewis, & Torres, 2015). The purpose of Triple Aim is to (1) improve the patient experience of care (including quality and satisfaction), (2) improve the health of populations, and (3) reduce the per capita cost of healthcare (IHI, 2015d).

The Triple Aim framework acknowledges that all three aims must be pursued together, as they are interdependent, and HCOs should clarify responsibilities for these aims. Meeting these aims requires a system approach to change.

The Triple Aim considers constraints that require a balance in the CQI process—for example, when considering costs and who gets care, there should be equity of care. As Berwick, Nolan, and Whittington (2008) state, "The gain in health in one subpopulation ought not to be achieved at the expense of another subpopulation. But that decision lies in the realms of ethics and policy" (p. 760). Diversity and disparities in healthcare remain a critical concern, and when one gets into this area, ethics becomes even more important. Berwick and colleagues comment that the United States has the technical methods for data collection, measurement, and analysis to monitor and improve care to meet the

Triple Aim, but the biggest barrier is whether or not there is drive to make changes in HCOs and maintain them. Meeting the Triple Aim requires organization transformation, and to accomplish this it is important to do the following: make paradigm change, not little changes; plan; be proactive; involve staff as a whole—one or a few is not enough; and have a clear purpose (Feeley, 2019).

There has been discussion about changing the Triple Aim, and some healthcare organizations have done this. What does the originator, Donald Berwick, M.D., think about changes in the Triple Aim? "People sometimes now talk about the quadruple aim with joy in work as the fourth part. You can't get to better care for individuals, better health for populations, and lower costs with a demoralized workforce. It won't work. We must have the energy to work together and confidence that we can succeed. It's too hard in a stressed environment with burnout and people losing confidence. As President Emerita and Senior Fellow Maureen Bisognano says, 'You can't give what you don't have.' We can't have the Triple Aim without joy in work, but I've resisted the label "quadruple aim" for a technical reason: the original idea of the Triple Aim is to define what society wants from us, which is external. Joy in work is internal. It's important, but it's not quite on the same playing field as the social need, though I recognize that it's essential for meeting the social need. The Triple Aim isn't biblical. It's not chiseled in tablets and people are certainly entitled to do anything they want with the term. But sometimes people say, 'The Triple Aim is better care, better satisfaction, and lower cost.' No, the satisfaction of patients is part of the first aim. I've heard people talk about it as quality, safety, and service. Anyone can list three aims and go ahead and do it. I'm not saying there's one right definition, but if you want to go back to the origins, it's very clear: It's better care for individuals, better health for populations, and lower per capita cost while maintaining the first two" (Berwick, 2019).

## Structure, Process, Outcomes Model

The *Quality Chasm* reports' definition of quality care incorporates the model of healthcare quality discussed many years ago by Donabedian (1980). This model, described in **Figure 5-1**, focuses on three aspects of the healthcare delivery system: structure, process, and outcomes. Most types of healthcare settings have used this model to understand and evaluate quality. Structure focuses on how the organization is organized—the system and its parts, including its facilities, finances, supplies and equipment, informatics (hardware and software), staff and staffing, clinical expertise, and so on. Process considers how the parts interact and function and also the interaction with patients and healthcare providers, including assessment and diagnosis, coordination, patient education, delivery of care, and use of HIT. Outcomes should indicate that care meets the STEEEP® criteria and should include long-term outcomes to improve functioning and quality of life (Lawless & Proujansky, 2006). As stated by Donabedian (1988), "Good structure increases the likelihood of good process, and good process increases the likelihood of good outcomes" (p. 1147).

## Continuous Quality Improvement (CQI): A Systematic Approach

CQI is the approach that is now recommended for all HCOs and providers. Sollecito and Johnson (2013) define CQI as "a structured organizational process for involving personnel in planning and executing a continuous flow of improvements to provide quality healthcare that meets or exceeds expectations" (p. 4). They go on to define the following characteristics of CQI:

- A link to key elements of the organization's strategic plan
- A quality committee made up of the institution's top leadership
- Training programs for personnel
- Mechanisms for selecting improvement opportunities
- Formation of process improvement teams
- Staff support for process analysis and redesign; staff engagement and commitment
- Personnel policies that motivate and support staff participation in process improvement
- Application of the most current and rigorous techniques of the scientific method and statistical process control (pp. 4–5)

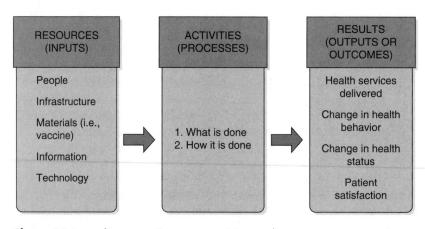

**Figure 5-1** Inputs/Structure, Processes, and Outputs/Outcomes

The goal of CQI is to improve or streamline activities, which should be a continuous process. This model focuses on data, leadership, and active participation from all relevant staff levels. Applying CQI means the HCO manages its performance, motivates improvement among staff, and learns from its experiences. As the HRSA (HHS, HRSA, 2011) describes CQI, "it is an ongoing effort to improve the efficiency, effectiveness, quality, or performance of services, processes, capacities, and outcomes." The following key strategies are often used in CQI (Draper, Felland, Liebhaber, & Melichar, 2008):

- Having supportive hospital leadership and keeping them actively engaged in the work
- Setting expectations for all staff—not just nurses—that quality is a shared responsibility
- Holding staff accountable for individual roles and responsibilities
- Inspiring and using physicians and nurses to champion efforts
- Providing ongoing, visible, and useful feedback to engage staff effectively (p. 3)

The main elements of this model are to first know the customer (patient) well and connect this understanding with the daily functions of the HCO. Second, there is need to develop the HCO culture through leadership emphasizing commitment, pride in the HCO, and use of scientific thinking. The third element is to use organized methods to collect and analyze data and make decisions based on this measurement (Berwick, 1999). Empowerment of staff is critical, as is controlling variation. Healthcare professionals usually like to be in control, which sometimes makes coping with patient variations difficult, impacting reliability and quality.

## Culture of Accountability

HCOs want to effectively use evidence-based practice (EBP) and evidence-based management (EBM) to support individual staff in learning and engaging in CQI. To do this, HCOs must adopt a culture of accountability. Establishing a no-blame culture does not meet all the requirements needed to be successful in improving care (Moriates & Wachter, 2015). **Accountability**, or being responsible for what you do and the outcomes, should be integrated in the HCO and supported in performance requirements, orientation and staff education, and ongoing performance measurement. Increasing staff accountability means the staff is more tuned into value and costs, such as working toward reducing overuse, misuse, and underuse of resources. Change is present and the staff should deal with change routinely. "Deciphering accountability and determining when individuals and systems are culpable are challenges. None of us—nurses, physicians, nor administrators—learned our craft working in collaborative teams, but today the public, policymakers, and payers expect us to practice as a synchronized whole. It is time to join forces and develop principles for healthcare accountability that serve the public, clinicians, and the system" (Goeschel, 2011, p. 30) "Who is accountable? For which issues are they accountable? What are the appropriate methods for holding them accountable? All quality issues are not the same, and different types of accountability apply to various aspects of health-care delivery" (p. 32).

Active engagement of staff in development of safety cultures and organizations increases accountability. "Today's challenges are to discern the dimensions of individual and team accountability within the context of systems accountability, to develop cross-discipline principles that minimize the risk of disproportionate responses after an error, and to disseminate this knowledge widely" (Goeschel, 2011, pp. 32–33).

## STEEEP®: Pursuit of Excellence

**STEEEP®** is a framework that is based on the six aims identified in the *Quality Chasm* series

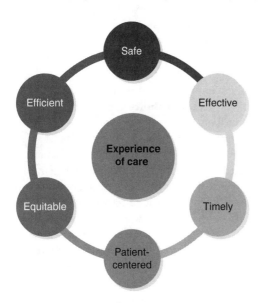

**Figure 5-2** STEEEP®

(safety, timeliness, effectiveness, efficiency, equity, patient-centeredness) (IOM, 2001). This framework was developed and trademarked by Baylor Scott & White Health (Texas). It integrates Kotter's change model, discussed in this text, and applies PDSA (Ballard, 2014). It is based on four principles: Develop a strong customer focus, apply CQI, engage staff, and use data to improve decision making. Performance improvement teams are used to ensure accountability and improvement. Resources on the website for this framework provide support to implement the framework (Ballard). The implementation plan includes the plan itself, organization or structure to meet the plan, communication, required staff education, motivation strategies, and measurement and review of performance. **Figure 5-2** describes STEEEP®.

## The Lean Approach to Quality Improvement

The **lean approach** in healthcare quality improvement focuses on value to the customer (the patient), with efforts made to reduce waste in time, effort, and cost—doing more with less (Lawal et al., 2014). This approach was adopted from Toyota and later applied to healthcare delivery. It focuses on the "application of lean principles in healthcare settings to improve quality of care, increase efficiency, lower costs, and provide better patient outcomes. Lean is an organizational redesign approach focused on elimination of waste, which is defined as any activity that consumes resources (e.g., staff, time, money, space) without adding value to those being served by the process" (HHS, AHRQ, 2014). A concern that staff may have with this model is its emphasis on reducing costs, and this might have major implications for staffing, equipment and supplies, staff education, and the work environment. It might also result in healthcare systems that are more structured and less flexible. To avoid this response, HCOs must assess themselves periodically to ensure that they are not overemphasizing reducing cost while failing to view the larger perspective and needs. A published review of 34 studies on the use of the lean approach with Transforming Care at the Bedside (TCAB) examined the impact of eliminating non-value-added activities on direct care or time at the bedside, noting that "although Lean and TCAB processes may be effective in the improvement of specific outcomes, there is no direct relationship with the implementation of these processes and time spent at the bedside. Furthermore, it is evident that organizations must be in a position to commit valuable time and resources to the implementation of these strategies" (Brackett, Comer, & Whichello, 2013, p. 13).

If the lean model is used, leaders need to be open about its purpose and provide opportunity for staff to discuss their fears, which may not be based on reality. The typical wastes within HCOs that must be assessed are unnecessary motion, unnecessary transportation (movement of supplies, equipment, people, information throughout the HCO), defects and errors, waiting (e.g., for supplies, for discharge), inadequate inventory, extra-processing, overproduction, and unused human talent potential (Six Sigma, 2019a). Within every process, there are opportunities to eliminate lean waste. The acronym DOWN-TIME illustrates these wastes—for example, waste during the hospital discharge process may exist in these eight forms (HHS, AHRQ, 2011):

- *Defects, or failure modes.* Examples: omission of discharge order, omission of follow-up appointment, incorrect selection of medication, failure to provide discharge prescriptions, incomplete discharge instructions, failure to assess patient comprehension, and omission of home medical equipment order
- *Overproduction.* Example: overproduction of printed discharge teaching sheets that are not individualized or then become outdated
- *Waiting.* Examples: wait times for patient information prior to discharge; staff waiting for medications for discharge patients
- *Non-value-added processing.* Examples: rework and redundancies (staff checking for supplies, order, and so on)
- *Transportation.* Example: too few wheelchairs creating discharge delays
- *Inventory.* Examples: over- or undersupply of medical treatment supplies needed to prepare patients for discharge
- *Motion.* Examples: having to go to another location to retrieve discharge materials instead of having them nearby or at the point of service; stooping, stretching, pulling, or pushing inappropriately
- *Employee.* Example: underutilizing or not using staff-based knowledge; not having staff who are part of the problem-solving process perform the actual work

The lean approach does not support use of workarounds, a subject discussed in other chapters, and looks to resolve problems at their root (Brackett et al., 2013). It is believed that inefficient processes can be improved by going to the root of the problem.

## Six Sigma

**Six Sigma** is a measurement-based strategy, and it is another approach that began outside of healthcare. This approach "provides organizations tools to improve the capability of their business processes. This increase in performance and decrease in process variation helps lead to defect reduction and improvement in profits, employee morale, and quality of products or services. Six Sigma quality is a term generally used to indicate a process is well controlled" (American Society for Quality [ASQ], 2019). This framework focuses more on statistical methods that are used to identify and remove errors.

A defect is an outcome that does not meet the requirements of its customers (Six Sigma, 2019b). Reducing process variability increases opportunity to reduce defects. Examples of defects might be long wait times for an appointment, long wait time in the emergency department for inpatient admission, medications not arriving on time from the pharmacy, and communication barriers. DMAIC is used for improving existing projects (define, measure, analyze, improve, control), and DMADV (define, measure, analyze, design, verify) is used in creating new improvement projects to guide development of new processes (Graves, 2019). These methods are discussed in other chapters. Some HCOs combine the lean model with Six Sigma, calling it Lean Six Sigma, with both models using small changes tested over time, focusing on analyzing processes and use of mapping to achieve improvement.

## High-Reliability Organization

**High-reliability organizations (HROs)** have become more common in healthcare. HROs are HCOs that use a three-step approach to reach and maintain high reliability (HHS, AHRQ, PSNET, 2019a). The six dimensions of quality healthcare (STEEEP®) are integrated into HROs. What is **reliability**? It is the state of being failure free that develops in an environment over time, with persistent effort to cultivate resilience. "Over time," as mentioned here, is a critical aspect, as it is not a one-time view of quality but rather consistent, effective performance, which ties in with CQI. The concept of "over time" also applies to the HCO and individual

patient trajectories. To implement and retain reliability requires concentrated effort. Leaders in HROs must commit to actively developing and maintaining CQI. **Table 5-1** provides information about critical characteristics of HROs and related strategies used to prevent the characteristics that interfere with maintaining an HRO.

**Table 5-1** Characteristics of High-Reliability Organizations

| Characteristic | Description |
| --- | --- |
| Preoccupation with failure | Everyone is aware of and thinking about the potential for failure. People understand that new threats emerge regularly from situations that no one imagined could occur, so all personnel actively think about what could go wrong and are alert to small signs of potential problems. The absence of errors or accidents leads not to complacency but to a heightened sense of vigilance for the next possible failure. Near misses are viewed as opportunities to learn about systems issues and potential improvements rather than as evidence of safety. |
| Reluctance to simplify | People resist simplifying their understanding of work processes and how and why things succeed or fail in their environment. People in high-reliability organizations (HROs) understand that the work is complex and dynamic. They seek underlying rather than surface explanations. While HROs recognize the value of standardization of workflows to reduce variation, they also appreciate the complexity inherent in the number of teams, processes, and relationships involved in conducting daily operations. |
| Sensitivity to operations | Based on their understanding of operational complexity, people in HROs strive to maintain a high awareness of operational conditions. This sensitivity is often referred to as "big picture understanding" or "situation awareness." It means that people cultivate an understanding of the context of the current state of their work in relation to the unit or organizational state—that is, what is going on around them—and how the current state might support or threaten safety. |
| Deference to expertise | People in HROs appreciate that the people closest to the work are the most knowledgeable about the work. Thus, people in HROs know that in a crisis or emergency the person with greatest knowledge of the situation might not be the person with the highest status and seniority. Deference to local and situation expertise results in a spirit of inquiry and deemphasis on hierarchy in favor of learning as much as possible about potential safety threats. In an HRO, everyone is expected to share concerns with others, and the organizational climate is such that all staff members are comfortable speaking up about potential safety problems. |
| Commitment to resilience | Commitment to resilience is rooted in the fundamental understanding of the frequently unpredictable nature of system failures. People in HROs assume the system is at risk for failure, and they practice performing rapid assessments of and responses to challenging situations. Teams cultivate situation assessment and cross-monitoring so they may identify potential safety threats quickly and either respond before safety problems cause harm or mitigate the seriousness of the safety event. |

Reproduced with permission from AHRQ Patient Safety Network. (2019). Patient safety primer: High reliability. Retrieved from https://psnet.ahrq.gov/primer/high-reliability

Other chapters discuss CQI measurement and improvement interventions/strategies in more detail; however, to provide a better description of HROs, one might ask this: What would this organization do to meet the three-step approach? HCOs that emphasize HRO use systems thinking throughout the organization, with recognition that the HCO is not static and change is ongoing. The goal is to create and maintain an environment "in which potential problems are anticipated, detected early, and virtually always responded to early enough to prevent catastrophic consequences" (HHS, AHRQ, PSNet, 2019b).

Accomplishing these strategies requires HCO leadership, an active safety culture, and an effective improvement process initiative that supports reliability. Since reliability was first used in non-healthcare industries, this is another example of applying methods and approaches used by other industries. In an HRO, management and staff might use standardization—for example, by using checklists and actively providing staff feedback. The HCO also uses structured communication methods with patients and staff, such as calling patients to remind them of appointments or making sure communication is clear when using abbreviations and numbers to avoid errors. The organization might apply failure modes and effects analysis (FMEA) as a method to improve structure and processes, which is discussed in other chapters.

Chassin and Loeb (2011) discuss the complex nature of care delivery and its impact on reliability: "As new devices, equipment, procedures, and drugs are added to our therapeutic arsenal, the complexity of delivering effective care increases. Complexity greatly increases the likelihood of error, especially in systems that perform at low levels of reliability" (p. 563). HROs are driven to ensure that the organization functions at its best level despite this complexity. Many new approaches to improve care have been developed and applied. In this text, many of these approaches are discussed. The field requires more collective

mindfulness, with every individual, the HCO as a whole, and all its parts working to identify potential failures that can lead to adverse events. In summary HROs are "organizations that achieve safety, quality, and efficiency goals by employing five central principles: (1) sensitivity to operations (e.g., heightened awareness of the state of relevant systems and processes); (2) reluctance to simplify (e.g., the acceptance that work is complex, with the potential to fail in new and unexpected ways); (3) preoccupation with failure (e.g., to view near misses as opportunities to improve rather than proof of success); (4) deference to expertise (e.g., to value insights from staff with the most pertinent safety knowledge over those with greater seniority); (5) and practicing resilience (e.g., to prioritize emergency training for many unlikely, but possible, system failures)" (Veazie, Peterson, & Bourne, 2019).

## The Agency for Healthcare Research and Quality (AHRQ): Quality Improvement Process

The AHRQ is the major agency in the HHS that guides national efforts toward improving quality. The NQS, discussed in other chapters, is the current national major initiative that it is expected to guide efforts to meet this goal. The AHRQ not only sets a model or framework but also works with stakeholders in implementation efforts to improve care through NQS and other initiatives. The agency is also concerned with ensuring that evidence from research is implemented in practice when appropriate—to fill the gap in knowledge (EBP and EBM). With the expansion of research and the concern for use of best-practice evidence falling through the cracks, this in itself is a major effort. The AHRQ supports the development of HROs and the CQI process based on STEEEP®, and it provides CQI recommendations for various healthcare settings, such as the hospital. The process uses administrative and clinical data to assess quality, identify problems or concerns that require more examination, and determine what needs to be monitored over time. When implementing the CQI process, the AHRQ recommends applying the following, which are not only supported by the federal government but also healthcare professional groups (HHS, AHRQ, 2019a):

- *Place a priority on encouraging communication, engagement, and participation.* Include the stakeholders involved with or affected by the changes required by your CQI work. Look for ways to help them embrace the changes and begin to take ownership of them.
- *Start your implementation of improvements with small-scale demonstrations.* Small-scale demonstrations are easier to manage than are large-scale changes. They also allow you to refine the new processes, demonstrate their impact on practices and outcomes, and build increased support by stakeholders. Some HCOs refer to this as pilot testing.
- *Keep in mind and remind others that CQI is an iterative process.* You will be making frequent corrections along the way as you learn from experience with each step and identify other actions to add to your strategy.

---

**STOP AND CONSIDER 5-1**

There are multiple theories and models about quality improvement that an HCO can choose to apply.

---

# The Blame Culture and Its Impact

The *Quality Chasm* reports noted problems not only with the quality of care but also with responses to errors. The reports indicated that HCOs emphasized a work culture that focused on blame, and that is a major barrier to improvement.

# Organizational Culture

Organizations have their own cultures, and the culture impacts how the organization is structured and functions. **Organizational culture** is the values, beliefs, traditions, and communication processes that bring a group of people together and characterize the organization. The culture also impacts teams and teamwork within the HCO. As explained by Heathfield (2020), culture "is a powerful element that shapes your work enjoyment, your work relationships, and your work processes. However, culture is something that you cannot actually see, except through its physical manifestations in your workplace."

An organization's culture is complex. There is the overall organizational culture, such as the culture of a hospital. Internally an organization typically has some differences in culture within its units, divisions, or departments and with staff groups, such as nurses, physicians, nonclinical staff, management, and so on. Ideally, all should reflect the overall organizational culture, but this may not be the case. Lack of an overall organizational culture may actually lead to conflict if there are major differences in values, attitudes, and behaviors. Sometimes these differences are due to differences in leadership style, and sometimes it comes more from the staff. Organizational culture does change over time and is influenced by changes in high-level leadership and the organization's vision, mission, and goals. Communication is a critical element in an organization's culture, and it is complex, with many staff levels and a great number of staff and services. Organizational culture includes language, decision making, symbols/communication, stories and legends, and daily work practices (Heathfield, 2020).

Organizational culture may be described as consonant and dissonant. A **consonant culture** implies that the organization's culture is effective. A **dissonant culture** acts as a block to effectiveness and thus has a negative impact on the development of a collaborative team environment. How does one identify a dissonant organization? The following characteristics of a dissonant culture were identified in Sovie (1993) and described again in Jones & Redman (2000, p. 605). Added to these dissonant characteristics are comments about the current relevance of the characteristics:

- *Focus on serving the providers and not the patients.* This focus would be in conflict with the movement today to increase patient-centered care.
- *Lack of clarity about individual and department expectations.* Staff members who do not know what is expected may become frustrated, and this lack of clarity may also impact staff burnout, productivity, and outcomes.
- *Failure to regularly measure quality of services.* There is more measurement of quality today with the increased emphasis and concern about problems in quality of care; however, the effectiveness of the measurement and response varies. We have need for much improvement and development of more effective measurement.
- *Lack of patient involvement in decision making.* Patient-centered care requires patient involvement in decision making; however, we have much to do to improve. Some providers are not as committed as they should be to ensuring patient participation, or there may be other barriers to patient involvement.
- *Limited concern about employee satisfaction.* This can be a major problem and lead to problems of staff frustration and burnout, recruitment and retention issues, lower productivity, and a culture that is not seen as caring of staff.
- *Limited education/training programs for employees.* This can lead to the same problems noted for employee satisfaction but may also have a major impact on quality of care and increasing errors.
- *Frequent turf battles.* This is a sign of an organization that is not functioning well, demonstrating lack of cohesiveness (i.e., no clear vision, mission, and goals), poor communication, conflict, and lack of collaboration.
- *Failure to recognize staff accomplishment.* This leads to poor relationships between upper and middle management and staff, decreasing trust and commitment to the organization. (p. 605)

Improving the culture so that the organization is a place where people want to work makes a major difference in how the organization functions and its outcomes. However, this is not something that is solely in the hands of upper or even middle management. All staff must work to improve the organization's culture, including eliminating bullying and reducing stress. This requires taking risks, being clear about perspectives, and communicating needs and goals effectively. Effective teams exist in effective organizational cultures.

## Description of a Blame Culture

The publication of *To Err Is Human* led to significant consideration of the approach HCOs had been taking toward errors (IOM, 1999). The report suggested a tendency of HCOs to examine errors with a focus on assigning blame to individuals. This approach results in what is often referred to as a **blame culture**. It is clear that this approach has not worked; errors continue to rise, and quality care continues to decrease. The blame culture has led to a work environment in which staff may fear they will be blamed when "things go wrong." Being assigned blame may lead to punishment, such as forcing staff to attend a medication administration course when staff knowledge may not be the cause of an error. In some situations individuals are the reason for an error, but many errors are system errors, and individual staff are merely involved in the system. Effective CQI requires that both system and individual factors be considered.

# Culture of Safety

Following the identification of a healthcare system that uses a blame culture to respond to errors in HCOs, the *Quality Chasm* reports and other experts recommended a change to a culture of safety, also known as a no-blame culture or a just culture.

## Description

Bashaw, Rosenstein, and Launsbury (2012) describe a **culture of safety** as "a system of shared accountability that supports the safest hospital environments for patients, staff, and visitors. Organizations that adopt the just culture model accept that errors will occur, with or without negative outcomes. Each type of error is equally important to disclose because error identification and reporting promote trust, transparency, high-quality care, and patient safety across disciplines. . . . [A culture of safety] embraces system failures, errors, and weaknesses for the purpose of turning them into opportunities for improvement and learning" (p. 38). A related term is **just culture**. According to the AHRQ's Patient Safety Network, this culture recognizes that "traditionally, medical errors were often met with blame and shame for the responsible clinician. This approach to mistakes was an ineffective strategy for preventing further patient safety mishaps, particularly considering that the majority of errors are committed by well-meaning, dedicated clinicians working in broken or unsupportive systems" (HHS, AHRQ, PSNet, 2015).

A just culture as compared to a no-blame culture supports staff behaviors throughout the HCO that result in "safe, reliable, and productive performance," meeting four critical dimensions of a culture of safety (Drenkard, 2011):

- A strategic focus at the top levels in the organization on cultural improvements and error reduction
- A comprehensive assessment of past, present, and future human performance leading to a prioritized improvement plan
- Systematic implementation of improvement initiatives using proven prevention, detection, and correction methods
- An appreciation that maintaining a strong safety culture is a lifelong endeavor for the organization (pp. 28–29)

Some refer to the culture of safety as a no-blame culture because the focus moves away from individual blame; however, this reluctance to assign blame can go too far. This type of work culture should not imply that there is no individual accountability. Healthcare providers are still responsible for following their professional standards and regulatory requirements, such as their state nurse practice act and HCO standards, policies, and procedures, and they need to acknowledge when they lack knowledge or expertise. The goal is to develop leadership and staff commitment to quality care. Within this culture, strategies are used to increase staff self-awareness; improve staff education about quality, errors, and error reporting to improve performance; and meet standards set by healthcare professions, government, accreditors, and insurers. Meeting these objectives requires effective communication and interprofessional teamwork. Developing a just culture is so important that The Joint Commission included a sentinel event alert entitled "Developing a Reporting Culture: Learning from Close Calls and Hazardous Conditions" (2018). An effective just culture decreases staff fear of punishment.

The American Nurses Association (ANA) entered the discussion about just culture in 2010 when it published a position statement on this topic (ANA, 2010). The goal was to understand the concept and implications for nurses. The ANA supports the use of just culture in HCOs and initiatives to support its use. There is recognition that a threatening and punitive approach to errors results in limited staff reporting of errors. The ANA position statement emphasizes system errors and recognizes the importance of individual accountability. A culture of safety or just culture views errors from three perspectives (ANA, 2010):

1. Human error, which refers to inadvertently making an error or doing something that should not have been done
2. At-risk behavior that may lead to errors
3. Behavior that does not consider standards and expectations

The focus should be on reducing errors in an environment that is open and allows staff to discuss issues. Nurses should be actively involved in the culture of safety and serve as leaders. Nurses should have input into the HCO structure, processes, and outcomes—for example, ensuring staffing levels for more effective care, participating in policy and procedure development that is based on EBP, engaging in CQI responsibilities as an individual provider, and participating in HCO-organized CQI activities. Individual staff members need to feel comfortable reporting concerns, which relates to the staff's sense of accountability for system improvement. The overall result for the HCO should be "an organization-wide mindset that positively impacts the work environment and work outcomes" (ANA, 2010, p. 6). The 2018 database "includes data from 630 hospitals, 306 of which provided data for both the 2018 and 2016 databases. Notable changes since 2016 include improvement in the overall perception of safety, with most participating hospitals reporting positive perceptions of management support for safety, teamwork within units, and organizational responses to errors. In contrast, handoffs, staffing, and nonpunitive responses

to error remained patient safety concerns for nearly half of respondents, with little to no improvement since 2016" (HHS, AHRQ, 2018b).

As with all of the content on QI, it is important to consider its relevance to nursing students. "Just culture" can be viewed as a catchy term that may not have meaning in the real world of practice. It requires continual effort and cannot be just a term found in healthcare organization documents. Even students have a responsibility to participate and support a culture of safety within all the organizations where they practice. This is not something that just applies to post-prelicensure education. Schools of nursing should also address the issue of a culture of safety and how it applies to students and faculty (Penn, 2014). Learning to practice in a QI environment begins before graduation or completion of a degree. Consider now how this applies to each student daily.

## System and Individual Concerns

An example of a system concern can be found in the AHRQ decision to update its Hospital Survey of Patient Safety Culture (2019d), which was initially developed in 2004. After feedback and further development, a pilot test of the revised survey was conducted in 2016. There are also surveys for nursing homes, ambulatory outpatient medical offices, community pharmacies, and ambulatory surgery centers. The AHRQ provides a database so that HCOs can compare their data with data from similar HCOs. Using this comparative approach provides information about the HCO's strengths and helps to identify opportunities for improvement of the patient safety culture. The survey asks staff questions, including to identify the number of patient safety events they have reported over the previous 12 months (HHS, AHRQ, 2018b). The survey includes many hospitals—for example, the 2018 survey included 630 hospitals ranging from 22 to 299 beds. The following describes the areas commented on in the survey (HHS, AHRQ, 2018b):

- Teamwork within units
- Supervisor/manager expectations and actions promoting patient safety
- Organizational learning–continuous improvement
- Management support for patient safety
- Feedback and communication about error
- Frequency of events reported
- Overall perceptions of patient safety
- Communication openness
- Teamwork across units
- Staffing
- Handoffs and transitions
- Nonpunitive response to error

The development, implementation, and revision of this survey offered through the AHRQ illustrate the importance of having a culture of safety in HCOs and assessing the culture routinely. Hospitals are provided with guidance to compare their results with other hospitals and what they might do with the results to improve.

The North Carolina Board of Nursing's culture of safety assessment instrument, the Complaint Evaluation Tool (CET), is an example of the impact of individual nursing concerns and recognition of the importance of a culture of safety (North Carolina Board of Nursing, 2018). Why did a board of nursing develop this type of tool or even have interest in a culture of safety? Regulation and performance are associated with one another. Traditionally, when errors and performance concerns have been reported to a board of nursing, the response has been similar to the blame culture found in some HCOs, with individual nurses identified at fault for the error followed by some type of punitive measure. The purpose of the CET is different. It is a collaborative initiative with nursing education, a board of nursing, and healthcare organizations providing a framework for accountability and need to treat nurses fairly and with respect

(Burhans, Chastain, & George, 2012). The CET identifies several views of human error. A human error may result when a staff member has had no prior supervisory issues related to practice. It may also occur when a staff member has a lack of required knowledge, skills, or ability, and in these cases the event could be described as accidental or an oversight. The third type of human error occurs when there is no policy, standard, or requirement that staff should have followed, in which case the error is considered to be unintentional. A rating scale is used to rate at-risk behavior and reckless behavior.

A culture of safety requires that HCOs be transparent systems reporting errors and openly discussing and considering types of errors, analysis of errors, and steps taken to prevent errors (IOM, 2001). This transparency not only communicates that it is acceptable to be open about errors so that they can be understood and care improved, but it also leads to individual staff learning more about safety and how to prevent errors—how to identify and analyze errors in a manner that leads to a more effective healthcare system. Each nurse is tuned in to practice actions as they occur and focused on assessing quality patient outcomes.

# Dangers of a Code of Silence

As noted, the ANA and other organizations joined together to examine the HCO culture and its connection to patient and staff safety. In 2005, the American Association of Critical Care Nurses and the Association of periOperative Registered Nurses joined with VitalSmarts® to conduct a study (Maxfield, Grenny, Lavandero, & Groah, 2011; Maxfield, Grenny, McMillan, Patterson, & Switzler, 2005). The conclusions from the study noted that tools and warnings about safety are helpful, but if staff do not feel safe in speaking up even when staff members know something is wrong and do not get others to act to improve, then the culture will not really be changed.

This **code of silence** exists in HCOs and acts as a major barrier for improvement, setting up a work environment that is not positive or healthy for the staff. Recognizing that nurses need to assume greater responsibility and leadership in CQI includes standing up and speaking out when an organizational culture requires improvement.

## Diversity Within a Culture of Safety

As noted in other parts of this text, the *National Healthcare Quality Report* and the *National Healthcare Disparities Reports* are now combined into one report, the *National Healthcare Quality and Disparities Report* (QDR) (HHS, AHRQ, 2019b). The *QDR* is an important data resource used to track quality care and disparities. A culture of safety must consider the impact of diversity on its functioning and the outcomes. The World Health Organization (2019a) defines the **social determinants of health** as the "conditions in which people are born, grow, live, work, and age, including the health system. These circumstances are shaped by the distribution of money, power, and resources at global, national, and local levels, which are in and of themselves influenced by policy choices. The social determinants of health are mostly responsible for health inequities." This definition recognizes the importance of culture and diversity. Other key definitions that help to understand culture and disparities include the following:

- **Health inequality** is the difference in health status or in the distribution of health determinants between different population groups (WHO, 2019b).
- **Healthcare disparity** relates to "differences in the quality of health care that are not due to access-related factors or clinical needs, preferences, and appropriateness of interventions. These differences would include the role of bias, discrimination, and stereotyping at the individual

(provider and patient), institutional, and health-system levels" (IOM, 2003, p. 32).

- **Health equity** is attainment of the highest level of health for all people. Achieving health equity requires valuing everyone equally, with focused and ongoing societal efforts to address avoidable inequalities, right historical and contemporary injustices, and eliminate health and healthcare disparities (WHO, 2019b, 2019c).
- **Cultural competence** is a set of congruent behaviors, attitudes, and policies that come together in a system or agency or among professionals, enabling effective work in cross-cultural situations (HHS, Office of Minority Health [OMH], 2016).
- **Linguistic competence** is the capacity of an organization and its personnel to communicate effectively and convey information in a manner easily understood by diverse audiences, including persons of limited English proficiency, those who have low literacy skills or are not literate, and those with disabilities (HHS, OMH, 2016).

"The consistent and compelling evidence concerning how social determinants shape health has led to a growing recognition throughout the health care sector that improvements in overall health metrics are likely to depend—at least in part—on attention being paid to these social determinants. The shift in the health care sector toward value based payments that incentivize prevention and improved health and health care outcomes for persons and populations rather than service delivery alone has made possible expanded approaches to addressing health-related factors that may be upstream from the clinical encounter. And there is increasing interest in the role of the health care sector in mitigating adverse social determinants (termed 'social risk factors' and including a lack of access to stable housing, nutritious food, or reliable transportation) in order to achieve more equitable health outcomes. The combined result of these trends has been a growing emphasis on health care systems paying attention to upstream factors and addressing the **social determinants of health** (SDOH). Taking social risk factors into account is critical to improving both primary prevention and the treatment of acute and chronic illness because social contexts influence the delivery and outcomes of health care" (NAM, 2019, p. 1). The healthcare system can improve social care by focusing on awareness as the critical activity and also on activities related to adjustment, assistance, alignment, and advocacy (NAM, 2019). **Table 5-2** provides some definitions of terminology important in communication and cultures of safety.

**Table 5-2** Patient Safety Culture Composites and Definitions

| | |
|---|---|
| 1. Communication openness | Staff freely speak up if they see something that may negatively affect a patient and feel free to question those with more authority. |
| 2. Feedback and communication about error | Staff are informed about errors that happen, are given feedback about changes implemented, and discuss ways to prevent errors. |
| 3. Frequency of events reported | Mistakes of the following types are reported: (1) mistakes caught and corrected before affecting the patient, (2) mistakes with no potential to harm the patient, and (3) mistakes that could harm the patient but do not. |
| 4. Handoffs and transitions | Important patient care information is transferred across hospital units and during shift changes. |
| 5. Management support for patient safety | Hospital management provides a work climate that promotes patient safety and shows that patient safety is a top priority. |
| 6. Nonpunitive response to error | Staff feel that their mistakes and event reports are not held against them and that mistakes are not kept in their personnel file. |
| 7. Organizational learning— Continuous improvement | Mistakes have led to positive changes and changes are evaluated for effectiveness. |
| 8. Overall perceptions of patient safety | Procedures and systems are good at preventing errors and there is a lack of patient safety problems. |
| 9. Staffing | There are enough staff to handle the workload, and work hours are appropriate to provide the best care for patients. |
| 10. Supervisor/manager expectations and actions promoting patient safety | Supervisors/managers consider staff suggestions for improving patient safety, praise staff for following patient safety procedures, and do not overlook patient safety problems. |
| 11. Teamwork across units | Hospital units cooperate and coordinate with one another to provide the best care for patients. |
| 12. Teamwork within units | Staff support each other, treat each other with respect, and work together as a team. |

Famolaro T, Yount N, Hare, R, et al. Hospital Survey on Patient Safety Culture 2018 User Database Report. (Prepared by Westat, Rockville, MD, under Contract No. HHSA 290201300003C). Rockville, MD: Agency for Healthcare Research and Quality; 2018. AHRQ Publication No. 18-0025-EF., p. 4. Retrieved from https://www.ahrq.gov/sites/default/files/wysiwyg/sops/quality-patient-safety/patientsafetyculture/2018hospitalsopsreport.pdf

What can we do to improve? We need to develop partnerships with stakeholders to arrive at best strategies to improve and decrease health inequities. HCOs and healthcare professional education programs must integrate cultural and linguistic competencies in health professions education (academic programs and staff education) and in practice, including adding this information to position descriptions and performance evaluation. There is now recognition that this screening should be done—for example, particularly related to poverty, food insecurity, violence, unemployment, and housing problems (Anderson, 2019).

Health literacy has become a critical component of quality improvement frameworks due to the need to respond to healthcare disparities problems. The *Health Literacy* report discusses three intervention points in its framework describing the impact of health literacy on health outcomes and costs (IOM, 2004b). The first intervention point is multifactorial: Culture and the society in which a person lives and works impact the ability to understand, think, and respond. Factors such as age, ethnicity, gender, race, socioeconomic status, education, native language, and so on are important to consider. The second intervention point is the health system, and the third is the education system. Health literacy impacts the health system: patient–provider interactions and communication, individual patient and HCO outcomes, access to care, and so on. The education system and its outcomes are crucial to individual literacy and numeracy skills, which impact health literacy. The following are examples of interventions or strategies that may be used to improve health literacy; healthcare diversity within communities, HCOs, and the healthcare delivery system in general; and health outcomes (HHS, OMH, 2011).

1. Develop and disseminate health and safety information that is accurate, accessible, and actionable.

2. Promote changes in the healthcare system that improve health information, communication, informed decision-making, and access to health services.

3. Incorporate accurate, standards-based, and developmentally appropriate health and science information and curricula in childcare and education through the university level.

4. Support and expand local efforts to provide adult education, English language instruction, and culturally and linguistically appropriate health information services in the community.

5. Build partnerships, develop guidance, and change policies.

6. Increase basic research and the development, implementation, and evaluation of practices and interventions to improve health literacy.

7. Increase the dissemination and use of evidence-based health literacy practices and interventions. (pp. 1–2)

The AHRQ provides extensive resources about health literacy (HHS, AHRQ, 2019c, 2017). Some of the topics are tools for healthcare professionals, patient education resources, assessing patient experience, health information technology, case studies, podcasts and videos, and other relevant information. TeamSTEPPS® is a resource that addresses the need for greater team efforts in healthcare to do the following: "The TeamSTEPPS® Limited English Proficiency module is designed to help you develop and deploy a customized plan to train your staff in teamwork skills and lead a medical teamwork improvement initiative in your organization from initial concept development through to sustainment of positive changes. This evidence-based module will provide insight into the core concepts of teamwork as they are applied to your work with patients who have difficulty communicating in English. Comprehensive curricula and instructional guides include short case studies and videos illustrating teamwork opportunities and successes" (HHS, AHRQ, 2017).

# Barriers to a Culture of Safety

Developing and maintaining a culture of safety or a just culture is not easy. Barriers exist in all HCOs. A lack of understanding of the meaning of a culture of safety or just culture is a significant barrier. Key leaders within the HCO need to understand it to ensure that it is communicated effectively to all staff, and all need to be committed to the culture of safety. It is easy to emphasize sharing this concept with clinical staff; however, all staff within the organization (e.g., staff from housekeeping, office support, dietary, maintenance, informatics technology) need to be engaged or efforts will fail. Leadership must actively plan and support a culture of safety recognizing six domains: establish a compelling vision for safety; build trust, respect, and inclusion; select, develop, and engage the board; prioritize safety in selection and development of leaders; lead and reward a just culture; and establish organizational behavior expectations (American College of Healthcare Executives [ACHE] and IHI/NPSF Lucian Leape Institute, 2017, p. 2). These domains apply to nurse leadership at all levels in all types of healthcare organizations (Kennedy, 2016). Related to this approach leaders must also develop and support learning systems. "Zero harm to patients and the workforce is only possible with both a robust culture of safety and an embedded organizational learning system (ACHE & IHI/NPSF, 2017, p. 3).

It is also easy for some staff to view a just culture as an opportunity for individual staff members to relinquish accountability for actions, and this is not the case. This misperception can represent a major barrier. We still must be able to ask staff to explain what they did and why. There are times when a staff member's performance, not the system, may be the reason for an error, even though most events are system based.

Many staff members may feel that the HCO's culture is fine and does not need to be changed, or that things have been done one way for so long that there is no chance the HCO will actually change. In some situations, surface changes are made, but underneath the HCO still has a blame culture. HCO factors such as major budgetary problems, lack of effective leadership or too many management positions in flux, inadequate staffing levels and/or inadequate expertise, major organizational changes such as merging with other organizations, the addition or elimination of services, the need for major facility improvements such as renovation, and so on impact changing organizational culture.

The central feature of a culture of safety is the recognition that events or incidents are opportunities for improvement. We know there will be events that are not acceptable, but this does not mean we treat all who might be involved negatively. Dekker (2016) recommends strategies to better ensure a just culture or culture of safety and other strategies that have been recognized as important, such as the following:

- Focus the culture on concern for system factors that impact CQI; however, recognize that there is need for accountability and times when cause may relate primarily to individual performance.
- Remove all penalties that have been associated with events or incidents.
- Monitor stigmatization of staff who are involved in these events; prevent stigmatization when possible.
- Provide support to staff involved in an event.
- Institute debriefing; if already using it, then evaluate it and make changes as needed to support a culture of safety or just culture.
- Develop an effective quality improvement program with staff committed to a culture of safety or just culture and ensure that it is demonstrated in actions throughout the HCO.

- Include the culture of safety or just culture as an important part of staff orientation, orientation for healthcare professions students who are at the HCO for clinical experiences, and routine staff education.
- Ensure that staff know their rights and responsibilities related to events or incidents.
- Include implementation and engagement in the culture in all position descriptions and performance appraisal.
- Build trust at all levels of the organization.
- Identify clear descriptions of roles and responsibilities, including who makes decisions when events or incidents occur.
- Integrate local, state, federal, and healthcare professional requirements and standards into the culture of safety or just culture. Clearly demonstrate how this integration is accomplished.
- Determine the HCO policy and procedure for patient disclosure, and consult with HCO legal experts as needed.

Establishing a just culture has been a healthcare initiative for some years. Does it make a difference? A study examined this question in hospitals applying the AHRQ Hospital Survey of Patient Safety Culture (Edwards, 2018; HHS, AHRQ, 2019d). The results indicated that 211 of 270 respondents (76%) noted that their hospitals initiated a just culture, with more than half identifying a positive impact. The conclusions indicated that establishing a just culture approach did not necessarily reduce staff concerns about reporting errors or the use of blame—these continue to be problems in some hospitals. A just culture must support staff members who speak up about concerns. This includes active response by letting staff know this is what should be done, thanking staff for speaking up, and informing staff of outcomes. Staff must take responsibility, be accountable, and do this in a positive, constructive manner. Blame can come not only from management but also can originate from peers. Respect and trust are part of an effective just culture.

## Leadership to Support a Culture of Safety

Leadership is required for effective CQI. This includes developing and maintaining a culture of safety. Leadership in an HCO includes the board of directors, senior management, and all other levels of managers. Assessing the effectiveness of a culture of safety is not easy to accomplish. More research is required to better understand effective methods for assessment of the culture of safety.

Clear communication has a positive impact on the culture of safety. Leadership within an HCO must ensure that communication at all levels is clear and should ensure improvement when necessary. This includes formal procedures such as incident reporting, sharing of feedback (from management to staff and vice versa), ensuring that orientation includes information about the culture of safety, and a transparent HCO. The culture of an HCO cannot be changed without effective communication and leadership. Part of this effort must be a discussion with all staff about the need for a culture of safety, their views of what this culture might entail, management and staff roles and responsibilities, and methods that will be used to ensure that a culture of safety is maintained over time. Leaders in the HCO need to drive this effort and maintain it.

### STOP AND CONSIDER 5-3

A culture of safety requires much effort to implement and maintain.

## Summary

There are many theories and models used to describe quality improvement, several of which are discussed in this chapter. Along with greater development of approaches to CQI, the culture of safety or just culture is now a critical aspect of CQI and the CQI process. This is a change from the view of the blame culture, moving away from individual blame to greater consideration of system factors. There is a question that needs to be considered: Do we make QI too complicated (Baldoza, 2019)? This chapter and others provide considerable information about quality improvement that can make it appear to be a complicated area, and it is—but do we treat this complexity as a barrier? The basic issue is preparing staff and the organization to do their jobs and improve when necessary. We all do this in our everyday life: unconsciously some of the time, and at other times we are very aware of the process. As will be discussed more, data are important in QI, and now we have access to more and more data. This is positive, but it can be negative as we sift through the data and also in decisions we make in planning QI—for example, how do we determine which data to collect and so on? Many things we do daily in our work are improving care, and in many cases staff do not realize it. We need to recognize the importance our many efforts—understanding QI models, frameworks, and such—but this should not be seen as a barrier to doing our jobs in the best way possible. Exemplars of quality improvement roles and responsibilities for staff nurses, nurse managers, and APRNs are found in **Exhibit 5-1**.

---

**Exhibit 5-1** Exemplars: Quality Improvement Roles and Responsibilities

**Staff Nurse**

A new staff nurse joined the staff on a maternity unit 9 months ago. The nurse is preparing medications and administers them. An error is made in the dosage, which the nurse realizes after giving the medication. She is very stressed and decides not to complete an incident report since no harm was done to the patient. Where she worked before, this was not an uncommon response to an error. This is called a Code of Silence.

**Nurse Manager**

The staff nurse had heard from other staff nurses in the hospital that the nurse managers typically responded rapidly to medication errors by assigning the involved nurse to a medication administration review course that was offered by the staff education department. The nurses complain about this as they wonder why an intervention is used before anyone knows the cause. This is a blame culture and not a culture of safety.

**Advanced Practice Registered Nurse***

The APRNs who work in an ambulatory care setting have been asked by the director to examine CQI and how it might be improved. At a meeting to discuss this problem, one of the APRNs suggests that there needs to be more emphasis on STEEEP® in the center's CQI efforts. The group decides to first focus on applying the elements to the admission process—safety, timeliness, effectiveness, efficiency, equity, and patient-centeredness. They realize they need to include management, clerical staff, the center's pharmacist, the source used for laboratory testing, and the electronic medical record system. The group of APRNs then turns their attention to staff education for clinical and nonclinical staff. They need to understand STEEEP® and the plan to apply it to the admissions process. They also include a plan to monitor outcomes—Is STEEEP® applied? Patient feedback must be part of this evaluation as patient-centered care is included.

*Advanced Practice Registered Nurse includes APRN, Clinical Nurse Specialist, Clinical Nurse Leader, and nurses with DNP.

# APPLY CQI

## Chapter Highlights

- There are many visions of quality improvement; some integrate multiple views of quality.
- The science of improvement focuses on innovation, rapid-cycle testing of change, and lessons learned from changes.
- The Triple Aim (to improve the patient experience, improve the health of populations, and reduce the per capita cost of healthcare) is now used in many quality improvement models/theories.
- Models built around structure (how organizations are organized as a system), process (how organization functions), and outcomes (results) were introduced in the 1980s and continue to influence quality improvement models/theories.
- CQI emphasizes a systematic approach that is ongoing.
- STEEEP® is based on the Triple Aim and the *Quality Chasm* reports. The focus is on customers/patients and CQI; data are important in making decisions.

- The lean approach emphasizes value and cost.
- Six Sigma is a measurement-based strategy.
- High-reliability organizations emphasize reducing operation failure and errors to reduce harm. Redesign of processes is used when necessary.
- The blame culture led to a healthcare work environment in which individual staff members were blamed for errors and system issues were not effectively addressed in improving care and reducing errors.
- A culture of safety or just culture is now recommended to replace the blame culture. Though it still recognizes individual accountability, it turns the focus to systems.
- Diversity (patients and staff) is an important factor in a culture of safety.
- Leadership is required to guide the development and maintenance of a culture of safety.

## Critical Thinking and Clinical Reasoning and Judgment: Discussion Questions and Learning Activities

1. Compare and contrast the examples of theories and models described in this chapter. Summarize your comparison in a visual format such as a figure, table, poster, and so on. Discuss your visual with a group of your classmates.
2. What is your opinion of the change from a blame culture to a culture of safety or just culture?

3. Assess a clinical organization in which you are working, or have previously worked, for clinical experiences. How would you describe its culture of safety? If it is not a culture of safety, why does it not meet the criteria for this type of culture? Is it a culture in which you would like to work? Why or why not?

## Connect to Current Information

- Graphics of models of improvement
  http://www.bing.com/images/search?q=
  graphics+of+models+of+improvement&
  qpvt=graphics+of+models+of+
  improvement&qpvt=graphics+of+
  models+of+improvement&FORM=IGRE
- AHRQ improvement resources

  http://www.ahrq.gov/professionals
  /quality-patient-safety/quality-resources
  /index.html
- Surveys on Patient Safety Culture (SOPs)
  http://www.ahrq.gov/professionals/quality
  -patient-safety/patientsafetyculture/index
  .html

---

### Connect to Text Current Information with the Author

Go to the update for this text to review the Blog, QI News, and Literature Review. Access this regular update at: http://nursing.jbpub.com/Finkelman/QualityImprovement/2e.

---

## EBP, EBM, and Quality Improvement: Exemplar

Flynn, R., Scott, S., Rotter, T., & Hartfield, D. (2017). The potential for nurses to contribute to and lead improvement science in health care. *Journal of Advanced Nursing, 73*(1), 97–107.

This is a discussion paper about the role of nurses in improvement science.

### Questions to Consider

1. What background information is provided? Is it helpful to your understanding of the issue discussed?
2. What are the implications for nursing discussed in the paper?
3. What is your opinion of the conclusions? What might you change or add to the paper? Provide your rationales for these changes or additions?

---

# EVOLVING CASE STUDY

After conducting a survey about the hospital culture and CQI, your hospital has moved to developing a culture of safety. There are broad guidelines for this change, but ultimately each unit must make the adjustment. As nurse manager of the obstetrical service, you are confronted with where to begin. Your services cover pre-delivery admissions, labor and delivery, nursery care, postpartum care, and clinics. It is a very busy specialty with overworked staff, and there is a problem with registered nurse retention and turnover. You have been manager for 2 years. Errors have increased by 10% in those 2 years, and the staff has become more reluctant to report incidents through the required system. They complain that staff members are penalized when they make errors. This complaint is also common within other areas of the hospital. You go to the following website to get information and resources: http://www.ahrq.gov/professionals/quality-patient-safety/patient-safety-resources/resources/esrd/cultureofsafety.html

## Case Questions A

*You first need to understand more about the change.*

1. What is a culture of safety, and how does it compare to the current culture?
2. How will you demonstrate and convince your staff that this change is real and will make a positive difference?

## Case Questions B

*After you understand the problem better, you move to planning.*

1. Develop a plan to foster a culture of safety. Specify tools you will use and the reason for their use. Develop your process. (See online resources and the chapter content for help.)
2. How will you engage staff in the development of the plan and its implementation? Be specific.
3. How will you assess your outcomes? Be specific.

# References

American College of Healthcare Executives (ACHE) and IHI/NPSF Lucian Leape Institute. (2017). *Leading a Culture of Safety: A Blueprint for Success.* Boston, MA: American College of Healthcare Executives and Institute for Healthcare Improvement.

American Nurses Association (ANA). (2010). *Position statement: Just culture.* Retrieved from https://www.nursingworld.org/practice-policy/nursing-excellence/official-position-statements/id/just-culture/

Anderson, A. (2019). Screening for social determinants of health in clinical care: Moving from margins to mainstream. *Public Health Review, 39,* 19. Retrieved from https://www.ncbi.nlm.nih.gov/pmc/articles/PMC6014006

American Society for Quality (ASQ). (2019). What is Six Sigma? Retrieved from https://asq.org/quality-resources/six-sigma

Baldoza, K. (2019). Do we make QI too complicated? Retrieved from http://www.ihi.org/communities/blogs/do-we-make-qi-too-complicated

Ballard, D. (2014). *The guide to achieving STEEEP® healthcare: Baylor Scott & White Health's quality improvement journey.* Boca Raton, FL: CRC Press/Proactivity Press.

Bashaw, E., Rosenstein, A., & Launsbury, K. (2012). Culture trifecta: Building the infrastructure for Magnet® and just culture. *American Nurse Today, 7*(9), 35, 38, 41.

Berwick, D. (1999). Controlling variation in health care: A consultation with Walter Shewhart. *Medical Care, 29*(12), 1212–1225.

Berwick, D. (2019). The Triple Aim: Why we still have a long way to go. Retrieved from http://www.ihi.org/communities/blogs/the-triple-aim-why-we-still-have-a-long-way-to-go

Berwick, D., Nolan, T., & Whittington, J. (2008). The Triple Aim: Care, health, and cost. *Health Affairs, 27*(3), 759–769.

Brackett, T., Comer, L., & Whichello, R. (2013). Do lean practices lead to more time at the bedside. *Journal for Healthcare Quality, 35*(2), 7–14.

Burhans, L., Chastain, K., & George, J. (2012). Just culture and nursing regulation: Learning to improve patient safety. *Journal of Nursing Regulation, 2*(4), 43–49.

Chassin, M., & Loeb, J. (2011). Ongoing quality improvement journey: Next stop, high reliability. *Health Affairs, 30*(4), 559–568.

Dailey, M. (2013). Overview and summary: Health care and quality: Perspectives from nursing. *OJIN: The Online Journal of Issues in Nursing, 18*(3). Retrieved from http://www.nursingworld.org/MainMenuCategories/ANAMarketplace/ANAPeriodicals/OJIN/TableofContents/Vol-18-2013/No3-Sept-2013/OS-Healthcare-and-Quality.html

Dekker, S. (2016). *Just culture. Restoring trust and accountability in your organization* (3rd ed.). Boca Raton, FL: CRC Press.

Donabedian, A. (1980). *Explorations in quality assessment and monitoring, Volume 1: The definitions of quality and approaches to its assessment.* Ann Arbor, MI: Health Administration Press.

Donabedian, A. (1988). The quality of care. How can it be assessed? *JAMA, 260*(12), 1743–1748.

Draper, D., Felland, L., Liebhaber, A., & Melichar, L. (2008). The role of nurses in hospital quality improvement. Center for Studying Health System Change. *Research Brief,* (3), 1–8.

Drenkard, K. (2011). Magnet momentum: Creating a culture of safety. *Nurse Leader, 9*(4), 28–31, 46.

Edwards, M. (2018). An assessment of the impact of just culture and quality and safety in U.S. hospitals. *American Journal of Medical Quality, 33*(5), 502–508.

Feeley, D. (2019). The five Ps of Triple Aim transformation. Retrieved from http://www.ihi.org/communities/blogs/the-five-ps-of-triple-aim-transformation

Galt, K., Paschal, K., & Gleason, J. (2011). Key concepts in patient safety. In K. Galt & K. Paschal (Eds.), *Foundations in patient safety for health professionals* (pp. 1–14). Burlington, MA: Jones & Bartlett Learning.

Goeschel, C. (2011). Defining and assigning accountability for quality care and patient safety. *Journal of Nursing Regulation, 2*(1), 28–32.

Graves, A. (2019). Six sigma fundamentals. DMAIC vs. DMADV. Retrieved from https://www.sixsigmadaily.com/six-sigma-basics-dmaic-vs-dmadv

Heathfield, S. (2020, March). Culture: Your environment for people at work. Retrieved from https://www.thebalancecareers.com/culture-your-environment-for-people-at-work-1918809

Institute for Healthcare Improvement (IHI). (2015a). New directions in patient safety. Retrieved from http://www.ihi.org/communities/blogs/_layouts/ihi/community/blog/ItemView.aspx?List=0f316db6-7f8a-430f-a63a-ed7602d1366a&ID=51&Web=1e880535-d855-4727-a8c127ee672f115d

Institute for Healthcare Improvement (IHI). (2015b). Science of improvement. Retrieved from http://www.ihi.org/about/Pages/ScienceofImprovement.aspx

Institute for Healthcare Improvement (IHI). (2015c). Improvement capability: Overview. Retrieved from http://www.ihi.org/Topics/ImprovementCapability/Pages/Overview.aspx

Institute for Healthcare Improvement (IHI). (2015d). The IHI Triple Aim. Retrieved from http://www.ihi.org/Engage/Initiatives/TripleAim/Pages/default.aspx

Institute of Medicine (IOM). (1999). *To err is human*. Washington, DC: The National Academies Press.

Institute of Medicine (IOM). (2001). *Crossing the quality chasm*. Washington, DC: The National Academies Press.

Institute of Medicine (IOM). (2003). *Unequal treatment*. Washington, DC: The National Academies Press.

Institute of Medicine (IOM). (2004a). *Keeping patients safe: Transforming the work environment of nurses*. Washington, DC: The National Academies Press.

Institute of Medicine (IOM). (2004b). *Health literacy: A prescription to end confusion*. Washington, DC: The National Academies Press.

Jones, K., & Redman, R. (2000). Organizational culture and work redesign: Experiences in three organizations. *Journal of Nursing Administration, 30*(12), 604–610.

Kennedy, S. (2016). A culture of safety starts with us. We need to follow the evidence and own up to our role. *AJN, 116*(5), 7.

Lawal, A., Rotter, T., Kinsman, L., Sari, N., Harrison, L. Jeffery, C., . . . Flynn, E. (2014). Lean management in health care: Definition concepts, methodology, and effects reported (systematic review protocol). *Systematic Review, 3*, (1), 103–106.

Lawless, S., & Proujansky, R. (2006). The provider's role in quality improvement. In D. Nash & N. Goldbarb (Eds.), *The quality solution* (pp. 135–154). Sudbury, MA: Jones & Bartlett Publishers.

Maxfield, D., Grenny, J., Lavandero, R., & Groah, L. (2011). The silent treatment: Why safety tools and checklists aren't enough. Retrieved from https://www.psqh.com/analysis/the-silent-treatment-why-safety-tools-and-checklists-arent-enough

Maxfield, D., Grenny, J., McMillan, R., Patterson, K., & Switzler, A. (2005). Silent treatment study. Provo, UT: VitalSmarts. Retrieved from https://www.vitalsmarts.com/resource/silent-treatment

Moriates, C., & Wachter, R. (2015). Accountability in patient safety. Retrieved from https://psnet.ahrq.gov/perspective/accountability-patient-safety

National Academy of Medicine (NAM). (2019). *Integrating social needs care into the delivery of health care to improve the nation's health*. Washington, DC: The National Academies Press.

North Carolina Board of Nursing. (2018). Complaint evaluation tool (CET). Retrieved from https://www.ncbon.com/discipline-compliance-employer-complaints-complaint-evaluation-tool-cet

Penn, C. (2014). Integrating just culture into nursing student error policy. *Journal of Nursing Education, 53*(9), S107–S109.

Six Sigma. (2019a). 8 wastes. Retrieved from https://goleansixsigma.com/8-wastes

Six Sigma. (2019b). Defect. Retrieved from https://www.isixsigma.com/dictionary/defect

Sollecito, W., & Johnson, J. (2013). The global evolution of continuous quality improvement: From Japanese manufacturing to global health services. In W. Sollecito & J. Johnson (Eds.), *McLaughlin and Kaluzny's continuous quality improvement in healthcare* (4th ed., pp. 1–48). Burlington, MA: Jones & Bartlett Learning.

Sovie, M. (1993). Hospital culture: Why create one? *Nursing Economics, 11*(2), 69–75.

Stiefel, M., & Nolan, K. (2012). A guide to measuring the Triple Aim: Population health, experience of care, and per capita cost. IHI Innovation Series white paper. Cambridge, MA: Institute for Healthcare Improvement (IHI). Retrieved from http://www.ihi.org/resources/Pages/IHIWhitePapers/AGuidetoMeasuringTripleAim.aspx

Storme, T. (2013). Healthcare analytics for quality and performance improvement. Hoboken, NJ: John Wiley & Sons, Inc.

The Joint Commission. (2018). Sentinel Event Alert 60. Developing a reporting culture: Learning from close calls and hazardous conditions. Retrieved from https://www.jointcommission.org/sentinel_event_alert_60_developing_a_reporting_culture_learning_from_close_calls_and_hazardous_conditions

U.S. Department of Health and Human Services (HHS), Agency for Healthcare Research and Quality (AHRQ).

(2011). Defining lean waste and potential failure modes. AHRQ Project RED (Re-Engineered Discharge) Training Program. Retrieved from http://archive.ahrq .gov/professionals/systems/hospital/red/leanwaste.html

U.S. Department of Health and Human Services (HHS), Agency for Healthcare Research and Quality (AHRQ). (2014). Improving care delivery through lean: Implementation case studies. Retrieved from https://www .ahrq.gov/practiceimprovement/systemdesign/lean casestudies/index.html

U.S. Department of Health and Human Services (HHS), Agency for Healthcare Research and Quality (AHRQ). (2017). Patients with limited English proficiency. Retrieved from https://www.ahrq.gov/teamstepps/lep /index.html

U.S. Department of Health and Human Services (HHS), Agency for Healthcare Research and Quality (AHRQ). (2018a). Understanding quality measurement. Retrieved from https://www.ahrq.gov/professionals/quality -patient-safety/quality-resources/tools/chtoolbx /understand/index.html

U.S. Department of Health and Human Services (HHS), Agency for Healthcare Research and Quality (AHRQ). (2018b). Hospital survey on patient safety culture: 2018 user database report. Retrieved from https://www .ahrq.gov/sites/default/files/wysiwyg/sops/quality -patient-safety/patientsafetyculture/2018hospital sopsreport.pdf

U.S. Department of Health and Human Services (HHS), Agency for Healthcare Research and Quality (AHRQ). (2019a). Section 4: Ways to approach the quality improvement process. (Three tips for facilitating the quality improvement process.) Retrieved from http://www .ahrq.gov/cahps/quality-improvement/improvement -guide/4-approach-qi-process/index.html

U.S. Department of Health and Human Services (HHS), Agency for Healthcare Research and Quality (AHRQ). (2019b). 2018 National healthcare quality and disparities report. Retrieved from https://www.ahrq.gov /research/findings/nhqrdr/nhqdr18/index.html

U.S. Department of Health and Human Services (HHS), Agency for Healthcare Research and Quality (AHRQ). (2019c). Health literacy. Retrieved from https://www .ahrq.gov/topics/health-literacy.html

U.S. Department of Health and Human Services (HHS), Agency for Healthcare Research and Quality (AHRQ). (2019d). Surveys on patient safety culture (SOPS) hospital survey. Retrieved from https://www.ahrq.gov /sops/surveys/hospital/index.html

U.S. Department of Health and Human Services (HHS), Agency for Healthcare Research and Quality (AHRQ),

Patient Safety Network (PSNet). (2015). Accountability in patient safety. Retrieved from https://psnet.ahrq .gov/perspective/accountability-patient-safety

U.S. Department of Health and Human Services (HHS), Agency for Healthcare Research and Quality (AHRQ), Patient Safety Network (PSNet). (2019a). IHI white papers: High reliability. Retrieved from http://www .ihi.org/resources/Pages/IHIWhitePapers/Improving theReliabilityofHealthCare.aspx

U.S. Department of Health and Human Services (HHS), Agency for Healthcare Research and Quality (AHRQ), Patient Safety Network (PSNet). (2019b). Culture of safety. Retrieved from https://psnet.ahrq.gov/primer /culture-safety

U.S. Department of Health and Human Services (HHS), Health Resources and Services Administration (HRSA). (2011). Quality improvement. Retrieved from http:// www.hrsa.gov/quality/toolbox/508pdfs/quality improvement.pdf

U.S. Department of Health & Human Services (HHS), Office of the National Coordinator for Health Information Technology (ONC). (2019). How do I use a rapid -cycle improvement strategy? Retrieved from https:// www.healthit.gov/faq/how-do-i-use-rapid-cycle -improvement-strategy

U.S. Department of Health & Human Services (HHS), Office of Minority Health (OMH), National Partnership for Action to End Health Disparities. (2011). National stakeholder strategy for achieving health equity. Retrieved from https://minorityhealth.hhs.gov/npa/files /Plans/NSS/CompleteNSS.pdf

U.S. Department of Health & Human Services (HHS), Office of Minority Health (OMH). (2016). Cultural and linguistic competency. Retrieved from https://minority health.hhs.gov/omh/browse.aspx?lvl=1&lvlid=6

Veazie, S., Peterson, K., & Bourne, D. (2019). Evidence brief. Implementation of high reliability organization principles. U.S. Department of Veterans Affairs. Retrieved from https://www.ncbi.nlm.nih.gov/books/NBK542883

Whittington, J., Nolan, K., Lewis, N., & Torres, T. (2015) Pursuing the triple aim: The first seven years. *Milbank Quarterly, 93*(2), 263-300.

World Health Organization. (WHO). (2019a). About social determinants of health. Retrieved from https:// www.who.int/social_determinants/sdh_definition/en

World Health Organization. (WHO). (2019b). 10 facts on health inequities and their causes. Retrieved from https:// www.who.int/features/factfiles/health_inequities/en

World Health Organization. (WHO). (2019c). Health equity. Retrieved from https://www.who.int/topics/health _equity/en

# Patient and Family Engagement in Quality Improvement

## CHAPTER OBJECTIVES

At the conclusion of this chapter, the learner will be able to:

- Examine the relationship of patient-centered care and patient/family engagement in continuous quality improvement (CQI).
- Explain the need to consider reimbursement when reviewing patient-centered care and CQI.
- Summarize the role of the patient in CQI.
- Apply methods to increase patient/family engagement in CQI.
- Explain the importance of technology to patient-centered care.
- Examine efforts to monitor and measure patient satisfaction and engagement in CQI.
- Critique examples of patient-centered initiatives.

## OUTLINE

## KEY TERMS

Advocacy
Collaboration
Collaborative care model

Coordination
Disclosure

Patient-centered care
Self-management

# Introduction

Patient-centered care became more important when the *Quality Chasm* reports brought it to the forefront. The reports identified ten rules to describe an improved health system, and four of them are directly related to patient-centered care. These rules are as follows: "Care is based on continuous health relationships; care is customized according to patient needs and values; the patient is the source of control; and knowledge is shared and information flows freely" (IOM, 2001, p. 8). These rules also apply directly to continuous quality improvement (CQI). This chapter discusses the need for patient-centered care and its relationship to CQI. The Institute for Patient- and Family-Centered Care (IPFCC) notes that every encounter in all settings with patients and families should support their strengths and increase patient and family confidence and competence (IPFCC, 2019). As this content is discussed, it is important to recognize that "first and foremost, patients are experts in their own care and the care of their loved ones. They consistently identify adverse events not detected through other means. Engaged patients

are also more satisfied and report higher quality communication with providers. Patient engagement can improve outcomes but only when their expertise is effectively mobilized" (Stern & Sarkar, 2017).

# Patient-Centered Care Supports Patient/ Family Engagement in CQI

Patient-centered care is a critical element of effective quality care and is described as a dimension of quality in which care is individualized and customized to patients and families. This perspective recognizes that patients, not healthcare providers, have control over their healthcare decisions (Berwick, 2009). As discussed in other sections of this text, the Institute of Medicine (IOM) emphasized **patient-centered care** in 2001 in the second of the *Quality Series* reports (IOM, 2001). "The principles of patient-centered care include respect for patients' values, preferences, and expressed needs; coordination and integration of care; and providing emotional support alongside the alleviation of fear and anxiety associated with clinical care" (Bau et al., 2019, p. 4).

It is important for healthcare organizations (HCOs) to incorporate patient-centered care in their views and application of CQI. This issue was introduced because patients expressed concern about their role and inability to participate in decision making. Healthcare has long advocated for patient rights; however, this approach had not been implemented very effectively. In 1993, critical dimensions describing quality care were identified, and the following dimensions were later applied in the *Quality Chasm* reports (Gerteise, Edgman-Levitan, Daley & Delbanco, 2002):

- *Respect for patients' values, preferences, and expressed needs.* What does the patient think is important? To make effective decisions and participate in planning, the patient needs to be informed. Terms used to describe this effort include *customized* and *individualized care.* Cultural factors are also part of patient-centered care, as they impact who the patient is, what the patient needs and prefers, how capable the patient is in understanding informed consent information, and how much a patient may or may not want to participate and make decisions. A patient's preferences may change over time, and healthcare providers need to adapt to changes.

- *Coordination and integration of care.* Coordination is also not a new concept in healthcare, but implementing it has not always been effective. In addition, the patient should be involved, but in many circumstances, the patient is not. Coordinating services to make sure they happen as they should and when they should is critical for positive outcomes. The patient and family need to be able to depend on effective coordination. Transitions from one healthcare provider and setting to another (handoffs) should occur with limited problems, clear communication to reduce errors, and involvement of the patient.

- *Information, communication, and education.* Patients need accurate information, particularly related to their diagnoses, instructions on how to stay well, and their prognosis, including details about what can be done to change or manage the prognosis. Patient diversity requires that this information be shared so that care meets individual patient needs. Patients want information they can trust from healthcare providers who are focused on helping them. Confidentiality and privacy are critical components.

- *Physical comfort.* Patients do not always receive the care they need to help with major symptoms such as pain. This care may be given, but it may not be timely, and thus patients suffer unnecessarily.

- *Emotional support—relieving fear and anxiety.* In addition to physical needs, patients have emotional needs. Often these needs are not met. When patients feel disconnected from their care and decisions, this may have a negative impact on patient responses.

- *Involvement of family and friends.* In many situations, the patient's family and significant others are involved with their ongoing care and care decisions, but this is not always the case—and should not be assumed. Including patients in care planning and seeking their approval of decisions have a positive impact on patient outcomes. (pp. 5–10)

These dimensions are recurrent themes in healthcare and are integrated throughout this text. Nurses and nursing care are critical in ensuring that these dimensions are part of each patient's care.

## Quality Improvement: Relationship to Patient-Centered Care

Patient-centered care is important to CQI for a number of reasons. An involved patient has a greater chance of having positive care outcomes. This patient will be more willing to share information with care providers, discuss concerns openly, and be engaged in treatment. The patient and provider relationship will be based more on trust. Patients vary a great deal, as do their needs and preferences. The degree to which they want to be involved is highly variable and changes. However, healthcare providers should not assume anything about what the patient wants and should not proceed in the care process without including the patient.

Because patients are more involved today, they will most likely be more aware of quality care issues; however, one should not assume the involved patient is a demanding or difficult patient but rather a patient who wants to express his or her needs, preferences, and concerns. To call this patient demanding would deny the relevance of patient-centered care. As Johnson and colleagues (2008) explain, "Patients and families have experience, expertise, insights, and perspectives that can be invaluable to bringing about transformational change in health care and enhancing quality and safety" (p. 1). The physician is responsible for diagnosis and recommending treatment options, and the patient is responsible for identifying goals and concerns, followed by communicating any decision regarding treatment choice to the physician. Today, advanced practice registered nurses (APRNs) in a variety of specialty areas are also involved in diagnosis and treatment decisions. The physician or the APRN then implements the plan.

For patients to actively participate in their health decisions and make their own decisions, they need to have clear information that they can understand; time to consider the information and concerns, such as risks and benefits of treatment; and interaction with healthcare providers so that they can discuss the information, their questions and concerns, and their own goals or outcomes. These elements are not always important for all patients; however, all healthcare providers need to recognize that patients need the opportunity to consider their health and care carefully and fully within

the existing time parameters (Fowler, Levin, & Sepucha, 2011).

The Nursing Alliance for Quality Care (NAQC) considers patient engagement to be critical to effective patient care quality, particularly to nursing care. This is based the belief on the following assumptions (Johnson, 2012):

1. There must be a dynamic partnership among patients, their families, and the providers of their healthcare, which at the same time respects the boundaries of privacy, competent decision-making, and ethical behavior.

2. This relationship is grounded in confidentiality, where the patient defines the scope of the confidentiality. Patients are the best and ultimate source of information about their health status and retain the right to make their own decisions about care.

3. In this relationship, there are mutual responsibilities and accountabilities among the patient, the family, and the provider that make it effective.

4. Providers must recognize that the extent to which patients and family members are able to engage or choose to engage may vary greatly based on individual circumstances. Advocacy for patients who are unable to participate fully is a fundamental nursing role.

5. All encounters and transactions with the patient and family occur while respecting the boundaries that protect recipients of care as well as providers of that care.

6. Patient advocacy is the demonstration of how all of the components of the relationship fit together.

7. This relationship is grounded in an appreciation of patient rights and expands on the rights to include mutuality.

8. Mutuality includes sharing of information, creation of consensus, and shared decision making.

9. Healthcare literacy is essential for the patient, family, and providers to understand the components of patient engagement.

Providers must maintain awareness of the healthcare literacy level of the patient and family and respond accordingly. Acknowledgment and appreciation of diverse backgrounds are essential to the engagement process.

Consider how each of these assumptions might impact nursing practice on a daily basis. Each assumption relates to important aspects of care, and all are interrelated to provide a positive care trajectory for the patient. The assumptions also focus on similar issues such as those found in the rules and description of patient-centered care dimensions mentioned in this chapter.

## Informed Decision Making: Impact on Quality Care

According to Fowler and colleagues (2011), the healthcare industry has a long way to go in including patients in the decision-making process: "Consumer rights are also more important today in health care, and the Institute of Medicine's identification of patient-centered care supports consumer or patient rights. Good-quality care requires that procedures, treatments, and tests be not only medically appropriate, but also desired by informed patients. Current evidence shows that most medical decisions are made by physicians with little input from patients" (p. 699). This type of practice is directly opposite the view of patient-centered care and patient rights, but it is gradually changing. Patients themselves are demanding more. Patients have rights to informed consent and unbiased information. Withholding information is not up to the healthcare provider and is appropriate only if the patient does not want to receive the information. If staff cannot answer patient questions, either because the staff member does not know the answer or because the staff member is not in a position to inform the patient, then the staff member needs to tell the patient that

someone will respond later. The staff member needs to inform the appropriate staff member of the patient's questions and follow up to make sure the patient receives the requested information.

## Privacy and Confidentiality: Relationship to Quality Improvement

The Health Insurance Portability and Accountability Act (HIPAA) of 1996 is a law that focuses on patient privacy and confidentiality. HIPAA identifies protected health information or any information about a patient that connects to an individual patient (e.g., demographic information). Only minimum necessary information may be shared without patient permission. Disclosure of information to others must be monitored. This law and patient rights have an impact throughout the care process, sometimes in ways that staff may think do not relate.

Other patient rights are also identified in HIPAA (U.S. Department of Health and Human Services [HHS], OCR, 2019). The patient has the right to access medical records, and the healthcare provider must respond within 30 days. If the patient does not think the information is correct or complete, then the patient has the right to amend the medical record. This does not mean the medical record information must be changed but rather the patient's comments must be added to the record.

## Patient Makes the Decision About Family Engagement

In some cases, the Health Insurance Portability and Accounting Act (HIPAA) has become a barrier to the exchange of information with the patient's family (HHS, OCR, 2019). In the past it was common for healthcare providers to share information with family members without asking the patient for permission, sometimes not even sharing the same information with the patient. This approach negates patient-centered care. HIPAA, which applies to any patient-related information, now makes such practices illegal. If, however, the patient does not state restrictions to healthcare providers, the HCO or healthcare provider may reveal the information. The best approach, however, is to ask the patient directly, preferably with family or significant other present so that the patient may openly inform healthcare providers. Many patients do not realize they can request restrictions. Patients may request that steps be taken to ensure privacy—for example, they may request information not be shared by telephone messaging, email, or postal mail to the patient's home. These requests must be reasonable. If the patient thinks his or her privacy has been violated, then the patient has the right to report the incident to the healthcare provider (individual or organization), the state licensure board, and the Office of Civil Rights (OCR) of the U.S. Department of Health and Human Services (HHS) through its website. Providers may be charged a fine for not following HIPAA.

Clarifying sharing of information prevents problems. An exception applies if a family member is the legal guardian for the patient. Staff may find it difficult to obey patient requests to not share information with family, as they may view not including family as being in conflict with patient-centered care, but in reality it strongly supports patient-centered care: The patient decides who gets information and who is involved in the patient's healthcare decisions.

## Disclosure of Errors and Patient-Centered Care

In the past, HCOs were hesitant to disclose errors to patients, mostly due to legal advice that did not support disclosure. This, however, is changing, and many HCOs now encourage or may require disclosure of errors to patients and, when the patient agrees, to the patient's family (Banja, 2005). Why is disclosure of errors now recommended? As discussed in this text, errors are inevitable even when great effort is made to reduce them. Prevention is important, but it is not enough, as we need to also understand errors and address methods to respond to errors when they occur. Being involved in an error is an emotional experience for the healthcare provider. We do not go into healthcare to harm the patient, but we are not perfect and neither are systems. These incidents leave us with a critical decision to make as to whether we should inform a patient that an error occurred, assuming the patient does not already know. Doing so is referred to as **disclosure**.

Disclosure of errors has always been a problematic issue. HCOs have worried that informing patients and families that an error almost occurred or did occur increases the risk of malpractice lawsuits, and as a result staff have often erred toward withholding the information. However, there has been a change in how healthcare providers approach errors with patients. Patient-centered care implies that there is a contract between the patient and the provider, with the patient making decisions about his or her care. If this is the case, then disclosure of errors is a factor that impacts this decision process and errors must be openly discussed. If we want patients to trust us, then we must reveal the negative events along with the positive. There are increased efforts to describe (1) methods for disclosing errors, (2) by whom, and (3) when. The Agency for Healthcare Research and Quality (AHRQ) provides information on disclosure and notes that the following should be considered by healthcare providers and HCOs (HHS, AHRQ, PSNet, 2019a):

- Disclosure of all harmful errors
- An explanation as to why the error occurred
- Minimization of errors
- Physician steps to prevent recurrences

Disclosure is connected to both legal and ethical concerns; both are discussed in other chapters. The content of an error disclosure is important. *Full disclosure* of an error incorporates the components found in **Exhibit 6-1**, as well as "acknowledgement of responsibility and an apology by the physician" (Gallagher et al., 2006, p. 1587); however, full disclosure is not always so straightforward: "There may be a disconnect between physicians' views of ideal practice and what actually happens. For example, most physicians agree that errors should be fully disclosed to patients, but in practice many "choose their words carefully" by failing to clearly explain the error and its effects on the patient's health" (p. 1587).

While *full disclosure* is an explicit statement, and *partial disclosure* mentions an adverse event but not an error, *no disclosure* indicates that the patient is not told anything about an adverse event or error. In a study on disclosure, it was noted that 56% of the physicians used partial disclosure, 42% full disclosure, and 3% no disclosure (Gallagher et al., 2006).

In addition to what should be shared, it is critical to consider how this information should be communicated. The decision to share information about an error with a patient would not be the nurse's responsibility. This responsibility belongs to the physician but should include team input. If the HCO has a policy and procedure on disclosure, and ideally it should, then the policy and procedure must be followed, including any documentation that might be required. This process should also include follow-up—going back to the patient to check on response and concerns that may develop. The following is a summary of guidelines for implementing disclosure of errors (Banja & Amori, 2005):

- Plan what will be said (including content, who will inform the patient, best location with privacy, time and patient status, whether the family will be included, and so on).
- Be clear and concise; answer questions truthfully.
- Stop and listen; give the patient time to respond.
- Evaluate response as it develops.
- Respond empathetically.
- Avoid being defensive or identifying blame.
- A meaningful apology may be made.

One should not assume that disclosure of errors always prevent lawsuits. Disclosure is not used to prevent a lawsuit, although it may make some patients reconsider whether they will sue the healthcare provider, as they may feel more trust in the healthcare provider who is honest with them. Disclosure is about

---

**Exhibit 6-1** Content to Include in a Full Disclosure

- A description of the nature of the error and the harm it could cause or caused
- A description of when and where the error occurred
- Consequence of the harm
- Clinical and institutional actions taken to diminish the gravity of the harm
- Identification of who will manage the patient's continuing care
- Identification of systematic elements that contributed to the error
- Identification of who will manage ongoing communication
- Associated costs of the error to be removed from the patient's bill (assuming these costs are known to be related to the error and risk management has been consulted)
- Offer of counseling and support

Banja, J. & Amori, G. (2005). Banja, J. (2005). The empathic disclosure of medical error. In J. Banja (ed.), *Medical errors and medical narcissism* (pp. 173-192). Sudbury, MA: Jones & Bartlett Learning. ISBN 0-7637-8361-7

professional responsibility, accountability, and patient-centered care. Why is patient-centered care important here? Patient-centered care emphasizes the right of patients to know about the care process and outcomes in order to participate in decisions about their health and care, and this patient involvement has an impact on care improvement.

## Patient Advocacy

Patient **advocacy** is "the act of pleading for or supporting a course of action on behalf of individuals, families, communities, and population" (Finkelman, 2019, p. 41). The American Nurses Association (ANA) *Code of Ethics for Nurses* supports the professional responsibility of each nurse to the patient (ANA, 2015a). The *Scope and Standards of Practice* is also critical in supporting the patient and patient-centered care (ANA, 2015b). The standards of professional practice include the nursing process with the patient at the center of this process. Another standard on coordination of care emphasizes that effective coordination requires patient involvement. Standards of professional performance also focus on a number of factors that influence advocacy and patient-centered care, such as culture, communication, collaboration, quality, evidence-based practice, and leadership.

Staff need to feel empowered to advocate for patients and, in the process, to empower the patient. Providing clear information should be part of the process. The goal is not to make the patient dependent on the healthcare provider but rather to work collaboratively with the patient. Effective advocacy requires understanding of patient needs and preferences and recognizing the importance of putting the focus on the patient. The nurse acts as the patient's advocate when the nurse speaks for the patient (individual patient, family, communities/populations). This does not mean the nurse tells the patient what to do but rather represents the patient—for example, in the CQI process, the nurse acts as the patient's

advocate in ensuring that procedures are followed or procedures are improved to reflect best practice. A nurse who stops a surgical procedure due to concern that the wrong site has been identified is serving as the patient's advocate, and a nurse serving on an HCO's quality improvement (QI) committee is serving as patient advocate for all HCO patients to ensure quality care. Nurses act as patient advocates every day in many ways.

### STOP AND CONSIDER 6-1

Patient-centered care must be part of an effective QI program.

## Reimbursement, the Patient, and CQI

For the healthcare consumer, reimbursement and the cost of healthcare have long been concerns. Consumers are also concerned about their out-of-pocket costs. As noted in other chapters in this text, cost and quality are interrelated; however, spending more money on care does not necessarily mean that the care is better. There are countries that spend less on care than does the United States, and yet they are ranked higher in health, access, and healthcare services. Another aspect is the cost of QI programs and methods used by these programs—funding, staffing, technology, and so on. CQI increases costs for HCOs, as well as on the macrolevel (local, state, federal).

There has been an increase in pay-for-performance (P4P) initiatives. This type of approach may improve care, but it is noted that some providers may view P4P as an incentive to use workarounds and limit reporting of problems to give the appearance that outcomes are met. It is important to recognize that most of what would be considered patient-centered care is not reimbursable: Healthcare providers and HCOs do not receive payment for many strategies used to ensure patient-centered care. This may have an impact on the HCO's commitment to make significant changes unless the HCO can see real value in doing so. The consumer (i.e., the patient) no longer is holding back on complaints about healthcare quality and cost, and in the future this outspokenness will most likely increase, particularly if costs continue to rise and quality remains a problem.

# Patient, Family, and Staff Responses to a Patient/Family Quality Improvement Role

HCO, government, and nongovernment initiatives to (1) improve care and (2) increase emphasis on patient-centered care developed during the same period. This led to greater recognition that the two goals were connected. A critical question was, and continues to be, what is the patient's role in CQI? One perspective is that the patient simply "gets the rewards" from a system that provides quality care, and this is certainly important to the patient and patient's family. There is, however, another important question: Is there a more active role that patients should assume?

## Roles and Responsibilities

Many now agree that there should be an active patient role in CQI, if the patient wants to assume it. Several factors influence this role. First, the healthcare provider and HCO must commit to accepting active participation from the patient and the family in the CQI process. This must be more than verbal acceptance; it must be demonstrated in actions taken and listening to the patient. Given that historically there has been a more "paternalistic" attitude toward patients, it is not easy for healthcare providers and HCOs to involve the patient, although this has changed over the years.

HCOs must take active steps to include the patient in HCO QI programs and plans. How might this be done? Sometimes patient representatives are included on various committees and task forces focused on improving care. Patients are frequently asked to complete satisfaction surveys (discussed later in this chapter). The newest method is the most direct: Ask patients to speak up when they have questions or concerns and when they notice problems. This active role puts the patient, and in many cases the family, right in the middle of the care process and the CQI process—stopping care to identify or question something. This patient empowerment can be threatening to staff, so staff education is necessary to improve understanding of the need for this approach and how best to respond. Ignoring patient comments or saying broadly "We will look into it" is not enough. Patients should be encouraged to participate, although they cannot be forced to do so. Assisting patients in understanding why their involvement is important is critical, requiring that staff follow the HCO approach of active patient engagement in CQI. Communicating to patients that the HCO is committed to CQI, describing CQI, and noting the value of input from all parties, including the patient, are vital steps toward engaging patients.

Patients also need examples of their role in CQI. Although staff cannot cover all possible scenarios, examples include the following:

- When a staff member does not wash their hands, the patient should refuse care until hands are washed.
- The patient should ask questions about medications or procedures that may not be in sync with the patient's understanding of his or her treatment.
- The patient should tell staff when there is clutter in the patient's room that makes

it difficult for the patient to walk safely, and the patient should ask for it to be removed or moved.

- The patient should identify potential flaws in the discharge plan that will make it difficult to implement the plan in the patient's home.
- The patient should note that informed consent has not been given.

Why might it be difficult for patients to speak up about quality care? Some patients are afraid they will offend staff and that then they may not get the best care or response from staff. Whether or not this concern is justified, this fear is present for many patients.

Coordination and **collaboration** are important aspects of care delivery, and patient feedback ensures better outcomes. The National Academy of Medicine (NAM, 2015) defines collaboration as follows: "Collaboration is an active and ongoing partnership, often involving people from diverse backgrounds who work together to solve problems, provide services, and enhance outcomes. Collaborative patient-centered practice is a type of arrangement designed to promote the participation of patients and their families within a context of collaborative practice" (p. xi).

This chapter focuses on how errors impact patients, how patients might respond to errors, and how patients might help to reduce errors; however, patients also have a role in precipitating errors. This may seem like an unusual statement, but consider the following insight from the AHRQ: "[Patient] errors may arise from the same underlying causes that contribute to clinicians' errors—while patients may engage in intentionally unsafe behavior, more commonly, patient errors are attributable to the difficulties inherent in an individual's interaction with a complex system. One study classified patient errors into *action errors*, which are errors of patient behavior such as failure to attend a scheduled appointment, and *mental errors*, which include thought process errors such as failing to take a medication as prescribed" (HHS, AHRQ, PSNet, 2019b).

Examples of factors that might impact this type of error are health literacy problems and ineffective patient–provider communication. As errors are analyzed, it is important to consider the patient's role, not to blame the patient, but to understand the error, respond to it, and if possible to prevent future errors for the patient and even for other patients. Later in this chapter, strategies to increase patient engagement in care and CQI are discussed. These strategies are also important in reducing errors in which the patient is more involved in the situation that led to the error.

# Effective Communication

Communication is an element in all that is done during the healthcare process. Staff who listen to the patient, respect the patient, and clearly communicate information the patient needs are much more successful in engaging the patient in CQI with the patient at the center. The patient also needs time to ask questions and feel that staff are listening and willing to answer questions. Both verbal communication and nonverbal communication are important in effective communication. Staff need to make sure that their nonverbal communication is in sync with their verbal messages. Active listening is critical in the communication process.

Sometimes it may seem that the simple issues are unimportant, but they can be very important. For example, admission staff often have the first encounter with the patient, and if they begin by addressing the patient with the patient's first name without asking permission to do so, it may have a negative impact. Staff tend to think that calling patients by their first name is more patient centered, but it is not. What is more patient centered is asking the patient what he or she wants to be called and using the correct title—for example, "Mr.," "Dr.," and "Ms." Assumptions get in the way of asking the patient and listening to the patient. The staff needs to know details about the patient, such as religion and ethnic factors. This information can impact communication with the patient and care.

The following is an example of multiple non–patient-centered communication problems with patients: A patient is recovering from anesthesia after open-heart surgery. The patient's wife is in the room and hears the staff calling her husband "honey" and "baby" as they provide care. The two nurses, including an advanced practice nurse, then try to get the patient to respond by calling him Mr. —. He does not respond, and they appear concerned. The patient is a physician. The patient's wife gets very irritated by the manner of communication and tells the staff not to refer to her husband as "honey" and "baby" as this is insulting, and that it would help if they called her husband Dr. —, as they might get more of a response from him since their voices are not familiar to him and he is still heavily medicated. The nurses reluctantly follow her instructions, and the patient responds immediately. They had no idea the patient was a physician, although this was in the medical record.

## The Patient and Diagnosis

In other chapters, diagnostic errors are discussed; however, in this chapter, the focus is on the patient. Developing strategies to reduce these errors should also involve the patient and communication with the patient, including during the process of diagnosis. The patient might help to reduce diagnostic errors, and therein greatly improve care, by doing the following (Graber, 2014, p. 26):

1. Be a good historian. Patients should keep records of their symptoms, when they started, and how they have responded (or not) to treatment.
2. Take advantage of cancer screening.
3. Know test results and keep accurate records of these results. Patients should not assume that no news is good news. They should follow up if they do not receive copies of the results of tests and consults.

4. Speak up! Patients should ask the following questions: (1) What else could it be? (2) What should I expect? (3) When and how should I follow up if symptoms persist or worsen? (4) What resources can I use to learn more? (5) Is this test worthwhile? Can we wait? (More testing does not always mean better care!)
5. Do not assume that the healthcare system will adequately coordinate care. Patients should keep their own records and help coordinate their own care.
6. Provide feedback about diagnostic errors to providers and organizations—for example, about past diagnosis errors.
7. Understand that diagnosis always involves some element of uncertainty.
8. Get a second opinion regarding a serious diagnosis or unresolved symptoms.
9. Take advantage of help and support—for example, support groups, patient safety staff, patient advocates.

It may seem obvious that the patient is the center of the diagnosis process, but in reality during this stage, healthcare providers tend to focus more on laboratory tests, exams, history, procedures, and so on. Patients need to be empowered to ask for second opinions and question diagnoses. If errors are made, patients need to report them so that this type of error can be tracked and steps can be taken to improve diagnosing and reduce these errors.

## Typical Patient and Family Responses to Engagement in CQI

Patients may respond emotionally as they participate more in their care. If they are concerned about care quality, they may respond with anger or frustration. They may also praise staff for their work and feel that they are getting the best of care. The range can vary. The patient's condition and past healthcare experiences are factors that may influence patient responses as well as the relationship they have with healthcare providers and responses they get from healthcare providers. Families, too, may vary in their responses. Patients and families need to feel that they can say what they think or feel and ask questions without staff responding defensively and negatively.

## Staff Responses to Patient Engagement in CQI

Every staff member, clinical and nonclinical, needs to commit to patient-centered care and take steps in their work to focus on the patient. We tend to focus on clinical staff, but nonclinical staff can make a difference, too. Consider the following nonclinical staff interactions with the patient:

- The dietary staff focus on patient dietary needs, including religious and ethnic factors, and make special arrangements to meet those needs.
- The admissions staff typically is the first staff patients and families encounter and are key to establishing the HCO as a patient-centered environment. How do they communicate and respond to the patient and family? Are they rushed? Do they answer questions? Do they recognize personal needs and respond? So much can be done with this interaction to make patients feel they are the center from the beginning of the experience.
- All staff may listen and respond to feedback in all areas of the HCO—for example, staff who clean the patient's room have a lot of contact with the patient and family and many opportunities to interact and personalize care for the patient.
- Staff transporting patients during admission or discharge, and to and from procedures, interact with patients during potentially stressful moments.

These are just a few of the many potential nonclinical staff interactions that may contribute to the patient's experience.

All staff should speak to the patient with respect and recognize when the patient does not want to converse. Acting defensively or with anger is not helpful. It is also easy to "put the patient off"—saying you will get back to the patient or family member later. If staff need to delay a response, then they need to go back to the patient or family member to follow up. Not doing so decreases trust and does not support an effective patient–provider relationship.

### STOP AND CONSIDER 6-3

Patients should be encouraged to participate in CQI, but they cannot be forced to participate.

## Methods to Increase Patient/Family Engagement in CQI

Patients, and their families when patients approve, have roles in the HCO's culture of safety. Many of the elements associated with patient-centered care are described at the beginning of this chapter; however, there are other elements to consider. Implementing patient-centered care in the healthcare delivery system is not easy to accomplish and takes time. It needs to impact the entire culture of the HCO regardless of the type of setting, such as acute care, ambulatory care, urgent care, physician practices, long-term care, home health, and hospice. A critical factor that impacts implementation, as noted, is that much of what is considered to be patient-centered care is not reimbursable; it is considered to be just a part of expected care. Strategies and interventions to support patient-centered care take time and expertise. There are also program costs associated with effective integration of patient-centered care and creating partnerships with patients and families to redesign healthcare and improve quality. Examples of costs are interpreters, staff training, signage to ensure patients can find their way around, personal attention requiring more staff time, and effective use of an HCO website and other technology to share information with patients and families and improve communication.

## Barriers to Patient Engagement

Barriers to engaging the patient and focusing on patient-centered care are typically related to lack of HCO and/or staff commitment to patient-centered care. This may take more time and initiative to accomplish. Staff are busy and stressed, so they may perform their jobs with minimal concern for the patient as a person—not listening and not responding to make changes. Nurses have a major role in supporting patient-centered care, but if they are stressed and understaffed, these factors impact whether or not they are able to support patient-centeredness in daily practice. Common barriers include inadequate staffing, lack of staff knowledge and understanding of patient-centered care, poor communication, fear that the patient will identify errors, view of patient-centered care as a nuisance, and failure to understand staff or patient roles in patient-centered care and CQI.

## Strategies to Increase Engagement

The Institute of Health Improvement also strongly supports a patient-centered approach to healthcare. This healthcare improvement model integrates patient-centered care in five CQI focus areas (Balik, Conway, Zipperer, & Watson, 201):

- *Leadership.* Governance and executive leaders demonstrate that everything in the culture is focused on patient- and family-centered care, practiced everywhere in the HCO. Patient-centered care needs to be a critical driver at the individual level, at the microsystem level (unit, department, service), and across the organization.

- *Hearts and minds.* The hearts and minds of staff are fully engaged through respectful partnerships with everyone in the organization and a commitment to the shared values of patient- and family-centered care.
- *Respectful partnership.* Every care interaction is anchored in a respectful partnership, anticipating and responding to patient and family needs (e.g., physical, comfort, emotional, informational, cultural, spiritual, and learning needs).
- *Reliable care.* Healthcare systems deliver reliable, quality care when needed.
- *Evidence-based care.* The care team instills confidence by providing collaborative, evidence-based care. (p. 8)

HCOs are providing more patient educational materials to explain and motivate patients to engage in CQI. As Schwappach, Hochreutener, and Wernli (2010) explain, "We cannot just expect patients to participate in quality improvement without some information and support in doing so, nor can we require patients to participate. We can encourage and provide the information needed. Some patients will choose not to participate" (p. E85). As HCOs plan what information to share with patients to increase their engagement, HCOs should consider the following about patient-centered care and CQI (Finkelman, 2019):

- Provider–patient communication
- Patient educational materials about health concerns
- Self-management tools to help patients manage their illness or condition and make affirmed decisions
- Access to care (e.g., timely appointments, off-hour services) and use of information technology (e.g., automated patient reminders, patient access to electronic medical records)
- Continuity of care
- Post-hospital follow-up and support
- Access to reliable information about the quality of healthcare providers (e.g. physicians, APRNs, nurses, and other providers

and staff) and HCOs, with opportunity to give feedback (p. 275)

It is also important to get routine patient feedback on patient material—helpfulness of the information and so on. Ask patients if it was easy to get information and understand it.

HCOs use many other methods to integrate patient-centered care into practice and care delivery systems, including the following examples:

- *Patient participation in care planning.* The patient participates in care planning and agrees to the plan. Patient values, needs, preferences, and cultural factors should be part of the planning. If the patient agrees, family may participate.
- *Staff etiquette.* This may seem to be a strange topic, but it is very important. It relates directly to patient-centered care. All staff need to follow good etiquette, including the following practices: Knock when entering the patient's room; introduce yourself by name and identify your role; ask for the patient's permission to talk with the patient or to provide care; never call the patient by first name unless the patient agrees; recognize that patients and families need private time; and never assume that the family can be told anything about the patient unless the patient agrees, unless the patient's condition does not allow the patient to provide consent.
- *Care coordination.* Ensure that patient needs are met by coordinating providers, functions, activities, and sites over time. Coordination also implies patient involvement in care decisions and covers the continuum of care required by the patient—multiple providers and settings over time.
- *Self-management of care.* Self-management of care is an element of care that is recognized in the *Quality Chasm* reports as a critical component. Self-management programs include educative process and outcomes (McGowan, 2005). Today, with the growing number of patients with chronic

illness, self-management is more important than ever. Even though self-management is particularly important for chronic illness, it can apply to any type of patient. **Self-management** is "the systematic provision of education and supportive interventions to increase patients' skills and confidence in managing their health problems, including regular assessment of progress and problems, goal setting, and problem-solving approach" (IOM, 2003, p. 52). The patient accepts much of the responsibility for the care. Teach-back is a method used to better ensure patients have understood information shared—to ask patients to repeat the information in their own words to improve self-management (HHS, AHRQ, PSNet, 2019c; Prochnow, Meiers, & Scheckel, 2019).

- *Primary Care.* This setting also requires strategies to increase patient engagement. Examples are using teach-back as mentioned for other healthcare settings; applying the AHRQ program "Be Prepared to Be Engaged" (HHS, AHRQ, 2017), using programs that explain medication management, and greater emphasis on sharing information during handoffs.

The healthcare system is not set up to easily accommodate self-management, but this needs to change. A major step is to consider how the patient can assume more responsibility when it makes sense for the patient's needs and preferences. Today, more care takes place in the home, requiring more self-management even if the patient is receiving home health services. Actively including the patient in planning sets the stage for a discussion about self-management. In many cases, an interprofessional team is used to ensure that the patient's complex, varied needs are met. There is also increasing use of electronic personal health records (EPHRs) to support the patient and self-management (Mitchell & Begoray, 2010). Use of EPHRs requires adequate patient health literacy, software, and technological support.

Self-management is also a time of high risk, particularly if the patient does not have preparation for self-management or support resources. The highest time of risk is when a patient who is actively involved in self-management requires professional intervention and may not realize it or deny the need for this action. Nurses need to work with the patient and, when the patient agrees, also include the family to develop acceptable plans.

- *Patient education.* Patient education has long been part of healthcare; however, its effectiveness is not always clear. Methods used to provide patient education must be updated to consider different patient needs, changes in healthcare delivery, and health informatics. Today, patients in the acute care setting are sicker and are discharged sicker than in the past. This impacts the effectiveness of patient education. Is the patient really able to understand information enough to apply the information to his or her needs? In other settings, such as outpatient clinics, the patient may not be as sick, but healthcare providers have less time with patients, which is also true in acute care settings. The tendency is to rely on printed material and assume we have provided patient education; however, patients need time to discuss the information with healthcare providers. We are also not taking full advantage of informatics, such as smartphones, computers, the Internet, and other new technology that could be used to provide information when the patient really needs it. Providing patients with information that means something to them and their health emphasizes patient-centered care and patient advocacy.
- *Human resources and patient-centered care.* Human resources should also recognize cultural issues that can impact hiring, performance, and personnel policies, as well as patient-centered care. Is patient-centered care discussed with job applicants? Is patient-centered care commented on in position descriptions and performance evaluation? Staff orientation and education sessions should incorporate patient-centered care. Staff meetings should include patient-centered care as staff discuss issues and problems at all levels in the HCO.
- *Health promotion and wellness and disease prevention.* Today, there is greater emphasis on health promotion and wellness and disease prevention. Many healthcare providers now incorporate screening of disease in their services. Community or public health services are particularly concerned with health promotion, wellness, and disease prevention. Even within the community, healthcare providers must consider individual needs, health history, and so on, and these considerations apply, too, for the community at large (population health).

  In the end, as with all health decisions, it really is the individual patient's choice. The 2010 healthcare reform legislation mandated the establishment of the National Prevention, Health Promotion, and Public Health Council within the HHS. The National Prevention Strategy for the United States focuses on increasing the number of people who are healthy at every stage of life. To meet this goal requires empowered people, healthy and safe community environments, clinical and community preventive services, and elimination of health disparities (HHS, National Prevention, Health Promotion, and Public Health Council, 2011). An example of this council's activity is the Surgeon General's report *Healthy Aging in Action* (HHS, ODPHP, National Prevention, Health Promotion, and Public Health Council, 2020).
- *End-of-life.* End-of-life care, palliative care, and hospice care are patient-centered approaches. The philosophy behind these services emphasizes the patient's individual needs and preferences.

- *Bedside rounds.* Some hospitals include patients and families (the latter with patient permission) in patient rounds rather than just "doing rounds" and offering the patient a minimal role. Rounds are part of planning and evaluating care, and if patient-centered care considers the patient to be the most important part of care, then the patient's inclusion is critical. These rounds provide patients with more information and time for staff to listen to the patient's feedback. Rounds are also used to educate patients about current needs, treatment, and post-discharge treatment when in transition to another setting, including the home. Ensuring privacy and confidentiality during rounds can be difficult when the patient is not in a private room. Alternative arrangements must be made if sharing of information should be private—there is no privacy in the typical room situation. Staff and healthcare profession students who participate in rounds need to understand the rounds procedure, integration of the patient (family), and all relevant privacy and confidentiality issues. Rounds are discussed further in other content as they are an important part of CQI.

- *Discharge and transition planning.* Patients have shorter lengths of stay in acute care today, and as a consequence they tend to go home sicker than in the past to continue recovery at home. Some go to other HCOs for continuation of their care, such as short-term rehabilitation or long-term care; others go home and receive home health services. Handoffs are times of increased risk of errors. Patients and their families need to be vigilant during these times and participate in identifying possible errors. Asking questions is a critical part of this process (patient to staff, staff to patients, and staff to staff). Patients should be involved in the planning. At all times, patients should be encouraged. Staff should ask "Does this make sense to you in your situation?" If healthcare providers hear the patient say that it does not make sense, if the patient asks questions that make the healthcare provider wonder about the plan's feasibility, or if the healthcare provider thinks that the patient and/or family are not committed to the plan, then they should consider whether the plan needs to be reviewed and possibly revised. For the plan to have a chance of success, the patient and family must feel the plan is appropriate and commit to it. Discharge planning without the patient runs a high risk of problems and failure. With increasing concerns about the level of readmissions, using effective patient-centered discharge planning helps to reduce readmission.

- *Visiting policies and procedures.* Structuring visiting hours can limit patient and family interactions. Many hospitals are changing visiting hours to allow for more opportunities for visits. The patient needs to be able to say when visitors are a problem, but the staff must also assess patient stress levels. If the patient is not able to set limits, then staff need to talk with the patient to plan effective visiting times. Changes have been made even in intensive care—the service that has traditionally had the most rigid visiting policies. Having family visit more frequently and in a reasonable number, such as one or two at a time, may bring more comfort to the patient. In some cases, family members are allowed to be present during codes, when the patient's life is at risk. There is also more flexibility now in the surgical arena, with some HCOs allowing families to stay with a patient longer prior to surgery and also to see the patient sooner after surgery. Privacy of other patients must always be considered. The emergency department is another area where there may be more flexibility, if the patient wants family present and family members do not interfere with required treatment.

- *Patient- and family-centered facility design.* The design of any HCO should consider the needs of the patients and families who use the services. Consideration must be given to the physical layout. For example, does the layout facilitate ease of access, does the flow of services make sense in the design, does the environment appear clean and well lit to reflect openness, are color tones welcoming and calming, is noise managed and interventions used to reduce noise, is carpeting safe and easy to clean, is temperature regulated, are appropriate waiting areas available for visitors, and are general patient areas available for sitting? More HCOs are now providing wi-fi so that patients, families, and visitors can use digital devices. Another issue is facilities that make it easier for family members and significant others to stay overnight, with the patient requiring consideration of furniture (e.g., chairs) so that visitors can rest and be near the patient. The facility should be welcoming from the time the patient enters the HCO. Privacy should be part of all aspects of the facility. Patients and families should feel as comfortable as possible in the facility. The design should also support staff collaboration, providing private space for discussions and making it easier for staff to reach one another. The diversity of patients and families should also be considered, with clear signage that all visitors can understand, use of color codes that make it easy to get around the facility with minimal need to read signs, and information stations with staff prepared to assist regardless of language. Facilities for special populations—such as children, the elderly, disabled persons, and patients with mental health concerns—should reflect the needs and characteristics of these patients.
- *Staff preparation.* All staff need information and ongoing updates about patient-centered care—what it means and how to implement it. This information should be provided during orientation so that all new staff understand the importance of patient-centered care. Staff education on the topic should be scheduled regularly for all staff, and staff should be asked to identify topics related to patient-centered care that they think should be included in staff education. Including patient and family representatives in orientation to share their experiences and thoughts about patient-centered care is an effective tool for emphasizing the commitment to patient-centered care.
- *Teams.* Teams are also important in supporting patient-centered care, particularly interprofessional teams. There is greater emphasis today on interprofessional education to improve effectiveness of interprofessional teams (NAM, 2015). Teams should focus on the patient and engage the patient in the team process, increasing communication, coordination and collaboration, effective decision making, and more. Additional information about teams and CQI are found in other chapters.

**Exhibit 6-2** highlights additional examples of strategies that might be used by healthcare providers to increase patient participation.

## STOP AND CONSIDER 6-4

It is easy to assume that patients do not understand CQI and that their engagement is not really an important part of patient-centered care.

# Technology to Support Patient Engagement

Technology also impacts the caring process in patient-centered care, and in some situations it can get in the way of this process. If, however, nurses are vigilant and recognize the risk of reduced caring, then they are more able to

**Exhibit 6-2** Strategies to Help Healthcare Providers Encourage Patient Participation in the Critical Thinking Process

- Do not talk to patients from the doorway. Stay in the room.
- Pay attention to your body language and to the patient's body language.
- Sit down so that you are at eye level with the patient.
- Use open-ended questions and comments, such as "Tell me about . . ." instead of closed questions that imply you expect a short answer.
- Touch patients, but be respectful of their space and cultural norms, as sometimes patients do not want to be touched or want others close to them.
- Use collaborative thinking language, such as "We should think this through," "Let's look at some possible conclusions," and "Can we analyze this together?"
- Use phrases that let the patient know that the patient's situation is not so unusual that the patient cannot discuss it—for example, "Some people feel anxious when. . . ."
- Address patients respectfully. Ask if they prefer Mr. or Mrs., Mrs. or Ms., Doctor, Professor, Reverend, and so on.
- Do not use affectionate terms to address the patient, such as "sweetheart," "dear," and so on.
- Do not look at your watch, no matter how busy you are.
- Be direct and honest—for example, tell patients when the schedule is backed up and why.
- If you feel like avoiding a patient, reflect on why you feel that way.

ensure, as care is given, that active methods are used to ensure that technology and informatics do not become barriers but rather support patient-centered care—for example, if a nurse is using an electronic device in the patient's room, the nurse needs to actively interact with the patient by looking at the patient and asking questions rather than just focusing on the screen. If a nurse is setting up infusion equipment, it is important to talk with the patient during the procedure but to still ensure that the equipment is used in a safe and effective manner and that orders are followed in a timely manner.

Informatics is a part of all types of consumerism today, including healthcare. Patients now check the Internet for information, although they may not always know the most reliable sources or how to evaluate them. They can prepare themselves for medical appointments and hospitalization. By using the many benchmarking and report card methods available through the Internet, patients can get important information to help them compare healthcare providers and make knowledgeable

decisions; however, as discussed in other chapters, these reports do not always reflect clear information about quality.

Patients use various types of technology (e.g., smartphones, tablet computers) to access the Internet and get health information and information about HCOs and providers. Integrating all of this information puts the focus on the patient, who should be the decision maker. Some HCOs are using electronic methods to identify "decision windows" or times when a patient has a decision to make (Fowler et al., 2011). In this case, symptoms are tracked through an electronic rating scale. When certain symptoms occur or symptoms get worse, an alert is sent to the provider, indicating that it may be time for evaluation and/or a change in treatment and thus a patient decision, or it might alert the patient to contact the healthcare provider. This type of method integrates patient-centered care with informatics, healthcare providers, and the patient.

The AHRQ now offers an app to help patients and families with their visits to healthcare providers (HHS, AHRQ, 2019a), known as the AHRQ QuestionBuilder App, which is free and can be downloaded on a variety of devices. The patient can prepare questions, organize them, and even take photos of, for example, skin, pills, and so on. The data are only accessible to the patient who has downloaded the app. The AHRQ provides information on the use of the app.

Some methods are focused on assisting caregivers. One new product is e-Caregiving Solutions (e-Caregiving, 2019), a web-based education and support system providing information to families and significant others so that they can be better care coordinators, advocates, and communicators. The system also provides a caregiving checklist to help guide caregivers. This method may improve quality of care for a large part of the patient population who are cared for primarily outside a structured healthcare organization.

Traditionally medical records have been used only by healthcare providers; however, this is changing. The use of OpenNotes is engaging informal caregivers to participate more actively, as noted in a study that obtained 7,053 surveys from caregivers who used this method (Chimowitz, Gerard, Fossa, Bourgeois, & Bell, 2018). The following are examples of information collected from the data: reading notes assisted in understanding of testing and referrals, reminder to get a test done, reminder for appointments, providing information about prescriptions and taking prescriptions correctly, increased trust in the healthcare provider, improved teamwork, and some mistakes noted by patients.

Electronic methods are used more and more for patients to communicate with HCOs and healthcare providers, and vice versa. To date, there is not enough evidence supporting the positive impact of electronic methods on healthcare outcomes, but today clearly many people are engaged in electronic communication and access information through these sources. As Carayon, Hoonakker, Cartmill,

and Hassol (2015) report, this new arena of communication is promising: "Some evidence indicates that these health IT applications may improve process measures, such as greater adherence, better self-care, improved patient–provider communication, and patient satisfaction. The results of this study support the findings in the literature that patients sharing their information with clinicians electronically can facilitate communication, improve the organization of work, reduce workload, and increase patient satisfaction" (p. ES-1).

Implementing and maintaining electronic methods are not simple to accomplish, and there are barriers to effective outcomes, such as time commitment, interference with workflow, and increases in healthcare provider workload. Other issues that come up are patient access to their own medical records, patient self-reported data (i.e., accuracy and timeliness), secure messaging, and use of online reminders. As more emphasis is placed on digital communication methods, the healthcare system will experience benefits but also problems that relate to technology use. There will be need for more strategies to make communication more secure, safe, accessible, and effective in healthcare delivery.

## STOP AND CONSIDER 6-5

Technology can improve patient-centered care, but it also can act as a barrier to patient-centered care.

# Monitoring and Measuring Patient Satisfaction and Patient-Centered Care

An HCO may proclaim itself to be patient centered, but actually demonstrating this care approach daily is a much different matter. So how do you know if an HCO demonstrates patient-centered care? A place to start is to determine how the HCO views patient-centered care. Does the HCO's culture and philosophy actually reflect patient-centered care (IPFCC, 2019)? There is no standard method to meet the goal, but there are some guidelines about the HCO that can be used in self-assessment. The following questions might guide an assessment of an HCO's commitment to patient-centered care:

- Are the concept and related principles clearly found in the organization's written vision, mission, and goals?
- Does the organization's definition of "quality healthcare" include the patient and family?
- Has this priority been communicated to patients, families, and the community, and in what way?
- Is the care provided effective?
- Do the organization's policies, procedures, standards, programs, and other aspects of the organization consistently include patients and families as partners?
- Do all staff, clinical and nonclinical, understand and apply patient-centered care? How is this demonstrated?
- What is demonstrated in documentation? For example, do medical records indicate how the patient participates?
- Is the patient actively considered in collection of CQI data and root cause analysis? For example, are patient surveys used?
- Is patient-centered care demonstrated in the physical environment? If so, how?

"The adoption of an integrated measure of health literacy, language access, and cultural competence would enable hospitals and health systems, as well as health consumer leadership organizations, to address specific as well as broader patient-centered framework issues in health equity" (Bau et al., 2019, p. 8).

The Planetree model is used by many HCOs to provide a framework to ensure that the HCO demonstrates patient-centeredness; supporting respect, inclusion, and compassion; and creating a standard of patient-centered care (Planetree International, 2018). HCOs that use this model consider the following elements to ensure that the model is applied: organization structure and functions, including patient and family feedback; human interactions that focus on continuity, consistency, and accountability to personalize care; patient education and access to information; nutrition program with 24-hour access; healing environment both in architecture and interior design; arts program to offer therapeutic distractions; spirituality and diversity to meet these needs; healthy communities to improve community health; and measurement to determine satisfaction.

## Patient Satisfaction Surveys

HCOs include patient satisfaction in their QI programs. Often HCOs use surveys developed and managed by external sources, such as Press Ganey®. The HCO pays for this service, and then it has access to a tested survey and often the ability to compare data with other similar HCOs.

It is important to get the data, but there are potential problems with the process and the data. A factor that has an impact on results of patient satisfaction surveys is concern about accepted definitions (Finkelman, 2019). How a patient views quality care is often different from an HCO's view or an individual provider's view of quality care, meaning patient responses to surveys may be difficult to interpret or not relevant to provider objectives. It is not uncommon for patients to complete satisfaction surveys and never hear anything from the HCO, though the patients may have commented on negative experiences. This lack of response communicates that the feedback may not be important. Including patients in CQI data collection and assessment is a critical source of valuable information. In a study that included 979 patient interviews, 386 or 39.4% indicated that they experienced at least one breakdown in care, with 4 out of 10 hospitalized patients reporting this type of experience in the U.S. (Fisher et al., Smith, Gallagher, Burns, Morales, & Mazor, 2017). The types of concerns related to sharing of information, medications, admission delays, communication, healthcare provider manner, and discharge. If one reviews this list, it covers the entire process of care, although it does not specifically address diagnosis and other areas of treatment that are connected with the areas identified.

There are myths about patient satisfaction and data collected. The following list explores some of these myths and the realities of measuring patient satisfaction, which continue to be of concern today (Zimmerman, 2001, pp. 255–256).

- *Patient satisfaction is objective and straightforward.* Surveys are difficult to develop, and they are often poorly designed.
- *Patient satisfaction is easily measured.* Satisfaction is complex and not easily measured. Patient expectations play a major role in the process, and many factors can affect patient responses that are not always easy to identify, such as past experiences.
- *Patient satisfaction is accurately and precisely measured.* This is not possible at this time. Attitudes are being measured, and this is complex.
- *It is obvious who is the customer.* An HCO actually has many different types of customers beyond the patient, including families, healthcare providers, insurers, and internal customers. To complicate matters, the staff within the HCO are often customers to other staff—for example, the laboratory provides services to the units, and, thus, the nursing staff is the laboratory's customers. A complete customer satisfaction analysis should include all relevant HCO customers.

# Monitoring Patient-Centered Care

In addition to monitoring patient satisfaction, monitoring patient-centered care should be part of HCO QI programs. One cannot assume that because it is written in the HCO's vision, mission, and goals and included in position descriptions, staff orientation, and staff education that patient-centered (family-centered) care is fully integrated in the HCO. In summary, the HCO needs to consider the following in its CQI data collection and analysis as part of its QI plans:

- Is there shared decision making with the patient? If so, how is this objective accomplished?
- Is there coordination and continuity of care? If so, how is this objective accomplished?
- Do patients have access to care that meets their individual needs and in a timely manner?
- Do care documentation methods demonstrate patient-centered care?
- What does patient satisfaction data indicate? Trends?
- What is the level of communication with the patient (content, with whom, timeliness)?
- How is the patient (and family) involved in the QI program?
- Are the patient's emotional and physical comfort needs met? How?
- Are there disparities in the system, and what are they? How are they resolved?
- Is evidence-based practice used to meet the patient's individual needs?

CQI data collection should routinely include data on patient-centered care and should be reported in the HCO's CQI reports for discussion and development of improvement strategies. In order to do this, "reducing disparities requires attention to the essential components of equitable, patient-centered, high-quality care—that is, to culturally and linguistically appropriate care as well as attention to health literacy" (Blau et al., 2019, p. 2).

**STOP AND CONSIDER 6-6**

Patient satisfaction data are not always reflective of quality care.

# Examples of Patient-Centered Initiatives

Local, state, and federal government and nongovernmental organizations (NGOs) have developed initiatives to support patient-centered care. The AHRQ is very involved in initiatives to support patient-centered care and patient engagement in CQI. For example, "Questions Are the Answers" provides patient or consumer information to increase patient and provider communication (HHS, AHRQ, 2019b). Another example is "Taking Care of Myself: A Guide for When I Leave the Hospital" (HHS, AHRQ, 2018a). The following discussion describes some of these initiatives, and the Connect to Current Information section at the end of this chapter provides links to other information on the Internet.

## Collaboration and Care Coordination

An example of an initiative to increase patient engagement is the **collaborative care model**, which focuses on managing the health of a population rather than on treating a specific diagnosis. The goal is to reduce risks and cost of care through **coordination**, "deliberately organizing patient care activities and sharing information among all of the participants concerned with a patient's care to achieve safer and more effective care. This means that the patient's needs and preferences are known ahead of time and communicated at the right time to the right people, and that this information is used to provide safe, appropriate, and

effective care to the patient" (HHS, AHRQ, 2018b). Medicaid uses this model to integrate physical and mental healthcare. Coordination is one of the six National Quality Strategy (NQS) priorities. As Craig, Eby, and Whittington (2011) explain, "Care coordination delivers health benefits to those with multiple needs, while improving their experience of the care system and driving down overall healthcare (and societal) costs" (p. 2). The Centers for Medicare and Medicaid (CMS) also promotes coordinated care and provides resources for Medicare accountable care organizations (ACOs). "Some ACOs focus on facilitating the exchange of data between primary care providers and emergency departments, whereas others establish networks of post-acute care partners to support their mission of improving the quality and effectiveness of care. Others developed initiatives that focus on managing the care of individual beneficiaries, such as launching a home visit program or using information technology to streamline referrals to community organizations" (HHS, CMS, 2019a).

The annual *National Healthcare Quality and Disparities Report* (QDR) includes tracking and analysis of care coordination. Several models of care now emphasize patient-centered care, coordination, collaboration, and interprofessional teams and are important for an effective healthcare delivery system. Examples of some of these models are ACOs mentioned above and also medical homes and nurse-managed health centers. The AHRQ notes the following: "Care coordination involves deliberately organizing patient care activities and sharing information among all of the participants concerned with a patient's care to achieve safer and more effective care. This means that the patient's needs and preferences are known ahead of time and communicated at the right time to the right people, and that this information is used to provide safe, appropriate, and effective care to the patient." (HHS, AHRQ, 2018b).

# Consumer Assessment of Healthcare Providers and Systems

There is no federally required system for collecting patient satisfaction data and public reporting of the data. The Consumer Assessment of Healthcare Providers and Systems (CAHPS®) is a system that does this, but it is not a required program. It was developed and maintained by the HHS and AHRQ and the CMS (HHS, AHRQ, CAHPS®, 2019). Surveys and tools for collecting patient evaluation data are provided and accessible on the Internet. Multiple surveys are provided that focus on specific healthcare delivery settings and services: health plans, clinicians and groups, patient-centered medical homes, hospitals, and experience of care and health outcomes. The CAHPS® database is a repository of the data collected from the surveys, providing detailed benchmark data per type of survey, and used by patients and consumers, healthcare providers, regulators, health plans, community collaborators, and public and private purchasers of healthcare. The CAHPS® defines the patient experience as "the range of interactions that patients have with the healthcare system, including their care from health plans, and from doctors, nurses, and staff in hospitals, and other healthcare facilities. The terms patient satisfaction and patient experience are often used interchangeably, but they are not the same thing" (HHS, AHRQ, CAHPS®, 2019).

## Partnership for Patients Campaign

The Partnership for Patients Campaign is composed of physicians, nurses, hospitals, employers, and patients and their advocates. It is maintained by the CMS (HHS, CMS, 2019b). Its purposes are to make care safer and to improve care transitions. The Partnership uses several initiatives to meet its purposes. The Hospital Engagement Network helps identify solutions to solve the problem of hospital-acquired conditions (HACs) across the country. The Community-Based Care Transitions Program identifies sites to participate in this program. The sites must meet criteria and use a collaborative approach, with a variety of HCOs and other agencies serving patient needs in the community. This program is particularly focused on reducing Medicare beneficiary 30-day unplanned readmissions. Other methods are used to improve patient and family engagement. Both the HAC and the readmission initiatives are discussed in more detail in other chapters.

# Patient-Centered Outcomes Research Institute

The Patient-Centered Outcomes Research Institute (PCORI) is a nongovernmental, nonprofit organization in Washington, DC, that was authorized by Congress in 2010. The PCORI vision and mission are stated as follows (PCORI, 2019):

- *Vision.* Patients and the public have information they can use to make decisions that reflect their desired health outcomes.
- *Mission.* PCORI helps people make informed healthcare decisions and improves healthcare delivery and outcomes by producing and promoting high-integrity, evidence-based information that comes from research with decisions guided by patients, caregivers, and the broader healthcare community.

PCORI's focus is on evidence-based research using comparative effectiveness research (CER) to support decisions and recommendations. The national priorities in the PCORI research agenda are assessing prevention, diagnosis, and treatment options; improving healthcare systems; undertaking communication and dissemination research; addressing disparities; and accelerating PCORI and methodological research.

## Quality Improvement Organization Program

According to the HHS, CMS (2019c), healthcare complexity drives the need for patient-centered care: "Health care is personal. Every individual's experience with the health care system is different—influenced by preferences and values, family situation, cultural traditions, and lifestyle. Because these factors strongly affect health outcomes, patient-centered care is increasingly a top priority in every health care setting." The Quality Improvement Organization (QIO) program focuses on better patient care, better individual and population health, and lower care costs through improvement (Triple Aim). QIOs are located in all states and coordinate with the CMS. The CMS (2019c) states, "Medicare beneficiaries, caregivers, and healthcare providers are encouraged to join in local and national initiatives to increase patient and family engagement. Beneficiaries and families also will have the opportunity to contribute to local QIO improvement initiatives." Collaborative initiatives provide opportunities to respond to concerns, increase communication with Medicare beneficiaries, and identify strategies to increase patient and family engagement emphasizing the CMS commitment to patient-centered care.

## Speak Up™

Speak Up™ is a patient safety program developed by The Joint Commission, a nongovernmental organization. The name Speak Up™ is an acronym for the following patient advocacy acts (The Joint Commission, 2019):

- **S**peak up if you have questions or concerns.
- **P**ay attention to the care you get.
- **E**ducate yourself about your illness.
- **A**sk a trusted family member or friend to be your advocate (advisor or supporter).
- **K**now what medicines you take and why you take them.

- **U**se a healthcare organization that has been carefully checked out.
- **P**articipate in all decisions about your treatment.

The program offers free information in multiple forms, such as infographics, animated videos, brochures, and posters. The resources are offered in multiple languages and used globally. The focus of the program is on the patient and providing patients with information and tools to support them in speaking for themselves and empowering them as they interact with the healthcare system and healthcare providers. Examples of topics are anesthesia and surgery, the doctor's office, follow-up care, pain, prevention of medical errors, depression, at-home care, and antibiotics.

## Patient Safety Awareness Week

Each year the United States, along with other countries, celebrates Patient Safety Awareness Week. It is a time to recognize the need for improvement and to engage all stakeholders, including patients and families in the process. A key emphasis is encouraging patients to speak up and ask questions. It is also important that nursing education participate in this recognition. However, as is common with recognizing an issue for a week, the recognition should not just be for one week—it needs to be ongoing.

---

### STOP AND CONSIDER 6-7

The federal government supports patient-centered care.

---

## Summary

This chapter focused on patient-centered care as a critical element of effective care and healthcare systems. The patient is not only the center of care but also needs to actively

---

**Exhibit 6-3** Exemplars: Quality Improvement Roles and Responsibilities

---

**Staff Nurse**

A staff nurse discusses the plan of care with a patient. The nurse reviews the plan and asks the patient's opinion. The patient comments that it is difficult for the patient to sleep at night routinely. The nurse then looks at some of the schedule and how the patient can be assisted to read late or listen to music.

**Nurse Manager**

The nurse manager asks all staff to do an objective appraisal of comfort for family visitors and then to discuss this information at the next staff meeting along with suggestions for improvement.

**Advanced Practice Registered Nurse***

A patient informs an APRN that he does not want to be cared for by an APRN but rather an MD. The APRN explains her role and background but recognizes that the patient has not changed his view. The APRN makes arrangements for the patient to be seen by an MD. The APRN is respectful toward the patient.

*Advanced Practice Registered Nurse includes APRN, Clinical Nurse Specialist, Clinical Nurse Leader, and nurses with DNP.

participate in CQI. Patients, and when appropriate their families, can help to identify care concerns that need to be improved immediately and/or long term. Staff and HCOs need to include them in their QI programs and plans and accept that this engagement is necessary for CQI.

Exemplars of quality improvement roles and responsibilities for staff nurses, nurse managers, and APRNs are found in **Exhibit 6-3**.

# APPLY CQI

## Chapter Highlights

- Patient-centered care is not a new approach, but it is now recognized as a critical element of an improved healthcare system.
- Patient rights and privacy are critical elements in ensuring patient-centered care. HIPAA supports this philosophy throughout the healthcare system by mandating requirements.
- Disclosure of errors to patients is connected to ethics and legal issues but also demonstrates patient-centered care, as it emphasizes the right of the patient to know about the care process and outcomes and to participate in decisions to improve care.

- Patients are concerned about the cost of care and reimbursement, and both are connected to CQI.
- The patient, and when appropriate the family, should assume an active role in CQI, and HCOs and healthcare providers need to communicate the importance of this role to patients and families.
- Many methods are used to engage the patient and family in CQI, such as asking patients to speak up when they have concerns about quality.

- Staff need to respect patients and allow them to actively communicate during the care process. The patient makes the decisions about his or her care, unless the patient chooses not to do so.
- Technology provides many opportunities to increase patient-centered care and patient inclusion in CQI.
- Government and nongovernmental organizations now offer programs to HCOs, healthcare providers, and patients as consumers that support patient-centered care. Examples are care coordination and collaborative models, the Consumer Assessment of Healthcare Providers and Systems (CAHPS®) surveys, the Partnership for Patients campaign, the Patient-Centered Outcomes Research Institute (PCORI), the Quality Improvement Organization (QIO) program, Speak Up™, and other efforts.

## Critical Thinking and Clinical Reasoning and Judgment: Discussion Questions and Learning Activities

1. Review the article "A Trail of Medical Errors Ends in Grief, But No Answers," an account of one patient's experience: https://www.propublica.org/article/patient-safety-medical-error-hospital-no-answers

   Provide a summary of errors and other experiences that should be noted for this patient. Share your results in a discussion group in the classroom or online. The group should select at least three of the incidents and develop strategies that an HCO might use to resolve these problems or prevent them from reoccurring.

2. Keep a log for one day of clinical. The log should have two columns. In one column, identify all the examples you observe or are involved in during the day that reflect positive patient-centered care. In the second column, identify examples that reflect negative patient-centered care. Share this information with a discussion group in the classroom or online, and compare and contrast examples. Next, identify solutions that might be used to prevent the negative examples and improve patient-centered care. (Do not specify any names or any identifiers, such as patient, staff, healthcare organization, student.)

3. For one week, keep a log of all CQI examples that you observe or are involved in during your clinical experiences. Identify how your examples are related to patient-centered care. (Do not specify any names or any identifiers, such as patient, staff, healthcare organization, student.)

4. The National Academy of Medicine has a new report that has relevance to nursing: *Integrating Social Care into the Delivery of Health Care: Moving Upstream to Improve the Nation's Health* (2019). Access the report here: https://www.nap.edu/catalog/25467/integrating-social-care-into-the-delivery-of-health-care-moving

   Students can review the executive summary and the report. Teams of students could divide up the report for review and then discuss the content using the following questions as a guide:
   - What is meant by social care?
   - How should the healthcare system workforce integrate social care? How does this relate to nursing practice?

- Consider the following, which are addressed in the report: leveraging data and digital tools, financing social care, and strategies.

- What is your opinion of the recommendations? How do they relate to nurses and nursing practice?
- Search for other literature on this topic and review.

## Connect to Current Information

- Information for reporting HIPAA violations http://www.hhs.gov/hipaa/filing-a-complaint/what-to-expect/index.html
- CMS: Person and Family Engagement https://www.cms.gov/Medicare/Quality-Initiatives-Patient-Assessment-Instruments/QualityInitiativesGenInfo/Downloads/Person-and-Family-Engagement-Strategy-Summary.pdf
- CAHPS®: Surveys and Tools to Advance Patient-Centered Care https://cahps.ahrq.gov
- Planetree International http://planetree.org

- Effective Health Care Program: Information on comparative effectiveness research https://www.ahrq.gov/topics/comparative-effectiveness.html
- PCORI https://www.ahrq.gov/topics/patient-centered-outcomes-research.html http://www.pcori.org
- The Joint Commission: Speak Up™ Initiatives http://www.jointcommission.org/speakup.aspx
- CMS: Quality Improvement Organizations https://qioprogram.org/about
- Institute for Patient- and Family-Centered Care https://www.ipfcc.org/about

## Connect to Text Current Information with the Author

Go to the update for this text to review the Blog, QI News, and Literature Review. Access this regular update at: http://nursing.jbpub.com/Finkelman/QualityImprovement/2e.

## EBP, EBM, and Quality Improvement: Exemplar

Schenk, E., Bryant, R., Van Son, C., & Odom-Maryon, T. (2019). Perspectives on patient and family engagement with reduction in harm: The forgotten voice. *Journal of Nursing Care Quality*, 34(1), 73–79.

### Questions to Consider

1. What is the objective of this study?
2. What is the study design? Why is this type of design effective for this

research problem? Describe the methods used.
3. What are the results?
4. Discuss the implications of this study to practice and quality improvement?

# EVOLVING CASE STUDY

You have been working for 4 years on a medical unit with 20 beds. You serve as the unit's CQI representative, working with the nurse manager and the entire staff to improve care. During a meeting with the nurse manager, you are reviewing the data from the last 6-month patient satisfaction survey that you are routinely sent by the QI program. Both of you are concerned about a 10% decrease in patient satisfaction, particularly noting problems with patient education and staff sharing information with patients, such as lack of information about medications. This CQI information is shared in the next unit staff meeting. Staff decide more data on the issue should be examined and then they will determine strategies to improve. All of the staff agree to immediately focus more on sharing information with patients and families.

## Case Questions
1. What other data should be reviewed?
2. What specific measures/indicators should be used to track this problem?
3. What specific strategies should be used to engage the patients in their care?

# References

American Nurses Association (ANA). (2015a). *Code of ethics for nurses with interpretive statements*. Silver Spring, MD: Author.

American Nurses Association (ANA). (2015b). *Nursing scope and standards of practice* (3rd ed.). Silver Spring, MD: Author.

Balik, B., Conway, J., Zipperer, L., & Watson, J. (2011). *Achieving an exceptional patient and family experience of inpatient hospital care*. IHI Innovation Series White Paper. Cambridge, MA: Institute for Healthcare Improvement.

Banja, J. (2005). *Medical errors and medical narcissism*. Sudbury, MA: Jones & Bartlett Publishers.

Banja, J., & Amori, G. (2005). The emphathic disclosure of medical error. In J. Banja (Ed.), *Medical errors and medical narcissim* (pp. 173–192). Sudbury, MA: Jones & Bartlett Publishers.

Bau, I., Logan, R., Dezii, C., Rosof, B., Fernandez, A., Paasche-Orlow, M., and Wong, W. (2019). Paient-centered, integrated health care quality measures could improve health literacy, language access, and cultural competence. *NAM Perspectives*. Discussion Paper, National Academy of Medicine, Washington, DC. Retrieved from https://nam.edu/patient-centered-integrated-health-care-quality-measures-could-improve-health-literacy-language-access-and-cultural-competence

Berwick, D. (2009). What "patient-centered" should mean: Confessions of an extremist. *Health Affairs, 28*(4), w555–w565.

Carayon, P., Hoonakker, P., Cartmill, R., & Hassol, A. (2015). Using health information technology (IT) in practice redesign: Impact of health IT on workflow. Patient-reported health information technology and workflow. (Prepared by ABT Associates under Contract No. 290-2010-00031I). AHRQ Publication No. 15-0043-EF. Rockville, MD: Agency for Healthcare Research and Quality.

Chimowitz, H., Gerard, M., Fossa, A., Bourgeois, F., & Bell, S. (2018). Empowering information caregivers with health information: OpenNotes as a safety strategy. *Joint Commission Journal Quality and Safety, 44*(3), 130–136.

Craig, C., Eby, D., & Whittington, J. (2011). Care coordination model: Better care at lower cost for people with multiple health and social needs. Institute for Healthcare Improvement Innovation Series White Paper. Cambridge, MA: Institute for Health Improvement.

e-Caregiving Solutions. (2019). E-Caregiving. Retrieved from http://www.e-caregiving.com

Finkelman, A. (2019). *Professional nursing concepts: Competencies for quality leadership* (4th ed.). Burlington, MA: Jones & Bartlett Learning.

Fisher, K., Smith, K., Gallagher, Burns, L., Morales, C., & Mazor, K. (2017). We want to know: Eliciting hospitalized patients' perspectives on breakdowns in care. *Journal of Hospital Medicine, 12*(8), 603–609.

Fowler, F., Levin, C., & Sepucha, K. (2011). Informing and involving patients to improve the quality of medical decisions. *Health Affairs, 30*(4), 699–706.

Gallagher, T., Garbutt, J., Waterman, A., Flum, D., Larson, E., Waterman, B., . . . Levinson, W. (2006). Choosing your words carefully: How physicians would disclose harmful medical errors to patients. *Archives of Internal Medicine, 166*(15), 1585–1593.

Gerteis, M., Edgman-Levitan, S., Daley, J., & Delbanco, T. (2002). Introduction: Medicine and health from the patient's perspective. In M. Gerteis, S. Edgman-Levitan, & J. Daley. (Eds.), *Through the patient's eyes: Understanding and promoting patient-centered care* (pp. 1–18). Hoboken, NJ: Wiley Publishing Company.

Graber, M. (2014). Diagnostic error: 10 things you could do tomorrow. Lists for physicians, healthcare organizations, and patients. *Inside Medical Liability* (first quarter), 22–26. Retrieved from https://flbog.sip .ufl.edu/risk-rx-article/minimizing-diagnostic-error -10-things-you-could-do-tomorrow-lists-for-physicians -patients-and-healthcare-organizations

Institute for Patient- and Family-Centered Care. (IPFCC). (2019). Partnering with patients and families to enhance safety and quality. About us. Retrieved from https://ipfcc.org/about/index.html

Institute of Medicine (IOM). (2001). *Crossing the quality chasm*. Washington, DC: The National Academies Press.

Institute of Medicine (IOM). (2003). *Health professions education: A bridge to quality*. Washington, DC: The National Academies Press.

Johnson, B., Abraham, M., Conway, J., Simmons, L., Edgman-Levitan, S., Sodomka, P., . . . Ford, D. (2008). *Partnering with patients and families to design a patient- and family-centered healthcare system*. Bethesda, MD: Institute of Family-Centered Care in collaboration with the Institute for Health Improvement.

McGowan, P. (2005). Self-management: A background paper. University of Victoria: Centre on Aging. Retrieved from http://www.selfmanagementbc.ca/uploads /Support%20for%20Health%20Professionals/Self -Management%20support%20a%20background%20 paper%202005.pdf

Mitchell, B., & Begoray, D. (2010). Electronic personal health records that promote self-management in chronic illness. *OJIN, 15*(3). Retrieved from https: //ojin.nursingworld.org/MainMenuCategories/ANA Marketplace/ANAPeriodicals/OJIN/TableofContents /Vol152010/No3-Sept-2010/Articles-Previously-Topic /Electronic-Personal-Health-Records-and-Chronic -Illness.html

National Academy of Medicine (NAM). (2015). *Measuring the impact of interprofessional education on collaborative practice and patient outcomes*. Washington, DC: The National Academies Press.

Patient-Centered Outcomes Research Institute (PCORI). (2019). About us. Retrieved from http://www.pcori .org/about-us

Planetree International. (2018). Who we are. Retrieved from https://www.planetree.org/who-we-are

Prochnow, J., Meiers, S., & Scheckel, M. (2019). Improving patient and caregiver new medication education using an innovative teach-back toolkit. *Journal of Nursing Care Quality, 34*(2), 101–106.

Schwappach, D., Hochreutener, M., & Wernli, M. (2010). Oncology nurses' perceptions about involving patients in the prevention of chemotherapy administration errors. *Oncology Nursing Forum, 37*(2), E84–E91.

Stern, R., & Sarkar, U. (2017). Patient engagement in safety. Retrieved from https://psnet.ahrq.gov/perspective /patient-engagement-

The Joint Commission (2019). Speak Up™. Retrieved from https://www.jointcommission.org/resources/for -consumers/speak-up-campaigns/facts-about-speak-up

U.S. Department of Health and Human Services (HHS), Agency for Healthcare Research and Quality (AHRQ). (2017). Be prepared to be engaged: Intervention Retrieved from https://www.ahrq.gov/patient-safety /reports/engage/interventions/prepared.html

U.S. Department of Health and Human Services (HHS), Agency for Healthcare Research and Quality (AHRQ). (2018a). Taking care of myself: A guide for when I leave the hospital. Retrieved from https://www .ahrq.gov/patients-consumers/diagnosis-treatment /hospitals-clinics/goinghome/index.html

U.S. Department of Health and Human Services (HHS), Agency for Healthcare Research and Quality (AHRQ). (2018b). Care coordination. Retrieved from https:// www.ahrq.gov/ncepcr/care/coordination.html

U.S. Department of Health and Human Services (HHS), Agency for Healthcare Research and Quality (AHRQ). (2019a). QuestionBuilder app. Retrieved from https:// www.ahrq.gov/patient-safety/question-builder/index .html

U.S. Department of Health and Human Services (HHS), Agency for Healthcare Research and Quality (AHRQ). (2019b). Tips & tools: Questions are the answers. Retrieved from https://www.ahrq.gov/patients-consumers /patient-involvement/ask-your-doctor/tips-and-tools /index.html

U.S. Department of Health and Human Services (HHS), Agency for Healthcare Research and Quality (AHRQ), Consumer Assessment of Healthcare Providers and Systems (CAHPS). (2019). About CAHPS®. Retrieved from https://www.ahrq.gov/cahps/about-cahps/index .html

U.S. Department of Health and Human Services (HHS), Agency for Healthcare Research and Quality. (AHRQ), Patient Safety Network (PSNet). (2019a). Patient safety primer: Disclosure of errors. Retrieved from https://psnet.ahrq.gov/primer/disclosure-errors

U.S. Department of Health and Human Services (HHS), Agency for Healthcare Research and Quality (AHRQ), Patient Safety Network (PSNet). (2019b). Patient engagement and safety. Retrieved from https://psnet .ahrq.gov/primer/patient-engagement-and-safety

U.S. Department of Health and Human Services (HHS), Agency for Healthcare Research and Quality (AHRQ), Patient Safety Network (PSNet). (2019c). Health literacy universal precautions toolkit, 2nd Edition: Use the teachback method: Tool #5. Retrieved from https:// www.ahrq.gov/health-literacy/quality-resources/tools /literacy-toolkit/healthlittoolkit2-tool5.html

U.S. Department of Health and Human Services (HHS), Centers for Medicare and Medicaid (CMS). (2019a). CMS releases care coordination toolkit for Medicare ACOs. Retrieved from https://www.aha.org/news/headline/2019-04-11-cms-releases-care-coordination-toolkit-medicare-acos

U.S. Department of Health and Human Services (HHS), Centers for Medicare and Medicaid (CMS). (2019b). Welcome to the partnership for patients. Retrieved from https://partnershipforpatients.cms.gov

U.S. Department of Health and Human Services (HHS), Centers for Medicare and Medicaid (CMS). (2019c). Quality improvement organizations. Retrieved from www.cms.hhs.gov/qualityimprovementorgs

U.S. Department of Health and Human Services (HHS), National Prevention, Health Promotion, and Public Health Council. (2011). National prevention strategy. Washington, DC: Retrieved from https://www.hhs.gov/sites/default/files/disease-prevention-wellness-report.pdf

U.S. Department of Health and Human Services (HHS), Office of Civil Rights Headquarters (OCR). (2019). Health information privacy. Retrieved from https://www.hhs.gov/hipaa/index.html

U.S. Department of Health and Human Services (HHS), Office of Disease Prevention and Health Promotion (ODPHP), National Prevention, Health Promotion, and Public Health Council. (2020). Healthy aging in action. Retrieved from https://www.hhs.gov/sites/default/files/healthy-aging-in-action-final.pdf

Zimmerman, P. (2001). The problems with healthcare customer satisfaction surveys. In J. Dochterman & H. Grace (Eds.), *Current issues in nursing* (6th ed.), pp. 255–260). St. Louis, MO: Mosby.

## CHAPTER 7

# Quality and Safety: Basic Understanding

## CHAPTER OBJECTIVES

At the conclusion of this chapter, the learner will be able to:

- Examine key models, types, and risks related to errors.
- Analyze the impact of staffing levels and workloads on outcomes.
- Examine frontline safety as an element of healthcare safety.
- Explain how human factors impact healthcare quality.
- Discuss workplace safety and implications for continuous quality improvement.

## OUTLINE

## KEY TERMS

| | | |
|---|---|---|
| Active error | Latent conditions | Red rules |
| Adverse event | Latent error | Root cause analysis |
| Bullying | Lateral violence | Sentinel event |
| Compassion fatigue | Mental fatigue | Slip |
| Errors of execution | Missed care | Standardization |
| Errors of planning | Mistake | Stress |
| Frontline safety | Misuse | Swiss cheese model |
| Frontline staff | Near miss | Technical failure |
| Human error | Omission | Underuse |
| Human factors and ergonomics | Organizational failure | Workplace mobbing |
| Human failure | Overuse | Workplace violence |
| Incivility | Physical fatigue | |
| Lapse | Presenteeism | |

# Introduction

According to Classen and colleagues (2011), "Identification and measurement of adverse medical events is central to patient safety, forming a foundation of accountability, prioritizing problems to work on, generating ideas for safer care, and testing which interventions work" (p. 581). The healthcare system has been undergoing major transformation to address the critical need to improve care. Are frontline nursing staff ready for this focus on continuous quality improvement (CQI)? In many cases, they are not. How are staff nurses, nurse managers, and advanced practice registered nurses (APRNs) participating in CQI? As noted in other chapters, nursing education must assume some of the responsibility to ensure that nurses are better prepared to engage in CQI. We need to recognize that good care should be based on good science (Larkin, Lorenz, Rack, & Shatzer, 2012). This insight applies to all the content in this text. Evidence-based practice

(EBP) and management is a critical theme and, when used, increases the opportunity to reach effective outcomes.

The landmark report *Keeping Patients Safe: Transforming the Work Environment for Nurses* (Institute of Medicine [IOM], 2004) indicated that the work nurses do has a major impact on quality care, but the work environment must be improved so that nurses can effectively meet patient outcomes. Hughes and Clancy (2005) state the following in response to this critical report that continues to influence nursing and quality improvement: "Caring for patients relies heavily on human decision-making and action. Nurses are vulnerable to being part of errors because the process of patient care leaves them exposed to the inevitable results of human fallibilities that occur throughout the entire process of care, the complexity of health care, or a combination thereof" (p. 289).

This chapter expands the discussion about CQI by examining errors and factors that impact the occurrence of errors. It is important to understand this content before examining CQI measurement and responses to quality problems and errors. We need to view CQI as an opportunity to improve work and outcomes.

# Understanding Errors

Understanding errors requires in-depth examination of the types and causes along with strategies to prevent and respond when errors occur. Nurses need to be involved in all aspects of this effort to improve and reduce errors.

## Models Used to Understand Errors

There are many models that healthcare organizations (HCOs) and the government might apply to understanding errors. The following discussion focuses on three of the more commonly used models.

### The Swiss Cheese Model

Reason's work on errors is a model that is frequently used (Reason, 2000). This model is called the **Swiss cheese model**. It focuses on system failure and recognizes that there is potential for errors in any process. Reason compared this situation to a stack of slices of Swiss cheese. The holes in the slices are opportunities for errors, and all processes have them, just like all slices of Swiss cheese have holes. The slices represent defenses to prevent errors. Sometimes an error goes through a hole, yet there is no serious problem or harm because the next slice prevents the error from passing further, thus avoiding a major problem or error. When the holes are aligned, an error may go straight through consecutive slices, and a major error occurs. The Agency for Healthcare Research and Quality (AHRQ) describes the model as follows: "[E]rrors made by individuals result in disastrous consequences due to flawed systems—the holes in the cheese. This model has not only tremendous explanatory power but it also helps point the way toward solutions—encouraging

personnel to try to identify the holes and to both shrink their size and create enough overlap so that they never line up in the future" (HHS, AHRQ, PSNet, 2019a).

In healthcare it is recognized that some errors are not acceptable, such as operating on the wrong site or wrong person. Such incidents represent times when the holes align, which is infrequent. As discussed elsewhere in this text, an emphasis on the system is of growing concern to CQI. Reason and others have also noted the importance of system problems, as the AHRQ articulates: "Many of the system problems discussed by Reason and others—poorly designed work schedules, lack of teamwork, variations in the design of important equipment between and even within institutions—are sufficiently common that many of the slices of cheese already have their holes aligned. In such cases, one slice of cheese may be all that is left between the patient and significant hazard" (HHS, AHRQ, PSNet, 2019a). Healthcare organizations (HCOs) may use failure modes and effects analysis (FMEA) as one method to analyze failure modes or error-prone situations, and this method is discussed in this text. The Connect to Current Information section at the end of this chapter provides a link to figures that illustrate the Swiss cheese model.

### Enthoven Classification of Causes of Errors

Another example of a model for understanding and responding to errors such as near misses is the Enthoven model. This model focuses on three sources of errors and is described in **Figure 7-1** (Henneman et al., 2010; Henneman & Gawlinski, 2004):

1. **Technical failure** or *active error, a system failure*. Examples of related factors are physical equipment not available or not working adequately and computer and software availability.
2. **Organizational failure** or *latent error, a system failure*. Examples of related factors

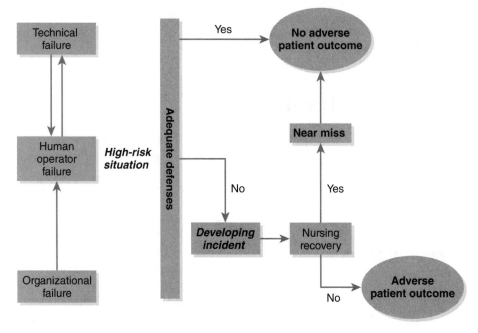

**Figure 7-1** Near-Miss Model

Reproduced from Henneman, E., & Gawlinski, A. (2004). A "near-miss" model for describing the nurse's role in the recovery of medical errors. *Journal of Professional Nursing, 20*(3), 196–201. Copyright 2004, with permission from Elsevier.

are staff orientation and training, policies, procedures, and use of clinical pathways or protocols. Enthoven also combined technical and organizational error and referred to these dynamics as latent error or condition.

3. **Human failure** or *individual failure*. Examples of related factors are staff knowledge and competencies. This type of error is also referred to as an *active failure*.

Enthoven also included a category he called "other" for errors that did not fall into his major error categories.

An effective CQI system provides defenses for responding when a risk situation occurs that could result in an error. If the defense works, then there is no error; however, if the defense does not work, then an error may be in process. It is at this time that nursing recovery may stop the error and thus a near miss may occur, in which case there is no adverse patient outcome. What this means is that

the nurse or other staff involved in direct care identifies, interrupts, and corrects the error. This intervention on the part of the nurse is a critical aspect of improving care and one that each nurse needs to apply in practice.

## Generic Error-Modeling System

Reason also developed the generic error-modeling system (GEMS) to pinpoint key concerns when examining errors. He notes that there seem to be several common types of errors. **Human error** is "a generic term to encompass all those occasions in which a planned sequence of mental or physical activities fails to achieve its intended outcome, and when these failures cannot be attributed to the intervention of some chance agency" (Reason, 1990, p. 7). The following error types are identified in the GEMS model (Van Metre, Slovensky, & McLaughlin, 2013):

- *Skill-based performance* is directed by the individual's education and expertise.

- *Rule-based performance* occurs when there are "familiar problems in which solutions are governed by stored rules of the 'if-then' type. These rules are based on previous experiences and are called into play when a trigger event or situation occurs" (p. 317). An example would be a cardiac arrest procedure that is not applied correctly.
- *Knowledge-based performance* occurs in situations that require the provider to think about what needs to be done and how best to do it. In this case, planning errors may occur.

Classification of an error begins with determining if the error results from action or inaction. If inaction, then there is little, if any, physical evidence, and often the event is not viewed as an error and thus not reported as one. Inaction errors may be of two types: knowledge based and rule based. If the error is an action error, then one has to determine if it is related to planning, execution, or intention. Most errors fall into the area of execution. For both planning and execution errors, the GEMS type of performance error is identified. Intention may also be a concern and is related to violations, such as staff not following a procedure in order to reduce their work time. Individual accountability is important in this category; even though systems are emphasized, there are circumstances in which accountability and blame are considered as errors and are assessed.

## Types of Errors

There are many different types of errors. As noted in other chapters, an error is "the failure of a planned action to be completed as intended or the use of [a] wrong plan to achieve an aim" (IOM, 1999, p. 28). Broadly, errors can be described as **errors of planning** (e.g., including the wrong intervention in a plan for a patient.); this may also be referred to as an *error of judgment*. Care begins with the patient, and the provider uses knowledge and expertise along with clinical judgment and reasoning to plan care and implement that plan. Anywhere in the process errors can occur and are referred to as **errors of execution** (e.g., using an intervention at the wrong time.). The most frequent error is leaving a step out of a planned sequence of activities (Gawande, 2010; Reason, 2002).

HCO management and staff may focus so much on avoiding failure or errors that they become preoccupied with this step rather than considering the full picture and developing effective response strategies (Clark & Bramble, 2013). It is not uncommon for managers and staff to ignore the smaller errors and even to view them as disruptions and nothing more. This scenario then is a lost opportunity to learn more about potential errors. For example, a nurse takes the wrong intravenous fluids to the patient's room and realizes they are the wrong fluids, requiring a search for the correct fluids. Even as the nurse is complaining about how long this is taking, the nurse may be ignoring or may not understand that this is a near miss that should be analyzed to determine why the wrong fluids were selected. Was the order not clear? Was the label on the fluid wrong or difficult to read? Was the storage area confusing, making it easy to select the wrong item? Did the nurse read or interpret the order incorrectly because she is at the end of a long shift—exhausted, stressed, preoccupied? Was the nurse interrupted and distracted from what she was doing? Finally, what made the nurse stop and realize the wrong fluids had been selected? **Figure 7-2** identifies some of the types of medical errors.

### Underuse, Overuse, Misuse

Three common types of errors are underuse, overuse, and misuse, and all are found in a variety of HCO settings and may involve a variety of staff (Finkelman, 2019):

- **Underuse**. This error is a failure to provide a service that would have produced a favorable outcome for the patient. It may

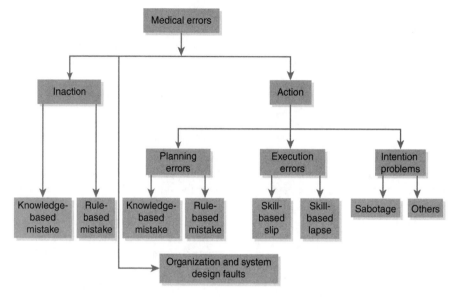

**Figure 7-2** Potential Classification of Human Medical Errors

Reproduced from Van Metre, J., Slovensky, D., & McLaughlin, C. (2013). Classification of medical errors. In *McLaughlin & Kaluzny's Continuous quality improvement in health care*, (4th ed., pp. 312–334). Burlington, MA: Jones & Bartlett Learning.

be due to lack of access to needed services or resources that are recognized as important in meeting the outcomes (Sadeghi, Barzi, Mikhail, & Shabot, 2013). Example: The patient is not able to get specialty service needed for cancer treatment because of the distance from resources, or the patient's insurer will not cover a medication for arthritis that could make the patient more mobile.

- **Misuse**. This error is an avoidable event that prevents patients from receiving the full potential benefit of a service. Misuse may relate to incorrect diagnoses, medical errors, or avoidable complications (Sadeghi et al., 2013). Example: The patient receives a medication that is not prescribed and conflicts with the patient's allergies; the patient experiences anaphylaxis.
- **Overuse**. This error occurs when the potential for harm from the provision of a service exceeds the possible benefit. In this situation, risks outweigh benefits (Sadeghi et al., 2013). Example: An elderly patient is on multiple medications, and

the patient's multiple healthcare providers do not know the medications that have been prescribed by different specialists. Overuse can result in several negative outcomes. The most obvious is cost. If more services are provided than needed, healthcare costs may increase. Other examples of possible problems are overtesting, overdiagnosis, and overtreatment, all of which may increase risk for patient harm such as more risk for complications and more opportunities for errors (Gawande, 2015, p. 384).

### Active Errors

An **active error** is an error that results from noncompliance with a procedure that involves a frontline worker (i.e., direct care worker). Another term that refers to this type of error is *error at the sharp end*. *Sharp end* refers to staff or parts of the system that come in direct contact with the patient, while the *blunt end* refers to factors that impact the sharp end. Active errors are errors that are obvious, or at the sharp end.

## Latent Errors

**Latent errors** are associated with errors that are caused by system problems or **latent conditions** that then impact a frontline worker and are less apparent failures. Latent conditions are not immediately apparent: "[T]he blunt end refers to the many layers of the health care system not in direct contact with patients, but which influence the personnel and equipment at the sharp end that come into contact with patients. The blunt end thus consists of those who set policy, manage healthcare institutions, or design medical devices, and other people and forces, which—though removed in time and space from direct patient care—nonetheless affect how care is delivered" (HHS, AHRQ, PSNet, 2019a). There are two of latent errors types: slips and mistakes (HHS, AHRQ, PSNet, 2019a). A **slip** happens when something is not clear. For example, the nurse may write the wrong date and time because she is not focused on what she is doing, or she may have lapses in concentration, often due to sensory or emotional distractions, fatigue, or stress. A **lapse** happens when the nurse fails to check something that is part of the procedure, something that should be monitored during implementation of a procedure. **Mistakes** relate to wrong decisions, often associated with inexperience, inadequate training, or even negligence. For example, we practice and learn how to do a procedure, and nurses might then experience a lapse or a slip. Another example might be when staff are not informed about a change in a procedure. Staff then do not follow the new procedure, and an error occurs. Factors that may lead to latent errors are identified in **Table 7-1**.

**Table 7-1** Factors That May Lead to Latent Errors

| Type of Factor | Example |
|---|---|
| Institutional/regulatory | The hospital was under regulatory pressure to improve pneumococcal vaccination rates. |
| Organizational/ management | A nurse detected a medication error, but the physician discouraged her from reporting it. |
| Work environment | Lacking the appropriate equipment to perform hysteroscopy, operating room staff improvised using equipment from other sets. During the procedure, the patient suffered an air embolism. |
| Team environment | A surgeon completed an operation despite being informed by a nurse and the anesthesiologist that the suction catheter tip was missing. The tip was subsequently found inside the patient, requiring additional surgery. |
| Staffing | An overworked nurse mistakenly administered insulin instead of an anti-nausea medication, resulting in hypoglycemic coma. |
| Task related | An intern incorrectly calculated the equivalent dose of long-acting MS Contin® for a patient who had been receiving Vicodin®. The patient experienced an opiate overdose and aspiration pneumonia, resulting in prolonged care on the intensive care unit. |
| Patient characteristics | The parents of a young boy misread the instructions on a bottle of acetaminophen, causing their child to experience liver damage. |

Reproduced with permission from AHRQ Patient Safety Network, Ranji, S., Wachter, R., & Hartman, E. (2014). Patient safety primer: Root cause analysis. Retrieved from https://psnet.ahrq.gov/primers/primer/10.

## Near Misses

A **near miss**, a common occurrence, is a situation during which an error almost happened, but staff caught it before it became an error. Near misses should not be ignored, as much can be learned from them. This is a weak area of monitoring, with many HCOs not tracking near misses, staff not reporting them, or staff and management not even knowing they occurred.

## Adverse Events

An **adverse event** is an injury resulting from a medical intervention, not from the patient's underlying condition. It is an untoward, undesirable event, usually not expected, and it may have a long-term effect. This event may be due to errors or be preventable. The World Health Organization (WHO) identifies the following as situations of greatest burden of harm (2019):

- Medication errors
- Healthcare-associated infections
- Unsafe surgical care procedures
- Unsafe injection practices
- Diagnostic errors
- Unsafe transfusion practices
- Radiation errors
- Sepsis
- Venous thromboembolism

Though the situations/factors listed here are the most common, adverse events can happen during any number of other situations. Causes of adverse events are also broad, and the following areas have greater potential for an adverse event outcome:

- Care planning
- Communication
- Continuum of care
- Coordination and collaboration
- Human factors
- Health information management
- Organization culture

- Patient assessment
- Patient identification
- Patient involvement and education
- Inadequate physical resources

Root cause analysis, discussed in other chapters, is often used to identify and understand causes and may result in identifying multiple causes.

If the adverse event is related to drugs or medical equipment and the event is serious, it should be reported to the Food and Drug Administration (FDA) when the patient outcome is any of the following (HHS, FDA, 2016):

- *Death.* Report if you suspect that the death was an outcome of an adverse event, and if known, include the date of the event.
- *Life threatening.* Report if it is suspected the patient was at substantial risk of dying at the time of the adverse event, or report if use or continued use of a device or other medical product might have resulted in the death of the patient.
- *Hospitalization (initial or prolonged).* Report if admission to the hospital or prolongation of hospitalization was a result of an adverse event. Emergency room visits that do not result in admission to the hospital should also be evaluated for one of the other serious outcomes (e.g., life threatening, required intervention to prevent permanent impairment or damage, other serious medically important event).
- *Disability or permanent damage.* Report if an adverse event resulted in substantial disruption of a person's ability to conduct normal life functions (e.g., a significant, persistent or permanent change, impairment, damage, or disruption in the patient's body function/structure, physical activities, and/or quality of life).
- *Congenital anomaly/birth defect.* Report if you suspect that exposure to a medical product prior to conception or during pregnancy may have resulted in an adverse outcome in the child.

- *Required intervention to prevent permanent impairment or damage (devices).* Report if you believe that a medical or surgical intervention was necessary to preclude permanent impairment of a body function or prevent permanent damage to a body structure; report if either situation is suspected to be due to the use of a medical product.
- *Other serious outcome (important medical events).* Report when the event does not fit the other outcomes, but the event may jeopardize the patient and may require medical or surgical intervention (treatment) to prevent one of the other outcomes. Examples include allergic bronchospasm requiring treatment in an emergency department, serious blood dyscrasias, seizures/convulsions that do not result in hospitalization, or the development of drug dependence.

**Table 7-2** provides additional examples of serious reportable events as identified by the National Quality Forum.

**Table 7-2** List of National Quality Forum Serious Reportable Events (SREs)

### 1. Surgical events

**1A. Surgery or other invasive procedure performed on the wrong site (updated)**
Applicable in: hospitals, outpatient/office-based surgery centers, ambulatory practice settings /office-based practices, long-term care/skilled nursing facilities

**1B. Surgery or other invasive procedure performed on the wrong patient (updated)**
Applicable in: hospitals, outpatient/office-based surgery centers, ambulatory practice settings /office-based practices, long-term care/skilled nursing facilities

**1C. Wrong surgical or other invasive procedure performed on a patient (updated)**
Applicable in: hospitals, outpatient/office-based surgery centers, ambulatory practice settings /office-based practices, long-term care/skilled nursing facilities

**1D. Unintended retention of a foreign object in a patient after surgery or other invasive procedure (updated)**
Applicable in: hospitals, outpatient/office-based surgery centers, ambulatory practice settings /office-based practices, long-term care/skilled nursing facilities

**1E. Intraoperative or immediately postoperative/postprocedure death in an ASA Class 1 patient (updated)**
Applicable in: hospitals, outpatient/office-based surgery centers, ambulatory practice settings /office-based practices

### 2. Product or device events

**2A. Patient death or serious injury associated with the use of contaminated drugs, devices, or biologics provided by the healthcare setting (updated)**
Applicable in: hospitals, outpatient/office-based surgery centers, ambulatory practice settings /office-based practices, long-term care/skilled nursing facilities

**2B. Patient death or serious injury associated with the use or function of a device in patient care, in which the device is used or functions other than as intended (updated)**
Applicable in: hospitals, outpatient/office-based surgery centers, ambulatory practice settings /office-based practices, long-term care/skilled nursing facilities

**2C. Patient death or serious injury associated with intravascular air embolism that occurs while being cared for in a healthcare setting (updated)**
Applicable in: hospitals, outpatient/office-based surgery centers, long-term care/skilled nursing facilities

*(continues)*

**Table 7-2** List of National Quality Forum Serious Reportable Events (SREs) *(continued)*

### 3. Patient protection events

**3A. Discharge or release of a patient/resident of any age, who is unable to make decisions to other than an authorized person (updated)**
Applicable in: hospitals, outpatient/office-based surgery centers, ambulatory practice settings /office-based practices, long-term care/skilled nursing facilities

**3B. Patient death or serious injury associated with patient elopement (disappearance) (updated)**
Applicable in: hospitals, outpatient/office-based surgery centers, ambulatory practice settings /office-based practices, long-term care/skilled nursing facilities

**3C. Patient suicide, attempted suicide, or self-harm that results in serious injury, while being cared for in a healthcare setting (updated)**
Applicable in: hospitals, outpatient/office-based surgery centers, ambulatory practice settings /office-based practices, long-term care/skilled nursing facilities

### 4. Care management events

**4A. Patient death or serious injury associated with a medication error (e.g., errors involving the wrong drug, wrong dose, wrong patient, wrong time, wrong rate, wrong preparation, or wrong route of administration) (updated)**
Applicable in: hospitals, outpatient/office-based surgery centers, ambulatory practice settings /office-based practices, long-term care/skilled nursing facilities

**4B. Patient death or serious injury associated with unsafe administration of blood products (updated)**
Applicable in: hospitals, outpatient/office-based surgery centers, ambulatory practice settings /office-based practices, long-term care/skilled nursing facilities

**4C. Maternal death or serious injury associated with labor or delivery in a low-risk pregnancy while being cared for in a healthcare setting (updated)**
Applicable in: hospitals, outpatient/office-based surgery centers

**4D. Death or serious injury of a neonate associated with labor or delivery in a low-risk pregnancy (new)**
Applicable in: hospitals, outpatient/office-based surgery centers

**4E. Patient death or serious injury associated with a fall while being cared for in a healthcare setting (updated)**
Applicable in: hospitals, outpatient/office-based surgery centers, ambulatory practice settings /office-based practices, long-term care/skilled nursing facilities

**4F. Any Stage 3, Stage 4, and unstageable pressure ulcers acquired after admission/presentation to a healthcare setting (updated)**
Applicable in: hospitals, outpatient/office-based surgery centers, long-term care/skilled nursing facilities

**4G. Artificial insemination with the wrong donor sperm or wrong egg (updated)**
Applicable in: hospitals, outpatient/office-based surgery centers, ambulatory practice settings /office-based practices

**4H. Patient death or serious injury resulting from the irretrievable loss of an irreplaceable biological specimen (new)**
Applicable in: hospitals, outpatient/office-based surgery centers, ambulatory practice settings /office-based practices, long-term care/skilled nursing facilities

**4I. Patient death or serious injury resulting from failure to follow up or communicate laboratory, pathology, or radiology test results (new)**
Applicable in: hospitals, outpatient/office-based surgery centers, ambulatory practice settings /office-based practices, long-term care/skilled nursing facilities

## 5. Environmental events

**5A. Patient or staff death or serious injury associated with an electric shock in the course of a patient care process in a healthcare setting (updated)**
Applicable in: hospitals, outpatient/office-based surgery centers, ambulatory practice settings /office-based practices, long-term care/skilled nursing facilities

**5B. Any incident in which systems designated for oxygen or other gas to be delivered to a patient contains no gas, the wrong gas, or are contaminated by toxic substances (updated)**
Applicable in: hospitals, outpatient/office-based surgery centers, ambulatory practice settings /office-based practices, long-term care/skilled nursing facilities

**5C. Patient or staff death or serious injury associated with a burn incurred from any source in the course of a patient care process in a healthcare setting (updated)**
Applicable in: hospitals, outpatient/office-based surgery centers, ambulatory practice settings /office-based practices, long-term care/skilled nursing facilities

**5D. Patient death or serious injury associated with the use of physical restraints or bedrails while being cared for in a healthcare setting (updated)**
Applicable in: hospitals, outpatient/office-based surgery centers, ambulatory practice settings /office-based practices, long-term care/skilled nursing facilities

## 6. Radiological events

**6A. Death or serious injury of a patient or staff associated with the introduction of a metallic object into the MRI area (new)**
Applicable in: hospitals, outpatient/office-based surgery centers, ambulatory practice settings /office-based practices

## 7. Potential criminal events

**7A. Any instance of care ordered by or provided by someone impersonating a physician, nurse, pharmacist, or other licensed healthcare provider (updated)**
Applicable in: hospitals, outpatient/office-based surgery centers, ambulatory practice settings /office-based practices, long-term care/skilled nursing facilities

**7B. Abduction of a patient/resident of any age (updated)**
Applicable in: hospitals, outpatient/office-based surgery centers, ambulatory practice settings /office-based practices, long-term care/skilled nursing facilities

**7C. Sexual abuse/assault on a patient or staff member within or on the grounds of a healthcare setting (updated)**
Applicable in: hospitals, outpatient/office-based surgery centers, ambulatory practice settings /office-based practices, long-term care/skilled nursing facilities

**7D. Death or serious injury of a patient or staff member resulting from a physical assault (i.e., battery) that occurs within or on the grounds of a healthcare setting (updated)**
Applicable in: hospitals, outpatient/office-based surgery centers, ambulatory practice settings /office-based practices, long-term care/skilled nursing facilities

National Quality Forum (2020). Serious SREs. Retrieved from http://www.qualityforum.org/Topics/SREs/List_of_SREs.aspx

## *Sentinel Events and Alerts*

**Sentinel events** are unexpected events that happen to patients and result in major negative outcomes, such as an unexpected death or a critical physical or psychological complication that can lead to major alteration in the patient's health. The term "sentinel" is used for these events because the events indicate the need for immediate response and analysis (The Joint Commission, 2019). Examples of sentinel events are suicide, wrong-site surgery, and serious operative and postoperative complications. These events may be quite unique and unexpected. For example, in 2016 in a pediatric hospital, parents of a hospitalized baby took heroin in their baby's hospital room. One parent died in the room, and the other required medical treatment. The father had a gun in his pocket (Seelye, 2016). This is not a typical event, and it put the parents at risk as well as their baby, other patients and their families, and the staff. This type of event requires immediate response and analysis to ensure safety of all along with long-term response to prevent similar occurrences. Factors that should be assessed in the analysis include the status of the pediatric patient admission assessment, including the parents, and the presence of active surveillance so that changes in behavior might have been noticed. Guns in hospitals are a major risk, although most hospitals in the United States do not have security that would identify when guns are brought in. Psychiatric hospitals are usually more alert to drugs and weapons and consider bringing them into a hospital a sentinel event.

Not all errors are sentinel events, but when errors are sentinel events, they should not be ignored. It is also important that staff involved in a sentinel event get support. It can be extremely traumatic and lead to staff experiencing physiological and psychological problems (The Joint Commission, 2019). A systematic review of studies indicates that there are a high number of second victims (staff) from errors, with data identifying more than two-thirds of staff from 98 studies experiencing bad memories of the event, anger, remorse, and distress (Busch et al., 2019).

The Joint Commission distributes sentinel alerts to its accredited HCOs and identifies them on its website. The alerts are classified based on the type of healthcare site and information provided to The Joint Commission for review. When HCOs report these events, information should include a plan identifying action(s) the HCO will take, as well as responsibilities, timelines, and strategies for evaluation and sustaining the change. The plan is, of course, useful to the individual HCO, but it also provides important data that can be used to alert other HCOs about potential risks and possible responses (Sorbello, 2008; The Joint Commission, 2019). **Root cause analysis** is used to analyze sentinel events to better understand events and steps that might be taken to respond to and prevent these events. All of these efforts provide opportunities for HCOs and healthcare providers to learn more about the trajectory of care. Many HCOs then benefit from self-reporting to The Joint Commission in the following ways (The Joint Commission, 2019):

- Allows The Joint Commission to provide support and expertise during the review of a sentinel event.
- Enables collaboration with a patient safety expert in The Joint Commission's Sentinel Event Unit of the Office of Quality and Patient Safety.
- Raises the level of transparency in the organization and promotes a culture of safety.
- Conveys the HCO's message to the public that it is doing everything possible, proactively, to prevent similar patient safety events in the future.

### Omissions and Missed Care

Errors may also be classified as **omissions**. This type of error occurs when effective assessment, planning, and interventions are not provided, and it may lead to problems for the patient and interfere with reaching expected outcomes. Nurses care for many patients and have many responsibilities, all of which can lead even the best practice to errors of omission (Kalisch, 2015). Research indicates that some of the common reasons for omissions are communication problems, difficulties getting material resources, such as supplies or equipment that are not available when needed, unavailability of needed drugs, equipment not working effectively, and inadequate staffing (Kalisch, Landstrom, & Williams, 2008).

**Missed care** is not something nurses typically consider, but it is omission of care and should also be considered an error. Nursing care that is delayed, partially completed, or not completed is missed care (HHS, AHRQ, PSNet, 2019a). This is the opposite of commission of an error when a a mistake is made. A missed care event is associated with higher rates of adverse events and lower patient satisfaction (Jones, Hamilton, & Murray, 2015). This event is primarily identified by staff self-report and patient report. The AHRQ reports that in a review of 42 studies, 55 to 95% of nurse respondents reported missed care for one or more items (HHS, AHRQ, PSNet, 2019a). Factors that increase risk for missed nursing care are ineffective culture of safety; high nursing workload and staffing that does not meet the need (Dabney & Kalisch, 2016), such as high patient-to-nurse ratio, resource inadequacy; and overall problems with work environment (Ball, Murrells, Rafferty, Morrow, & Griffiths, 2014). Ineffective teamwork between nurses may also lead to missed nursing care (Kalisch & Lee, 2010). In summary, the AHRQ notes that there are several predictors of missed care (HHS, AHRQ, PSNet, 2019a):

- Missed nursing care is primarily a problem of time pressure, competing demands, and adequate nurse staffing needed to prevent it.
- Organizational and unit culture influence missed nursing care.
- The organization of nursing work and the organization of the supply chain that supports nursing work may contribute to preventing missed care.

With concern about missed nursing care, some nurse experts developed a model of missed nursing care that is based on the structure-process-outcome framework (also described by others as "unfinished nursing care" and "care left undone") (HHS, AHRQ, PSNet, 2019a; Kalisch, 2015; Kalisch, Landstrom, & Williams, 2008; Kalisch, Xie, & Dabney, 2014). When assessing missed nursing care, staff need to examine structure factors, such as labor resources (e.g., number and types of nursing staff, nursing staff competence level, staff education and experience), material resources (e.g., availability of necessary medications, supplies, and equipment), and teamwork and communication (e.g., among patient care team members, between nurses and physicians, between nurses and support staff). The model suggests that when one or more of these resources is missing in an organization or during a work period, nurses need to prioritize their care activities, and this may then lead to delayed or omitted nursing care activities. When a nurse has limited resources, the common response is for the nurse to identify priorities; the nurse may then decide to delay care, which may result in omission of care. This decision process is influenced by four individual-level factors (HHS, AHRQ, PSNet, 2019a; Kalisch, Landstrom, & Williams, 2008; Kalisch, Xie, & Dabney, 2014):

1. The nurse's perceptions of team or group norms
2. The nurse's judgment about the importance of various aspects of care relative to the conditions of multiple patients under the care of the nurse
3. The nurse's values, attitudes, and beliefs
4. The nurse's usual practice

## Risk of Errors

Due to the *Quality Chasm* reports on quality, more attention has been placed on risk of errors in order to better understand reasons for errors and also when possible to develop strategies to prevent errors. Communication dysfunction is the number-one risk factor. Poor communication can occur between the healthcare provider and patient, among staff members, between staff and management, or more generally from an organizational perspective. Verbal and written communication that is not clear or timely may lead to error risk. Problems with the flow of information—someone left out of the communication process, for example—increases risk.

Another risk factor is staff preparation. This relates directly to the *Quality Chasm* report, *Health Professions Education* (IOM, 2003) that examined professional education and identified the five healthcare professions core competencies. HCOs need to have competent healthcare providers applying for positions. On the other end, HCOs need to focus on effective orientation for new staff and knowledge transfer and continuing staff education for all levels of staff. Improved knowledge and competence reduce risk of errors. HCO standards, policies, and procedures provide consistency, effective communication, and greater ability to measure care outcomes based on the criteria identified in these documents. These efforts decrease risk.

As healthcare becomes more technical, risk is increasing—not only in the use of informatics but also in the use of complex equipment needed for complex patient care. This equipment needs to be as new as possible and maintained. When working with equipment, staff and patients can be injured. Staff members need to recognize when equipment is not functioning at the level required or when it might cause harm. HCOs need to have experienced staff knowledgeable in the use of medical equipment and provide staff training in effective and safe use of equipment. Maintenance of equipment, both routine and following unexpected malfunctions, is also critical, and access to this assistance should be timely. Another technology-related issue of increasing relevance is use of passwords, which are sometimes required for equipment use, particularly if associated with computers. Timely and easy access to current passwords and methods to obtain passwords in emergencies are necessary to avoid errors and inability to provide care when needed. **Figure 7-3** describes five drivers and related elements that influence clinical quality and patient safety.

**STOP AND CONSIDER 7-1**

There are many types of errors, such as missed care, which many staff may not recognize as an error.

# Staffing Levels, Workloads, and Outcomes

Staffing levels have long been a concern. HCOs need the right staff with the right preparation and experience in positions and need the number of staff required to provide care effectively. **Human factors** are also important to consider in the staffing process. Many HCOs have problems with staffing levels, overscheduling of staff, use of temporary staff, and other staffing challenges that impact knowledge of the situation, consistency, communication, and teamwork. These staffing dynamics all impact the risk of errors. Unit nurse staffing plans must take into consideration all these factors and their impact on the unit's quality improvement. The ANA *Principles for Nurse Staffing* (American Nurses Association [ANA], 2019a) focus on health care consumers in all types of settings, teams, particularly interprofessional, workplace culture and environment, and need for evaluation of staffing to reach effective outcomes.

Some nursing staff and leaders have questioned whether it is best to legislate mandatory staffing levels—for example, Massachusetts

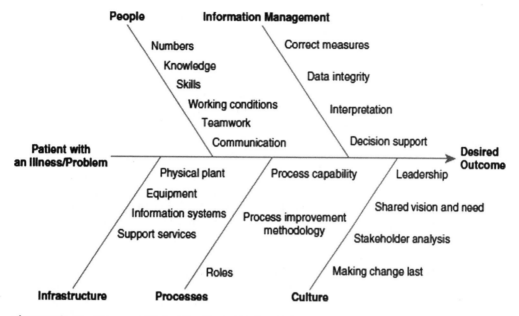

**People**  **Information Management**

Numbers

Correct measures

Knowledge

Skills

Data integrity

Working conditions

Interpretation

Teamwork

Communication

Decision support

**Patient with
an Illness/Problem**

**Desired
Outcome**

Physical plant

Process capability

Leadership

Equipment

Information systems

Shared vision and need

Process improvement
methodology

Support services

Stakeholder analysis

Roles

Making change last

**Infrastructure**    **Processes**    **Culture**

**Figure 7-3** Five Drivers of Clinical Quality and Patient Safety

Ettenberg, W. (2006). Basic tools for quality improvement. In D. Nash & N. Goldfarb, *The quality solution*, (pp. 115–132). Burlington, MA: Jones & Bartlett Learning.

and its hospital association decided to take a different approach that did not include mandatory ratios but rather provided flexibility, recognizing that HCOs and units within HCOs vary (Gale & Noga, 2013). This approach is called *PatientCareLink*, and it uses a dashboard to describe required staff skills, staffing per shift, staffing levels, and nurse management and support staff requirements along with the characteristics of the HCO and the unit. HCO participation is voluntary, but it has been very high (PatientCareLink, 2019). The initiative is based on five principles: (1) advancing healthcare quality and patient safety, (2) providing hospital staffing that meets patient needs, (3) making healthcare data and performance measures transparent and publicly available, (4) empowering patients and their families in their healthcare choices, and (5) promoting development/advancement of the healthcare workforce in a safe, respectful, and supportive work environment. Rhode Island HCOs and the state hospital association have joined this

initiative for patients, families, and healthcare providers. This information is now available to the public for comparison along with online quality data. Over time, quality has improved. Along with this type of statewide initiative, there is greater emphasis now on entry-level nursing education that supports the recommendations of *The Future of Nursing* report (IOM, 2010).

Nursing research has examined the impact of staffing on patient outcomes, but much more is needed. Several experts note that it is important to examine the influence of the intensity of patient needs and required nursing care (Aiken et al., 2010; Domrose, 2010; Rogers, Hwang, Scott, Aiken, & Dinges, 2004; Welton, 2007). These factors must be considered for mandatory staffing levels or any type of staffing that might be used. Who should provide care is important and should also be part of effective delegation decisions. Needleman, Liu, Shang, Larson, and Stone (2020) examined staff and inpatient hospital mortality, particularly looking at the cumulative effect of shifts with low registered nurse (RN) levels, low nursing support staff, and high patient turnover. This is a more complex analysis of staffing and its impact on patient outcomes. The conclusion from the study is low RN level and low nursing support staff are factors associated with increased patient mortality.

Other studies have examined work schedules (Trinkoff et al., 2010). What is it about work schedules and errors that we should be concerned about? Work schedules identify hours worked per day; hours worked per week; weekends worked per month; number of breaks lasting 10 minutes or more, including meals during a workday; and shift rotation. Weekend work schedules have been examined, recognizing that weekend staffing may have a different configuration and/or level impacting services and outcomes. Three factors may influence care during these times: lower-level and possibly less experienced staff, reduced or delayed access to some services for diagnosis or treatment, and patients in hospitals on weekend may be more acute (Ranji, 2017). The work schedule element that is most commonly associated with patient mortality is lack of nurse recovery time or time away from work, which often results in staff fatigue and injury. The researchers for this study also comment that HCOs should examine the impact of 12-hour shifts, as this might not be the best schedule, given the need for recovery time after working long hours. Today, this is a common shift configuration despite concerns about its impact on staff and patient care.

The Aiken et al. (2010) study examined the association between lower patient-to-nurse ratios and inpatient mortality to find that when the number of patients decreased, mortality rates decreased, as did failure to rescue. These hospitals also had effective work environments, but if the work environment was not effective, reducing the ratio did not decrease

mortality. This finding indicates that staffing may not be the only important factor.

Another study examined the relationship between nurse staffing in general and intensive care units and patient outcomes (Blegen, Goode, Spetz, Vaughn, & Park, 2011). This study also compared safety net and non-safety-net hospitals. A safety net hospital is "a hospital receiving adjustment payments to provide care to a significantly disproportionate share of low-income patients who are not paid by other payers, such as Medicare, Medicaid, the Children's Health Insurance Program, or other health insurance" (p. 407). In one study, it was thought that safety-net hospitals have higher rates of errors and greater need to improve quality of care because their patients are more complex (VanDeusen et al., 2015). The conclusion from the sample of 54 hospitals indicated that there was an association between higher staffing and lower hospital-acquired infections, lower failure to rescue events, lower mortality, and reduced hospital stay. The safety-net hospitals did experience higher rates of congestive heart failure, failure to rescue events, and decubitus ulcers, but the average staffing levels were not much different from non-safety-net hospitals. No specific explanation for this was identified, but it could be related to the long-term concern that the safety-net hospital patients are more complex and generally have poorer health status. There can be many other reasons, including how staffing is managed and the quality improvement programs in these HCOs.

Other studies also address staff turnover and patient outcomes (Bae, Mark, & Fried, 2009). Why is staff turnover a factor? When units lose staff familiar with the unit and HCO, they are losing expertise and consistency. Teams are also affected when staff members leave. Some units may have to use temporary staff until new staff members are hired, and temporary staff usually are not familiar with the unit, patients, policies, and other workplace dynamics and may not have the best level of expertise and practice. Teams are affected, as a temporary member may not be as welcome as regulars, and this may impact communication, collaboration, and decision making. In addition, when new staff are hired, an orientation period provides time for new team members to integrate and fully function. All of these changes are costly for the HCO. Bae and colleagues (2009) describe the situation as follows: "Workgroup processes mediate the nursing unit turnover–patient outcomes relationship. Nursing turnover leads to changes in workgroup processes such as decreased member attraction to the nursing unit, ineffective coordination, and inaccurate communication. Such inefficient workgroup processes in turn negatively affect patient outcomes" (p. 42). In addition to the importance of staffing levels or patient-to-nurse ratios, many other factors are related to staff and care quality, such as staff stress, burnout, job satisfaction, teamwork, nurse turnover, nursing leadership, the practice environment, and access to effective staff education.

Burnout is a frequent topic in the nursing profession. An important element of burnout is "emotional exhaustion, which is associated with emotional and cognitive detachment from work as a way to cope with work demands" (Cimiotti, Aiken, Sloane, & Wu, 2012, p. 486; Maslach, 2003). A 2019 report, *Taking Action Against Clinician Burnout: A Systems Approach to Professional Well-Being*, emphasizes the critical nature of burnout in the healthcare system that requires immediate response (National Academy of Medicine [NAM], 2019). Burnout is complex and not easily resolved. A nursing study that examined the impact of burnout on nurse staffing, specifically on hospital patient infections, concluded that there is an association between these factors (Cimiotti et al., 2012). **Figure 7-4** describes a model of clinician burnout and professional well-being and how the three system levels interact: frontline care delivery, healthcare organization, and external environment. Decisions made in all three levels have an impact on work factors and thus on clinician burnout.

When nurse burnout combines with high patient-to-nurse ratios, job dissatisfaction results, which has an impact on quality of care. It is important to note that other healthcare professionals such as physicians also experience burnout (Dzau, Kirch, & Nasca, 2018).

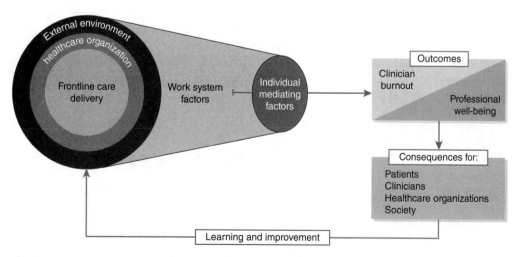

**Figure 7-4** A Systems Model of Clinician Burnout and Professional Well-Being

The AHRQ describes clinician burnout as follows: "[B]urnout is a syndrome of emotional exhaustion, depersonalization, and decreased sense of accomplishment at work that results in overwhelming symptoms of fatigue, exhaustion, cynical detachment, and feelings of ineffectiveness. Although it is difficult to determine causal relationships, burnout has been associated with increased patient safety incidents, including medical errors, reduced patient satisfaction, and poorer safety and quality ratings" (HHS, AHRQ, PSNet, 2019b). The 2019 reports notes that the following must be considered (NAM, 2019):

- Clinician burnout needs to be tackled early in professional development, and special stressors in the learning environment need to be recognized.
- Stakeholders in the external environment have an important role to play in preventing clinician burnout as their decisions can result in increased burden and other demands that affect clinician burnout. Every attempt at alignment and reduction of requirements to reduce redundancy is essential.
- Technology can either contribute to clinician burnout (e.g., poorly designed electronic health record technologies) or potentially reduce clinician burnout (e.g., well-functioning patient communications, clinical decision support) if it is well designed, implemented, and integrated into clinical workflow. The report reiterates several recommendations of previous IOM and National Academies of Sciences, Engineering, and Medicine reports to improve usability, workflow integration, and inter-operability of health information technology.
- Medical societies, state licensing boards, specialty certification boards, medical education and healthcare delivery organizations all need to take concrete steps to reduce the stigma for clinicians of seeking help for

psychological distress, and make assistance more easily available. (pp. xiv–xv)

Another factor that requires further examination is the impact of non–registered nurse (RN) staff on staff stress—for example, does the use of non-RN staff to do routine tasks give the RN more time for monitoring patients and providing more complex nursing care? Does this reduce staff stress, or does some staff experience stress from supervising others? Staffing must also consider supply. Are enough qualified nurses available to meet work demand? There have been times of shortages—some on the national level and some more localized. These experiences have led the nursing profession to recognize that prediction and preparation for future shortages are important. Some predictions that are important to consider are these: The RN workforce is expected to be 3.4 million by 2026, and it is currently the top occupation and is expected to continue to be. One million RNs are projected to retire by 2030, leading to not only loss in the number of nurses but also experience and knowledge; and this will lead to a shortage of nurses (American Association of Colleges of Nursing [AACN], 2019). This type of data can be helpful in designing local and national plans to address potential staff shortages.

## STOP AND CONSIDER 7-2

Staffing and workload are factors that should be part of error analysis.

# Frontline Safety

**Frontline staff** is direct care staff, and they often get lost in the big picture. However, in the end, it is the frontline staff who make the biggest difference in CQI, regardless of the type or size of the HCO. During direct care, **frontline safety** occurs when the staff considers patient afety and quality in their daily work. Nurses are represented in large numbers in the frontline staff, and to make an impact, they need to assume leadership and engagement in CQI.

## Impact on CQI

A study published in 2012 indicated that the safety culture is associated not only with patient and staff injuries but also with working conditions that increase risk, such as nursing hours per patient day and staff turnover (Taylor et al., 2012). This study describes safety as the perception of HCO commitment to safety and teamwork. Another critical factor is perception of the quality of collaboration. The study concludes that "patient and nurse safety may constitute linked outcomes rather than distinct silos. Traditionally, the fields of occupational and patient safety have been addressed separately, but regarding them as related components of an organization's safety culture might be more apt. Future healthcare safety research and intervention efforts should consider a new paradigm integrating lessons learnt from both disciplines to more comprehensively and efficiently reduce preventable injuries to both workers and patients" (p. 109). Energized and healthy staff members are more productive and provide more effective quality care.

## Red Rules: Do They Help?

Some HCOs have identified **red rules**, which are rules that must be followed to ensure CQI. This approach is used in other industries. A red rule must not be violated, and if it is, then staff must stop work (e.g., procedure, treatment). The goal is to empower staff to intervene; however, there is concern that this system can cause staff to fear that they will get in trouble. Red rules can also be problematic if they are used for situations that may at times make it difficult to follow the rules—for example, a red rule may require that bar coding always be used before medications are given, and yet there may be situations when they cannot be applied. Red rules represent situations in which nurses can directly influence quality. The Institute for Safe Medication Practice (ISMP, 2008) recommends the following criteria for red rules:

- It must be possible and desirable for everyone to follow a red rule every time in a process under all circumstances (i.e., red rules should not contain verbiage such as "except when . . ." or "each breach will be assessed for appropriateness").
- Anyone who notices that the red rule has been breached has the authority and responsibility to stop further progress of the patient care associated with the red rule while protecting the patient or employee from harm.
- Managers and other leaders (including the board of trustees) always support the work stoppage and immediately begin rectifying the problem and addressing the underlying reason for breaking the rule.
- The people who breached the red rule are given an opportunity to support their behavioral choices and then judged fairly based on the reasons for breaking the rule, regardless of rank and experience.
- The red rules are few, well understood, and memorable.

Examples of common red rules in healthcare are the following: Staff behavior related to patient abuse, sexual abuse, or practicing while under the influence of drugs or alcohol is unacceptable. Practice examples are reconciling sponges in surgery and taking time-outs before an invasive procedure.

## Standardizing

Safety, as described by Barach and Johnson (2018), is a "property of the clinical microsystem that can be achieved only through systematic application of a broad array of process, equipment, organization, supervision, training, simulation and teamwork changes" (p. 245). Systems will experience errors. There are, however, methods that might reduce this risk, but they will not totally eliminate it. Risk of adverse events can be controlled with strategies such as use of **standardization**, which focuses on making work consistent by regulating procedures, equipment, supplies, and so on "to increase reliability, improve information flow, and minimize cross training needs. Standardizing equipment across clinical settings . . . is one basic example, but standardized processes are increasingly being implemented as safety measures" (HHS, AHRQ, PSNet, 2019c).

Staff members best apply routines that can be learned, and risk for problems increases as the staff does fewer routine tasks/procedures. There is, however, a negative side to using routines. If routines lead to automatic responses, with staff not using effective thinking and problem solving, then routines such as procedures may lead to errors (Galt, Fuji, Gleason, & McQuillan, 2011). Staff may not be focused enough on details or catch things that should be noticed. Most human errors are difficult to stop; however, HCOs can develop systems that might decrease the risk of errors. On the one hand, there is a high rate of system errors, and on the other hand, it is recommended that systems should help identify when errors might occur and the steps to be taken to respond and improve. Other chapters discuss some of the methods used to assist staff, but here it is important to know that healthcare is complex and that human and system errors are related.

> **STOP AND CONSIDER 7-3**
>
> Red rules identify situations in which you must stop work and investigate what is happening; all staff members should be able to stop work for a red rule violation.

# Human Factors and Quality

**Human factors** are physical, cognitive, and organizational factors that can have an impact on errors. More attention is now given to staff, their work environment, and their relationship to errors and CQI. Human factors have a major impact on the quality of care. It is important for all staff to understand this impact, as it applies to all staff. The first step is for staff to recognize the factors in order to prevent problems or take steps to stop problems. **Presenteeism** refers to staff who are at work but not functioning at their fullest, often due to a medical problem—physical or psychological—such as stress at home, child care issues, and so on. This reduced functioning then impacts the quality of work. A Robert Wood Johnson Foundation, Nursing Research Network, summary of some studies on this topic notes that nurses who reported a high level of presenteeism were less likely to report high levels of quality on their units and reported higher levels of medication errors and patient falls during their work hours (HHS, AHRQ, PSNet, 2017). Assessing human factors has become a more important aspect of CQI. Errors will occur, but we must do our best to prevent them, and when they occur we must effectively respond to them.

## Types of Human Factors That Impact Quality Care

Human factors that impact care can be categorized as (1) environmental, (2) organizational and job, and (3) human and individual. Common examples of human factors that are of concern include the following:

- *Fatigue.* This factor impacts all the work that the staff does and can lead to staff injuries. Staff may experience mental fatigue, physical fatigue, or both. **Mental fatigue** is "a state that arises in response to increasing mental task demands and stresses (mental workload), and results in a perceived sense of weariness, reduced motivation, reduced alertness, and reduced mental performance in workers" (Pasupathy, & Barker, 2011, p. 22). **Physical fatigue** is "a state that develops throughout the body in response to increasing physical task demands and stresses (physical workload), as well as expectancy of work demands, and can lead to physical discomfort and a decreased capacity to generate force or power" (p. 22). As fatigue increases, staff experience decreased perceived performance. They have less ability to recognize that a change is occurring as they experience acute and chronic fatigue. When staff acute fatigue can be reduced, this does make a difference in reducing risk to performance.

- *Stress, hunger, and illness.* These factors interfere with work productivity due to decreasing energy and also impact effective thinking. An example is no time for a food break, which is a common problem in some work environments.
- *Unfamiliarity with task.* Not knowing how to complete a task can lead to errors, and a person may also then put off doing the task in a timely fashion or may not do the task at all; both approaches impact quality.
- *Inexperience.* New, inexperienced staff are at high risk for all types of errors and may not feel comfortable asking for help.
- *Shortage of time.* If the staff do not have enough time to complete an activity as it should be done and they feel rushed, patient care may be compromised and patients often feel dissatisfied. The staff member who does not have time to talk to patients may miss important information or observations.
- *Inadequate checking.* This factor can impact any staff member who needs to check orders, patient documentation, steps in a procedure, or patient identification.

- *Interruptions and noise.* This factor can affect, for example, a nurse who is preparing medications, a pharmacist preparing medications for a unit, or dietary staff identifying special diets.
- *Poor procedures to follow.* Policies and procedures need to be current and evidence based, clear, and accessible when the staff need them.
- *Limited memory capacity.* Situations that rely on memory increase the risk of errors, so efforts should be made to reduce reliance on memory by providing easy access to information or using methods to improve memory such as checklists.
- *Unwillingness or inability to ask for help.* No one can know everything, but it is difficult for many staff to admit this and ask for help. Doing something that one does not know how to do or does not understand is very risky.
- *Language and culture factors.* Diversity in staff and patients is a recognized fact; however, language and cultural differences can interfere with clear communication, leading to errors.

The AHRQ emphasizes that "the importance of human factors engineering is the discipline that attempts to identify and address these issues. It is the discipline that takes into account human strengths and limitations in the design of interactive systems that involve people, tools and technology, and work environments to ensure safety, effectiveness, and ease of use. A human factors engineer examines a particular activity in terms of its component tasks, and then assesses the physical demands, skill demands, mental workload, team dynamics, aspects of the work environment (e.g., adequate lighting, limited noise, or other distractions), and device design required to complete the task optimally. In essence, human factors engineering focuses on how systems work in actual practice, with real—and fallible—human beings at the controls, and attempts to design systems that optimize safety and minimize the risk of error in complex environments" (HHS, AHRQ, PSNet, 2019d).

The system and its processes need methods for responding to prevent errors when these human factors arise. Anything that interferes with effective performance must be considered in the CQI plan to reduce risk of errors due to human factors and ergonomics. HCO systems must be resilient and alert to factors that may lead to errors; this includes an understanding of how errors can be detected, mitigated, and resolved. These efforts are discussed in other chapters in more detail.

A 2014 study examined the relationship between sleep deprivation and occupational and patient care errors among staff nurses who worked the night shift (Johnson, Jung, & Brown, 2014). Night shifts are not uncommon in nursing. Sometimes the same staff work this shift permanently, and sometimes staff rotate in and out of the night shift or cover for other staff on a periodic basis. Working the night shift increases the risk of sleep deprivation. The results indicated that more than half of the 289 nurses who participated in this study were sleep deprived, and errors increased as hours of sleep decreased. The study concluded that sleep deprivation should also be considered one of the factors that impacts errors; however, collecting data on this topic is not always easy, as it requires staff to admit to sleep concerns and report errors and near misses. Staff may not be open about this information out of concern for how their employer may view them.

Another area of concern is staff working longer shifts, such as 10 and 12 hours, and often not getting off work as scheduled, errors and staff injuries are also more likely to occur. Occupational errors may seem insignificant to staff, but they may have significant implications, warning of fatigue and sleep deprivation. Failure of staff to get the amount of sleep they need to feel rested impacts both the personal and professional aspects of their lives. Examples

are an increase in car accidents to and from the workplace, staff infections and other illnesses, musculoskeletal injuries such as when lifting patients, and exposure to bloodborne pathogens. The ANA addresses staffing and fatigue, emphasizing the need for healthy work hours and avoidance of work when fatigued, as described in the Connect to Current Information section at the end of this chapter. Working when fatigued is an ethical issue, requiring decisions about whether a person is able to work safely and effectively. Stimpfel, Sloane, and Aiken (2012) note the following: "Working longer for fewer shifts may also attract nurses who work a second job. However, the strain of those three long work days and the rest and recovery time needed may offset any perceived benefit, if our survey results are any indication. When a three-day week turns into more days or additional, unplanned-for overtime, nurses' satisfaction appears to decrease" (p. 2507).

As is true for most of the studies on staffing, work environment, and patient outcomes, these studies are difficult to conduct, but more research is needed to better understand this area of healthcare delivery. In addition, research results may mean that HCOs, administrative staff, and healthcare professionals may need to make difficult decisions. Some of these changes may relate to 12-hour shifts, such as decreasing hours per shift, changing staffing levels to avoid overscheduling existing staff, and budgeting to allow for any increased costs to the HCO.

The Joint Commission's sentinel event alert on staff fatigue, which is based on evidence supported by a study reported in 2004, identifies the following factors that impact performance (Hughes & Clancy, 2005; The Joint Commission, 2011):

- Lapses in attention and inability to stay focused
- Reduced motivation
- Compromised problem solving
- Confusion

- Irritability
- Memory lapses
- Impaired communication
- Slowed or faulty information processing and judgment
- Diminished reaction time
- Indifference and loss of empathy

Consider how each of these factors might impact a nurse's thinking and practice.

## Staff Stress

**Stress**, as defined by Kuntz, Mennicken, and Scholtes (2014), "results from an imbalance between demands and resources, occurring when demand pressure exceeds an individual's perceived ability to cope" (p. 754). The biological response to stress is elevated hormone levels, particularly cortisol, and this impacts cognitive abilities such as memory, attention, and decision-making (Dickerson & Kemeny, 2004; Sonnentag & Fritz, 2006). In some cases, posttraumatic stress disorder may occur. Stress in some staff may be contagious—for example, when staff members complain frequently to one another that their workload is too heavy and work cannot be done safely, other staff may then complain about the stress of their own workload. The common reasons for stress among nurses are the following (HHS, Centers for Disease Control [CDC], National Institute for Occupational Safety and Health [NIOSH], 2014):

- Work overload
- Time pressure
- Lack of social support at work (especially from supervisors, nurse managers, and higher management)
- Staff incivility
- Exposure to infectious diseases
- Risk of needlestick injuries
- Exposure to work-related violence or threats
- Sleep deprivation
- Role ambiguity and conflict
- Understaffing

- Career development issues
- Dealing with difficult or seriously ill patients

Another factor is the impact of the system load on quality, as reported by a study done by Kuntz and colleagues (2014). This study indicates that clinical unit occupancy does not impact mortality rate until it reaches a "tipping point." Typical responses to changes in occupancy are to request more staff, such as from temporary staff pools; ask staff to work longer hours or overtime; admit patients to other units; or delay admissions from emergency department. As staff workload increases, staff may ration access to care—less time to do everything. This hurried care leads to increased staff and unit stress and patient dissatisfaction and errors.

**Compassion fatigue** is an "intense drain on the body, emotions, and spirit, and it adds to nurse stress" (Carpenter, 2011, p. 34). Today, more attention is focused on this problem. As mentioned, working long hours increases staff fatigue, but fatigue is also increased because of stress in the workplace. Staff are worn out and stressed when they leave work; as a result, they get less rest when off and then return reluctantly, still tired and stressed.

The NIOSH recommends the following strategies/interventions to assist HCOs in reducing staff stress (HHS, CDC, NIOSH, 2019). These strategies/interventions address many of the common causes of stress in nurses:

- Ensure that the workload is in line with workers' capabilities and resources.
- Clearly define workers' roles and responsibilities.
- Give workers opportunities to participate in decisions and actions affecting their jobs.
- Improve communication.
- Reduce uncertainty about career development and future employment prospects.
- Provide opportunities for social interaction among workers.

In addition to these strategies/interventions, HCOs are increasing their use of team processes and interprofessional teams. To be effective, the HCO needs to include staff in the development, implementation, and evaluation of strategies/interventions used to reduce staff stress. Stress management is also employed in some HCOs. Methods might include learning coping strategies such as progressive relaxation and biofeedback, improving time management, and expanding interpersonal skills. Some HCOs provide special benefits to staff, such as exercise, yoga, gym memberships, on-site child care, and other such perks. Reducing staff stress improves care quality and productivity and helps reduce incivility in the workplace.

The nursing profession has long recognized that stress is an important factor in retaining staff, and today more is known about its impact on patient outcomes. The ANA provides information on staff stress and emphasizes it as an issue. For example, in 2017, the theme for National Nurses week was "Nursing, The Balance of Mind, Body and Spirit" (ANA, 2017). In addition to employers, nursing education programs should also develop and implement strategies to prevent and reduce stress.

## Staff: At-Risk Attitudes and Behaviors

Disruptive behavior and incivility are a growing concern in healthcare. One might wonder why this topic is related to CQI. When this type of negative behavior occurs, communication is broken, which has an impact on staff stress, roles and responsibilities, and teamwork. Broken communication may be defined by unclear and confusing or mixed messages. Emotions may limit the ability to communicate, or there may be no communication at all. Ineffective communication is the most common type of problem that can increase risk of errors. When staff members have difficulties with one another and do not communicate effectively, teamwork is compromised, impacting care negatively. The relationship between

communication and near misses, errors, and quality care is clear. Improving staff communication has been one of The Joint Commission's annual patient safety goals.

**Incivility** may include rude and discourteous behavior, gossiping and spreading rumors, or refusing to help others in the work situation. **Bullying**, as defined by the ANA (2015a), is "repeated, unwanted harmful actions intended to humiliate, offend, and cause distress in the recipient"). Bullying may happen between peers as well as with staff from top to bottom or bottom to top within the HCO. **Workplace mobbing** may also occur when staff groups use bullying against a staff member. Research on incivility does not yet provide enough evidence to address this problem, but some studies indicate that education about workplace incivility and effective responses plus application of these responses can make a difference (Armstrong, 2018). This systematic review indicated that length of training and team building do not necessarily mean that a training program will be effective. There is a lack of consistency in training programs, and this has a negative impact on research.

In addition to incivility and other related behavior, violence initiated by staff, family members or external sources has increased. The NIOSH defines **workplace violence** as "physically and/or psychologically damaging actions that occur in the workplace or while on duty" (HHS, CDC, NIOSH, 2014). Staff training to prevent violence should include deescalation techniques, management of assaultive behavior, and how to prevent and prevention to avoid assaults (Robinson, 2019; U.S. Department of Labor [DOL], Occupational Safety and Health Administration [OSHA], 2016).

Inappropriate and disruptive nurse–physician interactions and communication must be stopped. As is true for any behavior that interferes with effective work, it is important to understand why it is happening and to respond in a positive manner using "I" language—for example, "I think" or "I observe"

(Gessler, Rosenstein, & Ferron, 2012). If the behavior cannot be stopped, then the staff need to use the designated HCO procedure for reporting problems, and management then should respond. **Lateral violence**, which refers to acts between coworkers (e.g., nurse to nurse), such as bullying, hostility, reprisals for speaking out, and so on, have also increased in HCOs (Daley, 2012).

Zero tolerance of incivility has become the norm in many HCOs and is supported by the ANA (2015a). These HCOs have clear policies that describe a code of conduct and acceptable behaviors. This topic should be part of orientation and staff education for managers and staff. Staff diversity issues (e.g., biases, differences in cultures, and differences in communication) must be handled with care, but all must follow the policy. Tracking these incidents helps to better understand the level of the problem and typical concerns that arise. Armed with this information, HCOs can better assess this culture, determine outcomes, and identify and implement strategies that will be used to prevent or respond to incivility.

Problems of incivility, bullying, and workplace violence are recognized by the ANA as critical concerns for the nursing profession and healthcare delivery. Such problems impact not just nurses but also patients and families and the overall quality of care delivered. This recognition led to the development of a position statement on these problems (ANA, 2015a) and also a position statement on zero tolerance. The incivility statement notes that these problems are not just problems for the nursing profession or for nurses to solve; rather, employers must also be involved and use an interprofessional perspective. The ANA's *Nursing: Scope and Standards of Practice* also includes information on the need for a healthy workplace (ANA, 2015b). Creating a healthy workplace requires a culture of respect. The ANA's *Code of Ethics* requires that nurses work to establish an ethical environment and culture of civility, which is connected to a culture of safety. This culture should consider

kindness and treating colleagues, coworkers, employees, students, and others with dignity and respect (ANA, 2015a, 2015c). The *Code of Ethics* provides the basis for our understanding of the meaning of "civility" and its relevance to the nursing profession.

Many HCO settings experience problems with staff incivility and workplace violence, and some are at greater risk, such as emergency departments, psychiatric hospitals, nursing homes, long-term care facilities, and acute care settings. These settings may also experience problems with security, weapons, drugs, and other threats. Risk is increased within the HCO—for example, employees who "float" or move from one unit to another frequently experience assault three times more often than do permanent employees (ANA, 2015a).

## Strategies to Improve: Eliminate or Reduce Problems with Human Factors

The best approach to reduce inappropriate behavior is prevention. The most effective prevention interventions are active listening; developing interpersonal relationships and teams; dealing with problems before they get out of control; engaging staff in decision making; developing clear communication; and offering training on communication, procedures, delegation, teamwork, conflict and conflict resolution, and other group dynamics. These interventions are the responsibility of the HCO and staff. The employer has obligations to provide leadership, support, resources, and education and develop plans and strategies to prevent and, if necessary, respond to incivility and workplace violence. Staff commitment to respecting others makes the difference in the HCO. When incivility, bullying, or workplace violence occur, staff need to feel comfortable confronting the situation in a respectful manner. The HCO needs to respond in a timely manner, clarify the situation, speak respectfully with involved staff, and support staff to reach a positive resolution.

It is not easy to speak up about a situation in which you have experienced or observed incivility or lateral violence. Many staff fear retaliation or even loss of their job. What can you do to respond in a professional and direct manner? Developing self-awareness is critical, and the following tips are helpful in managing your own emotions (Gessler et al., 2012):

- Communicate your concerns.
- Refuse to dwell on negative thoughts or emotions.
- Avoid negative behaviors.
- Admit to mistakes.
- Accept and act on valid feedback. (p. 42)

Taking care of yourself and reducing your personal stress gives you more energy to deal with negative situations at work and to avoid turning them into a negative reaction for yourself.

Supportive practice environments assist in nursing quality care (Flynn, Liang, Dickson, Xie, & Suh, 2012). Today it is recognized that when staff members are involved in errors, they may become the second victims due to the experience, the response from others, and their own personal response. "Multiple studies have found that 10%-20% of hospitalized patients experience adverse events, with approximately half of these events considered preventable" (HHS, AHRQ, PSNet, 2019e). To improve performance and view errors as opportunities to learn and not blame or feel guilty, HCOs need to put forth more effort to support staff and help them cope when they experience stress. Professional and personal self-esteem are factors that influence staff and their ability to cope in the work environment. What do clinicians consider to be supportive and helpful? The AHRQ reports the following: "A survey of 898 clinicians at the University of Missouri found that clinicians wanted a unit- or department-based support system that could relieve them of immediate patient care duties

for a brief period; provide one-on-one peer support, professional review, and collegial feedback, as well as access to patient safety experts and risk managers; and offer of crisis support and external referral when needed" (HHS, AHRQ, PSNet, 2019f).

Programs to reduce stress and burnout have been developed, and some have been tested. In one study, nurses were surveyed via a questionnaire to assess health-related consequences of stress and also related costs of absenteeism and turnover (Sallon, Katz-Eisner, Yaffe, & Bdolah-Abram, 2015). A program called Caring for the Caregivers used an 8-month course on stress reduction as an intervention. The course included multiple methods to reduce staff stress. Several reliable and valid rating scales, such as the Maslach Burnout Inventory, were used in the study. Among the participants, 97 improved, compared to 67 in the control group. For example, participants (staff) experienced fewer respiratory infections, doctor visits, and stress symptoms. The intervention was effective, although the length of the course may be problematic for many HCOs and their staff. This study does, however, indicate that organized strategies can assist staff.

The "I'M SAFE" checklist is one method that is taught to staff as a self-assessment tool to ensure safety. Staff determine if they have problems in any of the following areas, which may then limit their performance (HHS, AHRQ, 2013):

- **I**llness
- **M**edication
- **S**tress
- **A**lcohol and drugs
- **F**atigue
- **E**ating and **e**limination

If staff identify that they have a problem, they should seek support and recognize that not doing this increases the risk of errors. Mutual support among team members assists the team in working toward their goals together. As they work together, team member feedback should be respectful, timely, specific, directed toward improvement, and considerate.

# Workplace Safety

It is common to emphasize safety for patients, but there is another aspect of safety: safety for staff in the workplace. HCOs are settings where there is risk for staff everyday, such as the examples mentioned in the previous discussion on fatigue, incivility, violence, and stress. Workplace safety is concerned with many other factors that may lead to staff harm as they work.

## Importance of Maintaining Workplace Safety

Why is workplace safety so important? When the HCO makes workplace safety an important goal, it may result in reduced costs; safer care for patients, who may be injured when staff are injured or not able to function to full capacity when recovering from harm; consistent care when staff are not absent from work; and a decrease in staff stress (Finkelman, 2017). If staff members are unhealthy or injured while working, this may impact patient care. For example, if a staff member is using patient lift equipment in an unsafe manner or the equipment is not functioning correctly, both the staff member and the patient may be injured. Staff who miss work due to illness or injury cost the HCO money for paid sick time, disability payments (when appropriate), and the cost of finding coverage for the staff member, which may be more costly than paying the employee (e.g., temporary staff may get more pay). Error risk is also increased, as new staff or temporary staff may not be prepared for the position or may miss critical communication, and consistency might be affected.

HCOs are concerned about all of these considerations and thus often have staff health services or occupational health services on site to assist in ensuring that staff can function fully. Other issues that are managed through this service are required staff immunizations, staff education related to health and safety, and referrals to other health services as needed. The ANA website on workplace safety provides information on the major concerns of safe patient handling, needlestick injury prevention, staff drug and alcohol use, workplace violence, and environmental health.

## NIOSH and OSHA: Standards for Workplace Safety

NIOSH and OSHA provide important services to better ensure safe labor practices and a healthy workforce. HCOs must pay attention to the requirements from these two federal agencies, particularly to legislative mandates.

NIOSH is part of the HHS, Centers for Disease Control and Prevention. Some of the programs NIOSH leads are Prevention Through Design, which looks at how physical design impacts equipment and processes, improving total worker health, and health hazard evaluation in the workplace. NIOSH's mission is "to develop new knowledge in the field of occupational safety and health and to transfer that knowledge into practice" (HHS, CDC, NIOSH, 2019). Its goals are these: (1) Conduct research to reduce worker illness and injury and to advance worker well-being, (2) promote safe and healthy workers through intervention, recommendations, and capacity building, and (3) enhance international worker safety and health through global collaborations. The NIOSH website provides extensive information on many workplace health and safety topics. The Connect to Current Information section at the end of this chapter provides a link to this site.

The OSHA is part of the U.S. Department of Labor (DOL), so it is under different control than is the NIOSH. This agency "assures safe and healthful working conditions for working men and women by setting and enforcing standards and by providing training, outreach, education, and assistance" (DOL, OSHA, 2019). Federal law ensures that OSHA mandates on worker rights are enforced. One of these rights is that workers are entitled to working conditions that do not pose a risk of serious harm. To help ensure a safe and healthful workplace, the OSHA also provides workers with the right to the following (DOL, OSHA, 2019):

- Receive information and training about hazards, methods to prevent harm, and the OSHA standards that apply to their workplace. The training must be in a language that workers can understand.
- Get copies of test results used to identify workplace hazards.
- Review records of work-related injuries and illnesses.
- Get copies of their medical records.
- Ask OSHA to inspect their workplace.
- Use their rights under the law, free from retaliation and discrimination.

An employer cannot deny these rights to a worker, and if the employer attempts to do so, employees can complain to OSHA. Violating an OSHA mandate would be a serious situation for an HCO, as this would be breaking federal law. So not only must care be as safe as possible and of the best quality, but staff are also protected in the workplace to ensure their health and safety.

## Common Healthcare Workplace Concerns

Healthcare staff work in a variety of settings and circumstances that can increase their risks. Examples of common staff healthcare workplace safety concerns are the following (ANA, 2019b):

- *Infections.* Some infections are common, and some, such as Ebola, are not so common and very contagious such as COVID-19.
- *Bloodborne infections.* Needlesticks may expose nurses to bloodborne infections, such as HIV, hepatitis B, and hepatitis C.

This risk has been addressed by the use of safe needle devices, but also there is need to ensure there are human resources (staffing levels), equipment and supplies, policies and procedures, and training to ensure that the staff are safe. These precautions improve care and safety of patients. The ANA has position statements on these concerns on its website. The Needlestick Safety and Prevention Act of 2000 requires that employers do the following:
  - Identify, evaluate, and implement safer medical devices.
  - Maintain a sharps injury log.
  - Involve healthcare workers in device selection.
  - Implement engineering controls for sharps disposal containers, self-sheathing needles, safer medical devices, and use of engineering controls to eliminate or reduce employee exposure to pathogens.
  - Train employees in proper use of engineering and work practice controls.
- *Ergonomics and safe patient handling.* Addressing this concern may reduce injuries due to ergonomics. Nurses have to move patients, help them with mobility, and perform other activities, often using equipment that can lead to injuries and often without supportive equipment. Neck, shoulder, and back injuries are common. Factors that impact injury risk are staff age, height and weight, strength, health status, and knowledge and availability and use of safe ergonomics and assistive equipment. Patient factors are weight, strength to assist, age, medical problems, and needs. Safe Patient Handling and Mobility programs are important in identifying standards to protect staff and patients (ANA, 2019c). The Connect to Current Information section at the end of this chapter provides a link to the ANA website on safe handling and its resources and training materials. Schools of nursing and HCOs use this information to prepare students and staff.

- *Exposure to chemicals.* Chemicals that nurses should be concerned about include housekeeping chemicals, mercury-containing devices, latex, anesthetic gases, antiretroviral medications, chemotherapeutic agents, and some sterilization and disinfectant agents. Nurses need to know what chemicals are used in their area of practice and how to protect themselves. They should also protect against radiation exposure. When needed, the HCO should also provide training and protective equipment/supplies.

There are many causes of staff injuries, and settings and staff roles influence risk to staff. Common causes include the following (Gerwig, 2014):

- Lack of consistent, timely, and positive feedback for performance improvement
- Lack of employee engagement and empowerment
- Unresponsive systems (hazards go uncorrected)
- Miscommunication
- Information deficits
- Conflict between immediate and long-term goals (e.g., performance standards such as operating room turnover may conflict with adequate time to perform required tasks safely)
- Misaligned or conflicting goals among departments
- Lack of contingency planning and response
- Unclear allocation of responsibility
- Breakdown in coordination
- Lack of teamwork
- Inadequate training
- Poor supervision
- Inflexible policies
- Poor labor relations
- Cumbersome technology
- Undue time pressure
- Understaffing/overtasking
- Interruptions/distractions
- Inadequate policies and procedures
- "Drift" or noncompliance with policies and procedures

- Difficulty in speaking up when another staff member is doing something that is unsafe
- Lack of leadership engagement and sponsorship (p. 335)

### STOP AND CONSIDER 7-5

Workplace safety is a concern not only of HCOs but also of federal and state governments.

## Summary

This chapter examines quality healthcare by introducing safety and errors. Safety is not separate from quality; rather, it is a critical component of quality. In an integrative review of literature that included 20 studies focused on patient safety in nursing curricula, several key concerns are identified that nurses need to consider as they become active participants in the CQI process (Tella et al., 2014). These concerns are learning from errors, responsible individual and interprofessional teamwork, anticipatory action in complex environments, and patient-safety-centered nursing. Understanding basic factors influencing errors and terminology is required before you can appreciate CQI planning, measurement, analysis, and development of strategies to improve care. In summary, when examining events, there are three factors to remember that impact errors (Barach & Johnson, 2013; Perrow, 1984):

- All human beings, regardless of their skills, abilities, and specialist training, make fallible decisions and commit unsafe acts.
- All human-made systems possess latent (unseen) failures to some degree.
- All human endeavors involve some measure of risk.

Exemplars of quality improvement roles and responsibilities for staff nurses, nurse managers, and APRNs are found in **Exhibit 7-1**.

**Exhibit 7-1** Exemplars: Quality Improvement Roles and Responsibilities

**Staff Nurse**

A staff nurse is using special equipment to move a patient from a chair to the bed. Before the nurse begins she goes through the checklist to ensure that equipment is functioning properly. She notes that two aspects of the process seem to not be functioning properly. She asks another nurse to confirm her observations, and she does. The nurse stops the procedure and calls maintenance. They are told that the patient needs to be moved and the requirement for their services is immediate. They come and repair the equipment, and the patient is safely moved.

**Nurse Manager**

The nurse manager group has decided to conduct a review of staff assignments to the night shift and errors made. They ask for data from the HCO's Quality Improvement Program. One nurse manager suggests they should include staff stress and response as she has had two staff nurses involved in car accidents going home—no injuries were incurred but the incidents are enough to alert staff and the manager that this could be of concern.

**Advanced Practice Registered Nurse***

An APRN approaches a staff nurse in the hall and tells the nurse that her practice needs to improve and walks away. The staff nurse is confused and upset and leaves the unit for 15 minutes. Upon her return another staff nurse sees her and asks where she has been. She will not explain even though the tone of the question was one of concern.  The nurse manager hears about the incident and speaks with the APRN, who is new on the unit. She tells the APRN that this is a unit that does not tolerate incivility. Providing feedback to staff is an APRN responsibility, but this must be done in a professional manner—it should be done privately, with specifics and discussion of how improvement can occur. It must also include opportunity for the nurse to provide his or her viewpoint. The APRN agrees to make this change and to talk with the nurse again with the nurse manager present.

*Advanced Practice Registered Nurse includes APRN, Clinical Nurse Specialist, Clinical Nurse Leader, and nurses with DNP.

## APPLY CQI

## Chapter Highlights

- There are multiple models for understanding errors, including the Swiss cheese model, the Enthoven model, and the generic error-modeling system (GEMS). The Swiss cheese model is more commonly used by HCOs and some government initiatives.
- There are multiple types of errors that require tracking and analysis to improve care.
- Underuse, overuse, and misuse are common types of errors found in a variety of HCOs and involve a variety of staff.

- Active errors are associated with direct care providers.
- System factors impact latent errors, which are often not as apparent to staff.
- Near misses occur when staff members almost make an error but no actual error occurs. Staff may do something consciously or unconsciously to block the error.
- Adverse events are injuries resulting from medical interventions, not from the patient's underlying condition. They are untoward, undesirable events, usually

not expected, and may or may not have a long-term effect.

- Sentinel events are critical patient-related events that require a response; examples include a suicide, wrong-site surgery, and serious operative and postoperative complications.
- The Joint Commission issues sentinel alerts to share information about reported sentinel events to help HCOs learn from these events.
- Frontline safety focuses on direct-care staff and their impact on quality improvement.
- Red rules are used to identify events that the HCO does not consider to be acceptable performance. A red rule must not be violated, and if one is, staff must stop

work (e.g., procedure, treatment). The goal is to empower all staff to intervene.

- Standardizing care can reduce risk of quality problems; however, this cannot be done for all situations. Standards, policies, and procedures assist in ensuring greater standardization while still meeting individual needs.
- Human factors and ergonomics are physical, cognitive, and organizational factors that can have an impact on errors.
- Staff stress negatively impacts care quality, interfering with staff performance.
- Workplace safety focuses on direct care staff and their safety in the workplace.
- NIOSH and OSHA standards are important in supporting staff safety to ensure more effective quality improvement.

## Critical Thinking and Clinical Reasoning and Judgment: Discussion Questions and Learning Activities

1. Using the three error models described in this chapter create a visual (e.g., poster, PowerPoint slide, graphic) that highlights their key points. Compare your visual to those of your classmates.
2. What is your opinion of the use of red rules in frontline safety initiatives? Provide your opinion in one paragraph.
3. In a small group, compare and contrast the types of errors, and when possible, provide examples from clinical experiences. Summarize your discussion.

4. In a small group, discuss examples from your own clinical experiences relating to human factors and errors (or possible errors). Summarize your discussion.
5. Assess your own response to stress. Write down your assessment. How might your typical responses to stress impact your clinical practice? Provide examples of how your responses have affected your clinical practice as a student. How might you better cope with stress?

## Connect to Current Information

- Multiple graphics of the Swiss cheese model
  http://www.bing.com/images/search?q=swiss+cheese+model+health+care
- NIOSH: Workplace Safety Resources
  http://www.cdc.gov/niosh/topics/default.html
- OSHA: Workplace Safety Resources
  https://www.osha.gov/shpguidelines/additional-resources-by-topic.html

- OSHA: Healthcare Wide Hazards
  https://www.osha.gov/SLTC/etools/hospital/hazards/hazards.html
- AHRQ: Patient Safety Primers
  https://psnet.ahrq.gov/primers?f_topicIDs=412,503&most_recent=true
- ANA: Nursing Practice and Work Environment
  https://www.nursingworld.org/practice-policy/work-environment/health-safety

- ANA: Safe Patient Handling and Mobility
  http://www.nursingworld.org/MainMenu
  Categories/WorkplaceSafety/SafePatient
- ANA: Nurse fatigue
  https://www.nursingworld.org/~49de63
  /globalassets/practiceandpolicy/health-and
  -safety/nurse-fatigue-position-statement
  -final.pdf

- Action Collaborative on Clinician Well-Being
  and Resilience
  https://nam.edu/initiatives/clinician-resilience
  -and-well-being

## Connect to Text Current Information with the Author

Go to the update for this text to review the Blog, QI News, and Literature Review. Access this regular update at: http://nursing.jbpub.com/Finkelman/QualityImprovement/2e.

# EBP, EBM, and Quality Improvement: Exemplar

Riskin, A. et al. (2019). Incivility and patient safety: A longitudinal study of rudeness, protocol compliance, and adverse events. *Joint Commission Journal of Quality Patient Safety, 45*(5), 358–367.

This article describes a study that focuses on social interaction and patient safety.

### Questions to Consider

1. What is this study's design, including research question(s), sample,

interventions, data collection, and analysis?

2. What are the results of the study?
3. How might you apply these results to a clinical setting or your practice to improve care?

# EVOLVING CASE STUDY

In the unit's monthly staff meeting, staff stress is brought up as a growing problem. The staff complain that they are overworked and there is not enough staff. They are also tired of orienting new staff, and temporary staff members are not effective. Two nurses mention that they have personally experienced more near misses when administering medications. The unit experienced two sentinel events that resulted in complications for patients and extended their length of stay. One of the errors was due to overdose of medications that was not recognized before major complications occurred. The nurse manager tells the staff that he recognizes from the discussion that there is a lot of tension and this is a concern. The manager leaves the meeting, and in his office he begins to consider how he and the unit should respond to the problems.

### Case Questions

**1.** You want to better understand the impact of stress, workload, staffing, and quality care problems on your unit. How will you accomplish this?

**2.** You, as the nurse manager, arrange to have a staff meeting to increase staff knowledge of stress and stress responses. What will the presentation include? How will you engage the staff in the process to improve stress management?

**3.** What strategies might you use to decrease stress and improve care? Be specific.

# References

Aiken, L.. (2010). Implications of the California nurse staffing mandate for other states. *Health Services Research, 45*(4), 904–921.

American Nurses Association (ANA). (2015a). Incivility, bullying, and workplace violence. ANA position statement. Retrieved from https://www.nursingworld.org/practice-policy/nursing-excellence/official-position-statements/id/incivility-bullying-and-workplace-violence

American Nurses Association (ANA). (2015b). *Nursing: Scope and standards of practice* (3rd ed.). Silver Spring, MD: Author.

American Nurses Association (ANA). (2015c). *Code of ethics* (3rd ed.). Silver Spring, MD: Author.

American Nurses Association (ANA). (2017). American Nurses Association celebrates national nurses week, focuses on helping nurses get and stay healthy. Retrieved from https://www.nursingworld.org/news/news-releases/2017-news-releases/american-nurses-association-celebrates-national-nurses-week-focuses-on-helping-nurses-get-and-stay-healthy

American Nurses Association (ANA). (2019a). *Principles for nurse staffing* (3rd ed.). Silver Spring, MD: Author.

American Nurses Association (ANA). (2019b). Health & safety. Retrieved from https://www.nursingworld.org/practice-policy/work-environment/health-safety

American Nurses Association. (ANA). (2019c). Handle with care. Retrieved from https://www.nursingworld.org/practice-policy/work-environment/health-safety/handle-with-care

American Association of Colleges of Nursing (AACN). (2019). Nursing shortage. Retrieved from https://www.aacnnursing.org/News-Information/Fact-Sheets/Nursing-Shortage

Armstrong, N. (2018). Management of nursing workplace incivility in healthcare settings: A systematic review. *Workplace Health and Safety, 66*(8), 403–410.

Bae, S., Mark, B., & Fried, B. (2009). Impact of nursing unit turnover on patient outcomes in hospitals. *Journal of Nursing Scholarship, 42*(1), 40–49.

Ball, J., Murrells, T., Rafferty, A., Morrow, E., & Griffiths, P. (2014). Care left undone during nursing shifts: Associations with workload and perceived quality of care. *BMJ Quality Safety, 23*(2), 116–125.

Barach, P., & Johnson, J. (2018). Assessing risk and harm in the clinical microsystem. In W. Sollecito & J. Johnson (Eds.), *McLaughlin and Kaluzny's continuous quality improvement in health care* (5th ed., pp. 235–252). Burlington, MA: Jones & Bartlett Learning.

Blegen, M., Goode, C., Spetz, J., Vaughn, T., & Park, S. (2011). Nurse staffing effects on patient outcomes: Safety-net and non-safety-net hospitals. *Medical Care, 49*(4), 406–414.

Busch, I., Moretti, F., Purgato, M. Barbui, C., Wu, A., & Rimondini, M. (2019). Psychological and psychosomatic symptoms of second victims of adverse events: A systematic review and meta-analysis. *Journal of Patient Safety*, April 23. Retrieved from https://journals.lww.com/journalpatientsafety/Abstract/2020/06000/Psychological_and_Psychosomatic_Symptoms_of_Second.12.aspx

Carpenter, H. (2011). Environment, health, and safety. *American Nurse Today, 6*(11), 34–35.

Cimiotti, J., Aiken, L., Sloane, D., & Wu, E. (2012). Nurse staffing, burnout, and health care-associated infection. *American Journal of Infection Control, 40*, 486–490.

Clark, B., & Bramble, J. (2013). Safety improvement is achieved within organizations. In K. Galt & K. Paschal (Eds.), *Foundations in patient safety for health professionals* (pp. 71–78). Burlington, MA: Jones & Bartlett Learning.

Classen, D., Resar, R., Griffin, F., Federico, F., Frankel, F., Kimmel, N., . . . James, B. (2011). "Global trigger tool" shows that adverse events in hospitals may be ten times greater than previously measured. *Health Affairs, 30*(4), 581–580.

Dabney, B., & Kalisch, B. (2016). Nurse staffing levels and patient-reported missed nursing care. *Journal of Nursing Care Quality, 30*(4), 306–312.

Daley, K. (2012). Let's put an end to bullying and lateral violence. *American Nurse Today, 7*(3), 18.

Dickerson, S., & Kemeny, M. (2004). Acute stressors and cortisol responses: A theoretical integration and synthesis of laboratory research. *Psychology Bulletin, 130*(3), 355–391.

Domrose, C. (2010). States consider merits of mandated staffing rations. Retrieved from https://www.nurse.com/blog/2010/02/10/states-consider-merits-of-mandated-staffing-ratios

Dzau, V., Kirch, D., & Nasca, T. (2018). To care is human—collectively confronting the clinician-burnout crisis. *New England Journal of Medicine, 37*(4), 312–314.

Finkelman, A. (2017). *Teaching IOM/HMD: Implications of the Institute of Medicine and Health & Medicine Division reports for nursing education* (4th ed., Vol. I). Silver Spring, MD: American Nurses Association.

Finkelman, A. (2019). *Professional nursing concepts: Competencies for quality leadership* (4th ed.). Burlington, MA: Jones & Bartlett Learning.

Flynn, L., Liang, Y., Dickson, G., Xie, M., & Suh, D. (2012). Nurses' practice environments, error interception practices, and inpatient medication errors. *Journal of Nursing Scholarship, 44*(2), 180–186.

Gale, S., & Noga, P. (2013). Creating a transparent and dynamic view of staffing as a foundation for improving quality and efficiency. *Nursing Administration Quarterly, 37*(3), 129–135.

Galt, K., Fuji, K., Gleason, J., & McQuillan, R. (2011). Why things go wrong. In K. Galt & K. Paschal (Eds.), *Foundations in patient safety for health professionals* (pp. 107–120). Burlington, MA: Jones & Bartlett Learning.

Gawande, A. (2010). *The checklist manifesto: How to get things done right.* New York, NY: Metropolitan Books.

Gawande, A. (2015, May 11). Overkill: An avalanche of unnecessary medical care is harming patients physically and financially. What can we do about it? *New Yorker.* Retrieved from http://www.newyorker.com /magazine/2015/05/11/overkill-atul-gawande

Gerwig, K. (2013). When employees are safe, patients are safer. In B. Youngberg (Ed.), *Patient safety handbook* (2nd ed., pp. 333–346). Burlington, MA: Jones & Bartlett Learning.

Gessler, R., Rosenstein, A., & Ferron, L. (2012). How to handle disruptive physician behaviors. Find out the best way to respond if you're the target. *American Nurse Today, 7*(11), 8–10.

Henneman, E., & Gawlinski, A. (2004). A "near-miss" model for describing the nurse's role in the recovery of medical errors. *Journal of Professional Nursing, 20*(3), 196–201.

Henneman, E., Gawlinski, A., Blank, F., Henneman, P., Jordan, D., & McKenzie, J. (2010). Strategies used by critical care nurses to identify, interrupt, and correct medical errors. *American Journal of Critical Care, 19*(6), 500–509.

Hughes, R., & Clancy, C. (2005). Working conditions that support patient safety. *Journal of Nursing Care Quality, 20*(4), 289–292.

Institute for Safe Medication Practice (ISMP). (2008). Some red rules shouldn't rule in hospitals. Retrieved from https://www.ismp.org/resources/some-red-rules -shouldnt-rule-hospitals

Institute of Medicine (IOM). (1999). *To err is human.* Washington, DC: The National Academies Press.

Institute of Medicine (IOM). (2003). *Health professions education.* Washington, DC: The National Academies Press.

Institute of Medicine (IOM). (2004). *Keeping patients safe: Transforming the work environment of nurses.* Washington, DC: The National Academies Press.

Institute of Medicine (IOM). (2010). *The future of nursing: Leading change, advancing health.* Washington, DC: The National Academies Press.

Johnson, A., Jung, L., & Brown, K. (2014). Sleep deprivation and error in nurses who work the night shift. *Journal of Nursing Administration, 44*(10), 17–22.

Jones, T., Hamilton, P., & Murray, N. (2015). Unfinished nursing care, missed care, and implicitly rationed care: State of the science review. *International Journal of Nursing Studies, 52,* 1121–1137.

Kalisch, B. (2015). *Errors of omission: How missed nursing care imperils patients.* Chevy Chase, MD: American Nurses Association.

Kalisch, B., Landstrom, G., & Williams, R. (2008). Missed nursing care: Errors of omission. *Nursing Outlook, 57*(1), 3–9.

Kalisch, B., & Lee, K. (2010). The impact of teamwork on missed nursing care. *Nursing Outlook, 58,* 233–241.

Kalisch, B., Xie, B., & Dabney, B. (2014). Patient-reported missed nursing care correlated with adverse events. *American Journal Medical Quality, 29,* 415–422.

Kuntz, L., Mennicken, R., & Scholtes, S. (2014). Stress on the ward: Evidence of safety tipping points in hospitals. *Management Science, 64*(4), 754–771.

Larkin, J., Lorenz, H., Rack, L., & Shatzer, M. (2012). Good care, good science: Leveraging frontline staff for quality. *Nursing Administrative Quarterly, 36*(3), 188–193.

Maslach, c. (2003). Job burnout: New directions in research and interventions. Current Directions Psychological Science, *12,* 189-192.

National Academy of Medicine (NAM). (2019). Taking action against clinician burnout: A systems approach to professional well-being. Washington, D.C.: The National Academies Press.

Needleman, J., Liu, J., Shang, J., Larson, E., & Stone, P. (2020). Association of registered nurse and nursing support staff with inpatient hospital mortality. *BMJ Quality Safety, 29,* 10–18.

Pasupathy, K., & Barker, L. (2011). Impact of fatigue on performance in registered nurses: Data mining and implications for practice. *Journal for Healthcare Quality, 34*(5), 22–30.

PatientCareLink. (2019). About *Patient Care Link.* Retrieved from https://patientcarelink.org/about-patientcarelink

Perrow, C. (1984). *Normal accidents, living with the high-risk technologies.* New York, NY: Basic Books.

Ranji, S. (2017). The weekend effect: Annual perspective 2017. Retrieved from https://psnet.ahrq.gov /perspective/weekend-effect

Reason, J. (1990). *Human error.* Cambridge, UK: Cambridge University Press.

Reason, J. (2000). Human error: Models and management. *British Medical Journal, 320* (March), 768–770.

Reason, J. (2002). Combating omission errors through task analysis and good reminders. *Quality Safety Health Care, 11,* 40–44.

Robinson, I. (2019). Prevention of workplace violence among healthcare workers. *Workplace Health and Safety, 67*(2), 96.

Rogers, A., Hwang, W., Scott, L., Aiken, L., & Dinges, D. (2004). The working hours of hospital staff nurses and patient safety. *Health Affairs, 23*(4), 202–212.

Sadeghi, S., Barzi, A., Mikhail, O., & Shabot, M. (2013). *Integrating quality and strategy in healthcare organizations.* Burlington, MA: Jones & Bartlett Learning.

Sallon, S., Katz-Eisner, D., Yaffe, H., & Bdolah-Abram, T. (2015, November). Caring for the caregivers: Results of an extended, five-component stress-reduction intervention for hospital staff. *Behavioral Medicine,* 1–15.

Seelye, K. (2016, March 7). Use of heroin in public view across the U.S. *New York Times*, p. A1.

Sonnentag, S., & Fritz, C. (2006). Endocrinological processes associated with job stress: Catecholamine and cortisol response to acute and chronic stressors. In P. Perrewé & D. Ganster (Eds.), *Employee health, coping, and methodologies* (pp. 1–59). Bingley, UK: Emerald.

Sorbello, B. (2008). Responding to a sentinel event. *American Nurse Today, 3*(10). Retrieved from http://www.americannursetoday.com/responding-to-a-sentinel-event

Stimpfel, A., Sloane, D., & Aiken, L. (2012). The longer the shifts for hospital nurses, the higher the levels of burnout and patient dissatisfaction. *Health Affairs, 31*(11), 2501–2509.

Taylor, J. Dominici, F., Agnew, J., Gerwin, D., Morlock, L., & Miller, M. (2012). Do nurse and patient injuries share common antecedents? An analysis of associations with safety climate and working conditions. *BMJ Quality Safety, 22*(2), 101–111.

Tella, S., Liukka, M., Jamookeeah, D., Smith, N., Partanen, P., & Turunen, H. (2014). What do students learn about patient safety? *Journal of Nursing Education, 53*(1), 7–13.

The Joint Commission. (2011). Sentinel alert issue 48: Healthcare worker fatigue and patient safety. Retrieved from http://www.jointcommission.org/sea_issue_48

The Joint Commission. (2019). Sentinel events policy and procedures. Retrieved from https://www.jointcommission.org/sentinel_event_policy_and_procedures

Trinkoff, A., Johantgen, M., Storr, C. L., Gurses, A., Liang, Y., Han, K. (2010). Nurses' work schedule characteristics, nurse staffing, and patient mortality. *Nursing Research, 60*(1), 1–8.

U.S. Department of Health and Human Services (HHS), Agency for Healthcare Research and Quality (AHRQ). (2013). TeamSTEPPS® 2.0: Team strategies & tools to enhance performance and patient safety. Retrieved from https://www.ahrq.gov/sites/default/files/wysiwyg/professionals/education/curriculum-tools/teamstepps/instructor/essentials/pocketguide.pdf

U.S. Department of Health and Human Services (HHS), Agency for Healthcare Research and Quality (AHRQ), Patient Safety Network (PSNet). (2017). Healthcare worker presenteeism: A challenge for patient safety. Retrieved from https://www.psnet.ahrq.gov/perspective/health-care-worker-presenteeism-challenge-patient-safety

U.S. Department of Health and Human Services (HHS), Agency for Healthcare Research and Quality (AHRQ), Patient Safety Network (PSNet). (2019a). Patient safety primer: Missed nursing care. Retrieved from https://psnet.ahrq.gov/primer/missed-nursing-care

U.S. Department of Health and Human Services (HHS), Agency for Healthcare Research and Quality (AHRQ),

Patient Safety Network (PSNet). (2019b). Burnout. Retrieved from https://psnet.ahrq.gov/primer/burnout

U.S. Department of Health and Human Services (HHS), Agency for Healthcare Research and Quality (AHRQ), Patient Safety Network (PSNet). (2019c). Systems approach. Retrieved from https://psnet.ahrq.gov/primer/systems-approach

U.S. Department of Health and Human Services (HHS), Agency for Healthcare Research and Quality (AHRQ). Patient Safety Network (PSNet). (2019d). Human factors engineering. Retrieved from https://psnet.ahrq.gov/primer/human-factors-engineering

U.S. Department of Health and Human Services (HHS), Agency for Healthcare Research and Quality (AHRQ). Patient Safety Network (PSNet). (2019e). Patient Safety 101. Retrieved from https://psnet.ahrq.gov/primer/patient-safety-101U.S. Department of Health and Human Services (HHS), Agency for Healthcare Research and Quality (AHRQ), Patient Safety Network (PSNet). (2019f). Second victims: Support for clinicians involved in errors and adverse events. Retrieved from https://psnet.ahrq.gov/primer/second-victims-support-clinicians-involved-errors-and-adverse-events

U.S. Department of Health and Human Services (HHS), Centers for Disease Control and Prevention (CDC), National Institute for Occupational Safety and Health (NIOSH). (2014). Violence occupational hazards in hospitals. Retrieved from https://www.cdc.gov/niosh/docs/2002-101/default.html

U.S. Department of Health and Human Services (HHS), Centers for Disease Control and Prevention (CDC), National Institute for Occupational Health and Safety (NIOSH). (2019). About NIOSH. Retrieved from https://www.cdc.gov/niosh/docs/99-101/default.html

U.S. Department of Health and Human Services (HHS), Food and Drug Administration (FDA). (2016). What is a serious adverse event? Retrieved from https://www.fda.gov/safety/reporting-serious-problems-fda/what-serious-adverse-event

U.S. Department of Labor (DOL), Occupational Health and Safety Administration (OSHA). (2016). Guidelines for preventing workplace violence for healthcare and social service workers. Retrieved from https://www.osha.gov/Publications/osha3148.pdf

U.S. Department of Labor (DOL), Occupational Health and Safety Administration (OSHA). (2019). About OSHA. Retrieved from http://www.osha.gov/about.html

Van Metre, J., Slovensky, D., & McLaughlin, C. (2013). Classification and reduction of medical errors. In W. Sollecito & J. Johnson (Eds.), *McLaughlin and Kaluzny's Continuous Quality Improvement in Health Care* (4th ed., pp. 311–334). Burlington, MA: Jones & Bartlett Learning.

VanDeusen, L., Holmes, S., Koppelman, E., Charns M., Frigand, C., Gupte, G., Neal, N. (2015). System re-design responses to challenges in safety-net systems: Summary of field study research. Rockville, MD: Agency for Healthcare Research and Quality. AHRQ Pub. No. 15-0053-EF.

Welton, J. (2007). Mandatory hospital nurse to patient staffing ratios: Time to take a different approach. *The Online Journal of Nursing, 12*(3). Retrieved from http:// ojin.nursingworld.org/mainmenucategories/anamarket place/anaperiodicals/ojin/tableofcontents/volume12 2007/no3sept07/mandatorynursetopatientratios .htmlsep

World Health Organization (WHO). (2019). Patient safety. Retrieved from https://www.who.int/news-room/fact -sheets/detail/patient-safety

## CHAPTER 8

# Setting the Stage for Quality Improvement

## CHAPTER OBJECTIVES

At the conclusion of this chapter, the learner will be able to:

- Analyze the impact of fragmentation and variation in care.
- Examine the value of surveillance for nursing and continuous quality improvement.
- Compare and contrast examples of high-risk situations for errors and reduced quality care.
- Critique examples of two major national initiatives and strategies focused on response to potential risk of inadequate quality care: hospital-acquired conditions and 30-day unplanned readmissions.

## OUTLINE

## KEY TERMS

| | | |
|---|---|---|
| 30-day unplanned readmission | Harm | Point of care |
| Alarm/alert fatigue | High-risk | Surveillance |
| Diagnostic error | Hospital-acquired conditions | Workaround |
| Failure to rescue | (HACs) | |
| Handoffs | Medication error | |

# Introduction

This chapter examines the environment in which continuous quality improvement (CQI) is applied. Healthcare organizations (HCOs) and healthcare providers need to understand the care process, particularly the impact of fragmentation and variation in care. These are important factors that drive errors and difficulties in effectively meeting expected outcomes. Surveillance and measures/indicators are elements that impact the CQI environment and process. Consideration of these factors sets the stage for effective CQI initiatives. Two current major federal government initiatives that have a major impact on healthcare delivery and costs are described in this chapter. Research is ongoing to examine errors and strategies to resolve errors and these problems (e.g., hospital-acquired complications and unplanned 30-day readmissions). The Agency for Healthcare Research and Quality (AHRQ) funds numerous studies—for example, studies focused on medication errors and the electronic medical record; communication; policies to reduce pressure sores, falls, and so on; and teamwork (U.S. Department of Health and Human Services [HHS], AHRQ, 2018a). Understanding how the stage is set for effective CQI assists in the examination of the specific elements of CQI and how they may be applied in individual HCOs by healthcare providers and in macro-CQI initiatives on the state and federal levels.

# Impact of Fragmentation of Care and Variation in Care

As we continue to examine healthcare quality and how HCOs pursue the goal of improved care, it is important to recognize how the healthcare environment and care process impact CQI. HCOs must understand their own healthcare environment and care processes to better appreciate their strengths, weaknesses, and improvement needs. Some care process concerns commonly found in HCOs relate to point of care, fragmentation, and variation in care needs and approaches.

## Point of Care

**Point of care** refers to direct care experiences when the healthcare provider and patient intersect for care, such as for assessment and intervention. Ideally, this is the key place for CQI, as staff work toward effectively meeting the patient's needs and expected outcomes. At the point of care, staff can identify near misses and stop an action that might lead to an error or interfere with expected care outcomes. It is important that an HCO's quality improvement (QI) program and its plans emphasize the importance of CQI at the point of care. In doing so, there is a greater chance not only to identify problems early but also to increase direct care staff engagement in CQI. Direct care staff include physicians, nurses, nursing assistants, laboratory staff, radiology staff, transportation staff who take patients to other locations, and dietary staff.

## Fragmentation of Care

The early *Quality Chasm* reports noted that there were major problems in the healthcare systems, describing the system as dysfunctional (Institute of Medicine [IOM], 1999, 2001). Gaps in the continuum of care can have a negative impact on quality care—for example, medication reconciliation, which is discussed in this chapter, is a method used to address potential gaps in care related to problems with communication about medication needs and orders. Ineffective communication during transfer of care or handoff is another example that may lead to gaps in care. Gap analysis is a critical part of CQI and measurement, as discussed in more detail in other sections of this text. Here in this chapter, we recognize that fragmentation must be considered a barrier to effective care in the QI program and its plans. There is concern today about patient flow and emergency department crowding, both of which contribute to fragmentation of care, ineffective communication, handoff errors and workarounds, and reduced quality of care and patient satisfaction.

## Variation of Care

Care varies from one patient to another (even if they have the same diagnosis), from one individual healthcare provider to another, and from one HCO to another. To complicate matters, geographic areas may have different care practices and quality. A QI program has to account for the factors that may impact this variation—factors that are more than just individual patient differences. Care variation impacts performance comparisons or benchmarking (discussed in more detail in other areas of this text). It also impacts care planning. Furthermore, variation in care has implications for care interventions, which may result in different outcomes even when it appears the outcomes should be the same or similar. When such instances arise, HCOs are left to wonder if the best intervention was chosen? Was it possible to really identify and control factors that led to the variation? It is not always easy to make such determinations prospectively, but learning from retrospective results may assist in understanding variation in care and its influence on quality. Nurses should be actively involved in this analysis, as they work closely with patients and must respond to these variations daily. HCOs also must consider whether variations—as in patients and their health problems, providers, use of treatment, resource variability, access to care, and such—influence these differences and whether other factors are at play.

Do transient working conditions just prior to an adverse event or during the shift in which the event occurred affect occurrence rates (Grayson et al., 2014)? This is another type of variation in care. A study examined this question and potential triggers that were present when an adverse event occurred compared with a time when an adverse event did not occur. The results indicated that there is variation within a shift and across shifts for specific risk factors. Variation does impact event occurrence. An example is occurrence of unexpected, time-consuming events that then disrupt nurses from their tasks and increase workload. This study indicated that errors increase on busier, more demanding shifts and at times when information sharing is incomplete.

**STOP AND CONSIDER 8-1**

Care is complex, and its complexity and variation have a major impact on CQI.

## Surveillance

The report *Keeping Patients Safe* identifies the need for monitoring patient status or **surveillance** as one of the six major concerns related to direct care quality. The goal is "early identification and prevention of potential problems, which requires behavioral and cognitive skills" (IOM, 2004, p. 91). Assessment is typically done at one point in time, and surveillance is ongoing. Effective surveillance depends on staff competence, staffing levels, skill mix, communication, interprofessional issues and effective teamwork, limiting staff stress level and staff fatigue, use of evidence-based practice (EBP), equipment and supplies, health informatics, and leadership (Finkelman, 2017). If surveillance is not effective, then failure to rescue may occur, resulting in possible complications.

Surveillance is considered to be a critical performance measure, primarily focused on nurses and nursing care. Recognition of this process, data collection, identification of problems, and strategies to resolve should be integrated into the QI plan. Surveillance has an impact on when care is received, particularly identifying times of risk, such as variations in care and gaps in care. Effective surveillance

systems should meet the following objectives (Keroack & Rhinehart, 2012):

- Determine the overall magnitude of the problem relative to others.
- Decide whether the problem is increasing or decreasing in incidence.
- Identify which patient groups or care areas are most affected and therefore most in need of resources.
- Decide whether efforts to improve are succeeding. (p. 128)

**STOP AND CONSIDER 8-2**

Nurses have the primary responsibility for surveillance.

## Examples of High-Risk Situations for Errors and Reduced Quality Care

Risk is the chance that something will happen. An HCO cannot focus on all of its problems and must prioritize its CQI activities. A place to begin identifying CQI focus areas is with **high-risk** concerns. The term "high risk" applies to situations with a greater chance of near misses and errors occurring. In addition, there are barriers to reaching expected outcomes, thereby reducing care quality. Today, there is more concern about diversity and health literacy as factors that impact the risk for errors and reduce quality care.

High-risk situations may compromise quality care. Recognizing the possibility of such outcomes means the HCO and healthcare providers need to consider the possible consequences and then identify interventions. As Barach and Johnson (2018), state, "There is substantial evidence that the majority of harm caused by healthcare is avoidable and the result of systemic problems rather than poor performance or negligence by individual providers" (p. 250). With the growing concerns about errors, we know there is need for continuous improvement of care, and what has been done to date is not making a significant difference.

## Working in Silos

Working in silos means staff members are focused exclusively on their specific work area and concerns; they cannot see beyond their own work concerns. It is easy for this mentality to develop in healthcare, as there is a tendency to focus on specialties and even subspecialties—for example, a women's health department may be divided into gynecology and maternal–child (obstetrics) services. Gynecology may then be subdivided into gynecology patient care units, maybe oncology gynecology, and outpatient clinics; and maternal–child services may be subdivided into pregnancy support (usually through clinics), labor and delivery, neonatal and maybe neonatal intensive care, and postpartum care. In addition, there may be a variety of clinics within the women's health department. Nurses typically work in one specific unit or clinic. They often forget that staff are also located in other areas, and they may not feel connected to the department and the HCO. Nurses are also part of the nursing organization (department, service) within the HCO, which adds another level to nursing responsibilities.

Working in silos may lead to problems such as misunderstanding the trajectory of care, ineffective communication, inadequate coordination, inconsistency, and lack of commitment to the broader vision and goals. Staff may have fewer relationships and communication with staff outside their "silo" area. All of these factors impact outcomes, risk of errors, and CQI—for example, handoffs occur across silos, but when there is little routine connection and communication, communication and coordination may be limited.

Another factor that is important to consider when identifying risk is the opposite of working in silos. Today, with the increased use of teams, there is much more change even within work teams, such as team members coming and going, and these changes may increase risk (Wachter, 2008). HCOs must use strategies to increase communication and ensure that when people work alone they communicate effectively with others, they work within a team, and, when the team changes, they continue with clear, effective communication.

## Annual Joint Commission National Patient Safety Goals: Identification of High Risk Concerns

After the publication of several of the *Quality Chasm* reports, The Joint Commission began an initiative that now has a major impact on quality care. Annually, The Joint Commission identifies key safety goals (The Joint Commission, 2019). These goals are identified from the information The Joint Commission receives from its accredited HCOs. The goals are identified per specific type of HCO (e.g., acute care hospitals, ambulatory care). The 2020 hospital goals focus on patient identification, staff communication, medication safety, alarm safety prevention of infection, and prevention of mistakes in surgery (The Joint Commission). Current goals may be accessed through The Joint Commission link identified in the Connect to Current Information section at the end of this chapter.

HCOs accredited by The Joint Commission must now use the National Patient Safety Goals as one of their critical CQI guides. The goals provide information and alert staff to these high-risk concerns. Data about the goals are collected by individual HCOs and submitted to The Joint Commission, describing their results in aggregate form to assess progress in meeting the annual goals. Then the Joint Commission shares this information with HCOs and others to improve care. The goals apply to anyone who works in the HCO, including all healthcare professions students. Schools of nursing must stay up to date with the current goals, discuss them with students, expect students to be alert about the high-risk concerns, and initiate any interventions that the HCO requires to meet the goals. When students plan care for their assigned patients they should include relevant approaches to meet annual patient safety goals.

## Care Transitions and Handoffs

**Handoffs** are times when patients are transitioned from one form of care to another, such as from one clinical site (e.g., unit, department, HCO) to another, from one provider to another, or from a clinical site back to the patient's home (HHS, AHRQ, PSNet, 2019a). Patients report that a positive handoff experience is important to them (Ford & Heyman, 2017). HCOs and the government recognize these times as high risk. The Joint Commission requires that its accredited HCOs develop structured communication methods to address concern about the risk for errors during care transitions or handoffs, recognizing that an inadequate handoff is a contributing factor to adverse events (The Joint Commission, 2017). The Centers for Medicare and Medicaid Services (CMS) readmission program, which is discussed later in this chapter, focuses on increased risk with care transition during discharge. The electronic medical record/electronic health record (EMR/EHR) also assists in providing information during handoffs, particularly focusing on opportunity to share communication between care providers (e.g., from hospital to hospital, among individual providers, from hospital to a long-term care facility). Providing information across providers, such as hospitals or individual providers, is critical and a weak area. We now have a number of structured communication methods to assist staff during this transition. Multiple methods are discussed in this text, but more needs to be done to improve understanding of handoffs and communication during this time. For example, more information is needed to better identify high-risk patients, identify best time to intervene and best strategies/interventions, track outcomes, and then use this information to continue improvement (HHS, AHRQ, PSNet, 2019a).

Common barriers to effective handoffs are ineffective communication or no communication; lack of or misuse of time; stressful work environment; inconsistent information; environmental issues, such as interruptions; distractions, such as noise; multitasking; lack of standardization, such as standardized communication methods; problems sharing digital information; health informatics technology (HIT) equipment problems; leadership and management concerns, such as unclear policies and procedures; limited staff support and inadequate resources; lack of staff preparation and understanding of the transition process; inadequate staffing levels; and equipment problems (Risenberg, Leitzsch, & Cunningham, 2010; Welsh, Flanagan, & Ebright, 2010). Identification of barriers should then guide effective development of strategies/interventions to prevent or respond to handoff problems and should be used to prepare staff for this experience.

Nursing shift change is a time of handoffs: the handoff of all the patients on the unit to different nursing staff, typically done two to three times per 24 hours (Mayor, Bangerter, & Aribot, 2012). Staff may change multiple times on some units, with staff working individualized schedules. This approach increases the risk of problems during handoffs. Various types of reports may be used, such as a unit report, team report, bedside rounds, and written or audio report or a combination of methods. The purpose is to ensure greater communication and coordination of care. The type and amount of information shared varies from unit to unit. Management and staff influence how these methods are used. Patient condition also impacts how the handoff report is done and what information is included—for example, in a situation when the staff is overworked and in a hurry to get on with other tasks, there is higher risk of providing incomplete or incorrect information.

As mentioned in this text, some experts, including The Joint Commission, recommend the use of more structured and standardized shift handoff methods—for example, the standard might be to use the situation-background-assessment-recommendation (SBAR) approach discussed in other chapters. One study that examined a project using eSBAR, an electronic form of the approach, to reduce delays in an emergency and then reduce boarding times in the emergency room while patients waited for beds department increasing patient flow. "The tool provides an overview of patient information, including demographics, diagnosis, surgical/health history, medications, allergies, height, weight, vital signs, test/procedure results, intake, output, and multidisciplinary team documentation. The inpatient summary was organized in SBAR format" (Potts, Diegel-Vacek, Ryan, & Murchek, 2018, p. 434). Although it makes sense that these methods would improve communication, there is no strong evidence to indicate they make a difference in quality of shift handoffs (Mayor et al., 2012; Perry, Wears, & Patterson, 2008). In a study that examined shift handoffs, researchers hypothesized that uncertainty or variation drives the topics and communication during a shift change (Mayor et al., 2012). This means when patients are unstable and/or in critical condition, there is more uncertainty and handoff duration increases. In this study, the most common topics that did vary from different types of units and amount of uncertainty were the treatment, care process, and organization of work. Recommendations indicate that management needs to consider uncertainty and shift handoff to ensure that the units have resources to provide necessary information for efficient handoffs. More research is needed to better understand the importance of handoffs, something that occurs routinely throughout the healthcare delivery system every day and is a critical component of nursing care.

Bedside reports may improve effectiveness, efficiency, patient safety, patient-centered care, and patient satisfaction, thus impacting CQI. A study that examined the implementation of bedside reports identified some difficulties with using this method. Typically, reports are an opportunity for staff not only to discuss patients but also to interact with one another and build relationships, which is an important part of a work environment and provides time to discuss general work issues (Hagman, Oman, Kleiner, Johnson, & Nordhagen, 2013). This type of interaction and sharing is not typically part of a bedside report. Some staff also do not feel comfortable sharing all information in front of patients, even with the increased emphasis on patient-centered care. This study found other barriers that must be considered: frequent patient requests during the bedside report, concern for sleeping patients, patients in isolation, non–English-speaking patients, and lack of privacy in a multiple patient room. The staff were generally satisfied, but barriers must be addressed to improve bedside reporting. The staff need training to use this shift handoff method.

Problems with communication, such as missing information, require interventions focused on using more concise and accessible communication—for example, computer-generated summaries and standardized formats may facilitate more timely exchange of critical patient information (Kripalani et al., 2007). Handoff information should be timely and correctly dated. It should include clear information about diagnosis, testing, treatment, communication with the patient and family (as appropriate), and outcomes. The following strategies might be used to provide more effective handoff coordination and communication (Patterson, Roth, Woods, Chow, & Gomes, 2004).

- Use face-to-face verbal updates with interactive questioning.
- Provide additional updates relevant to other providers in addition to the major provider.

- Limit interruptions during updates.
- Incoming and outgoing staff should initiate topics for discussion or clarification.
- Discussion includes outgoing staff views about changes in plans.
- Information is read back to ensure it was accurately received.
- Outgoing staff write summary before handoffs completed.
- Incoming staff assess current status.
- Information is updated in the same order every time to ensure that all critical information is covered.
- Incoming staff scan historical data before update from outgoing staff.
- Incoming staff receive primary access to the most up-to-date information.
- Incoming staff receive paperwork that includes handwritten annotations.
- At a certain time, it is made clear to others at a glance which staff are responsible for which duties.
- The transfer of responsibility is delayed when there is concern about the status or stability of the process; such concerns should be clearly addressed as part of routine information during handoffs.

During report, staff need to ask questions and clarify both the written and the verbal information received. This process should not be rushed or viewed as just another task. How it is done and the content make a difference in patient care, outcomes, and CQI. The Joint Commission provides tips to improve handoffs (2018), providing strategies related to communication, electronic methods, type of information to share, sources of information, and so on. Examples of barriers to effective handoffs are highlighted in **Table 8-1**.

# Failure to Rescue

**Failure to rescue** (FTR) is missing an opportunity to prevent complications. Active surveillance is required to limit incidents of FTR. These are times of high risk for patients, impacting potential for errors and limiting

**Table 8-1** Examples of Barriers in the Handoff Process

**Technological Factors**
- Patient rosters (e.g., whiteboards)
- Electronic health records

**Team Factors**
- Shift schedules
- Physician compensation methods
- Peer relationships and power balances
- Failure to recognize importance of handoff
- Ambiguous moment during transfer of care

**Task Factors**
- Too much noise in background to hear communication
- Salience versus completeness
- Varied clinical volume, presentations, complexity
- Lack of standard approach
- Absence of "red flags"

**Patient Factors**
- Alertness
- Education
- Pain
- Language barrier
- Knowledge of own illness
- Unclear diagnosis

**Local and Institutional Environmental Factors**
- Location: loud, chaotic, lacking privacy
- Competing demands for time and attention
- Inpatient boarding
- Long emergency department lengths of stay

**Caregiver Factors**
- Fatigue, stress
- Inattention
- Poor memory
- Inexperience
- Knowledge deficit
- Cognitive bias
- Personal agendas after shift change

Data from Cheung, D., Kelly, J., Beach, C., Berkeley, R., Bitterman, R., Broida, R., . . . American College of Emergency Physicians Section of Quality Improvement and Patient Safety. (2009). Improving handoffs in the emergency department. *Annals of Emergency Medicine, 55*(2), 171–180.

reaching expected outcomes. One of the common steps taken when FTR occurs is to use rapid response teams (RRTs), discussed in other chapters, as a CQI strategy. The purpose of the FTR measure is to determine "the hospital's ability to rescue patients that have developed a serious complication" (Manojlovich & Talsma, 2007, p. 304). What constitutes an FTR situation is not universally accepted. The lack of a universal definition impacts collecting data about the event and comparing data with other HCOs. Even within one HCO, there can be different views of when FTR occurs.

To understand these events and then to initiate interventions to prevent them, HCOs need to analyze the events to examine causes and staff responses. HCOs often use root cause analysis to better understand causes such as problems with monitoring equipment, patient-staff interactions, assessment and communication, and the decision-making process (Jones, DeVita, & Bellomo, 2011).

## Diagnosis and Errors

The report *Improving Diagnosis in Health Care* focuses on quickly identifying, resolving, and reducing the incidence of diagnostic errors (National Academy of Medicine [NAM], 2015). "Each year an estimated 1 in 20 U.S. adults experiences missed, delayed, or incorrect diagnoses. Of the estimated 12 million Americans impacted, 4 million are believed to suffer serious harm. Diagnostic errors contribute to about 10 percent of patient deaths. They exact a painful financial toll as well. They are the single greatest source of medical malpractice claims, with an estimated cost of well over $100 billion a year, while the human cost is incalculably higher. Among a clinician's long list of responsibilities, perhaps none is more consequential than the act of diagnosis. The initial determination of a patient's condition sets in motion a series of steps that may include life-altering tests, referrals, and treatments. A correct diagnosis starts a patient on the path toward all that modern medicine has to offer. When errors occur, however, the consequences may range from merely wasted time and money,

to a patient who becomes sicker or is injured as a result. In worst cases, diagnostic error can directly lead to an otherwise preventable death" (Brady & Khanna, 2019).

Most people experience at least one diagnostic error in their lifetime. These errors may occur in all types of care. They are often related to malpractice claims, factoring into approximately 10% of patient deaths and between 6% and 17% of hospital adverse events (Kronick, 2013). National data indicate that diagnostic error is one of the most common errors and impacts an estimated 12 million patients each year, although HCOs do not commonly focus on this type of error (Singh, 2015). Diagnosis is a complex process that involves multiple providers and the patient. **Diagnostic error** is "a missed opportunity to make a correct or timely diagnosis based on the available evidence, regardless of patient harm" (Singh, 2014, p. 99). The recent national report addresses this important problem and identifies possible causes of diagnostic errors, such as ineffective collaboration and communication (healthcare providers/clinicians, patients, and families), healthcare system that is not supportive of an effective diagnosis process, need for greater feedback about performance related to diagnosis, and an HCO culture that does not support transparency and disclosure of these errors (NAM, 2015).

It is important to understand patients' perspectives regarding diagnosis, which include the interpersonal relationship and communications. Does the healthcare provider listen to the patient, respect patients, recognize that patients have important information, and engage the patient (Giardina et al., 2018). Ineffective patient-centered care has an impact on diagnostic errors (Kaplan, 2016). Patients may be reluctant to be open about their diagnosis and their concerns. Physicians and advanced practice registered nurses (APRNs) who diagnose may make assumptions and then not be able to consider other aspects of diagnosis. Past experience has an impact on how physicians view current patient problems and can interfere with objectivity. Physicians may also think they have the complete diagnosis and consider diagnostic errors to be rare situations. During the diagnosis process, it is best to take a diagnostic time-out to stop and reflect for at least a few minutes. Time may be needed to seek advice or a second opinion and discuss tests and radiology results with experts and others, all of which may expand on information that was in written reports (Society of Hospital Medicine [SHM], 2016).

The NAM examination of diagnostic errors also discusses possible strategies to prevent these errors, such as greater teamwork to improve collaboration and communication, use of AHRQ resources such as the Patient and Family Engagement Guide, toolkits on various topics to help HCOs (inpatient and ambulatory care) be more effective, and use of interventions to measure and better understand these errors. Despite this extensive report, it is still difficult to fully understand the extent of the problem. The report describes the Safer Diagnosis Framework, which can be used to improve strategies to prevent and respond to this type of error (NAM, 2015). This framework, accessible in the report *Improving Diagnosis in Health Care*, focuses on the patient and four diagnostic dimensions, which interact with one another: encounter with the patient and healthcare provider and the initial diagnostic assessment, diagnostic testing and interpretation, consultations and referrals, and follow-up and monitoring of diagnostic information. When diagnostic errors are measured, consideration should be given to reliability, validity, and retrospective and prospective views. Safer diagnosis should lead to improved value of healthcare and improved patient outcomes. The AHRQ provides numerous tools to help healthcare professionals prevent diagnostic errors—for example, related to patient and family engagement, laboratory testing, communication, and so on (HHS, AHRQ, 2019a).

Patients should also participate in reducing diagnosis errors—for example, they may inform healthcare providers of errors that providers may not know about, such as diagnosis problems from an emergency visit; ask for second opinions; keep track of their personal health information; ask about laboratory and other test results; and speak up—asking questions, requesting further information to understand the diagnosis, and stating when there is concern that care may not be effective (Graber, 2014).

Advanced practice registered nurses may diagnosis. Staff nurses and nurse managers, who do not make medical diagnosis, should, however, be involved in monitoring and responding to diagnostic errors. Graber (2014) recommends the following: "Empower nurses to become involved in improving diagnosis. Monitor for new or resolving symptoms, [and] facilitate communication between patients and providers" (p. 26). Other recommended strategies include use of morbidity and mortality conferences to better understand care provided and outcomes; use autopsies to learn more about diagnoses, although this is done less and less; get second opinions; provide best possible expertise for radiology and clinical laboratory testing; send laboratory test results to patients; monitor how many critical test results (including radiology) are acted upon within 30 days; empower patients to participate and speak up; and actively use root cause analysis, requiring clinicians to participate in the process (Graber). Many of these strategies should involve nurses.

## Medication Administration

Medication administration is a high-risk event for possible errors with multiple points for risks of errors. A **medication error** is defined by the U.S. Department of Health and Human Services (HHS, Food and Drug Administration [FDA], 2015) as a "preventable event that may cause or lead to inappropriate medication use or patient harm while the medication is in control of the healthcare professional, patient, or consumer." The FDA notes that these errors are related to factors such as professional practice, healthcare products, and procedures and systems, including prescribing, communication of medication order, product labeling, packaging, nomenclature, compounding, dispensing, distribution, and administration of the medication. Staff education and monitoring of the process are also critical factors.

## Medication Administration: A Process and Its Implications

Medication administration is a complex process. Interruptions cannot be eliminated, but nurses must recognize the risk involved and take whatever steps possible to reduce interruptions (Bavo, Cochran, & Barrett, 2016; Thomas, Donohue-Porter, & Fishbein, 2017). One strategy for dealing with interruptions is to establish "Do Not Interrupt" zones or times (Westbrook et al., 2017). There is also increased risk during transition of care—for example, transfer from intensive care to a non–intensive care unit. In one study nearly half the patients (sample of 985) experienced a medication error during handoff from intensive care to a non–intensive care unit although the errors did not cause harm (Tully, Hammond, Jarrell, & Kruer, 2019).

The Institute for Safe Medication Practices (ISMP) identifies the following key interrelated elements that affect what the ISMP refers to as the Medication Use System™ (ISMP, 2019):

1. *Patient information.* Obtaining the patient's pertinent demographic (age, weight) and clinical (diagnoses, allergies, lab results) information will assist practitioners in selecting the appropriate medications, doses, and routes of administration. Having essential patient information at the time of medication prescribing, dispensing, and administration will result in a significant decrease in preventable adverse drug events (ADEs).

2. *Drug information.* Providing accurate and usable drug information to all healthcare practitioners involved in the process reduces the amount of preventable ADEs. Not only should drug information be readily accessible to the staff through many sources (e.g., drug references, formulary, protocols, HCO-prepared information, dosing scales) but also it must be up to date and accurate.

3. *Communication of drug information.* Miscommunication among physicians, pharmacists, and nurses is a common cause of medication errors. To minimize the amount of medication errors caused by miscommunication, it is always important to verify drug information and eliminate communication barriers.

4. *Drug labeling, packaging, and nomenclature.* Drug names that look alike or sound alike, as well as products that have confusing drug labeling and non-distinct drug packaging, significantly contribute to medication errors. The incidence of medication errors is reduced with the use of proper labeling and the use of unit-dose systems within hospitals.

5. *Drug storage, stock, standardization, and distribution.* Standardizing drug administration times, regulating drug concentrations, and limiting the dose concentration of drugs available in patient care areas reduce the risk of medication errors or minimize their consequences should an error occur.

6. *Drug device acquisition, use, and monitoring.* Appropriate safety assessment of drug delivery devices should be made both prior to their purchase and during their use. Also, a system of independent double-checks should be used within the HCO to prevent device-related errors, such as selecting the wrong drug or drug concentration, setting

the rate improperly, or mistaking the infusion line for another line.

7. *Environmental factors.* Having a well-designed system offers the best chance of preventing errors; however, sometimes the environment in which we work contributes to medication errors. Environmental factors that often contribute to medication errors include poor lighting, noise, interruptions, and a significant workload.

8. *Staff competence and education.* Staff education should focus on priority topics, such as new medications used in the hospital; high-alert medications; medication errors that have occurred both internally and externally; and protocols, policies, and procedures related to medication use. Staff education can be an important error prevention strategy when combined with the other key elements for medication safety.

9. *Patient education.* Patients must receive ongoing education from physicians, pharmacists, and the nursing staff about the brand and generic names of medications they are receiving, their indications, usual and actual doses, expected and possible adverse effects, drug or food interactions, and how to protect themselves from errors. Patients have a vital role in preventing medication errors and should be encouraged to ask questions and seek answers about their medications before drugs are administered in an HCO, prescribed by a healthcare provider, or dispensed at a pharmacy.

10. *Quality processes and risk management.* The way to prevent errors is to redesign the systems and processes that lead to errors, rather than focus on correcting individuals who make errors. Effective strategies for reducing errors include making it difficult for staff to make an error and promoting the detection and correction of errors before they reach a patient and cause harm.

The ISMP encourages use of consensus-based practice for specific medication safety issues and updates this information for healthcare practitioners and healthcare organizations (ISMP, 2018). Some of the drugs included in the 2018–2019 best practice list are oral methotrexate, oral liquid medications, and vincristine, as well as specifics as to administration about certain drugs and storage of drugs. Using this type of guideline reduces risk of errors and patient harm, and this type of listing changes from time to time based on outcomes. Examples of common sources of medication errors are identified in **Table 8-2**.

The National Coordinating Council for Medication Error Reporting and Prevention (NCC MERP), a collaboration of 27 national organizations, recognized the need for a standardized categorization of errors and compared preventable ADEs with non-preventable ADEs, as describe in **Figure 8-1**.

The following are some of the key types of errors (NCC MERP, 2019).

- A *preventable ADE* is harm caused by the use of a drug as a result of an error (e.g., patient given a normal dose of a drug, but the drug was contraindicated for this patient). These events require examination to determine why they occurred.
- A *non-preventable ADE* is drug-induced harm occurring during appropriate use of medication (e.g., anaphylaxis from penicillin in a patient who had no previous history of an allergic reaction). While these events are currently non-preventable, future studies may reveal ways to prevent them.
- An *adverse drug reaction (ADR)* is any response to a drug that is noxious, unintended, and occurs at doses normally used for prophylaxis or diagnosis or for the modification of a physiological function.

Both the NCC MERP and the FDA provide online methods to report medication errors and concerns, identified in the Connect to

**Table 8-2** Common Sources of Medication Errors

| | |
|---|---|
| Ambiguous orders | Incorrect drug selected |
| Drug device use | Incorrect patient |
| Environmental stress | Insufficient drug information |
| Errors in communication or miscommunication of drug orders | Insufficient information about other drugs patient is on (therapeutic duplication) |
| Error-prone abbreviation | Insufficient laboratory information |
| Illegible handwriting | Known allergy |
| Improper dose | Limited patient education |
| Incomplete orders | Limited staff education |
| Incomplete or insufficient monitoring | Look-alike or sound-alike drugs |
| Incomplete patient information or unavailable patient information | Poor communication |

Reproduced from Youngberg, B. (2013). *Patient safety handbook* (2nd ed.). Burlington, MA: Jones & Bartlett Learning.

Current Information section at the end of this chapter. These resources help expand nurses' knowledge about medications and errors.

The five administration rights (right patient, right drug, right dosage, right time, right route) have long been the standard for nursing care. Applying these rights helps to reduce errors and keeps nurses alert to common medication risk areas. Other additional rights that are also important are right documentation, right to refuse medication, and right to evaluation and monitoring (Anderson & Townsend, 2010). Given the need for improvement, two other rights have been recommended: identify the right indication or reason for the medication and ensure the right documentation is completed (Walton, 2014).

HCOs and CQI initiatives tend to emphasize reliance on medication error rates; however, not all experts agree with the value of these rates. In 2002, the NCC MERP reported that it did not consider it helpful to rely on incidence rates for medication errors, and in

2008, it restated its belief (NCC MERP, 2008). Focusing on numbers is not enough, as there is need to gain better understanding of errors beyond numbers. The NCC MERP gives the following reasons for not over-relying on incidence rates when comparing results with other HCOs (NCC MERP):

- *Differences in culture* among HCOs can lead to significant differences in the level of reporting of medication errors.
- *Differences in the definition* of a medication error among HCOs can lead to significant differences in the reporting and classification of medication errors.
- *Differences in the patient populations* served by various HCOs can lead to significant differences in the number and severity of medication errors occurring among organizations.
- *Differences in the type(s) of reporting and detection systems* for medication errors among HCOs can lead to significant differences in the number of medication errors recorded.

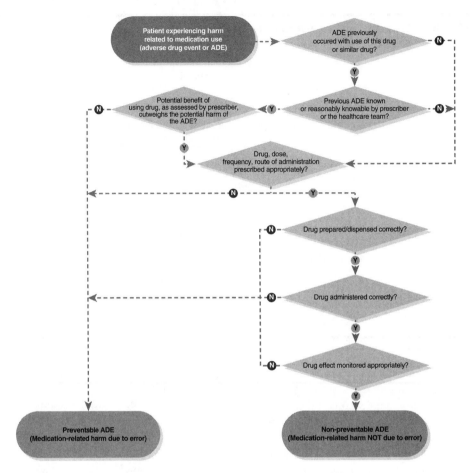

**Figure 8-1** Comparing Preventable Adverse Drug Event with Non-Preventable Adverse Drug Event

Reproduced from National Coordinating Council for Medication Error Reporting and Prevention. (2015). Contemporary view of medication-related harm. A new paradigm. Retrieved from http://www.nccmerp.org/sites/default/files/nccmerp_fact_sheet_2015-02-v91.pdf

The goal of every HCO should be to focus on CQI processes to prevent harm to patients due to medication errors (ISMP, 2018). Achieving this goal requires monitoring of actual and potential medication errors that occur within the HCO. The NCC MERP recommends that each HCO work to improve and prevent harm to patients within the organization. It defines **harm** as "impairment of the physical, emotional, or psychological function or structure of the body and pain or injury resulting therefrom" (NCC MERP, 2001). Focusing on the prevention of harm allows the HCO to identify limitations in its medication systems

and identify opportunities to learn from the experience. This should be done by using root cause analysis, as discussed in other chapters, to further understand medication errors and make changes as needed, recognizing that the number of errors is less important than the quality of the data.

Despite the fact that medication administration is one of the most common nursing interventions and also one with a high risk for errors, more still needs to be understood about this process—for example, it is recommended that nurses double check or have more than one nurse check the same information for some medications. Does this actually prevent errors? A systematic review, which included 13 studies, concluded that there was insufficient evidence from these studies that double-checking reduced errors. More research is required to understand the process and outcomes (Koyama, Maddox, Li, Bucknall, & Westbrook, 2019).

## Nursing Education and Medication Administration

Nursing education has a major role in reducing medication errors. Nurse educators need to consider the topic of medication administration as a critical part of content and experience, emphasizing with students that medication administration is a time in the care process when they must be engaged in CQI, both as students and after graduation. The most common student nurse medication errors are related to failure to follow administration rights, system issues, and lack of knowledge and understanding about medications (Cooper, 2014). These situations should be considered red flags for students, putting them on alert to be more careful. Students need to apply root cause analysis to errors both in simulation and if they should experience an error in clinical experiences (Dolansky, Druschel, Helba, & Courtney, 2013).

The focus of this text is primarily on CQI within HCOs, although the content does include the need to recognize core competencies that should be demonstrated not only by nurses in practice but also by those entering practice. Nursing students are involved in a variety of near misses and errors when they are in their clinical rotations. Simulated experiences provide a safe environment in which students can not only practice medication administration but also learn about medication administration risks, strategies to prevent errors, and how to respond and track near misses and errors. In a study conducted from 2011 to 2013 funded by the National Council of State Boards of Nursing (NCSBN),

the researchers collected and analyzed information about school of nursing practices and policies for student near misses and errors (Disch & Barnsteiner, 2014). A web-based survey was sent to 1,667 schools, and 557 (33%) responded. Of the responding schools, 86 (16%) had a tool or policy focused on student errors. This is a very small percentage, indicating a greater need for schools of nursing to examine CQI and how they handle student near misses and errors. There should be clear school of nursing policies and procedures related to these situations, and schools should also review and consider clinical agency policies and procedures. Schools of nursing must coordinate and share information with their HCOs so that there is effective CQI implemented within schools of nursing as well as collaboration with HCOs and their QI programs. It should be clear that when an error occurs in which a student and/or faculty is involved, there are procedures to follow at the HCO and at the school of nursing to ensure effective information sharing. Just as HCOs should avoid a blame environment, so should schools of nursing.

Following the first phase of the NCSBN-funded school of nursing study, a pilot was conducted in 10 schools of nursing. Using the survey form provided by the study, the sample submitted 70 error or near-miss reports in this period. The survey form identified the following types of incidents that would then be tracked in a new national database (Disch & Barnsteiner, 2014):

- Medication error
- Needlestick
- Inadequate preparation for providing patient care
- Blood/pathogen exposure
- Fall event
- Outside scope of practice
- Injury to body
- Change in patient condition
- Deviation in protocols
- Equipment or medical device malfunction

- Environmental safety for self, patient, and others
- Inappropriate or inadequate communication by faculty, preceptor, other student, healthcare team, patient, or visitor
- Breach of confidentiality (p. 7)

This survey includes not only data underlying the type of incident but also data about the recipient of the unsafe event, event demographics, event description in narrative form, location of the event, and follow-up action. The long-term goal of this study is to establish a web-based national data repository with anonymous reporting by students, faculty, or both to reduce student incidents. The repository is called Safe Student Reports (SSR) (NCSBN, 2019). Membership in the network allows members (schools of nursing) to access the data and track data for their students. It also provides opportunities to identify trends and additional information to better understand student learning needs related to safe medication administration.

This major study and the development of a national database support the need for schools of nursing to examine medication and medication administration content and learning experiences to ensure they are in line with current CQI information and recommendations for effective medication administration. Competence has a major impact on CQI. It is also important for students to appreciate the implications of effective and safe medication use for all patients in all settings—that is, in all situations, students should understand their role and responsibilities.

## *Examples of Strategies to Reduce Medication Errors*

It is vital that HCOs consider how their QI program and related CQI activities can reduce medication error risk. Examples of critical guidelines for safe medication administration include the following (Anderson & Townsend, 2010):

- Reading back and verifying medication orders given verbally or over the phone

- Asking a colleague to double-check medications when giving high-alert drugs
- Using an oral syringe to administer oral or nasogastric medications
- Assessing patients for drug allergies before giving medications
- Becoming familiar with the facility's "Do Not Use" list of abbreviations (p. 3)

It is common to use abbreviations in documentation and orders; however, risks are associated with this practice. The objective here is not to eliminate use of abbreviations but to caution staff to be careful when using them. HCOs should maintain an approved list of abbreviations, and staff must use only abbreviations that are on the list. Staff orientation and ongoing staff education should include this information, and when changes are made staff need to be informed. Electronic documentation programs provide more opportunities to alert staff to incorrect use of abbreviations and should block their use.

There is now greater use of unit-based dispensing devices that include storage for unit-dose and some multiple-dose options (decentralized automated dispensing devices). These devices are often connected in real time to the pharmacy so that staff can get assistance when needed, allowing for timely administration of medication with a safer dose method (Ehlert & Rough, 2013). The devices have also altered methods that were used for management of controlled substances, reducing time for staff to complete this more complex medication administration procedure, as well as providing a more effective, secure procedure.

Since the 1980s and 1990s, the dispensing devices have helped nurses during medication administration, reducing time and in some cases errors; however, potential problems with these devices must be considered in QI programs. HCOs must have the right equipment, maintained so that it functions correctly, and enough dispensing devices to cover workload and care needs. Problems with the equipment can lead to risk of errors and increased staff frustration, requiring more work when time is limited. However, using these devices does not ensure an error-free procedure. When a nurse opens a patient's medication container or drawer, there is still a risk of selecting the wrong drug and administering it—for example, the nurse may assume that all drugs in the container are correct according to the patient's orders without confirming. The HCO system must be consistent so that the same drugs and equipment are kept in the same place; however, there is the possibility that the nurse may be on autopilot and grab something that is misplaced. Policies and procedures related to a decentralized and automated dispensing device should be routinely reviewed, including staff feedback, and when changes are made, they should be shared with staff. New staff must be oriented to the system and supervised on initial use until the supervisor and the nurse feel comfortable with correct use, policies and procedures are followed, and the nurse has an understanding of the system.

Medication near misses have an impact on nurses' workloads. When nurses experience a near miss, they need to double-check orders and may need additional communication with the provider who ordered the medication. This process has an impact on other patients, too, as time is taken away from other care when staff are distracted. In the end, this situation increases risk for other problems and possibly results in more serious problems than a near miss—an outright error (Anderson & Townsend, 2010).

High-alert medications are drugs that have high potential to cause patient harm when misused (Ehlert & Rough, 2013). HCOs should develop a list of these medications. Examples are chemotherapy, heparin, and insulin. Typically, these drugs require double-checking with another licensed professional whenever the drug is taken from a multidose vial. Staff education should include information about these drugs, related policy and procedures, and also testing to ensure competency in administration of the drugs. If an automated dispensing device is used,

there should be clear labels and other methods to indicate that these drugs are included. The pharmacy must also use high-alert labels for the drugs—for example, specific labeling should be used when these drugs are used in infusion pumps. Intravenous infusions with these drugs should be handled carefully, such as reporting on their use at points of handoff and at shift change and when resetting the amount infused at each shift. The HCO should have a policy and procedure on this care issue. In a recent study, it was identified that 60% of the sample experienced one or more errors—for example, labeling error, bypassing of the smart pump (workaround), and violation of HCO policy (Schnock et al., 2016). Despite this high percentage, harm to patients was minimal. This type of result, however, should not be ignored, as it demonstrates that errors occur at a high rate and could be harmful.

Some changes to improve care may be viewed negatively and may lead to controversy. Not all changes are the right ones, and some may add complexity that makes work more difficult for staff and negatively impacts care—for example, a policy that medications should be administered within 30 minutes of the time ordered was supported by the CMS. This led to concerns that failure to meet this policy would then be classified as an error (Cipriano, 2011). The ISMP was not in favor of this policy (ISMP, 2010). The ISMP conducted a survey: "responses from almost 18,000 nurses. Respondents made it clear that changes to drug delivery methods and gradual increases in the complexity of care, number of prescribed medications per patient, and number of patients assigned to each nurse have made the long-standing CMS '30-minute rule' troublesome. Many nurses now feel the rule is unsafe, impossible to follow, and often unnecessary from a clinical perspective" (ISMP, 2011). What is the potential problem with this policy? If an order is written to administer a medication at 10:00 a.m. and the nurse is busy with an emergency or took longer with a procedure and does not administer the medication until 10:40 a.m., then the policy has not been met. But has an error occurred? Staff members frequently use workarounds, increasing the risk of errors, and this 30-minute policy creates just the scenario in which a nurse might use a workaround. Those who disagree with overemphasizing the 30-minute rule think it does not recognize that nurses should be able to use clinical reasoning and judgment—for example, does a 15-minute delay make a real difference in the effect of a specific drug or in the condition of an individual patient? In 2011, as a result of data that the ISMP collected about the increased risk of using workarounds during these situations, the CMS rescinded its support of the 30-minute policy. This is an example of how data can make an impact when collected in a structured manner and analyzed to determine outcomes. Now hospitals must identify specific time-critical scheduled medications rather than having a rule that applies to all medications. Medications that fall into the time-critical schedule are these (Hawkes, 2014):

- Antibiotics
- Anticoagulants
- Insulin
- Immunosuppressives
- Anticonvulsants
- Medications prescribed more frequently than every 4 hours
- Scheduled (not PRN) opioid pain medications

The most commonly identified incidents in anesthesia are drug administration errors. Medication administration has received a lot of attention, and many methods are used to prevent and respond to events, such as the use of safety checks, active pharmacy participation, and multiple nursing checks during medication administration. These efforts, however, are not extended to perioperative care. There is also a great difference in stress levels between the operating room (OR) and other units. All are stressful, but the OR may be much more stressful. This has an impact

on work and staff responses. Most of the data about the OR are self-reported, and this is not the most reliable method for studies. Although non-operative areas have seen a decrease in medication errors, this is not the case in the OR. In a study conducted in a large medical center with 40,000 operations annually in 64 ORs, it was concluded that approximately 1 in 20 perioperative medication administrations resulted in a medication error and/or adverse event (Nanji, Patel, Shaikh, Seger, & Bates, 2016). This was a prospective observational study, and when compared with retrospective studies the rate of these events was higher in this study. Of the 193 events identified in the study, 153 (79.3%) were thought to be preventable and 20.7% non-preventable. The events were not life threatening; the majority of the events were serious (68.9%) or significant (29.5%); 53% of the events occurred during induction (first 20 minutes of the anesthesia process). The problems identified with the events were labeling errors, wrong dose, omitted medication or failure to act, delay or failure to treat an adverse event, and error in monitoring. Longer procedures (more than 6 hours) and procedures with 13 or more medication administrations experienced more events. The researchers recommend greater use of point-of-care bar-coding anesthesia documentation systems and examination of the timing of documentation (e.g., using the bar coding to identify potential problems before drugs are administered and documented). Most drugs used in the OR are documented some time after they are administered and in some cases at the conclusion of the surgery. Areas in which improvements are needed include decreasing opportunities for workarounds, connecting infusions to the most proximal intravenous port, carefully selecting equipment, and provision of training on use of equipment.

When preparing and administering medications, disruptions are a major concern and increase the risk of errors. Nurses use multitasking all the time, and when they do this they often experience interruptions, distractions, lack of focus, and task switching (Clark & Flanders, 2012). Error recovery is something that nurses are involved in, and it can make a difference in the quality of care. Examples of error recovery strategies include knowing the plan of care, who is involved, and patient information; applying relevant policies and procedures; double-checking information and questioning; actively using surveillance; and using expected systematic processes (Henneman et al., 2010).

Clinical reasoning and judgment are important, but the nurse should be aware that interruptions and distractions might affect reasoning (Dickson & Flynn, 2012). In a study of nursing interruptions in the emergency department, it was noted that interruptions during patient care can come from other staff and may also be associated with the patient and the family (Cole, Stefanus, Gardner, Levy, & Klein, 2015). This study recommended that future research consider the impact of interruptions that are urgent versus routine or unnecessary. Better understanding of the nature of interruptions should guide nurses in determining their best response choice.

Admission is a time of increased risk for medication errors (Gleason et al., 2010). It is at this time that the patient's medication history should be obtained. There may be barriers to getting accurate and complete information. Examples of these barriers include the following:

- Older patients may not have good recall of medications they take.
- The patient's condition may make it difficult to get information.
- Look-alike or sound-alike medications may cause problems.
- Patients may have limited health literacy and/or language problems, be poor historians, and/or withhold information.

To complicate matters, staff may be busy with multiple admissions and other required work, leading to distractions and disruptions.

Handoffs, as mentioned, increase risk, and an admission may be a transfer—for example, a patient moving from the emergency department to inpatient services or from the hospital to a long-term care facility. Errors at the time of admission are influenced by factors that may impact obtaining an accurate medication history.

Medication administration is an important part of home care, and there is a risk for errors in the home. Most patients in home care are older adults, and this patient population has a higher risk for ADEs and ADRs, which might be due to under- or overprescribing (Anathhanam, Powis, Cracknell, & Robson, 2012). In the home environment, older adults are at risk for taking too much or too little medication and/or using the wrong medication. These medication errors may then lead to incidents such as sedation, falling, medical complications, and unintended overdose. In some cases, ADEs may lead to confusion of medication side effects with symptoms and an impact on diagnosis, and they may then lead to problems that require hospitalization. LeBlanc and Choi (2015) propose that the following strategies be considered to make the home a safe environment:

1. Increase the ability of patients to self-manage medications.
2. Identify and make necessary medication changes.
3. Create an accurate, up-to-date medication list to be available in the home.
4. Provide communication between the primary care provider, patient, and case manager. (p. 317)

Medication assessment should be completed prior to developing the care or treatment plan after discharge to ensure medication safety when the patient is discharged home. The GerontoNet ADR Risk Score can be used to identify hospitalized elderly patients who are at risk for ADEs (Onder et al., 2010). Having this assessment can then help the clinical team use interventions to prevent ADEs. The following factors are important to consider (Anathhanam et al., 2012):

- Identify prescribing omissions (underprescribing).
- Identify inappropriately prescribed medications.
- Develop methods for safer use of high-risk medications such as antipsychotics, anticoagulants for atrial fibrillation, and opioids.
- Improve safety in healthcare settings and across care transitions.

The ISMP provides guidelines and alerts for staff about medications; see the Connect to Current Information section at the end of this chapter for a link to this site. Practicing nurses should use this source to keep up to date with high-risk situations that may lead to medication errors. In summary, the following is a list of suggested strategies that may assist in decreasing risk of medication errors (Wachter & Gupta, 2018; Walton, 2014):

- Recognize and report errors.
- Review patient medication orders, considering patient outcomes, duplications, and drug interactions.
- Verify and ensure orders are complete.
- Verify the five (preferably the seven) medication administration rights.
- If there are any questions about an order, confirm before giving the medication, even if it means medication administration may be late.
- Double-check dosage and flow rate calculations with another staff member, especially if standard dose concentration or dosage charts are not available.
- Double-check orders with another staff member, such as when administering blood or for special drugs identified by the pharmacy or high-risk/alert or error-prone medications. HCOs may require that certain drugs be checked with a second nurse.
- Do not circumvent (work around) the medication delivery system by "borrowing" medications from one patient and administering to another even if the label indicates the same drug and dosage.

- If there is a question about a large dose, check this with prescriber and/or pharmacist.
- If using an infusion pump, know how to use it, monitor the equipment, and make sure any previously administered drugs are not in the tubing.
- Talk with the patient to determine if the patient understands prescribed medications and indications. If the patient questions a medication, then check the order.
- Consider your fatigue and stress levels and how these factors impact safe practice.
- Use acceptable abbreviations, and be particularly alert for abbreviations prone to causing errors; do not use any trailing zeros when transcribing dosages.
- Document administration immediately after giving medication.
- Follow HCO policies and procedures and keep up to date with changes.
- Do not guess on an order; double-check if in doubt.
- Be on alert when using look-alike and sound-alike medications.
- Use bar coding as required, following the procedure.
- Collaborate with the pharmacy to ensure stock medications are available; use the pharmacist as a source of information; ask about potential risk of medication error.
- Use the medication dispensing equipment correctly, and if you do not know how to use it or have questions, get assistance.
- Identify allergies and apply allergy alert system.
- Do not leave medication with the patient to take.
- Remind the patient about safety issues (e.g., call for help to get out of bed or chair), tell the patient to report if pain does not decrease within a certain time period, and otherwise encourage measures of patient self-advocacy. Reassess if need more medication or other intervention.

- Listen to the patient, who may alert you to problems with a medication.
- Complete medication reconciliation at time of admission and discharge, or when needed, such as for home care services.
- Provide patient education about medications; include family, with permission of the patient. (Permission is not required if the family is legal guardian.)
- Understand how computerized physician order entry (CPOE) works—if it is available.
- Maintain and increase knowledge about medications; this requires that nurses recognize when they do not know about a drug and need to get further information such as from the pharmacy or other resources. Some HCOs assign clinical pharmacists to provide direct consultation to unit clinical staff.
- Use sterile technique when required for administering drugs and infusions.
- Wash hands before preparing medications and before and after administering.
- Recognize, document, and apply guidelines for medications that require monitoring of data before administering (e.g., temperature, blood pressure, lab results).

## Alarm/Alert Fatigue

The problem of alarm/alert fatigue has increased so much that The Joint Commission issued a sentinel event alert for medical device alarm safety in hospitals (The Joint Commission, 2013). A number of devices are relevant to alarm safety, such as bedside physiologic monitors that include electrocardiogram machines, pulse oximetry devices, and monitors of blood pressure and other parameters; bedside telemetry; central station monitors; infusion pumps; and ventilators (HHS, AHRQ, PSNet, 2019b). In some cases, on a single unit there can be several hundred alarms per patient in a day. If you multiply this number by the number of patients on a unit, it is easy to see how over time these

alarms can stress staff and added to this is the problem that between 85% and 99% of the alarms are false, requiring no clinical intervention. The persistence of these (often false) alarms may lead to staff experiencing **alarm/alert fatigue**, which may mean staff respond by not rushing to respond or ignoring alarms. The following factors commonly impact alarm/alert sentinel events (The Joint Commission, 2013):

- Alarm fatigue—the most common contributing factor
- Alarm settings that are not customized to the individual patient or patient population
- Inadequate staff training on the proper use and functioning of the equipment (e.g., inconsistent team training, response, and interpretation of alarm signals)
- Inadequate staffing to support or respond to alarm signals
- Alarm conditions and settings that are not integrated with other medical devices
- Equipment malfunctions and failures (p. 2)

Three years after these recommendations were made, the problem continued. The Joint Commission 2014 Patient Safety Goals required that by 2016 HCOs accredited by The Joint Commission must do the following: designate alarm management as a patient safety priority, understand clinical alarm hazards, create an action plan, implement the plan, and identify best practices (The Joint Commission, 2016). Since nurses are the staff most involved in responding to alarms, nurses should assume leadership in meeting these requirements and improving effective responses.

In a systematic review of 24 studies on alarm characteristics, 8 studies focused on evaluating alarm fatigue interventions and noted that most of the time the alarm does not mean there is a problem; it is a false alarm. The review recommends additional strategies to address this problem: widening alarm parameters that set off the alarm, using alarm delays, and frequently changing telemetry electrodes and wires, which may impact alarm function (Paine et al., 2016). As this research and others demonstrate, HCOs are making efforts to understand alarm fatigue and resolve this problem.

In a study on drug allergy alerts integrated into EMR/EHRs, an overall increase in alert overrides by providers was noted, from 83.3% (2004) to 87.6% (2013 data) (Topaz et al., 2015). These overrides are dangerous and are not an effective response to increased alarms/alerts. The Joint Commission recommends that the culture of safety develop a shared sense of responsibility among all staff. HCOs are reluctant to remove alarms due to legal concerns, and alert override and removal of alarms compromise effective response for patients who require surveillance and effective, rapid response for their care needs. The following are examples of effective strategies that might be used to reduce problems with alarm fatigue (The Joint Commission, 2013):

- Tailor alerts to patient characteristics and critical integrated clusters of physiologic indicators.
- Tier alerts according to severity. Warnings could be presented in different ways in order for key clinicians to be alerted to more clinically consequential events.
- Make only high-level (severe) alerts interruptive.
- Apply human factor principles when designing alerts (e.g., format, content, legibility, color of alerts).

## Workarounds

A **workaround** occurs when a staff member avoids a problem without eliminating it (Lalley & Malloch, 2010). Workarounds are used in many different situations. Medication administration is one of them. In a study that examined 986 medication errors that were either reported through a trigger system or that staff voluntarily reported, approximately half of the errors were not prevented by information technology system

such as CPOE and/or bar codes (Stultz & Nahata, 2015). Staff used workarounds to avoid using the informatics systems that were established to avoid errors, and errors occurred in doing so.

Workarounds can result in positive or negative outcomes. Errors can result, which could be due to a lack of awareness of a risk of error and what should be done to prevent an error. Sometimes the use of workarounds may provide opportunities for creative change or improvement and may identify areas that must be improved. This all, however, requires acknowledgement of use of workarounds and examination of the workaround process.

## Health Informatics

More information about HIT is provided in other chapters. It is, however, important to note in this chapter that HIT is an important part of HCO QI programs and plans. The use of HIT can improve care outcomes by providing methods for data collection and analysis and can even provide strategies to prevent and respond to quality care problems. HIT, however, also increases risk of errors and problems with communication and documentation, the focus of this chapter.

## Staff Competence

Staff need to be competent in the work they are required to do. When staff are not competent, there is risk of harm to patients. Competence is the responsibility of individual nurses and employers, including direct supervisors and staff educators. Professional organizations and regulators, such as boards of nursing, and licensure requirements also have an impact on competence. The critical bottom line is all staff members must feel comfortable admitting they need help; they must be able to ask questions and seek out assistance to take steps to improve their practice. Other chapters discuss competence and staff continuing education required to improve care.

# Communication

Communication is mentioned frequently in this text and is a critical element of healthcare delivery. Problems with communication are the number one cause of errors and difficulties meeting expected outcomes, thereby increasing risk. The list of situations in which communication occurs is unending. Critical examples are patient–staff interactions, reports and rounds, delegation of responsibilities, handoffs, and performance evaluation. Interprofessional factors are important, such as work difficulties among staff (discussed in other content on teams in this text). During communication, nurses need to be aware of the significance of the facts as they relate to a situation in their practice to reduce errors and improve communication to meet outcomes of care. The process requires that information be updated and evaluated, and this must be an active process, not a passive one, to decrease risk of errors.

# Chronic Illness: Complex Patients

Chronic illness has an important impact on CQI and cost of care, with one in four Americans having multiple chronic conditions (MCC). This care consumes two-thirds of the U.S. healthcare costs (HHS, 2015). A commonly used chronic care model can be reviewed through the Connect to Current Information section at the end of this chapter. Embedded within this model are elements that relate to the five healthcare professions core competencies, and the model also reflects the aims (STEEEP®) to improve care. Chronic illness and complex treatment needs increase risk for patients, impacting patient outcomes and possible errors.

In 2010, the U.S. Department of Health and Human Services (HHS) developed a strategic framework to address MCC and risk of quality-care problems with this patient population. The framework goals are as follows (HHS, 2010):

- Strengthen the healthcare and public health systems.
- Empower the individual to use self-care management.
- Equip healthcare providers with tools, information, and effective interventions.
- Support targeted research about individuals with MCC and effective interventions.

In support of the framework and the need to improve care, the HHS provides training modules to improve healthcare profession knowledge of MCC. The reason for all of this activity is recognition that the quality of care for these patients has an impact on overall HCO CQI outcomes and cost of care with increased risk for quality-care problems.

# Pain Management

Pain is a common health problem that is complex (impacted by biological, behavioral, environmental, and societal factors), increasing risk of errors, and individuals respond differently to pain. Effectively managing pain is a critical element of patient-centered care. Patients expect that healthcare providers will help them with pain management to maintain or improve their quality of life, including activities of daily living. To meet this expectation, we must have a better understanding of pain and improve how we prevent, assess, and treat it, as reported in a major report on pain described in **Figure 8-2** (IOM, 2011).

Addiction has increased rapidly in the past few years. The opioid crisis has become a critical public health problem that impacts quality care. It is thought that the increasing use of prescription pain medication has led to people using other types of addictive drugs or using prescriptions for addictive drugs to provide a source of drugs for others (e.g., family members, friends). This represents a major healthcare problem and requires careful assessment (NAM, 2016; NAM, 2019; Volker & McLellan, 2016). There is also the danger of going too far in limiting pain medication due to concern about addiction and then not

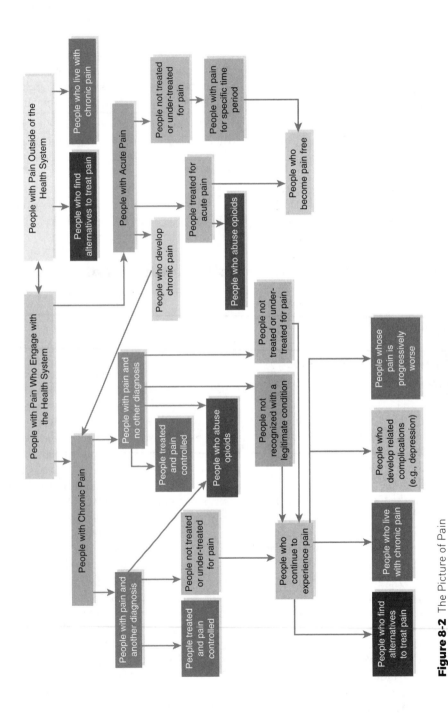

**Figure 8-2** The Picture of Pain

Reproduced from Institute of Medicine (IOM). (2011). *Relieving pain in America. A blueprint for transforming prevention, care, education, and research.* Washington, DC: The National Academies Press. Courtesy of the National Academies Press, Washington, DC.

assisting patients who need pain management. Undermedicating can impact health status. Staff need to be aware of this risk early in the process of pain management. Finding a balance in pain management is important. All of these factors are directly related to quality care for patients with pain, whether short term or long term.

Some of the barriers to improving pain management are the need for more knowledge, staff attitudes toward pain, system issues such as how medication is delivered, use of computerized records, staffing levels to respond to patients when they need help with pain, costs and access to medications, rehabilitative services, planning and coordination of care, and patient education about pain. Effective pain management requires effective teamwork and may require effective medication administration.

Nurses are involved directly in pain management in all types of settings. They can influence the quality of care for pain and reduce risk for errors and patient harm. Assessment and interventions, particularly medication administration, are used to ensure effective pain management. Use of pain intensity scales is common now and recommended by experts for assessment and effective treatment decisions.

## Responding to High-Risk Situations for Errors and Reduced Quality Care

In 2010, a study was undertaken to expand a 2005 study that was referred to as the Silence Kills study. Findings from more than 6,500 nurses and nurse managers were used to examine other aspects of the problem of communication and errors. The conclusion was that safety tools do not address a second category of communication breakdowns referred to as "undiscussables." These are topics we do not like to talk about or are not able to talk about, such as dangerous shortcuts, incompetence, and disrespect, which have a direct impact on CQI. Often, they represent risks that are widely known by staff but not discussed. For staff to fully engage in CQI

and share concerns, they need active support from other staff and management. As Maxfield, Grenny, Levandero, and Goah (2010) articulate, "Tools don't create safety; people do."

Several examples of high-risk situations when errors may occur and quality of care may be reduced are described in this chapter. This list is not complete, but it provides examples to think about and a basis for identifying other examples. In summary, nurses need to consider the following general guidelines related to high-risk situations:

- Every staff person has a role in ensuring quality care.
- Understand the many aspects to quality and risk and how they relate to your work daily.
- Understand why it is important for the HCO to commit to QI.
- Commit to participating in the CQI process daily in your work.
- Recognize higher-risk situations.
- HCOs and individual nurses need to commit to expanding their knowledge and understanding of risk for errors through staff education and continuing education.
- Patients and families need to be engaged in the process.

### STOP AND CONSIDER 8-3

Nurses are involved in all of the high-risk situations that lead to errors and reduce quality care.

## Examples of Two Major National Initiatives Focused on Potential Risks of Inadequate Quality Care

With the recognition that there are high-risk situations that may have an impact on quality care, more initiatives have been developed and implemented to focus on these concerns to decrease risk. The initiatives apply the CQI process and planning. Nongovernmental organizations (NGOs) and some governmental organizations at the state and federal levels have developed these initiatives. There are two major national initiatives directed by the HHS that have become very important to HCOs and nursing. These relate to hospital-acquired conditions and 30-day unplanned readmissions. Although both of these programs focus on Medicare patients and some Medicaid patients through the CMS, they have an impact on most, if not all, acute care hospitals. Few hospitals do not have Medicare-covered patients, and many have Medicaid-covered patients, and requirements for these patient populations then impact other patients. In addition, the requirements from these programs have influenced other third-party payer requirements and have a major impact on nursing practice and management.

## Hospital-Acquired Conditions

Use of "never events" began in 2001 as part of efforts to drive greater interest in CQI. The CMS defines **hospital-acquired conditions (HACs)** as "reasonably preventable conditions that were not present at the time of admission to the hospital" (Austin & Pronovost, 2015; HHS, CMS, 2019a). This is a pay-for-performance program in that hospitals with higher HAC rates are paid less for care. The National Quality Forum identified a list of these events; later The Joint Commission developed its sentinel event list; and then the CMS identified its list of events that would not be covered by CMS payment. Some third-party payers also have similar lists. Data on these events are used for more than determination of payment—for example, some states require reporting of these events, although individual HCOs may have different methods for collecting and reporting the data (Austin & Pronovost). These conditions

are classified by the CMS as follows (HHS, CMS, 2019a):

1. High cost, high volume, or both
2. Identified through the International Classification of Diseases as complicating or major complicating conditions that when present and included in secondary diagnoses may result in a higher-paying diagnosis-related group (DRG), the diagnosis classification system developed by the CMS
3. Conditions that are reasonably preventable through use of evidence-based guidelines

Patient care for these events are not covered by CMS, nor can Medicare and Medicaid patients be personally charged for additional care needs. This can lead to a significant financial problem for the HCO, and consequently, HCOs are now initiating efforts to reduce HACs. Quality management—including patient safety, teamwork, staffing effectiveness, and patient, staff, and physician satisfaction—has an impact on preventing HACs (Bartlett & Kelly, 2009). Since the HAC program focuses on effectiveness, it is considered to be a type of pay-for-performance program with incentive to improve.

### Types of HACs

The types of HACs change over time based on data collected and analysis of the data to determine if there is improvement and a need to change the list. The goal is to identify the most significant potential problems or high-risk events. Examples of HACs include the following, and the most current list can be found on the CMS website (HHS, CMS, 2019a):

- Adverse drug events
- Catheter-associated urinary tract infection
- Central line–associated bloodstream infections
- Clostridioides difficile infections
- Falls
- Obstetric adverse events

- Pressure ulcer/pressure injuries
- Surgical site infections
- Ventilator-associated pneumonias
- Venous thrombolisms
- All other infections (not including Clostridioides difficile infections)

What is the status of the implementation of the HAC program? Has it made a difference in decreasing HACs? Updated and new patient safety data for 2014 through 2017 continue to show a downward trend in the annual number of HACs (HHS, AHRQ, 2020a). Some research indicates that HACs have had an impact on quality improvement, but this is not yet clear enough, plus there is need for more research to understand the outcomes (Bae, 2017). These data, however, indicate movement toward improvement

To provide a basis for understanding the relevance of HACs to CQI, the following content discusses two HAC examples in more detail: falls and hospital-acquired infections.

### Examples of Strategies to Reduce Falls and Trauma

Falls can result in a number of adverse consequences for patients in a variety of HCOs, including reduced quality of life, increased fear of falling, restricted activities with decreased ability to function, serious injuries, and increased risk of death (HHS, AHRQ, 2020b). The factors that increase risk of falls are effects of aging on gait, balance, and strength; acute medical conditions and also chronic diseases that weaken the patient or impact function; deconditioning from inactivity; behavioral symptoms and unsafe behaviors; medication side effects; environmental hazards, such as poor lighting, improper footwear, and unsafe flooring/carpeting; spills; lack of support, such as handrails; clutter and unsafe furniture; and unsafe use of equipment, such as walkers, crutches, and wheelchairs.

In the past, HCOs that had an increase in patient falls typically made changes in how care was provided—for example, staff might identify patients at risk and increase paperwork to describe these incidents. Concern about the risk of lawsuits also increased, although the HCOs were more concerned about receiving payment for additional care that patients might need due to falls in the HCO. With the establishment of the HAC initiative, HCOs are changing their approaches and monitoring risks and events so that the HCO does not experience loss of CMS payment for care when falls occur. This acts as a very strong incentive to reduce falls.

When a patient is in an HCO, many interventions can be used to prevent falls, including the following (Quigley & White, 2014; Rodak, 2013; Volz & Swaim, 2013):

- Establish and reassess fall risk policy and procedure.
- Screen for high-risk patients, ensuring that the method used to identify risk is clear but does not embarrass the patient. Identify high-risk patients so staff is aware.
- Identify patients with recent fall or fall injury present at time of admission.
- Clarify and communicate patient interventions per patient with the team, noting changes as they occur.
- Assess patients on pain and sleep medications or any medications that may cause drowsiness and/or dizziness.
- Provide safety companions to attend to and assist high-risk patients.
- Consider impact of staff level and mix.
- Educate family and significant others about risks and interventions.
- Use bed and chair alarms, set for time interval so that when the patient gets out of bed, staff can get to the patient in time to prevent a fall.
- Implement safety rounds and hourly rounds to help patients with ambulation and toileting, and clear clutter in the room.
- Provide and encourage use of handrails.
- Keep beds low when there is no need for them to be higher.
- Use restraints per policy and procedure.

- Install bathroom safety features and explain use to patients.
- Keep call lights and personal items within reach of the patient.
- Assist patients with ambulation and when patients are out of bed with intravenous equipment and other equipment that might limit mobility.
- Suggest patient wear nonskid socks or appropriate shoes.
- Provide staff training about falls and prevention.
- Implement a safety culture that supports reporting of near-miss falls and falls.
- Track fall data and use analysis to identify improvement or need for improvement; engage staff in this process.

The Joint Commission considers falls with injuries—most of which occur in acute care hospitals but also occur in other HCOs, such as long-term care facilities—as important events and identifies them as sentinel events (The Joint Commission, 2015). Along with the preceding strategies, The Joint Commission recommends that HCOs also use the following overall strategies to reduce falls:

- Increase awareness.
- Establish an effective interprofessional falls injury prevention team.
- Implement use of a standardized, validated tool to identify risk.
- Develop individualized care plans based on risk and need.
- Apply standardized interventions such as handoff communication and patient education.
- Conduct post-fall management—post-fall huddle, transparent reporting, analysis and trending of falls to make decisions about care improvement. (p. 2)

A critical strategy to reduce falls is identifying patients at risk for falls. Identifying these patients allows HCOs to plan care that includes fall prevention. The AHRQ developed a fall self-assessment tool that covers the organization, healthcare providers, and patient

concerns (HHS, AHRQ, 2017). In addition to HAC monitoring by HCOs and the CMS, the National Database of Nursing Quality Indicators, the National Quality Forum, the AHRQ Patient Safety Indicators, and The Joint Commission all measure falls and include measures/indicators associated with the following (Quigley & White, 2014): fall rates, fall injury rates, fall assessment completed, repeat fall rates, injury rates with level of injury, and percentage of patients who fell. Some measures/indicators specify type of injury or trauma, such as hip fracture, dislocations, and intracranial injury, as noted in the list of HACs. An example of a tool used to identify fall risk: *Tool 3H: Morse Fall Scale for Identifying Fall Risk Factors.* Staff nurses use this tool along with regular clinical assessment and review of medications. The tool assists in identifying fall risk factors in hospitalized patients. The tool's total score can predict falls, but the best use of the scale is to integrate identification of risk factors in care planning. The AHRQ provides details about the scale and directions for its use. It is a simple scale that includes six categories of data: history of falling; secondary diagnosis; ambulatory aid, such as nurse assist, crutches, cane, walker, furniture; bed rest; gait; and mental status. Patients are ranked from no risk to low, moderate, or high risk (HHS, AHRQ, 2013). All of these efforts require understanding and a clear approach—assess the problem, develop a response plan to improve, implement the plan, and then evaluate the outcomes (Quigley, Barnett, Bulat, & Friedman, 2016). The Connect to Current Information section at the end of this chapter provides links to more detailed information about the tools.

### Examples of Strategies to Reduce Hospital-Acquired Infections

Hospital-acquired infections (HAIs) are a common concern in healthcare, and several infections (urinary tract, vascular catheter-associated, and various surgical site infections) are identified in the list of HAIs provided in this chapter (HHS, AHRQ, 2020a). Almost half of HAIs are associated with invasive procedures (Hessels, 2015). One of the most common HAIs is central line–associated bloodstream infections (CLABSIs). These infections can result in great harm to patients and are costly to treat. Nurses are in the primary position to reduce CLABSIs (Sandoval, 2015). The AHRQ provides tools to address this problem (HHS, AHRQ, 2018b). For a CLABSI to be considered an HAI it must occur after admission; however, whether the patient is admitted with an infection or gets an infection after admission, the risk for patient harm is still high. For the infection to be classified as an HAI, it must also be confirmed by laboratory test and not be due to any infection in another part of the body.

Surgical site infections (SSIs) are also a serious problem that puts patients at risk post-surgery, increasing costs, length of stay, and also readmission rates (Greene, 2015). More than 10 million inpatient surgical procedures are performed annually, putting all these patients at risk for HAIs (2% to 4%) (HHS, AHRQ, PSNet, 2019c). The most common type of hospital infection is SSI associated with pneumonia, representing 21.8% of total infections. Nurses are involved in the care of surgical patients during all phases of the surgical process and can help reduce the SSI risk.

Ventilator-assisted pneumonia (VAP) is a pneumonia that develops within 48 hours of endotracheal intubation; however, there is no clear definition, which makes it difficult to get a reliable rate (HHS, CDC, 2020). Prevention strategies should consider three causative mechanisms: bacterial colonization of the respiratory and upper gastrointestinal tracts, aspiration of contaminated secretions, and contaminated respiratory equipment.

Nurses should assume a major role in preventing catheter-associated urinary tract infection (CAUTI) and providing care for harm caused by CAUTIs. Three major strategies to accomplish these goals are to (1) use fewer catheters, (2) adhere to timely removal of catheters, and (3) follow effective procedures for insertion, maintenance, and post-removal

care. In *American Nurse Today*, Trevellini provides a care decision flowchart (Trevellini, 2015). Publications like this one demonstrate the critical nature of HAIs and nursing responsibilities, and they make the information widely available to nurses who need the information (ANA, 2015a).

Studies also indicate that education regarding infections is important in reducing HAIs. In a sample of 5 hospitals and 394 nurses, an AHRQ-funded study found inadequate nurse knowledge and application of correct procedures that impact CAUTIs (Jones, Sibai, Battjes, & Fakih, 2015). The results noted that recommended procedures were not followed—for example, over half of the respondents did not think that their peers complied with required procedures. The study also found that nurses were not commonly evaluated on their skills in placing and maintaining urinary catheters. This study demonstrates that there are major problems with nursing care that must be addressed. Other research focuses on using strategies such as algorithms to guide nursing process and decisions, resulting in a reduction in CAUTI incidents (Russell, Leming-Lee, & Watters, 2019). This demonstrates how nurses can lead in reducing HACs; can have an impact on quality improvement and reduction of healthcare costs; can improve patient recovery and functioning; but need to be competent and vigilant, which requires ongoing education.

Due to the growing concern about HAIs, the ANA published a special report on HAIs that includes information to help prevent HAIs, focusing on zero tolerance of HAIs and on the use of a CAUTI prevention tool (ANA, 2015b). The report also discusses the need to use other methods to prevent CLABSIs and SSIs. There is now greater emphasis on applying evidence-based strategies to prevent VAP. HAIs represent 6 of the 11 HACs listed in 2017 (HHS, AHRQ, 2020a). These infections are a major healthcare problem that has an impact on clinical and financial outcomes. Though infection control has long been emphasized in HCOs, with nurses assuming an active role, HCOs continue to have major problems with HAIs. Understanding the reasons for this outcome is critical to improving and thus reducing HAIs.

## Nursing and HACs

HACs are related to nursing care, and some of the burden for preventing and responding to HACs is a nursing responsibility (Kurtzman & Buerhaus, 2008). HACs require that more effort be spent on system improvements, and nursing services are often tasked with "fixing this." When HACs occur, nursing management and other staff examine the types of HACs, review data about incidence related to the measures/indicators, analyze possible causes, identify interventions, implement the interventions, monitor results, and make adjustments as needed. This is an ongoing process and is part of CQI. Should nursing alone be responsible for improving problems with HACs? If one accepts that more system issues are related to CQI than were recognized in the past and that there is greater need to consider interprofessional teams and practices, then nursing should not be solely responsible for HACs. If an HCO is committed to a culture of safety rather than blame, then this requires a more comprehensive response. Policies, procedures, processes, communication, documentation, staff competencies, and so on are part of this culture. As is relevant with all HACs, a better understanding of the impact of staffing on HACs is needed. A systematic review that included 54 studies noted that, even though the studies were not consistent, their results indicated that increased staffing does decrease risk of acquiring HAIs (Mitchell, Gardner, Stone, Hall, & Pogorzelska-Maziarz, 2018; Shang, Needleman, Liu, Larson, & Stone, 2019). This is an example of the need for both clinical and management assessment and interventions and also for use of evidence-based practice and evidence-based management. Achieving this comprehensive

approach requires strong nursing leadership that will stand up and agree that many, if not all, HACs relate directly to nursing care, but this is not enough for improvement. Engaging all critical healthcare professionals makes a difference in an effective response. Tools discussed in this text provide methods for staff to examine and respond to problems with HACs. The pressure of no payment is strong, but it should not drive the HCO to take limited steps in responding, such as just focusing on nurses and nursing care.

## Impact of the Centers for Medicare and Medicaid Services HAC Initiative

Hospital patient safety improved from 2010 to 2017, with a gradual decline in HACs. The "2014 rate started at 99 HACs per 1,000 discharges and is estimated at 86 HACs per 1,000 discharges for 2017" (HHS, AHRQ, 2020a). The HACs included in the data are ADEs, CAUTIs, CLABSIs, pressure ulcers, SSIs, and several other types of adverse events. Several initiatives targeted these problems and had a strong influence on this improvement. However, as promising as these statistics are, other recent studies indicate that if errors were identified as a disease, they would represent the third leading cause of death in the United States (Makary, 2016).

In fiscal year 2020, the CMS reduced its payments to 786 hospitals due to their HAC levels. These hospitals had unacceptable levels of potentially avoidable infections and other injuries (Ellison, 2020). In the 6 years that CMS has applied the HAC requirement to encourage improvement by reducing CMS payment, of the total hospitals, 16 have been penalized all 6 years. Seven of the penalized hospitals this year are included in the U.S. News Best Hospitals Honor Roll. This is an example of how complex ratings are in healthcare.

HAC data and analysis of the data are now an important part of CQI and are used in a variety of ways—for example, a study examined the relationship of receiving HAC penalties to factors such as HCO accreditation status and teaching hospitals, which typically care for more complex patients. Safety-net hospitals also have similar types of patients. Compared to non-safety-net and non-teaching hospitals, these hospitals received more HAC penalties. One of the results of this study identifies concerns that some experts predicted would be a problem with pay-for-performance approaches. HCOs that are not teaching hospitals or safety-net hospitals tend to attract and seek patients that are healthier with less complex health needs and socioeconomic problems. This then leads to controlling greater health disparities and selective treatment and is known as "cherry-picking" of healthier patients (Rajaram et al., 2015).

# 30-Day Unplanned Readmission

Discharge from hospital care usually does not mean the patient is fully recovered, and the full recovery may take a short time or a long time or may never be complete. As such, there is risk for problems following discharge that may lead to readmission. The AHRQ notes that some of the concerns or problems that occur are ADEs, the most common problem; infections; complications from procedures; and pending test results or testing scheduled post-discharge that may then require a change in treatment (HHS, AHRQ, 2014). After examination of the problem of readmissions, the CMS decided to initiate a change to reduce 30-day unplanned readmissions. According to the CMS, **30-day unplanned readmission** "measures are estimates of unplanned readmission for any cause to an acute care hospital within 30 days of discharge" (HHS, CMS, 2019b). Because readmissions over longer periods may be influenced by factors outside the hospital's control (e.g., other illnesses, the patient's behavior, lack of follow-up on treatment, or care provided or not provided to the patient after discharge),

the CMS decided it was best to measure unplanned readmission within 30 days instead of over longer periods.

The AHRQ identifies some of the common HCO barriers that may limit HCO success in reducing readmissions (HHS, AHRQ, 2014):

- "We're still studying the root causes of readmissions."
- "The senior leadership doesn't care about Medicaid readmissions because we don't get penalized by Medicaid."
- "We don't have the money to hire any FTEs [staff]."
- "Waiting for the new electronic medical record system to be implemented."
- "We have really limited access to primary care."
- "There's no peer-reviewed literature to support this readmission reduction strategy."
- "Our community has very limited resources." (p. 32)

The problem of readmissions does not apply only to Medicare patients—for example, adult Medicaid patients have a higher rate of 30-day discharge readmissions than do Medicare patients, and other patient populations also have risk of this type of readmission (HHS, AHRQ, 2014).

## *Examples of Strategies to Reduce Unplanned Readmission*

Discharge is a major example of transition of care and handoffs. It is at this time that the patient has the highest risk of disconnection from healthcare providers—for example, there may be system problems such as ineffective communication between the provider and patient, between a new provider and past provider, between the hospital pharmacist and the patient's community-based pharmacist, and so on. Obtaining medications needed after discharge may be a problem—for example, the patient may be unable to get a prescription filled due to economic reasons, lack of transportation, or lack of support to get the medication from the pharmacy. Admission, discharge, and readmission data should be shared with unit staff, and these data should provide a foundation for an open discussion of problems and sharing of ideas to solve the problems. Some hospitals are using the teach-back method to better prepare patients and families when the patient is at high risk for readmission and evaluating the use of this method to ensure it is meeting required outcomes (Peter et al., 2015).

Due to these potential events, the AHRQ recommends the following general strategies to prevent 30-day unplanned readmission (HHS, AHRQ, PSNet, 2019d; Institute for Healthcare Improvement [IHI], 2011):

- Use structured discharge communication that includes information about medications, pending tests, and follow-up, shared with the patient and with providers the patient will see post-discharge.
- Use medication reconciliation, checking all medications to ensure there are no conflicts and safety concerns with prescriptions given to the patient.
- Educate the patient (and when patient agrees, the family) so that there is understanding of diagnosis, follow-up, and whom to contact with questions or problems after discharge. Specific contact information in written form should be provided with directions for follow-up care.
- Focus on the patient, not the patient's diagnosis, to better understand needs such as patient education, transportation, nutrition, home care (e.g., equipment, bed, ambulatory assistive devices), and emotional support.
- Set outcomes for evaluation of discharges and readmission.
- Evaluate and improve the discharge process.
- Use interprofessional teams.
- Consider how to improve and develop new transitional interventions.

- Determine how to engage and listen to patients and families.
- Use readmission prevention programs to try to reduce this risk.
- Assess patients, focusing on the whole patient, not just the diagnosis—for example, consider psychological needs, home status, transportation to get prescriptions and to medical appointments, support after discharge, ability to function, and so on.
- Ask patients—and when the patient agrees, the family—what they need post-discharge.
- Ensure that the patient participates in discharge planning and agrees to the plan.
- Track data over time to understand types of patients who get readmitted and reasons, and then use this information to make changes.
- Establish a consistent policy and procedure for preparing patients for discharge.
- Provide greater support for high-risk patients.
- Ensure that the patient has medications (prescriptions), supplies, and equipment that may be needed immediately after discharge to allow time for the patient to get what is needed long term.
- Use follow-up telephone calls to check how the patient is doing.

HCOs should develop a specific readmission reduction program. Staff members then apply aspects of the program that meet individual patient needs. An effective readmission reduction program includes the following practices (HHS, AHRQ, 2014):

- *Analyze the root causes of readmissions.* Understand patterns and trends for the HCO and the local community for comparison; understand the patient's perspective (e.g., effectiveness of communication and coordination). Data should be tracked routinely.
- *Inventory and align the current readmission reduction efforts to meet the needs of the HCO's targeted patients.* This should be an

in-depth inventory; the AHRQ guide provides several tools (e.g., Hospital Inventory, Cross-Continuum Team Inventory, and Conditions of Participation Checklist) so that the HCO can understand what they currently do to prevent and/or respond to the problem to better plan changes.

- *Examine the extent to which the current readmission reduction efforts meet the needs of the HCO's targeted patients.* Combine previous information.
- *Improve hospital-based processes to better target and serve targeted patients' needs.* Using the preceding information, set aims and objectives, and then identify strategies that will be part of the program. Examples of strategies are using checklists, arranging for post-discharge follow-up, flagging in the chart patients who have experienced readmission more than 30 days post-discharge, developing transitional plans, engaging the patient and, if the patient consents, the family, and identifying high-risk patients based on HCO criteria.
- *Expand and strengthen cross-setting partnerships.* Implement strategies to increase collaboration with cross-setting partners.
- *Provide enhanced services to patients at high risk of readmission.* Implement strategies for high-risk patients. (p. 5)

The CMS developed the Community-Based Care Transitions Program (CCTP), which is focused on improving care transitions and handoffs, particularly to reduce readmission for high-risk Medicare beneficiaries (HHS, CMS, 2019c). The CCTP is part of the Partnership for Patients, which is a national public–private partnership that works to reduce errors in hospitals by 40% and to reduce hospital readmissions by 20%. As of September 2015, there were 72 participating CCTP sites. Approximately 2.6 million senior adults experience readmission within 30 days of discharge, costing $26 billion annually. Discharge planning is not new; however, it is clear that this planning has been inadequate in reducing readmissions. The

CCTP is a 5-year program that began in February 2012 to determine if this type of program can decrease the rate. As part of the CCTP, the government funds Community-Based Organizations (CBOs) to provide care transition services to assist Medicare patients and improve care. Acute care hospitals can partner with CBOs to provide transition services. The CMS requires that CBOs meet at least one of the following criteria (HHS, CMS, 2019c):

- Care transition services that begin no later than 24 hours prior to discharge
- Timely and culturally and linguistically competent post-discharge education to patients so patients understand potential additional health problems or a deteriorating condition
- Timely interactions between patients and post-acute and outpatient providers
- Patient-centered self-management support and information specific to the beneficiary's condition
- A comprehensive medication review and management, including, if appropriate, counseling and self-management support

To apply for CBO funding, CBO proposals must describe the applicant's community-specific root causes of readmissions, target population, strategies to identify high-risk patients, interventions and services, communication with providers, culturally appropriate strategies, set outcomes, budget, and prior experience with transition care.

## Readmission: Impact on Nursing

Process mapping is used to understand all steps that lead to discharge (Endo, 2015). The following questions might be included when applying this method to readmissions (SHM, 2015):

- What standardized processes already exist for care transitions?
- How often are steps in these processes actually followed?

- What other elements of the discharge process can/should we standardize?
- What elements of the discharge process need to be more customized to a specific patient population?
- What checks exist to ensure critical processes occur?
- Who owns each process?

By using this information, the HCO and its nurses can better develop strategies/interventions for the patient and family/caregiver to help them prepare for discharge, identify medication safety needs at the time of discharge, and plan follow-up care after discharge. Having greater understanding of discharge needs and how these needs might impact readmission risk provides information that should then be applied to staff education to ensure that staff are prepared to assess patients carefully, implement the interventions, and improve care transitions.

Inpatient nurses need to be aware of community resources for patients and maintain relationships with home health agencies and other service providers. Many HCOs have specific staff assigned to discharge planning; however, this does not mean that nurses working directly with patients are exempt from active participation in preparing patients for discharge. Leaving discharge preparations solely to designated staff relates back to the discussion of working in silos. If key staff do not lend input when patients are being prepared to leave the hospital, important information, needs, and problems may be missed. An effective discharge planning process includes all relevant members of the care team, the patient, and the family, when appropriate. Discharge is a critical handoff, and it is a time of risk for near misses, errors, and ineffective care and patient dissatisfaction.

Readmission data can be used to assist HCOs and nurses to be more alert and plan strategies to reduce unplanned readmissions. Important data to consider are the common types of diagnoses that result in readmission within 30 days post-discharge. Individual HCOs should track the data, but there is also national data from the Healthcare Cost and Utilization Project (HCUP). Data change over time and thus common diagnoses may change, but it is important to be alert and use the most current national and HCO-specific information to improve care. The HCUP website provides a new Nationwide Readmission Database (NRD), which offers a valuable source of data and trends, representing all types of insurers (Medicare, Medicaid, commercial payers) and the uninsured.

## *Impact of the Centers for Medicare and Medicaid Services Readmission Initiative*

There are now financial penalties for hospitals with above-average readmission rates within 30 days of discharge for target diagnoses. According to the AHRQ, as of 2014, "more than 2200 hospitals had up to two percent of their annual Medicare reimbursements withheld due to excess readmissions. Hospitals also receive 'bundled' payments for target illnesses that cover all costs associated with patient care for a 30-day period providing a financial incentive to ensure continuity of care" (HHS, AHRQ, 2014). Expected costs are used to determine the retrospective payment amount per patient. In this model, if a patient was admitted for treatment of a myocardial infarction, then the HCO would be paid a specific bundled amount for that diagnosis that would include all expected services, such as laboratory tests, medications, hospital room and food, nursing services, and so on. If the patient receives more care than was considered in the bundled payment established by the payer with the HCO, such as more medication or more laboratory tests, then there would be no additional payment for these services. Readmissions have decreased since the CMS initiative began, but the majority of hospitals are still penalized, as there is much more that needs to be done to reduce these unplanned readmissions. Some factors that may have an impact on outcomes, although more research is needed, are factors such as weekend discharge and discharges during July when changes in some medical staff occur. Same-hospital readmission or patient discharged and readmitted to the same hospital is the most common readmission scenario, but this varies from state to state and per condition.

CMS has developed initiatives to reduce readmissions for its beneficiaries. Medicare state-based Quality Improvement Organizations (QIOs) are groups of QI experts, healthcare providers, and consumers who have organized to assist Medicare patients and improve care. QIOs have made a difference in reducing hospital readmissions within 30 or fewer days after discharge.

## STOP AND CONSIDER 8-4

Some HCOs are now penalized financially if they do not meet certain care outcomes.

# Summary

Healthcare continues to be fragmented, with great variation due to patient characteristics and problems, differences in individual healthcare providers and HCOs, and differences from state to state, with healthcare systems struggling with improving care. This chapter sets the stage for greater examination of how CQI works: what is done to better understand CQI and then how best to improve. HCOs must plan an effective QI program, and other sections of this text offer greater detail on methods used to monitor and measure quality. The content focuses on high-risk events. Using this information helps HCOs and the staff take steps to prevent these problems when possible and also be prepared to respond if problems occur. The federal government has assumed more responsibility in trying to direct CQI efforts that identify high-risk events on a national basis. Two initiatives are part of these efforts; they relate to HACs and 30-day unplanned readmissions. "An unacceptably large proportion of patients experience preventable harm at the hands of the healthcare system, and even more patients experience errors in their care that (through early detection or sheer chance) do not result in clinical consequences. Considerable effort has been devoted to optimizing methods of detecting errors and safety hazards, with the goal of prospectively identifying hazards before patients are harmed and analyzing events that have already occurred to identify and address underlying systems flaws. Despite much effort, healthcare institutions are still searching for optimal methods to identify underlying system defects before patients are harmed and, when errors do occur, methods to recognize them as rapidly as possible to prevent further harm" (HHS, AHRQ, PSNet, 2019e). There is still much to be done to improve care and also to develop and improve methods for identifying, measuring, and addressing quality care problems. Exemplars of quality improvement roles and responsibilities for staff nurses, nurse managers, and APRNs are found in **Exhibit 8-1**.

---

**Exhibit 8-1** Exemplars: Quality Improvement Roles and Responsibilities

**Staff Nurse**
A pediatric intensive care staff nurse focuses much of her time on ongoing assessment and surveillance of assigned patients. She recognizes that this is an important part of her position and she is also vigilant in documenting this surveillance.

**Nurse Manager**

The nurse manager group meets regularly with the chief nurse executive (CNE). At the current meeting, the CNE reports that the 30-day unplanned readmission rate for the hospital is increasing. The hospital executive committee wants the nurse manager group to address this problem and present a plan. The nurse managers inform the CNE that they are willing to participate and would want to participate actively in working on this problem but that they do not "own" this problem. This is not just about nurses and nursing care. This requires collaboration and teamwork with physicians, pharmacy, laboratory, discharge office, medical records, and administration.

**Advanced Practice Registered Nurse***

The APRN in a medical intensive care unit reviews data with the nurse manager on HACs for the unit. They are concerned that VAP is showing a steady increase. The APRN reviews patient records for patients with VAP over the last 6 months, develops a summary of critical points, and uses this information to develop a discussion and education program with staff. He also works directly with staff who are caring for patients with risk of VAP.

*Advanced Practice Registered Nurse includes APRN, Clinical Nurse Specialist, Clinical Nurse Leader, and nurses with DNP.

# APPLY CQI

## Chapter Highlights

- Three major concerns in healthcare delivery are important in CQI. These are point of care, fragmentation of care, and variation of care. All impact risk of errors and occurrence of quality problems.
- Surveillance should be used throughout the care process in order to assess the patient and situations and allow for appropriate response—for example, to prevent failure to rescue. Surveillance also provides critical information for CQI and allows nurses providing direct care to initiate interventions to prevent or respond to CQI problems and errors.
- HCOs and healthcare providers experience many high-risk error situations and

reduced quality of care during care, and they need to be alert to these situations. This chapter highlights some of the high-risk situations: working in silos, application of the annual Joint Commission National Patient Safety Goals, care during transitions/handoffs, failure to rescue, diagnosis and errors, medication administration, alarm /alert fatigue, workarounds, health informatics, staff competence, communication, chronic illness, and pain management.

- Two national initiatives address two major types of high-risk events that apply to most hospitals: hospital-acquired conditions and 30-day unplanned readmission.

## Critical Thinking and Clinical Reasoning and Judgment: Discussion Questions and Learning Activities

1. How do you use surveillance in your practice to assist patients and support CQI? Provide specific examples.

2. Select one of the high-risk situations for errors and reduced quality care discussed in this chapter. Provide a brief

summary based on content and research of other information via the Internet and literature. Provide two examples that demonstrate why your selection is a high-risk area and two strategies/interventions you might use to improve

care and prevent problems with the two high-risk examples.
3. Discuss how HACs might impact your practice. Provide two specific examples.
4. Why are nurses involved in strategies to reduce 30-day unplanned readmissions?

## Connect to Current Information

- Institute for Safe Medication Practices http://ismp.org
- Using Self-Assessment to Improve Care: General High Alert Medications https://www.ismp.org/assessments/high-alert -medications
- National Coordinating Council for Medication Error Reporting and Prevention http:// www.nccmerp.org/report-medication-errors
- FDA: MedWatch Reporting Program http://www.fda.gov/Safety/MedWatch /default.htm
- The Joint Commission: National Patient Safety Goals http://www.jointcommission.org/standards _information/npsgs.aspx

- The Joint Commission: Patient Flow Resources https://store.jointcommissioninternational .org/managing-patient-flow-in-hospitals -strategies-and-solutions-second-edition/
- AHRQ: Tool 3H: Morse Fall Scale for Identifying Fall Risk Factors http://www.ahrq.gov/professionals/systems /hospital/fallpxtoolkit/fallpxtk-tool3h.html
- CMS: Hospital-Acquired Conditions https://www.cms.gov/Medicare/Medicare -Fee-for-Service-Payment/HospitalAcqCond /index.html?redirect=/HospitalACqCond 06_Hospital-Acquired_Conditions.asp
- CMS: Thirty-Day Unplanned Readmission https://www.medicare.gov/hospitalcom-pare/Data/30-day-measures.html
- The Chronic Care Model http://www.improvingchroniccare.org/index .php?p=The_Chronic_ CareModel&s=2

## Connect to Text Current information with the Author

Go to the update for this text to review the Blog, QI News, and Literature Review. Access this regular update at: http://nursing.jbpub.com/Finkelman/QualityImprovement/2e.

## EBP, EBM, and Quality Improvement: Exemplar

Prochnow, J., Meiers, S., & Scheckel, M. (2019). Improving patient and caregiver new medication education using an innovative teach-back toolkit. *Journal of Nursing Care Quality, 34*(2), 101–106.
This study describes a medication education program designed to improve care.

### Questions to Consider

1. What is the design used for this study, including purpose, research question(s), sample, interventions, data collection, and analysis?
2. What are the results of the study?
3. How might you apply these results in a clinical setting to improve care?

# EVOLVING CASE STUDY

As nurse manager for an intensive care unit, you have been sent data about HACs in your unit. You are particularly concerned with the following data about the CLABSI rate: 7 per 1,000 central-line days over the last year, resulting in 1 death and extended length of stay by 3 days. This represents a 10% increase in CLABSIs over the last year. You know you need more information, and then you have to figure out what to do to improve. You know that sources such as the CDC and the AHRQ offer important information and resources. You meet with the two APRNs who are associated with the unit to discuss the issue.

## Case Questions A

*You begin your process by gathering information about CLABSIs and your own situation regarding CLABSIs.*

1. What other data might you want from the QI program to better understand your unit's problem and how it has changed?
2. What method(s) might you use to describe the data? Provide an example of its use.

## Case Questions B

*You are now ready to address next steps using the information you have.*

1. Develop a plan with strategies/interventions to address this problem.
2. How will you engage your staff (staff nurses, APRNs, physicians, other providers on the unit such as physical therapists) in developing and implementing the plan? Be specific.

# References

American Nurses Association (ANA). (2015a). Special report: Infection prevention. Retrieved from http://www.americannursetoday.com/resources/special-report-infection-prevention

American Nurses Association (ANA). (2015b). Catheter-associated urinary tract infection prevention. *American Nurse Today, 10*(9), 3–4.

Anathhanam, S., Powis, R., Cracknell, A., & Robson, J. (2012). Impact of prescribed medications on patient safety in older people. *Therapeutic Advances in Drug Safety, 3*(4), 165–174.

Anderson, P., & Townsend, T. (2010). Medication errors: Don't let them happen to you. *American Nurse Today, 5*(3), 23–27.

Austin, J., & Pronovost, P. (2015). "Never events" and the quest to reduce preventable harm. *Joint Commission Journal of Quality Patient Safety, 41,* 279–288.

Bae, S. (2017). CMS nonpayment policy, quality improvement, and hospital-acquired conditions. *Journal of Nursing Care Quality, 32*(1), 55–61.

Barach, P., & Johnson, K. (2018). Assessing risk and harm in clinical microsystems. In W. Sollecito & J. Johnson (Eds.), *McLaughlin and Kaluzny's continuous quality improvement in health care* (5th ed., pp. 249–274). Burlington, MA: Jones & Bartlett Learning.

Barlett, M., & Kelly, K. (2009). Hospital-acquired conditions: A leadership challenge for nursing quality management and performance improvement. *Nurse Leader, 7*(6), 26–28.

Brady, J., & Khanna, G. (2019). Improving diagnosis: A vital patient safety frontier. Retrieved from https://www.ahrq.gov/news/blog/ahrqviews/vital-patient-safety-frontier.html

Cipriano, P. (2011). When medication regulations collide with common sense. *American Nurse Today, 6*(2). Retrieved from https://www.myamericannurse.com/when-medication-regulations-collide-with-common-sense

Clark, A., & Flanders, S. (2012). Interruptions and medication errors. Part II. *Clinical Nurse Specialist, 26*(5), 239–243.

Bavo, K., Cochran, G., & Barrett, R. (2016). Nursing strategies to increase medication safety in inpatient settings. *Journal of Nursing Care Quality, 31*(4), 335–341.

Cole, G., Stefanus, D., Gardner, H., Levy, M., & Klein, E. (2015). The impact of interruptions on the duration of nursing interventions: A direct observation study in an academic emergency department. *BMJ Quality Safety*. Published first online at http://qualitysafety.bmj.com/content/early/2015/08/20/bmjqs-2014

-003683.abstract?sid=161de7be-65a9-40a5 -b337 -74433203c93f

Cooper, E. (2014). Nursing student medication errors: A snapshot view from a school of nursing's quality and safety officer. *Journal of Nursing Education, 53*(3S), S51–S54.

Dickson, G., & Flynn, I. (2012). Nurses' clinical reasoning: Processes and practice in medication safety. *Quality Health Research, 22*(1), 3–16.

Disch, J., & Barnsteiner, J. (2014). Developing a reporting and tracking tool for nursing student errors and near misses. *Journal of Nursing Regulation, 5*(1), 5–7.

Dolansky, M., Druschel, K., Helba, M., & Courtney, K (2013). Nursing student medication errors: A case study using root cause analysis. *Journal of Professional Nursing, 29* (2),102–108.

Ehlert, D., & Rough, S. (2013). Improving the safety of the medication use process. In B. Youngberg (Ed.), *Patient safety handbook* (2nd ed., pp. 461–493). Burlington, MA: Jones & Bartlett Learning.

Ellison, A. (2020). CMS cuts payments to 786 hospitals over high rates of infection, injury. Becker's Hospital CFO Report. Retrieved from https://www.becker shospitalreview.com/finance/cms-cuts-payments -to-786-hospitals-over-high-rates-of-infection-injury .html?origin=CFOE&utm_source=CFOE&utm _medium=email&oly_enc_id=6777B2161145E3A

Endo, J. (2015). 5 steps for creating value through process mapping and observation. Retrieved from http://www .ihi.org/communities/blogs/_layouts/ihi/community /blog/itemview.aspx?list=7d1126ec-8f63-4a3b-9926 -c44ea3036813&id=166

Finkelman, A. (2017). *Professional concepts. Competency for quality leadership* (4th ed.). Burlington, MA: Jones & Bartlett Learning.

Ford, Y., & Heyman, A. (2017). Patients' perceptions of bedside handoff: Further evidence to support culture of always. *Journal of Nursing Care Quality, 32*(1), 15–24.

Giardina, T., Haskell, H., Menon, S., Hallisy, J., Southwick, F., Sarkar, U., . . . Singh, H. (2018). Learning from patients' experiences related to diagnostic errors is essential for progress in patient safety. *Health Affairs, 37*(11), 1821–1827.

Gleason, K., McDaniel, M., Feinglass, J., Baker, D., Lindquist, L., Liss, D., & Noskin, G. (2010). Results of the medications at transitions and clinical handoffs (MATCH) study: An analysis of medication reconciliation errors and risk factors at hospital admission. *Journal of General Internal Medicine, 25*(5), 441–447.

Graber, M. (2014). Minimizing diagnostic error: 10 things you could do tomorrow. Lists for physicians, healthcare organizations, and patients. *Inside medical liability* (first quarter), 22–26.

Grayson, D., Boxerman, S., Potter, P., Wolf, L, Dunagan, C., Sorock, G., & Evanoff, B. (2014, October).

Do transient working conditions trigger medical errors? Patient safety executive walkarounds. *Advances in Patient Safety*, 53–64.

Greene, L. (2015). Preventing surgical site infections. *American Nurse Today, 10*(9), 10–11.

Hagman, J., Oman, K., Kleiner, C., Johnson, E., & Nordhagen, J. (2013). Lessons learned from the implementation of a bedside handoff model. *JONA: Journal of Nursing Administration, 43*(6), 315–317.

Hawkes, B. (2014). What's the window for passing meds before it's considered late? Retrieved from http://nursecode.com/2014/12/whats-window-passing -meds-considered-late

Henneman, E., Gawlinski, A., Blank, F., Henneman, P., Jordan, D., & McKenzie, J. (2010). Strategies used by critical care nurses to identify, interrupt, and correct medical errors. *American Journal of Critical Care, 19*(6), 500–509.

Hessels, A. (2015). Moving toward zero hospital-acquired infections. *American Nurse Today, 10*(9), 2.

Institute for Healthcare Improvement (IHI). (2011). Reduced readmissions: Reform's low-hanging fruit. Retrieved from http://www.ihi.org/resources/Pages/Publications /ReducedReadmissionsReformsLowHangingFruit.aspx

Institute for Safe Medication Practices (ISMP). (2010). CMS 30-minute rule for drug administration needs revision. Retrieved from https://www.ismp.org/resources /cms-30-minute-rule-drug-administration-needs -revision

Institute for Safe Medication Practices (ISMP). (2011). Guidelines for timely medication administration: Response to the CMS "30 minute rule." Retrieved from https://www.ismp.org/resources/guidelines-timely -medication-administration-response-cms-30-minute -rule

Institute for Safe Medication Practices (ISMP). (2018). 2018–2019 targeted medication safety best practices for hospitals. Retrieved from https://www .ismp.org/sites/default/files/attachments/2019-01 /TMSBP-for-Hospitalsv2.pdf

Institute for Safe Medication Practices (ISMP). (2019). Key elements of medication use. Retrieved from https://www.ismp.org/ten-key-elements#

Institute of Medicine (IOM). (1999). *To err is human: Building a safer health system*. Washington, DC: The National Academies Press.

Institute of Medicine (IOM). (2001). *Crossing the quality chasm*. Washington, DC: The National Academies Press.

Institute of Medicine (IOM). (2004). *Keeping patients safe*. Washington, DC: The National Academies Press.

Institute of Medicine (IOM). (2011). *Relieving pain in America: A blueprint for transforming prevention, care, education, and research*. Washington, DC: The National Academies Press.

Jones, D., DeVita, M., & Bellomo, R. (2011). Rapid response teams. *New England Journal of Medicine, 365,* 139–146.

Jones, K., Sibai, J., Battjes, R., & Fakih, M. (2015). How and when nurses collect urine cultures on catheterized patients: A survey of 5 hospitals. *American Journal of Infection Control, 44*(2), 173–176.

Kaplan, M. (2016). Diagnosis is a process: Experts offer advice on diagnostic error and delays in patient safety. Institute for Healthcare Improvement. Improvement blog. Retrieved from http://www.ihi.org/communities/blogs/_layouts/ihi/community/blog/itemview.aspx?List=7d1126ec-8f63-4a3b-9926-c44ea3036813&ID=186

Keroack, M., & Rhinehart, E. (2012). The investigation and analysis of clinical incidents. In B. Youngberg (Ed.), *Patient safety handbook* (2nd ed., pp. 125–142). Burlington, MA: Jones & Bartlett Learning.

Koyama, A., Maddox, C., Li, L., Bucknall, T., & Westbrook, J. (2019, August 7). Effectiveness of double checking to reduce medication administration errors: A systematic review. *BMJ Quality Safety.* doi:10.1136/bmjqs-2019-009552

Kripalani, S., LeFevre, F., Phillips, C., Williams, M., Basaviah, P., & Baker, D. (2007). Deficits in communication and information transfer between hospital-based and primary care physicians. *JAMA, 297*(8), 831–841.

Kronick, R. (2015, September). New report outlines goals and recommendations to reduce diagnostic errors. Blog Agency for Healthcare Research and Quality. Retrieved from https://archive.ahrq.gov/news/blog/ahrqviews/092315.html

Kurtzman, E., & Buerhaus, P. (2008). New Medicare payment rules: Danger or opportunity for nursing? *AJN, 108*(6), 30–35.

Lalley, C., & Malloch, K. (2010). Workarounds: The hidden pathway to excellence. *Nurse Leader, 8*(4), 29–32.

LeBlanc, R., & Choi, J. (2015). Optimizing medication safety in the home. *Home Healthcare Nurse, 33*(6), 313–310.

Makary, M. (2016, May 3). Medical error—the third leading cause of death in the US. *BMJ.* Retrieved from http://www.bmj.com/content/353/bmj.i2139

Manojlovich, M., & Talsma, A. (2007). Identifying nursing processes to reduce failure to rescue. *Journal of Nursing Administration, 37*(11), 504–509.

Maxfield, D., Grenny, J., Levandero, R., & Goah, L. (2010). The silent treatment. American Association of Critical Care Nurses, AORN, VitalSmart. Retrieved from http://www.silenttreatmentstudy.com/Silent%20Treatment%20Executive%20Summary.pdf

Mayor, E., Bangerter, A., & Aribot, M. (2012). Task uncertainty and communication during nursing shift handovers. *Journal of Advanced Nursing, 68*(9), 1956–1966.

Mitchell, B., Gardner, A., Stone, P., Hall, L., & Pogorzelska-Maziarz, M. (2018). Hospital staffing and healthcare-associated infections: A systematic review of literature. *The Joint Commission Journal of Quality and Patient Safety, 44*(10), 612–622.

Nanji, K., Patel, A., Shaikh, S., Seger, D., & Bates, D. (2016). Evaluation of perioperative medication errors and adverse drug events. *Anesthesiology, 124*(1), 25–34.

National Academy of Medicine (NAM). (2015). *Improving diagnosis in health care.* Washington, DC: The National Academies Press.

National Academy of Medicine (NAM). (2016). *Pain management and prescription opioid-related harms: Exploring the state of the evidence.* Washington, DC: The National Academies Press

National Academy of Medicine (NAM). (2019). *Pain management for people with serious illness in the context of opioid use disorder epidemic.* Washington, DC: The National Academies Press.

National Council State Boards of Nursing (NCSBN). (2019). Safe student reports (SSR). Retrieved from https://www.ncsbn.org/safe-student-reports.htm

National Coordinating Council for Medication Error Reporting and Prevention (NCC MERP). (2001). NCC MERP index for categorizing medication errors algorithm. Retrieved from http://www.nccmerp.org/sites/default/files/algorBW2001-06-12.pdf

National Coordinating Council for Medication Error Reporting and Prevention (NCC MERP). (2008). Statement of medication error rates. Retrieved from https://www.nccmerp.org/statement-medication-error-rates

National Coordinating Council for Medication Error Reporting and Prevention (NCC MERP). (2019). Types of medication errors. Retrieved from http://www.nccmerp.org/types-medication-errors

Onder, G., Petrovic, M., Tangiisuran, B., Meinardi, M., Markito-Notenboom, W., Somers, A., . . . van der Cammen, T. (2010). Development and validation of a score to assess risk of adverse drug reactions among in-hospital patients 65 years or older: The GerontoNet ADR Risk Score. *Archives of Internal Medicine, 170,* 1142–1148.

Paine, C., Goel, V., Ely, E., Stave, C., Stemler, S., Zander, M., & Bonafide, P. (2016). Systematic review of physiologic monitor alarm characteristics and pragmatic interventions to reduce alarm frequency. *Journal of Hospital Medicine, 11*(2), 136–144.

Patterson, E., Roth, E., Woods, D., Chow, R., & Gomes, J. (2004). Handoff strategies in settings with high consequences for failure: Lessons for healthcare operations. *International Journal of Quality Health Care, 16*(2), 125–132.

Perry, S., Wears, R., & Patterson, E. (2008). High-hanging fruit: Improving transitions in health care. In K. Henriksen, J. Battles, E. Marks, & D. Lewin (Eds.), *Advances in patient safety: From research to implementation* (Vol. 2., pp. 159–267). Research Findings. AHRQ Publication No. 05-0021-1. Rockville, MD: AHRQ.

Peter, D., Robinson, P., Jordan, M., Lawrence, S., Casey, K., & Salas-Lopez, D. (2015). Reducing readmission using teach-back: Enhancing patient and family education. *JONA: Journal of Nursing Administration, 45*(1), 35–42.

Potts, L., Diegel-Vacek, L., Ryan, C., & Murchek, A. (2018). Improving patient flow from the emergency department utilizing a standardized electronic nursing process. *JONA: Journal of Nursing Administration, 48*(9), 432–436.

Quigley, P., & White, S. (2013). Hospital-based fall program measurement and improvement in high reliability organizations. *OJIN, 18*(2). https://ojin.nursingworld.org/MainMenuCategories/ANAMarketplace/ANAPeriodicals/OJIN/TableofContents/Vol-18-2013/No2-May-2013/Fall-Program-Measurement.html

Quigley, P., Barnett, S., Bulat, T., & Friedman, Y. (2016). Fall-related injuries in medical-surgical units. One year multihospital falls collaborative. *Journal of Nursing Care Quality, 31*(2), 139–145.

Rajaram, R., Chung, J., Kinnier, C., Barnard, C., Mohanty, S., Pavey, E., . . . Bilimoria, K. (2015). Hospital characteristics associated with penalties in the Centers for Medicare and Medicaid hospital-acquired condition reduction program. *JAMA, 314*, 375–383.

Risenberg, L., Leitzsch, J., & Cunningham, J. (2010). Nursing handoffs: A systematic review of literature. *American Journal of Nursing, 110*(4), 24–34.

Rodak, S. (2013). Prevent patient falls now: Five strategies. *Becker's infection control & clinical quality.* Retrieved from http://www.beckersasc.com/asc-quality-infection-control/prevent-patient-falls-now-5-strategies.html

Russell, J., Leming-Lee, T., & Watters, R. (2019). Implementation of a nurse-driven CAUTI prevention algorithm. *Nursing Clinics of North America, 54*, 81–96.

Sandoval, C. (2015). Preventing central line-associated bloodstream infections. *American Nurse Today, 10*(9), 8–9.

Schnock, K., Dykes, P., Albert, J., Ariosto, D., Call, R., Cameron, C., . . . Bates, D. (2016, February 26). The frequency of intravenous medication administration errors related to smart infusion pumps: A multihospital observational study. *BMJ Quality Safety*. doi:10.1136/bmjqs-2015-004465

Shang, J., Needleman, J., Liu, J., Larson, E., & Stone, P. (2019). Nurse staffing and healthcare-associated infection, unit-level analysis. *JONA: Journal of Nursing Administration, 49*(5), 260–265.

Singh, H. (2014). Editorial: Helping healthcare organizations to define diagnostic errors as missed opportunities in diagnosis. *Joint Commission Journal on Quality and Patient Safety, 40*(3), 99–101.

Singh, H. (2015). Measurement of diagnostic errors is a key first step to their reduction. Retrieved from https://www.researchgate.net/publication/325860531_Measurement_of_Diagnostic_Errors_Is_a_Key_First_Step_to_Their_Reduction

Society of Hospital Medicine (SHM). (2015). Overview project BOOST® implementation toolkit. Retrieved from http://tools.hospitalmedicine.org/Implementation/Workbook_for_Improvement.pdf

Stultz, J., & Nahata, M. (2015). Preventability of voluntarily reported or trigger tool-identified medication errors in pediatric institution by information technology: A retrospective study. *Drug safety, 38*(7), 661–670.

The Joint Commission. (2013). Sentinel event alert 50: Medical device alarm safety in hospitals. Retrieved from http://www.jointcommission.org/sea_issue_50

The Joint Commission. (2015). Sentinel event alert 55: Preventing falls and fall related injuries in health care facilities. Retrieved from https://www.jointcommission.org/sea_issue_55

The Joint Commission. (2016). National patient safety goals effective January 1, 2016. Retrieved from https://www.jointcommission.org/-/media/deprecated-unorganized/imported-assets/tjc/system-folders/topics-library/old---to-delete/2016_npsg_happdf.pdf?db=web&hash=23105C3839C69F741F877120E8183F51

The Joint Commission. (2017). Sentinel alert event 58: Inadequate hand-off communication. Retrieved from https://www.jointcommission.org/sentinel_event_alert_58_inadequate_handoff_communications

The Joint Commission. (2018). 8 tips for high-quality hand-offs. Retrieved from https://www.jointcommission.org/assets/1/6/SEA_8_steps_hand_off_infographic_2018.pdf

The Joint Commission. (2019). 2020 National patient safety goals. Retrieved from https://www.jointcommission.org/standards_information/npsgs.aspx

Thomas, L., Donohue-Porter, P., & Fishbein, J. (2017). Impact of interruptions, distractions, and cognitive load on procedure failure and medication administration errors. *Journal of Nursing Care Quality, 32*(4), 309–317.

Topaz, M., Seger, D., Slight, S., Goss, F., Lai, K., Paige, G., . . . Zhou, L. (2015). Rising drug allergy alert overrides in electronic health records: An observational retrospective study of a decade of experience. *Journal American Medical Informatics Association*. Retrieved from http://jamia.oxfordjournals.org/content/early/2015/11/17/jamia.ocv143

Trevellini, C. (2015). Operationalizing the ANA CAUTI tool in acute-care settings. *American Nurse Today, 10*(9), 5–7.

Tully, A., Hammond, D., Jarrell, A., Kruer, R. (2019). Evaluation of medication errors at the transition of care for an ICU to a non-ICU location. *Critical Care Medicine, 47*(4), 543–549.

U.S. Department of Health and Human Services (HHS). (2010). Multiple chronic conditions: A strategic framework. Retrieved from http://www.hhs.gov/ash/initiatives/mcc/mcc_framework.pdf

U.S. Department of Health and Human Services (HHS), (2015). HHS initiative on multiple chronic conditions. Retrieved from http://www.hhs.gov/ash/initiatives/mcc

U.S. Department of Health and Human Services (HHS), Agency for Healthcare Research and Quality (AHRQ). (2013). Preventing falls in hospitals. Tool 3H: Morse fall scale for identifying fall risk factors. Retrieved from http://www.ahrq.gov/professionals/systems/hospital/fallpxtoolkit/fallpxtk-tool3h.html

U.S. Department of Health and Human Services (HHS), Agency for Healthcare Research and Quality (AHRQ). (2014). Designing and delivering whole-person transitional care: The hospital guide to reducing Medicaid readmissions. Publiation No. 14-0050-EF. Retrieved from http://www.ahrq.gov/professionals/systems/hospital/medicaidreadmitguide/index.html

U.S. Department of Health and Human Services (HHS), Agency for Healthcare Research and Quality (AHRQ). (2017). The falls management program: A quality improvement initiative for nursing facilities. Retrieved from https://www.ahrq.gov/patient-safety/settings/long-term-care/resource/injuries/fallspx/manapb1.html

U.S. Department of Health and Human Services (HHS), Agency for Healthcare Research and Quality (AHRQ). (2018a). AHRQ-funded patient safety research on reducing medication, diagnostic errors. Retrieved from https://www.ahrq.gov/news/newsroom/press-releases/health-affairs-patient-safety-research.html

U.S. Department of Health and Human Services (HHS), Agency for Healthcare Research and Quality (AHRQ). (2018b). Guide: Purpose and use of CLABSI tools. Retrieved from https://www.ahrq.gov/hai/clabsi-tools/guide.html

U.S. Department of Health and Human Services (HHS), Agency for Healthcare Research and Quality (AHRQ). (2019a). Diagnostic safety and quality. Retrieved from https://www.ahrq.gov/topics/diagnostic-safety-and-quality.html

U.S. Department of Health and Human Services (HHS), Agency for Healthcare Research and Quality (AHRQ). (2020a). Hospital acquired conditions annual report. Retrieved from https://www.ahrq.gov/hai/pfp/hacreport.html

U.S. Department of Health and Human Services (HHS), Agency for Healthcare Research and Quality (AHRQ). (2020b). Falls prevention. Retrieved from https://www.ahrq.gov/topics/falls-prevention.html

U.S. Department of Health and Human Services (HHS), Agency for Healthcare Research and Quality (AHRQ), Patient Safety Network (PSNet). (2019a). Handoffs and signouts. Retrieved from https://psnet.ahrq.gov/primer/handoffs-and-signouts

U.S. Department of Health and Human Services (HHS), Agency for Healthcare Research and Quality (AHRQ), Patient Safety Network (PSNet). (2019b). Alert fatigue. Retrieved from https://psnet.ahrq.gov/primers/primer/28

U.S. Department of Health and Human Services (HHS), Agency for Healthcare Research and Quality (AHRQ), Patient Safety Network (PSNet). (2019c). Surgical site infections. Retrieved from https://psnet.ahrq.gov/primer/surgical-site-infections

U.S. Department of Health and Human Services (HHS), Agency for Healthcare Research and Quality (AHRQ), Patient Safety Network (PSNet). (2019d). Readmission and adverse events after discharge. Retrieved from http://psnet.ahrq.gov/primer.aspx?primerID=11

U.S. Department of Health and Human Services (HHS), Agency for Healthcare Research and Quality (AHRQ), Patient Safety Network (PSNet). (2019e). Detection of safety hazards. Retrieved from https://psnet.ahrq.gov/primer/detection-safety-hazards

U.S. Department of Health and Human Services (HHS), Centers for Medicare and Medicaid Services (CMS). (2019a). Hospital-acquired conditions. Retrieved from https://www.cms.gov/Medicare/Medicare-Fee-for-Service-Payment/HospitalAcqCond/Hospital-Acquired_Conditions.html

U.S. Department of Health and Human Services (HHS), Centers for Medicare and Medicaid Services (CMS). (2019b). Thirty-day unplanned readmission and death measures. Retrieved from https://www.medicare.gov/hospitalcompare/Data/30-day-measures.html

U.S. Department of Health and Human Services (HHS), Centers for Medicare and Medicaid Services (CMS). (2019c). Community-Based Care Transitions Program (CCTP). Retrieved from http://innovation.cms.gov/initiatives/CCTP/index.html

U.S. Department of Health and Human Services (HHS), Centers for Disease Control (CDC). (2020). Ventilator-associated event. Retrieved from https://www.cdc.gov/nhsn/PDFs/pscManual/10-VAE_FINAL.pdf

U.S. Department of Health and Human Services (HHS), Food and Drug Administration (FDA). (2015). Medication errors related to CDER-regulated drug products. Retrieved from http://www.fda.gov/Drugs/DrugSafety/medicationErrors/default.htm

Volker, N., & McLellan, T. (2016). Opioid abuse in chronic pain—Misperceptions and mitigation strategies. *New England Journal of Medicine, 374*, (13),1253–1263.

Volz, T., & Swaim, T. (2013). Partnering to prevent falls. *JONA: Journal of Nursing Administration, 43*(6), 336–441.

Wachter, R., & Gupta, K. (2018). *Understanding patient safety*. New York, NY: McGraw-Hill.

Walton, B. (2014). Are you prepared to prevent medication errors? *Ohio Nurse,* March, 10–15.

Welsh, C., Flanagan, M., & Ebright, P. (2010). Barriers and facilitators to nursing handoffs: Recommendations for redesign. *Nursing Outlook, 58*(3), 148–154.

Westbrook, J. et al. (2017). Effectiveness of a 'do not interrupt' bundled intervention to reduce interruptions during medication administration: A cluster randomized controlled feasibility study. *BMJ Quality & Safety, 26*(9). Retrieved from https://qualitysafety.bmj.com/content/26/9/734

## CHAPTER 9

# The Quality Improvement Plan

## CHAPTER OBJECTIVES

At the conclusion of this chapter, the learner will be able to:

- Examine the relevance of quality improvement (QI) programs and planning.
- Discuss the purpose of continuous quality improvement (CQI) programs and planning.
- Examine the planning and implementation necessary for effective quality improvement.

## OUTLINE

## KEY TERMS

Operational plan

Organizational readiness

Performance management

Performance measure

Performance measurement

Project plan

Quality improvement plan

Strategic plan

# Introduction

Previous content laid the groundwork for understanding continuous quality improvement (CQI) in healthcare organizations (HCOs), within states, and nationally. This information is critical background information that is related to quality improvement (QI) program planning and measurement. Developing, implementing, and maintaining an effective QI program requires planning at the strategic, operational, and project levels. Other chapters discuss the change process and planning for change, and this content applies to CQI planning. Following the development and implementation of plans, the QI program must then focus on measurement based on the plans. Measurement is discussed in other chapters.

# Quality Improvement Program: Structure to Support CQI

Each HCO typically has some type of structure within its organization that guides its CQI activities. The structure may have many different titles, but for this discussion the term *QI program* will be used. Integrated into the QI program is planning, a key function, to meet the CQI needs of the HCO.

HCOs need to consider their size and determine who will be on the QI program team and how leadership will be provided. Engagement at all levels of the organization is important, and this then impacts representation in the CQI process. Since the QI program is complex and ongoing, who participates, how, and when may vary. The HCO board of directors must have an understanding of CQI and participate in the discussion to identify overarching goals. Senior management is responsible for providing information and open discussion with the board so that it has an understanding of the importance of CQI and

factors that impact quality improvement. The board has ultimate responsibility for HCO actions and organization outcomes. The board also approves the budget, which impacts care delivery in many ways, including by allocating funds for initiatives such as the QI program. Not only does the HCO board need initial information and education about CQI, but board members also need ongoing reports of progress prepared by senior management.

Many HCOs have designated QI staff—for example, a QI program director (although the title may vary)—and other formal staff positions such as staff that collect and analyze data, develop CQI plans, and so on. Once the QI program is implemented, there is much work to be done, and relying only on committees/teams will not be effective. The organizational structure needs to be described for the QI program staff—for example, QI staff need to know to whom they report and their responsibilities. Ideally, the staff should have CQI experience. They are often also part of the organizational structure that is responsible for accreditation and regulatory issues and also risk management and utilization review/management. All of these activities relate to the same overarching goals.

CQI activities need to be integrated throughout the HCO, and it is the QI program that guides the activities. However, all senior management, such as the chief executive officer, chief nursing executive, chief operating officer, and chief financial officer (titles vary from one HCO to the other), must be committed and participate in key decisions regarding CQI, including development of plans; receive and respond to CQI information; and ensure that updated information on progress is shared with staff, the board, and other relevant stakeholders external to the HCO.

CQI communication must move both ways in the organization: down from the board and management and up from the staff. When CQI is solely directed and managed by management, it will not be effective. Teams, working with CQI program staff, are a critical aspect of the process. Various teams work on different parts of planning and implementation. A core team develops the overall QI program plan (strategic plan) and the operational plan. However, this team and all teams that get involved in CQI need to reach out to others for input and expertise, which later helps to engage other staff when their feedback and assistance may be needed.

Teams are discussed in several chapters, and they are relevant to this chapter's content. Team membership includes representatives from management and administration services such as finance, data management and information technology, and medical records; clinical support services such as pharmacy and laboratories; and medical and nursing representation. The consumer (patient) should be represented at some point during planning, as should community representatives. Membership and responsibilities need to be clearly defined. Support staff are needed to assist the QI program staff and CQI teams—for example, they help maintain documentation of meetings and CQI activities, track data, and so on. CQI work takes time, and staff members who participate need time to complete required work, which may require adjustment in position responsibilities.

### STOP AND CONSIDER 9-1

The QI program requires a structure within an HCO to support its functions.

# Purpose of CQI Program and Planning

QI program staff develop a CQI plan in collaboration with other HCO staff, and the plan should relate to current standards and benchmarks, performance appraisal, interprofessional assessment and improvement, and specific HCO CQI needs. Developing such a plan requires understanding of and effective

application of the change process (Fuji, Hoidal, Galt, Drincic, & Abbott, 2009). The **quality improvement (QI) plan**, or the strategic plan, is a detailed, organizational plan describing an HCO's CQI goals and proposed activities. The purpose of the HCO's QI plan is "to provide a formal ongoing process by which the organization and stakeholders utilize objective measures to monitor and evaluate the quality of services, both clinical and operational, provided to the patients" (U.S. Department of Health and Human Services [HHS]. Agency for Healthcare Research and Quality [AHRQ], 2017). The QI plan serves as a road map for all QI program activities and includes the following (HHS, AHRQ, 2017):

- A systematic process with identified leadership, accountability, and dedicated resources
- Use of data and measurable outcomes to determine progress toward relevant, evidence-based benchmarks
- Focus on linkages, efficiencies, and provider and patient expectations in addressing outcome improvement
- Continuous process that is adaptive to change and fits within the framework of other programmatic quality and CQI activities (e.g., JCAHO, Centers for Medicare and Medicaid Services [CMS], accreditation)
- Assurance that goals are accomplished and are concurrent with improved outcomes based on data collected

QI plans should address selection of performance measures, the performance measurement process, and performance management, focusing on core areas of clinical care, operations, and finance (HHS, Health Resources and Services Administration [HRSA], 2011a).

- **Performance measures** are designed to measure systems of care and are derived from clinical or practice guidelines. Data that are sorted into specific measurable elements provide an HCO with a meter to measure the quality of its care.

- **Performance measurement** is a process by which an HCO monitors important aspects of its programs, systems, and processes. In this context, performance measurement includes the operational processes used to collect data necessary to assess performance measures.
- **Performance management** is a forward-looking process used to set goals and regularly check progress toward achieving those goals. In practice, an HCO sets goals and evaluates its success in achieving those goals by reviewing the actual data of its performance.

Nurses should be involved in all of these focus areas as direct care providers and managers/leaders.

### STOP AND CONSIDER 9-2

The purpose of a QI program plan is similar to that of a nursing care plan.

# Planning and Implementation

Each HCO should develop and implement a QI plan and then evaluate and revise it on a scheduled basis. Change is a major concern throughout the process. Effective change requires leadership and also staff engagement. A QI plan that is dictated from management will not be effective. Proactive leadership is required for effective QI planning (Finkelman, 2020). Planning requires input from all levels of the staff—active participatory planning. When the CQI plan recognizes and integrates nurses in the planning, there is a greater chance that their involvement will be expected in all CQI process steps. Planning is a key competency for nurse leaders, who need to assume more active responsibility in QI planning. It is important for the HCO to have a structured process for approval of the plan and for plan modification. This ensures that planning changes are considered carefully, goals are reviewed, and commitment to CQI is maintained.

A QI program uses three types of planning: (1) strategic, (2) operational, and (3) project. The **strategic plan** is the overall plan; it considers CQI long-term goals and outcomes, noting the gaps or what needs to be improved over time. The **operational plan** describes detailed steps needed to ensure that outcomes are met; describes roles and responsibilities; identifies timelines, as well as interventions such as measurement and evaluation of plans; and describes the plan revision process. As the CQI strategic and operational plans are implemented, the QI program will need **project plans** focused on specific needs, such as implementing use of structured communication methods in the HCO or a change in the medication administration procedure for the emergency department. Many smaller initiatives or projects are undertaken to reach overall CQI goals. Data collection, measurement, and analysis must be integrated throughout all this planning.

An initial step is to clearly identify the HCO's overarching CQI goals or aims, which must connect with the HCO's vision, mission, and goals. Today, many HCOs apply the aims identified in the *Quality Chasm* reports discussed elsewhere in this text to the HCO's overarching goals or aims (Institute of Medicine [IOM], 2001)—safe, timely, effective, efficient, equitable, and patient-centered (STEEEP®)—and integrate the triple aim (better care, healthy people/healthy communities, affordable care). HCOs often apply one of the QI theories or models discussed in other chapters to their QI programs.

Planning is never static and requires ongoing review and revision as situations change, problems are resolved, and new problems are identified. QI plans are used to implement systematic CQI activities that incorporate processes, structure, outcomes, patients, teams and teamwork, and measurement.

# Assessment to Prepare for CQI Planning

In order to develop an effective QI program and plans, the HCO needs to complete a careful self-assessment. Clear goals and timelines require understanding of the current status of the organization. The QI team also needs to consider factors such as internal policies and procedures, healthcare trends, healthcare policies and legislation at the state and national levels, professional standards and other types of standards, state requirements, accreditation, national quality measurement and reporting systems, and third-party payer requirements such as those of the Centers for Medicare and Medicaid Services (CMS) relating to hospital-acquired conditions and 30-day unplanned readmissions. With the increasing importance of information management and technology in all phases of CQI, the QI program needs to consider the functioning of the HCO's health informatics technology (HIT). Can HIT provide effective support for CQI activities including data collection, measurement, and analysis? During self-assessment, the HCO may identify weaknesses in its system that may impact the QI plans, such as ineffective data management requiring a change in software.

As HCOs prepare to develop or expand and improve their QI programs, it is important to determine **organizational readiness**. As discussed in content relating to change, knowing when staff and the organization are better able to handle change is important to success. To determine HCO readiness for CQI, the HCO should undertake a "systematic analysis of an organization's ability to undertake a transformational process or change" (HHS, HRSA, 2011b, p. 1). What does the HCO gain from this analysis? It should have a better understanding of its processes, structures, and outcomes; its culture and environment; barriers; and gaps—what needs to be improved or better analyzed. There are two levels of readiness assessment—organizational QI program readiness and QI project readiness. The first level considers the overall organization and its readiness for CQI planning, implementation, and evaluation. The second is much more specific, and it is ongoing as new CQI projects are undertaken. HCO self-assessment should consider the following areas (HHS, HRSA, 2011b, pp. 2–3):

- *Organizational readiness.* Readiness is marked by high levels of executive commitment to the QI initiative from key decision makers; an understanding of the financial investment and time commitment that QI requires; consensus throughout the organization that the QI initiative is aligned with organizational goals, physicians, and clinicians who support the initiative and understand its value, as well as clinicians who enjoy a collaborative working environment.

- *Staff characteristics.* A critical staff characteristic is the provider's adoption of the CQI initiative. The provider may be considered supportive of adoption if the provider believes that it is relatively easy to care for patients at the facility and that the improvement strategy will improve this experience; the relationship between the provider and the organization's administration and other clinicians is open and collaborative; the provider actively participates in initiatives that promote evidence-based practice (EBP) and leading clinical practices; and the provider is willing to assume a leadership role while implementing an integrated care system by taking responsibility for key objectives and helping to promote the system to other providers within the organization.

- *Resource readiness.* The organization's ability to support the CQI initiative requires assessment to determine if healthcare decision makers are knowledgeable about the type and availability of organizational resources required for initial implementation of a CQI initiative/project and for ongoing support of CQI. Resource readiness encompasses a wide range of assets, such as, money, space, technology, training availability, supervisors, and sometimes consultation services.

There are many approaches an HCO could use in its planning, but this text focuses on the Agency for Healthcare Research and Quality (AHRQ) recommendations for CQI planning. AHRQ's QI resources for HCOs use an EBP approach. These resources include input from multiple stakeholders providing assessment tools or surveys for HCOs to use as they assess their CQI readiness and CQI activities, including tools for hospitals, nursing homes, ambulatory outpatient medical offices, community pharmacies, and ambulatory surgery services. Using these surveys also provides opportunities for HCOs to compare their results with those of similar HCOs. The AHRQ surveys are designed to meet the following goals for the HCO culture of safety (HHS, AHRQ, 2019a):

- Raise staff awareness about patient safety.
- Diagnose and assess the current status of patient safety culture.
- Identify strengths and areas for patient safety culture improvement.
- Examine trends in patient safety culture change over time.
- Evaluate the cultural impact of patient safety initiatives and interventions.
- Conduct internal and external comparisons.

## Strategic and Operational Plans

HCO self-assessment provides information needed to develop effective CQI strategic and operational plans that meet the current needs of the HCO. Typically, these plans include the following information, with the operational plans providing more details and covering a shorter period of time:

- Goals and objectives
- Establishment of a culture of safety, including consideration of how to accomplish and maintain it

- Description of the QI program structure and functions, including staff roles and responsibilities
- Identification of budgetary requirements
- Clarification of communication and engagement at all levels in the HCO structure—for example, executive, departmental, and unit meetings and meetings with clinical and nonclinical staff
- Reporting methods to ensure that all are informed of CQI status
- Description of required planning for QI projects, including consideration of what needs to be included and who determines when a project should be initiated
- Current analysis of quality status, including identification of best practices and problems (gaps) with prioritization of problems and actions to take
- Description of the process to be used to identify and develop measures/indicators with thresholds
- Description of measurement process and methods, including data required and data availability or need for new data collection methods
- Identification and prioritization of QI project plans, including consideration of the focus, teams, and timeline
- Description of staff education needs regarding CQI and a plan to meet these needs in orientation and other staff education activities
- Required evaluation of the QI program and project plans

Engaging staff in the QI program should be considered in planning, implementation, and evaluation of plans. The following are examples of methods that an HCO might use to increase staff engagement (Fallon, Begun, & Riley, 2012, p. 199):

- Screen new hires for attitudes toward practice, management, and CQI.
- Take advantage of management levers to enhance motivation—recognize, reward, and reinforce high motivation.
- Invest in employee learning.

- Experiment with creative forms of recognition.
- Search for and recognize positives in employee performance.
- Demonstrate the impact of the employee's work on patients and consumers.

## Impact of Analysis on CQI Planning

During data collection and analysis, an HCO examines its performance and often compares its performance to that of other HCOs. During this phase, the HCO analyzes data to determine if HCO performance meets the desired quality level based on the measures/indicators identified in the CQI plan. Following the collection of data, analysis and interpretation of data allow staff to better understand the meaning of data and its relevance to CQI (HHS, AHRQ, 2017). Based on analysis, a decision is made regarding the next step: (1) Continue the process as is, with the same measures/indicators and data monitoring, (2) continue the process with modifications (e.g., implement additional interventions/strategies), (3) add new measures/indicators, or (4) stop monitoring. There may need to be changes in measure/indicator thresholds, or the decision may be to maintain current targets. Adjustments to the plan are made as needed. This process is applied to clinical and administrative/management measures/indicators and should be ongoing.

## Project Plans

Project plans are a critical element, as this is where the HCO focuses on improving care for specific concerns or gaps in care quality. A project charter describes the rationale and roadmap for a team's improvement project. The Institute for Health Improvement (IHI) provides a template for a charter HCOs may develop to help guide the QI process (IHI, 2019). Plan-do-study-act (PDSA), discussed in other sections of this text, is one method that is commonly used in the planning process. **Figure 9-1** reviews the key PDSA elements.

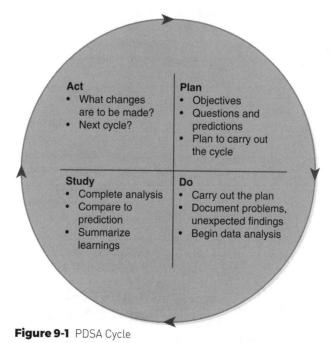

**Act**
- What changes are to be made?
- Next cycle?

**Plan**
- Objectives
- Questions and predictions
- Plan to carry out the cycle

**Study**
- Complete analysis
- Compare to prediction
- Summarize learnings

**Do**
- Carry out the plan
- Document problems, unexpected findings
- Begin data analysis

**Figure 9-1** PDSA Cycle

This approach identifies the problem based on analysis of data. Then the project team plans and implements a strategy/intervention for improvement. After implementation, results are measured and analyzed to evaluate whether outcomes were met. If so, then the strategy/intervention may be standardized in the HCO. An HCO may be implementing several CQI projects at the same time—for example, use of a new checklist to improve emergency department admissions, patient education on discharge needs for a postsurgical patient, ongoing evaluation of bar coding for medication administration, and use of hand washing in the clinic. The identification and prioritization of these projects depend on data and data analysis. Since data and outcomes change, these projects are revised or new projects are begun. Key project plan questions include the following (Sollecito & Johnson, 2013, pp. 38–39):

1. What are we trying to accomplish?
2. What changes can we predict will be an improvement?
3. How will we know when the change (strategy/intervention) is an improvement?
4. What do we expect to learn from the test run (pilot)?
5. As the data come in, what have we learned?
6. If we get positive results, how do we hold on to the gains?
7. If we get negative results, what needs to be done next?
8. When we review the experience, what can we learn about doing a better job in the future to improve our CQI processes?

A CQI project plan typically includes the following elements (and HHS, HRSA, 2011c):

1. Problem(s) identified through a variety of sources (e.g., patient and other stakeholder complaints, providers, over- or underutilization, clinical quality or safety gaps and errors, administrative problems, changes in third-party payer requirements such as monitoring of 30-day discharge readmissions, changes in standards and regulations, accreditation concerns)
2. Identification of issues with the greatest impact on the selected population based on demographics, utilization and cost of care, and so on (use of prioritization)
3. Development or selection of measures/indicators related to the problem(s) (e.g., what will be measured), including thresholds
4. Description of data needed and data source(s) per measures/indicators
5. Detailed data collection plan, including identification of data collection methods and who will collect data, training for data collectors, data recording methods, methods to describe data, and timelines
6. Identification of data collection barriers and if possible resolution before data collection
7. Description of data analysis methods
8. Ongoing evaluation of plan implementation to ensure work is done and the plan is effective in collecting and analyzing data

After an appropriate time, new data may be gathered to assess the success of the plan and may be collected at regular intervals on an ongoing basis for continuous assessment of performance. For example, patient safety culture surveys can be used to identify opportunities for improvement. When plans are made, goals should be specific, achievable, measurable, realistic, and time bound (HHS, AHRQ, 2018).

It is important to recognize that sometimes a QI project can become a research study (Gandhi, 2017). Consulting with researchers may assist QI staff in identifying potential research studies. It is not always clear how a QI project and a research study differ; however, this should be clarified before implementation of a project or a research study.

# Patient-Centered Care and CQI Planning

Patient-centered care is the core of healthcare delivery today and thus needs to be the core element in the QI program. The patient's needs and expectations are part of CQI, and services that are typically used to meet patient needs should be considered in planning. Examples include the following (HHS, HRSA, April 2011d):

- Systems that affect patient access
- Care provision that is evidence based
- Patient safety
- Support of patient engagement
- Coordination of care with other parts of the larger healthcare system
- Cultural competence, including assessing health literacy of patients, patient-centered communication, and linguistically appropriate care

## Evaluation of Planning and Plans

The QI program and its plans should be reviewed according to a schedule, which should be identified in the plans. Evaluating its own processes and plans is often a weak part of the QI program. Objective feedback should be obtained, such as data and feedback from all levels of staff. Evaluation of whether the HCO met its goals is typically done annually; however, throughout the implementation of the QI program, leaders need to be attuned to ongoing evaluation to ensure that the program is functioning effectively. An ineffective CQI process should not be allowed to continue. This will lead to flawed data and analysis, which then impacts decision making, often leading to incorrect decisions. As noted elsewhere in this text, change is difficult enough, but if not done well it will be a barrier to future effective change. Effective QI programs should also look ahead. QI programs are often able to predict trends and problems. In doing so, they can be proactive in their responses to problems.

In summary, it is important to note that the AHRQ, under its mandate to focus on healthcare quality for the nation, provides many resources for HCOs to use in QI planning, including implementation and evaluation. It recommends steps that should be taken. The AHRQ tools may be used to help HCOs develop action plans based on the analysis of an HCO's self-assessment and assessment of its culture of safety (HHS, AHRQ, 2019b). One of the AHRQ tools is a template focused on the critical elements that should be considered: goals, planned initiatives, needed resources, process and outcome measures, and timelines. The AHRQ identifies the following questions as a guide for HCOs to use as they develop their plans (HHS, AHRQ, 2017):

1. *Understand your AHRQ survey results.* It is very important for HCOs to recognize that collecting data about CQI status and analyzing data are not endpoints but rather critical first steps in planning effective CQI. The following are important questions for staff to initially consider:
   - Which areas were most and least positive?
   - How do your HCO results compare with the results from the database hospitals?

   Next, consider examining your AHRQ survey data broken down by work area/unit or staff position. (The AHRQ provides surveys for specific types of HCOs.) Questions to consider include the following:
   - Are there different areas for improvement for different HCO units (e.g., departments, services, clinical units)?
   - Are there different areas for improvement for different HCO staff?
   - Do any patterns emerge?
   - How do your HCO results for these breakouts compare with the AHRQ hospital database (or other survey setting you have selected)?

   If your HCO administered a survey more than once, compare your most recent results with your previous results to examine change over time. Consider the following:

- Did your HCO have an increase in its scores on any of the survey composites or items?
- Did your HCO have a decrease in its scores?
- When you consider the types of patient safety actions that your hospital implemented between each survey administration, do you notice improvements in those areas?

Then review your results and select two or three areas for improvement. Focusing on too many at one time is not effective.

2. *Communicate and discuss survey results.* To engage staff at all levels, it is important to share results from the survey and also identify decisions made based on the results and analysis and input on planning.

3. *Develop focused action plans.* These plans should be SMART: specific, measurable, achievable, relevant, and time bound. A typical major barrier is lack of resources, including expertise and staff (e.g., number, levels, mix).

4. *Communicate action plans and deliverables.* All aspects of the plans need to be shared with staff who need to know and may be directly involved. Leaders/managers need to assume responsibility for ensuring that this communication occurs. Roles and responsibilities need to be clear to all who are involved in implementing the plan.

5. *Implement action plans.* This is the most difficult step. Many methods are used during this step, as discussed in other chapters on measurement.

6. *Track progress and evaluate impact.* Measures/indicators are used to review progress and evaluate the change. If this review indicates that outcomes are not being met, then adaptations in the plan need to be made. Assessing HCO culture can be overdone, as change takes time. If HCOs assess outcomes too soon, they may not be able to clearly identify the outcome results. If an HCO is using one of the AHRQ assessment surveys and different staff complete the survey from an earlier use of the survey, it will be difficult to compare the survey with earlier survey results.

7. *Share what works.* Once a strategy/intervention works and outcomes are met, typically the strategy/intervention is spread to other areas of the HCO, if this applies to the specific strategy/intervention or change. Throughout the process, results must be shared with staff and other stakeholders.

### STOP AND CONSIDER 9-3

An emphasis on patient-centered care should be integrated into all CQI planning.

## Summary

This chapter provides critical information about CQI planning that a QI program might use to develop its strategic, operational, and project plans. Nurses should be involved in all of the planning and assume active roles in implementing and evaluating the CQI plans. The CQI plans provide the framework for CQI measurement, discussed in other chapters.

Exemplars of quality improvement roles and responsibilities for staff nurses, nurse managers, and APRNs are found in **Exhibit 9-1**.

---

**Exhibit 9-1** Exemplars: Quality Improvement Roles and Responsibilities

---

**Staff Nurse**

Members of the staff nurses' organization in an HCO (500-bed hospital) meet to identify key goals for the coming year. The group discusses quality improvement in detail. The group concludes that not enough staff nurses are participating in QI projects, mostly because they are not asked to do this. A recommendation is sent to the nurse manager organization and the chief nurse executive stating that staff nurses have a professional responsibility to actively engage in QI and a critical place for this to occur is in QI projects. Given this responsibility, all QI projects that are connected to patient care should include at least one staff nurse and these nurses should be given time from their regular work activities to do this work.

**Nurse Manager**

All nurse managers are required to review the HCO QI plan and discuss it annually in a nurse manager meeting with the chief nurse executive. Written feedback should then be shared with the QI program.

**Advanced Practice Registered Nurse***

An APRN in the surgical department recommends that the department conduct a QI project related to surgical site infections. The APRN then participates in the project and at the conclusion is responsible for providing training to the staff on the recommended changes in practice.

* Advanced Practice Registered Nurse (APRN) includes APRN, Clinical Nurse Specialist, Clinical Nurse Leader, and nurses with Doctorate of Nursing Practice (DNP).

# APPLY CQI

## Chapter Highlights

- QI programs need to develop strategic, operational, and project plans to provide guidance for the CQI work that needs to be done. Nurses need to be involved in all phases of planning.
- The plans need to be detailed in order to meet outcomes.

- Preparing for planning requires an understanding of the organization and its readiness to develop, implement, and evaluate plans.
- Planning and implementing the plan must be done carefully. The AHRQ provides resources to assist HCOs.

## Critical Thinking and Clinical Reasoning and Judgment: Discussion Questions and Learning Activities

1. Compare and contrast the three types of QI planning, and identify when each is used.
2. Why is organizational readiness important in planning CQI?
3. Apply the CQI planning process to a clinical problem you select.
   Review AHRQ's Creating Quality Improvement Teams and QI Plans http://www.ahrq .gov/professionals/prevention-chronic-care /improve/system/pfhandbook/mod14.html
4. Make a list of information that would be useful to your understanding of QI planning. Compare your list with IHI's Project Planning Form noted in the following subsection.

## Connect to Current Information

- Images Quality Improvement Plan Templates
  https://www.google.com/search?sa=X&sxsrf=ACYBGNT2DlQmdane5_XhWGmyIf7oKmr0LA:1580399582294&q=quality+improvement+plan+template+2018&tbm=isch&source=univ&client=firefox-b-d&ved=2ahUKEwjqsNKd16vnAhUIuaQKHWyFDRMQsAR6BAgKEAE&biw=1551&bih=913

- AHRQ: Creating Quality Improvement Teams and QI Plans
  https://www.ahrq.gov/ncepcr/tools/pf-handbook/mod14.html

- Institute for Healthcare Improvement: Project Planning Form
  http://www.ihi.org/resources/Pages/Tools/ProjectPlanningForm.aspx

### Connect to Text Current information with the Author

Go to the update for this text to review the Blog, QI News, and Literature Review. Access this regular update at: http://nursing.jbpub.com/Finkelman/QualityImprovement/2e.

## EBP, EBM, and Quality Improvement: Exemplar

U.S. Department of Health and Human Services (HHS), Agency for Healthcare Research and Quality (AHRQ). (2018). Quality improvement (QI) toolkit with templates, instructions, and examples. Retrieved from https://www.ahrq.gov/evidencenow/tools/qi-essentials-toolkit.html

This website provides several tools, templates, and examples.

### Questions to Consider:

Select one of the toolkits. Summarize why it may be useful to an HCO. Develop a rationale for using the toolkit. This may be done in a PowerPoint slide presentation or using a visual method (e.g., figure, poster).

# EVOLVING CASE STUDY

As a nurse manager for a medical unit, you have been asked to serve on a CQI project committee to develop a plan to address an increase in the number of patient falls in the four medical units in the hospital. The committee includes you, representing the nurse managers; a staff nurse and a physician from the medical units; a QI program staff member; a staff educator; and an administrator.

### Case Questions:
1. Before you begin planning, what other plans should you review? Why is this important?
2. What data should you review as part of your planning?
3. What should be in the project plan? Provide an outline.
4. Describe how you will engage staff (clinical and nonclinical) in this CQI project.

# References

Fallon, L., Begun, J., & Riley, W. (2012). *Managing health organizations for quality performance*. Burlington, MA: Jones & Bartlett Learning.

Fuji, K., Hoidal, P., Galt, K., Drincic, A., & Abbott, A. (2009). Safe patient care systems. In K. Galt & K. Pascal (Eds.), *Foundations in patient safety for health professionals* (pp. 161–180). Burlington, MA: Jones & Bartlett Learning.

Finkelman, A. (2020). *Leadership and management for nurses* (4th ed.). Upper Saddle River, NJ: Pearson Education.

Gandhi, T. (2017). 5 tips for turning QI projects into research. Retrieved from http://www.ihi.org/communities/blogs/five-tips-for-turning-qi-projects-into-research

Institute for Health Improvement (IHI). (2019). QI project charter. Retrieved from http://www.ihi.org/resources/Pages/Tools/QI-Project-Charter.aspx

Institute of Medicine (IOM). (2001). *Crossing the quality chasm*. Washington, DC: The National Academies Press.

Sollecito, K., & Johnson, J. (2013). The global evolution of continuous quality improvement: From Japanese manufacturing to global health services. In W. Sollecito & J. Johnson (Eds.), *McLaughlin and Kaluzny's continuous quality improvement in health care* (4th ed., pp. 3–47). Burlington, MA: Jones & Bartlett Learning.

U.S. Department of Health and Human Services (HHS), Agency for Healthcare Research and Quality (AHRQ). (2017). Toolkit for using the AHRQ indicators. Retrieved from https://www.ahrq.gov/patient-safety/settings/hospital/resource/qitool/index.html

U.S. Department of Health and Human Services (HHS), Agency for Healthcare Research and Quality (AHRQ). (2018). SOPS action planning tool. Retrieved from https://www.ahrq.gov/sops/resources/planning-tool/develop-plan.html

U.S. Department of Health and Human Services (HHS), Agency for Healthcare Research and Quality (AHRQ). (2019a). Surveys on patient safety culture™ (SOPS®). Retrieved from http://www.ahrq.gov/professionals/quality-patient-safety/patientsafetyculture/index.html

U.S. Department of Health and Human Services (HHS), Agency for Healthcare Research and Quality (AHRQ). (2019b). Culture of safety. Retrieved from https://psnet.ahrq.gov/primer/culture-safety

U.S. Department of Health and Human Services (HHS), Health Resources and Services Administration (HRSA). (2011a). Performance management and measurement. Retrieved from http://www.hrsa.gov/quality/toolbox/508pdfs/performancemanagementandmeasurement.pdf

U.S. Department Health and Human Services (HHS), Health Resources and Services Administration (HRSA). (2011b). Readiness assessment and developing project aims. Retrieved from https://www.hrsa.gov/sites/default/files/quality/toolbox/508pdfs/readinessassessment.pdf

U.S. Department of Health and Human Services (HHS), Health Resources and Services Administration (HRSA). (2011c). Developing and implementing a QI plan. Retrieved from https://www.hrsa.gov/sites|/default/files/quality/toolbox/508pdfs/developingqiplan.pdf

U.S. Department of Health and Human Services (HHS), Health Resources and Services Administration (HRSA). (2011d). Quality improvement. Retrieved from https://www.hrsa.gov/sites/default/files/quality/toolbox/508pdfs/qualityimprovement.pdf

# A Toolbox to Monitor, Measure, and Analyze Care Quality

## CHAPTER OBJECTIVES

At the conclusion of this chapter, the learner will be able to:

- Examine the use of measurement in continuous quality improvement.
- Critique methods used to monitor care and collect data for continuous quality improvement.
- Critique methods used to analyze care quality.
- Compare and contrast examples of national healthcare measurement programs.
- Appraise roles of nurses in continuous quality improvement measurement, including monitoring, collecting data, and analyzing quality care.

## OUTLINE

**Examples of National Healthcare Measurement Programs**
    Centers for Medicare and Medicaid Services Quality Core Measures
    Patient Safety Organizations
    Healthcare Effectiveness Data and Information Systems
    National Healthcare Quality and Disparities Reports
    AHRQ QI™
    *Healthcare Cost and Utilization Project*
**Multiple Roles of Nurses in Quality Improvement Measurement: Monitoring, Collecting Data, and Analyzing**

**Summary**
**Apply CQI**
    Chapter Highlights
    Critical Thinking and Clinical Reasoning and Judgment: Discussion Questions and Learning Activities
    Connect to Current Information
    Connect to Text Current information with the Author
    EBP, EBM, and Quality Improvement: Exemplar Evolving Case Study
**References**

## KEY TERMS

Baseline data
Benchmarking
Check sheets
Common Formats
Core measure set
Dashboards
Data
Database
Deep dive
Define, measure, analyze, design, verify (DMADV)
Disease-specific measures/indicators
Enterprise data warehouse
Failure modes and effects analysis (FMEA)
Fishbone analysis

Flowcharts
Gap analysis
Generic measures/indicators
Global trigger
Healthcare delivery measures
Incidence
Incident reports
Indicators
Measure
Metrics
Morbidity
Mortality
Outcome measure/indicator
Pareto charts
Performance measures
Population health measure
Prevalence

Primary CQI data
Process measure/indicator
Qualitative data
Quantitative data
Reliability
Report cards
Risk management
Root cause analysis (RCA)
Run charts
Secondary CQI data
Sentinel measure/indicator
Structure measure/indicator
Tally sheets
Utilization review/management
Validity
Value stream mapping

# Introduction

Continuous quality improvement (CQI) has expanded with greater emphasis on measuring, monitoring, and analyzing care quality. Each healthcare organization (HCO) selects the methods it will use and identifies them in its quality improvement (QI) program planning, as discussed in other sections of this text. This chapter discusses measurement, providing nurses with a toolbox to understand the methods and their application. For nurses to be actively engaged in CQI, they must have this information and know how to use the methods effectively. Nurses may not actually use all the methods, but they need to understand the methods and their application in order to participate in analyzing results and making changes necessary to respond to problems and improve care.

# Measurement

With the increasing emphasis on CQI since the *Quality Chasm* reports were first published in 1999, there has been expansion in the

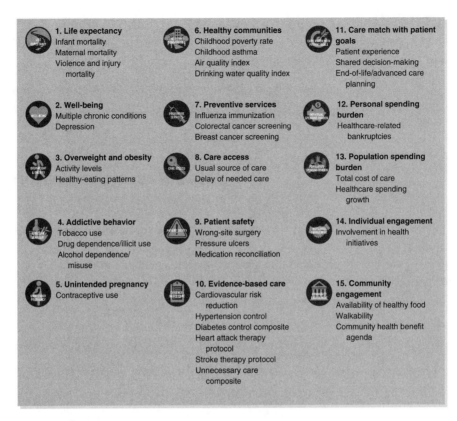

**Figure 10-1** Core Measure Set with Related Priority Measures

Reproduced from Institute of Medicine. (2015). *Vital signs: Core metrics for health and health care progress.* Washington, DC: The National Academies Press. Courtesy of the National Academies Press, Washington, DC.

development of measures; however, many of them are duplicative or similar. This expansion can get out of control and make the situation even more complicated. The report *Vital Signs: Core Measures for Health and Health Care Progress* describes a set of core measures to support measurement efficiency and effectiveness, as described in **Figure 10-1** (National Academy of Medicine [NAM], 2015). Collecting, analyzing, tracking, and storing data for multiple measure options are time-consuming and costly endeavors that have an impact on understanding performance.

## Description and Purpose

Why measure healthcare quality? Measures/indicators drive improvement by providing a structured process to collect performance data

to better understand actual practice, identify problems, and assist in best practice changes to improve. The Health Resources and Services Administration (HRSA) of the U.S. Department of Health and Human Services (HHS) describes the importance of measuring healthcare quality as follows: "Measuring a health system's inputs, processes, and outcomes is a proactive, systematic approach to practice-level decisions for patient care and the delivery systems that support it. Data management also includes ongoing measurement and monitoring. It enables an organization's CQI team to identify and implement opportunities for improvements of its current care delivery systems and to monitor progress as changes are applied. Managing data also helps a CQI team to understand how outcomes are achieved, such as[,] improved patient satisfaction with care, staff satisfaction with working in the organization, or an organization's costs and revenues associated with patient care" (HHS, HRSA, 2011a, p. 8). An important consideration today in quality improvement is the development of measures, and this has increased and in some cases has led to confusion and duplication of efforts. Trying to control these changes is important as it has an impact on CQI outcome efforts to provide reliable and valid data to best describe quality status and then to use this information for decision making to improve.

It is critical that an HCO's QI program and plans identify clear steps to be taken to ensure that the CQI activities have direction. This direction is provided by overall goals, which typically are fairly universal and often focus on the six aims: safety, timeliness, effectiveness, efficiency, equity, and patient-centeredness (STEEEP®); however, more specific direction is also required. Measures/indicators provide this direction to assist in reaching the

overarching goals, identifying topics that will be monitored to determine performance and expected outcomes. Data from monitoring are then used to identify potential quality concerns and areas that require more examination and to track changes over time (HHS, Agency for Healthcare Research and Quality [AHRQ], 2019).

## Measures and Indicators

A **measure** is a "standard used as a basis for comparison, a reference point against which other things can be evaluated" (HHS, AHRQ, 2016). **Indicators** are aggregate measures for a specific operation. **Metrics** allow HCOs to quantify some aspect of care by comparing it to a specified criterion in categories—for example, **Figure 10-2** describes a hierarchical view of quality measures, indicators, and metrics related to the major aims, STEEEP® (Sadeghi, Barzi, Mikhail, & Shabot, 2012). Comparison of data to a measure or indicator is critical to assessing quality care. Is the

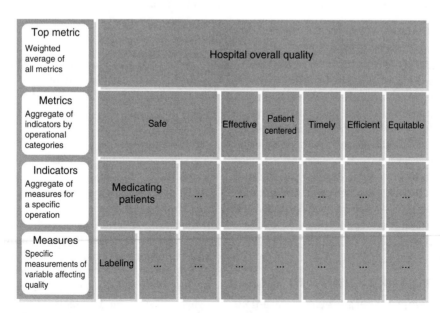

**Figure 10-2** A Hierarchical View of Quality Measures, Indicators, and Metrics

Reproduced from Sadeghi, S., Barzi, A., Mikhail, O., & Shabot, M. (2013). Integrating quality and strategy in healthcare organizations. Burlington, MA: Jones & Bartlett Learning.

result lower or higher than expected with the measure/indicator?

A measure/indicator provides a quantitative method for assessing care and has several parts: "proportions or rates, ratios, or mean values for a sample population" (Mainz, 2003, p. 524). The first part of the measure/indicator is the focus of the measurement: what will be measured—for example, it might measure performance of a procedure or a diagnosis outcome and may include specific patient identifier information, such as age, gender, diagnosis code, admission date, and provider. The numerator is the number of what is measured—for example, it may be number of admissions of patients diagnosed with pulmonary edema who experience need for rapid response team, number of patient falls while getting out of bed, or number of medication errors at time of discharge. The denominator is the population at risk—for example, it might be patients with pulmonary edema, number of patient falls regardless of cause or situation, or number of discharges. Observed rate is the numerator over denominator. A measure or indicator should identify a threshold/criterion, the preestablished level that should be achieved— for example, 100% of medical records should include information about allergies. If the result is less than the identified threshold level, then a problem is indicated.

Measures/indicators serve many purposes, one of which is to inform patients and others, such as policy makers and insurers, about quality care status. Publicly reported measures/indicators are now more accessible via the Internet. Measurement influences payment, and both public and private payers may use measures/indicators to determine payment. The overall result should be a better picture of the status of healthcare quality. Increased experience with measurement has influenced the development of government CQI initiatives, such as the hospital-acquired conditions (HACs) and 30-day unplanned readmission initiatives discussed in other chapters. As defined by the HHS, HRSA (2011b),

"**performance measures** are designed to measure systems of care. . . . Data that are defined into specific measurable elements provides an organization with a meter to measure the quality of its care" (p. 1).

Who determines what will be measured? Within HCOs, leadership and CQI staff or teams make this decision based on data and the needs of the HCO, its patients, and staff. HCOs should also use healthcare literature (evidence-based practice and evidence-based management), healthcare professional organization standards, accreditation and regulation requirements, and government resources (local, state, and federal). As NAM describes, however, current health measurement practices continue to need improvement: "A case can be made that, while the health measurement landscape today consists of a great many high-quality measures, meaningful at some level for their intended purpose, the effectiveness of the health measurement enterprise as a whole is limited by a lack of organizing focus, interrelationship, and parsimony in the service of truly meaningful accountability and assessment for the health system" (NAM, 2015, p. S-5).

Selecting what should be measured is a critical measurement step in the CQI process. Data should not be collected just to demonstrate that data are collected. There are general guides for what should be measured, and then each HCO must customize its QI program to meet its own CQI needs. Some of the guides include HAC incidence, 30-day unplanned readmission rate, STEEEP® or the six major CQI aims, Centers for Medicare and Medicaid Services (CMS) requirements and measures/indicators, and the National Quality Strategy (NQS). Quality measures/indicators relate to healthcare delivery concerns about accessibility, appropriateness, continuity, effectiveness, efficacy, efficiency, timeliness, patient perspectives, and safety. HCOs monitor clinical outcomes, such as mortality rates, complications, adverse events, patient/family satisfaction, and outcomes that relate to the HCO structure and functions, such as staffing levels, staff retention, reasons for staff turnover, budget goals, and staff satisfaction (Gottlieb, 2006).

Should HCOs continue focusing on broad-stroke measurement or blunt measures, such as measuring adverse events (Shojania, 2015)? After an HCO identifies its specific problems, it should focus more on them. To determine long-term effectiveness, the HCO should apply follow-up measurement to changes that have been made. For example, if the HCO changes its bar-coding procedure, then evaluating the new procedure should be the focus, not overall medication adverse events. This is a more efficient and effective approach for a QI program. As HCOs make plans for measuring CQI and identifying or developing their measures/indicators, they should consider questions such as the following (Casey, 2006):

1. What are the goals in attempting to measure outcomes? In other words, why bother?
2. What sort of outcomes management (OM) expertise is available to assist with the measurement of outcomes? OM is not for the amateur and requires specific prerequisite skills, knowledge, and experience.
3. What resources, especially computer software and hardware, are necessary and available to support the process of OM?
4. What are the costs and benefits of measuring outcomes?
5. Can other published or unpublished experiences be identified, consulted, and utilized that will assist in short-cutting the process of developing and measuring outcomes without sacrificing scientific accuracy? This effort includes identifying information that can be used in conjunction with or instead of information that might be generated by an expensive process.
6. What is the process for interpretation and identification of limitations of the OM that are generated? (p. 94)

The Joint Commission accreditation focuses on accountability measures, which are measures of evidence-based care closely linked to positive patient outcomes. The Joint Commission uses the following criteria to identify accountability measures (The Joint Commission, 2019):

1. *Research.* There should be strong evidence demonstrating that the evidence-based process improves health outcomes.
2. *Proximity.* Performing the process is closely connected to the patient outcomes, with few clinical processes occurring after the one that is measured before improved outcome occurs.
3. *Accuracy.* The measure accurately assesses whether the care process has actually been provided.
4. *No adverse effects.* Implementing the measure has little or no chance of inducing unintended adverse consequences.

The AHRQ Quality Indicators Toolkit also describes criteria that HCOs should consider in selecting measures, remembering that not everything can or should be measured (HHS, AHRQ, 2014):

- Processes, utilization, and outcomes measures
- Importance of the factor being measured—should focus on most important outcomes met for new processes implemented
- Ability to interpret and act on findings
- Feasibility of measurement—most efficient data collection is from existing automated information systems
- Identifiable and measureable denominators

This type of criteria system may be used in conjunction with the criteria used by The Joint Commission mentioned earlier. The critical point is that each QI program should approach selection of measures/indicators in a systematic manner and apply clear criteria.

Ideally, measures/indicators should be based on best evidence, and their validity and reliability are important so that results can be used to effectively improve care. Mainz (2003) describes these concepts as follows: "**Validity** is the degree to which the measure/indicator measures what it is intended to measure. . . . **Reliability** is the extent to which repeated measurements of a stable phenomenon by different data collectors, judges, or instruments, at different times and places, get similar results. Reliability is important when using a measure/indicator to make comparisons among groups or within groups over time. A valid measure/indicator must be reproducible and consistent" (p. 103). **Table 10-1** describes some attributes used to evaluate measures.

**Table 10-1** Attributes Used to Evaluate Measures

| Attribute | Definition |
|---|---|
| **1. Importance of topic area addressed by the measure** | |
|   **A.** High priority for maximizing health of population | For example, measure focuses on medical condition as defined by high prevalence, incidence, mortality, morbidity, or disability. |
|   **B.** Financially important | Measure focuses on clinical conditions or area of healthcare that requires high expenditures on inpatient or outpatient care; a condition is financially important if it has either high per-person costs or if it affects a large number of people. |
|   **C.** Demonstrated variation in care and/or potential for improvement | Measure focuses on an aspect of healthcare for which there is a reasonable expectation of wide variation in care and/or the potential for improvement; if the measure is used for internal QI and professional accountability, then wide variation in care across physicians is not necessary. |
| **2. Usefulness in improving patient outcomes** | |
|   **A.** Based on established clinical recommendation | Evidence indicates that process improves health outcomes; there are processes or actions that providers can take to improve the outcome. |
|   **B.** Potentially actionable by the user | The measure addresses an area of healthcare that potentially is under the control of the physician, other healthcare provider, HCO, or healthcare system that it assesses. |
|   **C.** Meaningful and interpretable to the user | The results of the measure are reportable in a manner that is interpretable and meaningful to the intended use—for example, results need to be of use to improve care, help make administrative decisions, compare health systems, and so on. |
| **3. Measure design** | |
|   **A.** Well-defined specifications | The following need to be well defined: numerator, denominator, sampling methodology, data sources, allowable values, methods of measurement, and method of reporting. |
|   **B.** Documented reliability | The measure will produce the same results when repeated in the same population and setting; use of test of reliability; inter-rater; and internal consistency. |
|   **C.** Documented validity | The measure has face validity—that is, it should appear to a knowledgeable observer to measure what is intended. The measure should also correlate well with other measures or the same measures. |

Modified from Casey, D. (2006). Fundamentals of outcomes measurement. In D. Nash & N. Goldfarb (Eds.), *The quality solution* (pp. 93–113). Sudbury, MA: Jones & Bartlett Publishers.

There are several different types of measures/indicators. A common approach is to use the three quality elements described by Donabedian (1980): structure (how work is organized), process (how work is done), and outcomes (results of work). The following are examples of the application of these elements of quality to measures/indicators (Mainz, 2003; National Quality Forum [NQF], 2019):

- **Structure measures/indicators.** Examples are access to specialists, clinical guidelines based on evidence-based practice, staffing level met as required per standard, access to procedure (specify) in timely manner (specify), and amount of admission wait time from emergency department to inpatient.

- **Process measures/indicators.** Examples are proportion of patients with infection who receive appropriate antibiotic, nurse assessment of newly admitted patients within half an hour of admission, rate and type of specific medication errors, and rapid response team called per guidelines when patient's blood pressure rapidly changes.

- **Outcomes measures/indicators.** Examples are blood pressure maintained per guidelines, blood sugar maintained per guidelines, mortality, morbidity, quality of life, patient satisfaction, and patient functional status. Multiple factors may impact outcomes, and these must be considered, particularly when comparing with other HCOs—for example, smoking and weight have an impact on health outcome, so if groups of patients where these factors vary are compared, then comparing outcomes is not really possible unless this factor is included in the sample.

Combining these measures/indicators provides a clearer picture of the status of healthcare quality and the organization.

Other types of measures/indicators are commonly used by HCOs. The **sentinel measure/indicator** "identifies individual events or phenomena that are intrinsically undesirable, and always trigger further analysis and investigation" (Mainz, 2003). The Joint Commission requires all its accredited HCOs to address all sentinel events. Examples would be the number of patients who die during labor or the number of suicides in the hospital. For this type of measure/indicator, the threshold is zero, as no sentinel event is acceptable. **Generic measures/indicators** are relevant to most patients—for example, the proportion of physicians to a population. **Disease-specific measures/indicators** focus on a disease and apply to patients with that disease—for example, the number of patients with lung cancer who have surgery or the number of patients receiving chemotherapy who require support for extreme nausea and loss of weight.

An example of a national program that includes indicators used by many hospitals is the Inpatient Quality Indicators, which includes 28 provider-level indicators established by the AHRQ and applied to hospital inpatient discharge data. These indicators provide aggregate data from multiple acute care hospitals and are grouped into the following four categories (HHS, AHRQ, 2016):

- *Volume indicators* are proxy, or indirect, measures of quality based on counts of admissions during which certain intensive, high technology, or highly complex procedures were performed. They are based on evidence suggesting that hospitals performing more of these procedures may have better outcomes.

- *Mortality indicators for inpatient procedures* include procedures for which mortality has been shown to vary across institutions and for which there is evidence that high mortality may be associated with poorer quality of care.

- *Mortality indicators for inpatient conditions* include conditions for which mortality has been shown to vary substantially across institutions and for which evidence suggests that high mortality may be associated with deficiencies in the quality of care.

- *Utilization indicators* examine procedures whose use varies significantly across hospitals and for which questions have been raised about overuse, underuse, or misuse.

CQI must focus on the goals of improved health status, care, quality, affordability, and public engagement; however, nationally there are differences in the domains of influence on health and healthcare, including disparities by race, ethnicity, income, education, gender, geography, and urban or rural populations (NAM, 2015). HCOs and organizations have developed and use many individual measures/indicators, many of which are very specific to HCO needs and may not provide broader data about CQI. The growth in measures/indicators is positive, but it has negative aspects as it has resulted in "a measurement system that lacks standardization for the assessment and reporting of data on commonly assessed health concepts" (NAM, 2015, p. S-5).

In 2012, the HHS decided that it was time to address the concern of expanding measurement and need for greater control. To address this concern, the HHS focused on clarifying criteria for measures, determining a strategic implementation plan that provides greater coordination, and developing measurement policy and management. This effort needed to be based on the three aims of better care, healthy people/healthy communities, and affordable care. This initiative was related to the development of the NQS, which is discussed in other chapters in more detail. Core measure sets have now been developed; however, these measures do not cover all areas of CQI. A **core measure set**, as defined by the NAM (2015), is a "set of measures that provide a quantitative indication of current status on the most important elements in a given field, and that can be used as a standardized and accurate tool for informing, comparing, focusing, monitoring, and reporting change, reducing reporting burden while improving impacts" (pp. S-8–S-9).

## Data

Healthcare is producing a large amount of **data**, which are "discrete entities described objectively without interpretation" (Finkelman, 2019, p. 430). The purpose of using data is to help identify potential quality concerns and describe problems, gaps, trends, patterns, and so on. **Primary CQI data** are found in original sources—information collected for the purpose of CQI. Examples are using observation to determine if the staff responds to patient call lights when needed and collecting information about medication errors. **Secondary CQI data** are found in secondhand sources, and in the case of CQI, these sources are often sources that are primarily used in care delivery, such as the electronic medical record/electronic health record (EMR/EHR) or a preoperative checklist. The data are collected routinely for other purposes and then may also be used for CQI data collection, although this was not the original intent of the documentation.

The medical record is a rich source of data for multiple measures/indicators. Many HCOs now use electronic records, making data collection easier and more accurate; quicker; and less costly, as such data collection takes less staff time. Electronic records also make the data accessible in real time. Hard copy records are often illegible, incomplete, and less accessible over time. Administrative data are also used, and most administrative records provide some secondary data for CQI purposes—for example, tracking utilization data about admissions and discharges is important for HCO financial and planning purposes, but the data can also be used in conjunction with CQI needs. Pharmacy records also provide valuable CQI data, although most of the data are not collected for the primary purpose of CQI.

Data are classified as quantitative or qualitative: (1) **Quantitative data** focus on numbers and frequencies so that measurable data can be obtained and statistics used to analyze the data—for example, calculating the average of a specific laboratory value, frequencies of read-missions, and percentages of patients who meet health screening standards. (2) **Qualitative data** provide information about descriptive characteristics, used to make inferences based observable data, not measurable data. **Baseline data** are collected prior to a change or an improvement. The data are then used to compare against data collected after a change is implemented to determine if outcomes were met (HHS, HRSA, 2010). HCOs and CQI initiatives use all of these types of data in their data collection efforts. With any data collection, it is important to be concerned about the quality of the data. Is it accurate, clear, and concise? Is information missing? Is the information accessible? Can it be accessed in a timely manner? As mentioned in this chapter, validity and reliability are important in evaluating the quality of CQI data and results.

## Databases

Due to the increase in data and complex, multidimensional data, there is a need for nurses to work with informatics specialists to provide methods for changing the data into formats that can lead to actionable information—particularly to improve outcomes (Nelson-Brantley, Jenkins, Chipps, 2019). Nurses also need to be trained for positions in informatics to actively engage in these processes and ensure that nursing perspectives are included. A **database** is a method used to organize data so that information is easy to store, manage, and access. Given the large amount of data used in QI programs, databases are critical, storing large amounts of data, typically computerized, and providing easier access to the data for analysis and for CQI decision making. The federal government has a number of healthcare databases used by the government, HCOs, healthcare providers, healthcare professional organizations, insurers, and accreditors. An example is the Healthcare Cost and Utilization Project (HCUP). Databases also are provided by nongovernment sources, such as the National Database of Nursing Quality

Indicators (NDNQI) (HHS, AHRQ, HCUP, 2019; Press Ganey, 2019). An **enterprise data warehouse** provides a collection of databases that can then be accessed and analyzed. This makes it easier to search for different data from multiple databases to gain access to more data and use data more effectively (HHS, AHRQ, Patient Safety Network [PSNet], 2019a). HCOs and healthcare professionals are inundated with data today. Methods that help to organize the data are critical to effective use of data in a QI program. The Connect to Current Information section at the end of this chapter provides links to sites with examples of healthcare databases.

Along with the development of the Network of Patient Safety Databases (NPSD), the AHRQ has developed **Common Formats**, which constitute a set of definitions and reporting formats that offer cross-HCO consistency when reporting data external to the HCO, such as to the AHRQ, and also may be used to compare HCOs. The NPSD was developed with input from multiple stakeholders, including the National Quality Forum (NQF) and the Food and Drug Administration (FDA). A common concern about reporting CQI data is consistency, particularly using the same terms with the same meanings when data are collected. Using common terms avoids comparing "apples to oranges." For a long time, the United States did not have a national system that provided CQI data and guidance, but now there are major efforts to develop and maintain an effective CQI system that considers the issue of consistency and the CQI reporting process. According to the AHRQ and its CQI initiative, three situations should be reported (HHS, AHRQ, PSO, 2019a):

- *Incidents* are patient safety events that reached the patient, whether there was harm or not.
- *Near misses or close calls* are patient safety events that did not reach the patient; they may be precursors to adverse events.
- *Unsafe conditions* are circumstances that increase the probability of a patient safety event.

The Common Formats "focus on generic common formats or all patient safety events and on event-specific common formats or frequently occurring and/or serious types of patient safety events, and the list expands as needed" (HHS, AHRQ, PSO, 2019b). Currently, the settings for application of the Common Formats are acute care and skilled nursing facilities; however, the plan is to expand into other healthcare settings. Types of information collected are circumstances of the event, patient information, and reporting, reporter, and report information. **Table 10-2** describes information the AHRQ recommends HCOs report for generic and event-specific events.

## Prevalence and Incidence

Prevalence and incidence rates are used in CQI. **Prevalence** is the rate of the number of cases at a given time divided by the number in the at-risk population. This rate provides a close-up of a particular concern. For CQI purposes, the goal is to understand how common something is, and then if an improvement intervention is implemented, it is possible to determine if there was a change in prevalence. **Incidence** is an

---

**Table 10-2** Information Required for Common Formats: Generic and Event-Specific Events

**Generic Common Formats**

### Type of Event

1. Class of patient safety concern being reported
   a. Incident
      i. Harm
      ii. No harm
   b. Near miss (close call)
   c. Unsafe condition
2. Category of patient safety concern

### Circumstances of Event

1. Date and time that the event was discovered
2. Where the event occurred or unsafe condition exists
3. Factors contributing to the event, known at the time of the initial report
4. Association of the event with a handover (handoff)
5. Preventability of the event, as noted at the time of the initial report
6. Reason the near miss did not reach the patient
7. Narrative descriptions (for facility and PSO use)
   a. Narrative by the initial reporter
   b. Summary comments by the patient safety manager

### Patient Information

1. Identifying information about the patient affected
2. Degree of harm—AHRQ's Harm Scale—including when the harm was assessed
3. Rescue—interventions made within 24 hours after discovery of an incident to reduce or halt the progression of harm to the patient
4. Increased length of stay attributed to an adverse outcome (hospital setting only)
5. Notification of the patient, patient's family, or guardian

### Reporting, Reporter, and Report Information

1. Unique identifier assigned to the event/condition
2. Report date
3. Reporter information

*(continues)*

**Table 10-2** Information Required for Common Formats: Generic and Event-Specific Events *(continued)*

**Event-Specific Common Formats**

**Definition of the Event**

1. Brief narration of the name of the event category, with specifications of the event.
2. Processes of care—delineation of process error(s) that caused/are the (defined) event; these can include near misses.
3. Patient outcomes—delineation of outcomes that are associated with/are the (defined) event; includes no-harm events; by definition, unsafe conditions do not result in patient outcomes.

**Scope of Reporting**

Separate Common Formats are developed for each overall type of setting, such as a hospital or skilled nursing facility. Furthermore, scope delineates the applicability of specific event descriptions to incidents, near misses, and unsafe conditions. For example, the description for *fall events* pertains to incidents only (not near misses or unsafe conditions), whereas the description for *medication and other substance events* pertains to incidents, near misses, and unsafe conditions.

**Risk Assessments and Preventive Actions**

Event-specific Common Formats list assessments, preventive actions, or other measures that should have been performed or established prior to the event to prevent or mitigate its occurrence. This includes the precise circumstances in which such actions should have been taken. The event-specific Common Formats do not include routine protocols that apply to all patients, such as the universal protocol (used in the operating room).

*Note:* If precise specification is not possible, such actions cannot be delineated in an event-specific Common Format; this type of information/opinion can be entered into a narrative field to assist in the analysis of any individual event.

**Circumstances of the Event**

1. Identifying or descriptive information pertaining to the category of patient safety concern (e.g., product name, drug name, ICD-9/ICD-10).
2. Risk factors specific to the event. Risk factors increase the probability of an event and are known in advance of its occurrence.
3. Contributing factors specific to the event. Contributing factors are determined only retrospectively, after the event has occurred. These factors are different from those that could apply to any event and that are found in the generic event descriptions.

To access the most current versions of the Common Formats, go to Connect to Current Information section at the end of this chapter. There, you will find the full list of event-specific formats for both acute care hospital settings and skilled nursing facility settings. Future versions of the Common Formats will be developed for ambulatory settings to include ambulatory surgery centers and physicians' and practitioners' offices.

**Common Formats for Surveillance—Hospital**

Most recently, AHRQ and the interagency Federal Patient Safety Workgroup released *Common Formats for Surveillance—Hospital*. Until now, Common Formats have been designed to support only traditional event reporting. *Common Formats for Surveillance—Hospital* are designed to provide, through retrospective review of medical records, information that is complementary to that derived from event reporting systems. These formats will facilitate improved detection of events and calculation of adverse event rates in populations reviewed. To view the Federal Register notice announcing *Common Formats for Surveillance—Hospital*, go to http://www.gpo.gov/fdsys/pkg/FR-2014-02-18/html/2014-03492.htm.

"estimate of how frequently new events, cases, etc., develop" (Strome, 2013, p. 13). These methods help HCOs identify occurrence patterns. To ensure arriving at an incident rate that provides a clear picture, the population at risk should be described as concisely as possible. This can be useful in CQI, but it should not be the only approach taken. There are many CQI reports, both from individual HCOs and from state and national sources. What is more critical is not how data are presented in the reports but whether the report is useful, accurate, timely, relevant to the question(s) asked, directed toward the best stakeholders, analyzed appropriately based on types of data and questions, and visualized in a way that is helpful (Keroack & Rhinehart, 2013).

---

**STOP AND CONSIDER 10-1**

CQI measurement must be individualized for each HCO.

---

# Monitoring Care Quality

There is a lot of information and discussion about errors, mostly with the focus on what happens after they occur—a retrospective review; however, more must be done to prospectively identify safety hazards. More methods to detect these hazards are needed. Transparency, public reporting, and benchmarking are now important aspects of healthcare delivery. Measurement systems are needed that are effective and meet the multiple needs of individual departments, HCOs, agencies, and programs; individual healthcare professions; accreditors; insurers; and government regulations and standards.

## Data Collection to Improve Care

In an HCO's QI program and its plans (strategic, operational, and project levels), a critical part of the work is to clearly identify measures/indicators, but the QI program must identify the data that are needed to assess the measures/indicators in a clear data collection plan. This task requires careful consideration of the data that are currently available, such as from secondary sources, and the need to develop new effective data collection methods. The CQI team and staff should avoid repetitive work, such as collecting data that are already available, and also should avoid collecting data that are not needed. An effective data collection plan must do the following for each measure/indicator (HHS, HRSA, 2011a, 2011b):

- Identify the measure/indicator.
- Describe the denominator in detail with inclusions and exclusions; this needs to clarify whom or what will be included in the sample/population.
- Identify the data source for the denominator and include any specific queries to be run or report parameters that must be entered in the digital system.
- Describe the numerator in detail with inclusions and exclusions (e.g., "Documentation in the medical record must note the date on which the laboratory test was performed and the results, or the record notates the date and results of a test ordered by another provider.").
- Use randomized sampling when possible. Randomized sampling is the most recommended method for performance improvement because it ensures every patient or selected event has an equal chance of inclusion in the sample without bias.
- Identify data sources for the numerator and include specific computer queries to be run, manual steps, or specific sampling parameters.
- Identify who collects each data element and calculates the measure.
- Describe the calendar for measure-performance reporting.
- Describe data collection procedures, timelines, and any required data collection training.

An important attribute of the AHRQ Quality Indicator Toolkit is that there is more than one way to develop a system of monitoring sustainability of performance. There are, however, some critical elements of effective monitoring that HCOs must consider in their CQI planning. According to the HHS (HHS, AHRQ, 2016), the HCO should choose a limited set of effective measures, establish a schedule for regular reporting, develop report formats for acting on problems identified, and assess sustainability on a periodic basis.

Human factors, as noted in other parts of this text, impact our understanding of risks and harms in healthcare delivery. In cultures of safety where the staff are recognized for their contributions, they can add important information to this understanding of care processes and the use of policies and procedures, thereby expanding the CQI prospective. This contribution, however, requires that management listen to staff and staff feel they can make comments without retribution. An effective CQI environment is one in which staff do not feel they must wait to be asked for feedback.

Data collection is typically retrospective, prospective, or a combination. There are no universally effective prospective and retrospective methods for detecting errors and safety hazards. Retrospective, the most common approach, reviews safety hazards typically focused on two types of methods (HHS, AHRQ, PSNet, 2019a):

- Screening large data sets for preventable adverse event evidence for further examination
- Screening and analyzing adverse events or strongly suspected adverse events, including use of trigger tools; screening administrative data sets; and using more in-depth methods such as root cause analysis and mortality reviews

Many methods are used for screening these data sets for evidence of adverse events. One of these methods is the AHRQ Patient Safety Indicators (PSIs). These screening measures/indicators identify potential problems within an HCO that require more analysis and should not be used to compare data from one HCO to another nor are they useful in estimating the overall incidence of adverse events—for example, if a hospital notes an increased incidence of postoperative sepsis PSI, then the specific HCO may have a systematic problem with failure to rescue (FTR) in postoperative patients with problems, but making a definitive determination of cause or intervention requires more examination (HHS, AHRQ, PSNet, 2019a).

Consideration of national CQI data and data collection methods notes that the first source of data is often the medical record. This source offers considerable data, but there are also barriers to obtaining accurate and relevant data from this source (Rosen, 2010). Collecting data is costly and labor intensive. Before the development of the electronic medical record/electronic health record (EMR/HER), it was even more difficult to get data from hard copies of records, although both types of documentation have potential problems. It is not legitimate to say that electronic methods are perfect—they are not. They present numerous problems, such as variation, inaccuracies, and missing information, but they are better than hard copy format. Electronic methods and use of technology are discussed further in other chapters.

This text discusses transfers or handoffs, situations that make it difficult to effectively maintain and share data. When patients move within a system or between systems, we do not always get the information we need in documentation that might be retrievable for CQI purposes and may not be accurate or timely. Once the data are collected, they must be put into some type of database so that the data can be analyzed, and sometimes this process also affects the quality of the data.

## Methods Used in Data Collection

HCOs and other organizations involved in CQI use a number of methods to collect data, which are discussed here. Staff may be involved in data collection, but even if not directly involved, they need to understand these methods in order to provide feedback and consider how the results impact their work.

### Check/Tally Sheets

**Check sheets** or **tally sheets** provide a simple way to collect data and document data. It is not difficult to develop a data collection check/tally sheet focused on a particular event. An example might be a check/tally sheet used to document data on observations of meeting hand-washing requirements. Check/tally sheets should be clear and easy to use. After data are collected, another method must be used to aggregate the data. The Connect to Current Information section at the end of this chapter provides a link to a site with examples of check/tally sheets.

### Questionnaires/Surveys

Questionnaires/surveys may be used by HCOs to collect data. It also takes time to develop effective surveys and then to analyze the data, although electronic methods have made this method easier to use. It also requires staff time and cooperation to complete the surveys. One needs to keep in mind data analysis—for example, data from narrative responses take much more time to summarize and analyze, and it may be difficult to be objective in this process compared to obtaining simple answers or numerical data. The HCO also must identify who should respond to the questionnaire and ensure that this is clearly communicated—for example, if the problem is the need to improve intensive care unit documentation, then data from staff who work in dietary services may not be relevant, but data from the nutritionist who works with intensive care unit patients might be important. Also, questionnaires/surveys are often used with patients, such as patient satisfaction surveys. These methods are discussed in greater detail elsewhere in this text.

### Interviews

Interviews may be used to learn more about care and how to improve care. Interviews may focus on individuals or may be done in a group, such as a focus group. Questions may be highly structured, using specific questions and no variation; structured questions may be used, adding more questions during the interview based on responses; or questions may be open ended, with the interviewer introducing the topic and then asking group members to share their thoughts. The interviewer needs to use a clear method for recording the responses so that data can then easily be used—for example, the interviewer might use a form listing the questions, then record the responses on the form. When using this method, it can be time consuming to collect, aggregate, and analyze the data.

### Observation

Observation is used to collect data, although it is a time-consuming method and thus can be costly. Observer subjectivity may be a potential barrier to obtaining objective data, although observer training and using consistent data-collection documentation methods reduces subjectivity. Management uses observation routinely to determine performance and identify situations that require immediate response as well as long-term concerns. When changes are made to improve care, observation might be used—for example, are staff members using the hand-washing procedure when required? Is the new staff call system effective? Is a change in a treatment or procedure improving outcomes?

## Examples of Methods Used to Describe Data

Before data collection is begun, it is important to determine how data will be described. What format or method best provides a visual of the data so that the data can be analyzed, understood, and applied? Since data serve a variety of purposes, understanding the purpose of the data collection is important so that the most effective data collection is used. The following are common methods (Kelly, Johnson, & Sollecito, 2013):

- *Flowcharts* enable reviewing or updating of information and help keep it current.
- *Cause and effect diagrams* stratify and examine causes.
- *Pareto diagrams/charts* stratify causes and demonstrate change.
- *Histograms (frequency distribution)* are used in presentations to provide a visual of data, assess patterns, and enable monitoring.
- *Run charts* relate data to changes and examine the relationship of improvement to change(s).
- *Control charts* relate data to changes and help determine if a process is or remains under control.
- *Regression analysis* helps assess strength of association and test hypotheses. (p. 93)

The Connect to Current Information section at the end of this chapter identifies links that provide visuals of some of the methods. Viewing these examples will help to better understand the methods and how they might be applied in a QI program.

## Run Charts

**Run charts** display data to illustrate or plot change and patterns over time. They assist in identifying problems and when they occurred. Other terms used for these charts are line graphs, trend charts, and time-series charts.

## Pareto Charts

**Pareto charts** are vertical bar graphs with bars ordered from the longest to the shortest. They are based on the Pareto principle that 80% of the output in a situation is due to 20% of the input. The chart prioritizes frequency of causes related to one another (Kelly et al., 2013).

## Flowcharts

**Flowcharts** are useful tools to gain a better understanding of a process and variations in the process. These charts may be used to display information prospectively—for example to describe an approach to a process such as a description of a unit's admission process. During the root cause analysis process, flowcharts may be used retrospectively to visualize steps that were taken in a specific process, such as a procedure for a specific patient; identify possible and potential causes of problems; examine handoffs; identify staff, teams, and departments that were involved in the process; and provide a view of current practice and consideration for improvement. Staff that understand the process are more effective in developing a flowchart, and typically this means an interprofessional team. The following questions might be considered when developing a flowchart (Kelly et al., 2013):

1. How effective is the process in meeting customer (patient) requirements?
2. Are there performance gaps or perceived opportunities for improvement?
3. Have the relevant stages of the process been represented? If not, what must be done to gather feedback and ideas?
4. What inputs are required for the process, and where do they come from? Are the inputs constraining the process or not? Which ones?
5. Are there equipment or regulatory constraints forcing this approach?
6. Is this the right problem process to be working on or to continue working on? (p. 97)

## Dashboards

**Dashboards** provide a clear visualization of data in one view: a compilation of run charts or a summary. Managers need quick information on CQI status, and dashboards can be used to communicate current status, sharing results with staff and offering a view of the performance of each measure over time.

# Examples of Monitoring Methods

In developing its QI plans, an HCO must decide not only what, specifically, it will monitor but also how it will consistently monitor performance in general to identify gaps or problems and key measures/indicators. Some monitoring methods may be determined by external sources, such as accreditors, third-party payers, and both state and federal government agencies (e.g., the CMS). Many potential methods could be used, including the examples found in **Table 10-3**.

## Benchmarking and Report Cards

**Benchmarking** refers to comparison—for example, consumers might compare hospital ratings, or an HCO might collect data prior to instituting an improvement change and then compare results after the change, with the initial data serving as the benchmark (NAM, 2015). Using benchmarking to compare data

**Table 10-3** Strategies for Measuring Patient Safety

| Measurement Strategies | Advantages | Disadvantages |
|---|---|---|
| **Retrospective chart review** (by itself or after use of a trigger tool) | Considered the "gold standard," contains rich detailed clinical information | Costly, labor intensive, data quality variable due to incomplete clinical information, retrospective review only |
| **Voluntary error reporting systems** | Useful for internal QI and case finding, highlights adverse events that providers perceive as important | Capture small fraction of adverse events that occur, retrospective review only based on provider self-reports, no standardization or uniformity of adverse events reported |
| **Automated surveillance** | Can be used retrospectively or prospectively, helpful in screening patients who may be at high risk for adverse events using standardized protocols | Need electronic data to run automated surveillance, high proportion of "triggered" cases are false positives |
| **Administrative/claims data** | Low cost, readily available data, useful for tracking events over time across large populations, can identify "potential" adverse events | Lack detailed clinical data, concerns over variability and inaccuracy of ICD-9-CM codes and ICD-10 codes across and within systems, may detect high proportion of false positives and false negatives |
| **Patient reports** | Can capture errors not easily recognized by other methods (e.g., errors related to communication between providers) | Measurement tools are still in development |

may act as an incentive to stimulate HCOs and individual healthcare providers to improve and also provides positive feedback and recognition of improvement. The process also helps to identify variations and gaps in care. In addition, measurement is a method used to determine if HCOs and individual healthcare providers are compliant with standards and regulations (NAM, 2015). It is important to evaluate the CQI process, and part of this is comparing performance with other similar providers. **Report cards** are summary reports of status, and in the case of CQI, they are reports on quality care status. Individual HCOs also must monitor their own CQI and may use a report card format for this purpose. Common data found in these reports are about admissions and discharges, diagnoses, procedures/treatments, patient satisfaction, staffing, patient outcomes, and more. Report cards are often published—for example, on the Internet—so that consumers and others can compare HCOs.

Do these rating systems offer clear, accurate, and helpful information? In a study that compared four major rating systems, it was found that none of the rated hospitals were rated as high performers by all four rating systems. Only 10% of the 844 hospitals rated as a high performer by one system were rated the same by one of the other three systems (Austin et al., 2015). This result is most likely due to differences in HCO methods, focus, measures of performance, and differences in measuring systems. Definitions of terminology may also differ, and this can have a major impact on data collected. For the consumer, this study result means there might not be clear and accurate views of an HCO for comparison, and when consumers search for this information, typically online, most consumers do not realize the ratings may not be all that valid and reliable. To decrease these problems, there is need for more consistency in the rating scales that are used, such as using the same definitions for patient safety. The goal should be greater transparency with effective information so that consumers can make more informed choices.

Some noted QI experts have questioned the direction CQI measurement is taking (Wachter, 2016). Dr. Wachter published his concerns in the *New York Times*, noting that there is now an overemphasis on targets, yardsticks, metrics, and outcomes. Such measures seek to determine whether something was or was not done, but often to the exclusion of important and clear CQI insights. There are many report cards for rating hospitals, and over 1,600 hospitals claim to be in the "top 100." This has led to questions about the value of HCO ratings and measurements. The EMR/EHR has had both a positive and a negative impact on healthcare and quality improvement—for example, in tracking physician computer use, physicians clicked the mouse 4,000 times in a 10-hour shift (Wachter, 2016). While all this clicking shows staff engagement in documentation and technology interfacing, it says very little about the quality of care they are providing. Understanding the sometimes arbitrary or misleading nature of poorly selected or applied CQI measurement methods, The Joint Commission is no longer reporting hospital ratings, and the CMS is reducing some of its measurement and reporting initiatives related to the electronic medical record/electronic health record (EMR/HER) (CMS Blog, 2016). Wachter (2016) expresses his concern for the state of CQI measurement as follows: "Measurement cannot go away, but it needs to be scaled back and allowed to mature. We need more targeted measures, ones that have been vetted to ensure that they really matter" (p. 5).

We moved into measurement and did not fully understand that it may have both positive and negative impacts on healthcare providers. Throughout the discussion on CQI in this text, it is important not to make the CQI process the sole focus or goal. The goal is always to focus on the patient, high-quality patient care, and effective performance that make a difference in outcomes. Each healthcare provider can do this daily in practice.

## Mandatory Versus Voluntary Reporting

The *Quality Chasm* reports recommend mandatory reporting, but how do major healthcare delivery organizations, organizations that focus on healthcare delivery, healthcare profession organizations, and government agencies view this recommendation? The American Hospital Association (AHA) is a major organization for hospitals. It is very involved in supporting CQI and reducing errors. It collaborates with the Institute for Safe Medication Practices (ISMP) to identify needs and develop solutions that will help HCOs reduce errors. The recommendation to provide legal protections for those who report errors is supported by the AHA; however, it is not in full agreement with some of the recommendations for reporting. The AHA supports voluntary rather than required reporting of errors, believing this approach best encourages staff reporting (Regenstein, 2013). The AHA does not believe that the AHRQ should be the reporting agency but rather it recommends that medication errors be reported to the ISMP and that errors related to devices should be reported to the FDA. This demonstrates how complex CQI is, involving multiple stakeholders who do not always agree. **Figure 10-3** describes the National Coordinating Council for Medication Error Reporting and Prevention (NCCMERP) Index for categorizing medication errors. This categorization of errors, which is important in reporting errors, represents a coordinated effort between nongovernmental and

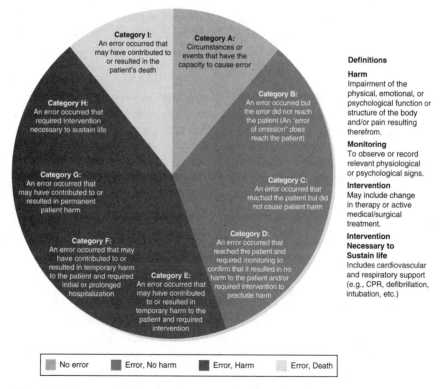

**Figure 10-3** National Coordinating Council for Medication Error Reporting and Prevention Index for Categorizing Medication Errors

government organizations and demonstrates the complexity of reporting errors.

The Joint Commission incorporates CQI in its accreditation process (Regenstein, 2013). It has not made a clear statement for or against mandatory or voluntary reporting of errors, although it does support the need for legal protections for those who report errors. However, it does require all of its accredited HCOs to report sentinel events, as discussed in this text. The Joint Commission has a major impact on HCOs, not only due to its role in accreditation but also due to its annual patient safety goals and reporting requirements for its accredited HCOs.

As Kizer and Stegun (2014) state, "HCOs and healthcare providers through their mission and ethical principles that support public accountability should provide information and transparency to consumers when there is concern about problems and actions taken" (p. 341). Disclosure to patients about errors has been discussed in this text, and there are conflicting views about its use. HCOs are also obligated to provide some information about their performance to external agencies (e.g., state and federal), insurers, and accreditors. The question that has become more important today is this: How much of this performance information should then be shared with the general public, and should this be mandatory? The HHS, Office of the Inspector General (OIG) (2010) summarizes this issue as follows: "Public disclosure of adverse event information offers potential benefits, yet may also lead to unintended negative consequences. For example, publicly disclosing adverse event information can educate healthcare providers about the causes of events potentially leading to improvements in patient safety, and assist patients making decisions about their care. However, there is concern that disclosure of event information could undermine patient privacy and that naming the hospital where an event occurred, or the individual providers involved, could discourage reporting of

events" (p. 6). With multiple viewpoints about a universal decision on mandatory reporting and to whom, this concern has not yet been resolved.

Two issues that are important to consider are the complexity of reporting and reporting data to multiple entities, such as accreditors, insurers, state agencies, and federal government agencies. Accountability means that all HCOs and staff should focus on improving patient care. Systematic reporting using standard definitions is critical if one is to compare data across HCOs and other entities to which reports are given, but at this time there is no systematic reporting that meets the needs of multiple organizations and state and federal governments.

## Incident Reports

**Incident reports** have long been used by HCOs, particularly hospitals, to report and track quality care issues. The AHRQ's Patient Safety Network describes an incident report as follows: "*Incident reporting* is frequently used as a general term for all voluntary patient safety event reporting systems, which rely on those involved in events to provide detailed information" (HHS, AHRQ, PSNet, 2019b). Although this reporting has been used for a long time, incident reporting has not done enough to improve care.

HCOs should have a policy that describes when the incident report should be completed and a procedure defining how it should be completed. Typically, HCOs use incident reports to track infections, pharmacy and medication errors, treatment procedure errors, patient complaints, falls, sentinel events, security issues, harm to staff, and regulatory compliance (Levinson, 2012). **Exhibit 10-1** provides an example of a list of serious reportable events.

It is not simple to develop and implement effective error reporting systems, and the process requires ongoing attention. Getting staff

## **Exhibit 10-1** Serious Reportable Events

1.  **Surgical or Invasive Procedure Events**

    **1A. Surgery or other invasive procedure performed on the wrong site (updated)**
    Applicable in: hospitals, outpatient/office-based surgery centers, ambulatory practice settings/office-based practices, long-term care/skilled nursing facilities

    **1B. Surgery or other invasive procedure performed on the wrong patient (updated)**
    Applicable in: hospitals, outpatient/office-based surgery centers, ambulatory practice settings/office-based practices, long-term care/skilled nursing facilities

    **1C. Wrong surgical or other invasive procedure performed on a patient (updated)**
    Applicable in: hospitals, outpatient/office-based surgery centers, ambulatory practice settings/office-based practices, long-term care/skilled nursing facilities

    **1D. Unintended retention of a foreign object in a patient after surgery or other invasive procedure (updated)**
    Applicable in: hospitals, outpatient/office-based surgery centers, ambulatory practice settings/office-based practices, long-term care/skilled nursing facilities

    **1E. Intraoperative or immediately postoperative/postprocedure death in an ASA Class 1 patient (updated)**
    Applicable in: hospitals, outpatient/office-based surgery centers, ambulatory practice settings/office-based practices

2.  **Product or Device Events**

    **2A. Patient death or serious injury associated with the use of contaminated drugs, devices, or biologics provided by the healthcare setting (updated)**
    Applicable in: hospitals, outpatient/office-based surgery centers, ambulatory practice settings/office-based practices, long-term care/skilled nursing facilities

    **2B. Patient death or serious injury associated with the use or function of a device in patient care, in which the device is used or functions other than as intended (updated)**
    Applicable in: hospitals, outpatient/office-based surgery centers, ambulatory practice settings/office-based practices, long-term care/skilled nursing facilities

    **2C. Patient death or serious injury associated with intravascular air embolism that occurs while being cared for in a healthcare setting (updated)**
    Applicable in: hospitals, outpatient/office-based surgery centers, long-term care/skilled nursing facilities

3.  **Patient Protection Events**

    **3A. Discharge or release of a patient/resident of any age, who is unable to make decisions, to other than an authorized person (updated)**
    Applicable in: hospitals, outpatient/office-based surgery centers, ambulatory practice settings/office-based practices, long-term care/skilled nursing facilities

    **3B. Patient death or serious injury associated with patient elopement (disappearance) (updated)**
    Applicable in: hospitals, outpatient/office-based surgery centers, ambulatory practice settings/office-based practices, long-term care/skilled nursing facilities

    **3C. Patient suicide, attempted suicide, or self-harm that results in serious injury while being cared for in a healthcare setting (updated)**
    Applicable in: hospitals, outpatient/office-based surgery centers, ambulatory practice settings/office-based practices, long-term care/skilled nursing facilities

4. **Care Management Events**

   4A. **Patient death or serious injury associated with a medication error (e.g., errors involving the wrong drug, wrong dose, wrong patient, wrong time, wrong rate, wrong preparation, or wrong route of administration) (updated)**
   Applicable in: hospitals, outpatient/office-based surgery centers, ambulatory practice settings/office-based practices, long-term care/skilled nursing facilities

   4B. **Patient death or serious injury associated with unsafe administration of blood products (updated)**
   Applicable in: hospitals, outpatient/office-based surgery centers, ambulatory practice settings/office-based practices, long-term care/skilled nursing facilities

   4C. **Maternal death or serious injury associated with labor or delivery in a low-risk pregnancy while being cared for in a healthcare setting (updated)**
   Applicable in: hospitals, outpatient/office-based surgery centers

   4D. **Death or serious injury of a neonate associated with labor or delivery in a low-risk pregnancy (new)**
   Applicable in: hospitals, outpatient/office-based surgery centers

   4E. **Patient death or serious injury associated with a fall while being cared for in a healthcare setting (updated)**
   Applicable in: hospitals, outpatient/office-based surgery centers, ambulatory practice settings/office-based practices, long-term care/skilled nursing facilities

   4F. **Any Stage 3, Stage 4, and unstageable pressure ulcers acquired after admission/ presentation to a healthcare setting (updated)**
   Applicable in: hospitals, outpatient/office-based surgery centers, long-term care/skilled nursing facilities

   4G. **Artificial insemination with the wrong donor sperm or wrong egg (updated)**
   Applicable in: hospitals, outpatient/office-based surgery centers, ambulatory practice settings/office-based practices

   4H. **Patient death or serious injury resulting from the irretrievable loss of an irreplaceable biological specimen (new)**
   Applicable in: hospitals, outpatient/office-based surgery centers, ambulatory practice settings/office-based practices, long-term care/skilled nursing facilities

   4I. **Patient death or serious injury resulting from failure to follow up or communicate laboratory, pathology, or radiology test results (new)**
   Applicable in: hospitals, outpatient/office-based surgery centers, ambulatory practice settings/office-based practices, long-term care/skilled nursing facilities

5. **Environmental Events**

   5A. **Patient or staff death or serious injury associated with an electric shock in the course of a patient care process in a healthcare setting (updated)**
   Applicable in: hospitals, outpatient/office-based surgery centers, ambulatory practice settings/office-based practices, long-term care/skilled nursing facilities

   5B. **Any incident in which systems designated for oxygen or other gas to be delivered to a patient contains no gas, the wrong gas, or are contaminated by toxic substances (updated)**
   Applicable in: hospitals, outpatient/office-based surgery centers, ambulatory practice settings/office-based practices, long-term care/skilled nursing facilities

   5C. **Patient or staff death or serious injury associated with a burn incurred from any source in the course of a patient care process in a healthcare setting (updated)**
   Applicable in: hospitals, outpatient/office-based surgery centers, ambulatory practice settings/office-based practices, long-term care/skilled nursing facilities

**5D. Patient death or serious injury associated with the use of physical restraints or bedrails while being cared for in a healthcare setting (updated)**
Applicable in: hospitals, outpatient/office-based surgery centers, ambulatory practice settings/office-based practices, long-term care/skilled nursing facilities

6. **Radiologic Events**

**6A. Death or serious injury of a patient or staff associated with the introduction of a metallic object into the MRI area (new)**
Applicable in: hospitals, outpatient/office-based surgery centers, ambulatory practice settings/office-based practices

7. **Potential Criminal Events**

**7A. Any instance of care ordered by or provided by someone impersonating a physician, nurse, pharmacist, or other licensed healthcare provider (updated)**
Applicable in: hospitals, outpatient/office-based surgery centers, ambulatory practice settings/office-based practices, long-term care/skilled nursing facilities

**7B. Abduction of a patient/resident of any age (updated)**
Applicable in: hospitals, outpatient/office-based surgery centers, ambulatory practice settings/office-based practices, long-term care/skilled nursing facilities

**7C. Sexual abuse/assault on a patient or staff member within or on the grounds of a healthcare setting (updated)**
Applicable in: hospitals, outpatient/office-based surgery centers, ambulatory practice settings/office-based practices, long-term care/skilled nursing facilities

**7D. Death or serious injury of a patient or staff member resulting from a physical assault (i.e., battery) that occurs within or on the grounds of a healthcare setting (updated)**
Applicable in: hospitals, outpatient/office-based surgery centers, ambulatory practice settings/office-based practices, long-term care/skilled nursing facilities

National Quality Forum. (2016). List of SREs. Retrieved from http://www.qualityforum.org/Topics/SREs/List_of_SREs.aspx and https://psnet.ahrq.gov /primer/never-events

to report actual events is not easy, and it is even more difficult to report potential events (Duffey, Oliver, & Newcomb, 2019). There must be an HCO culture where the staff feels empowered to report, and this requires better understanding of nurses' perceptions and attitudes toward reporting safety events. Dashboards may be used to routinely share incident report information with staff without inclusion of specific staff information and other identifiers so staff can see value in reporting and engaging in CQI.

Staff members who are at the point of care, rather than managers, usually identify error or near-miss information, although managers are also involved in some of these errors and near misses. Incident reporting is a passive form of surveillance as compared to active forms such as record reviews, observation of care delivery, and use of trigger tools (HHS, AHRQ, PSNet, 2019b). For the reporting system to be effective, the HCO should have a culture of safety that protects privacy when staff members report events, and the HCO should expect any staff involved in an event to use the required incident reporting procedure. The HCO should use structured methods to analyze the data, including root cause analysis, benchmarking, and development of action plans to respond when needed. Today, many HCOs have changed to electronic reporting methods, which make it easier for staff to report.

The reports and the data should be reviewed by CQI staff and management, as well as by risk management, to determine possible malpractice risk. This information is then used to develop needed changes to improve care. However, as stated, this process may not be effective. The incident reporting process has had a major impact on the development of the blame culture, with staff viewing the reports as a way for HCO administration to identify the staff member involved in an error and possibly "punish" that person. It is, however, necessary to have a documentation process for monitoring and examining errors and sharing with management and clinical staff. Attitudes toward monitoring should be positive, focused on identifying opportunities for improvement, not blame or punishment. Although an individual staff member typically completes the incident report, it is critical for error assessment to move away from just focusing on individuals and move to a system approach. The documentation then provides information for tracking errors and identifying errors that require examination and root cause analysis.

Management and staff attitudes toward incident reporting must be carefully monitored and evaluated long term. A negative attitude toward incident reporting is difficult to change to a positive one. HCOs must consider whether the use of incident reports limits reporting—for example, in one review of incident reports, the following was noted: "[H]ospital staff did not report 86 percent of events to incident reporting systems, partly because of staff misperceptions about what constitutes patient harm" (Levinson, 2012, p. i). When these events were identified, the HCOs investigated which events were considered to most likely lead to CQI problems. The review noted that few policy or practice changes resulted from data about incidents. **Table 10-4** describes the Common Format data elements that were included in the HHS review of incident reports.

Many common barriers affect staff voluntarily reporting events in their HCO system, including the following (Evans et al., 2006): no feedback on incident follow-up, confusing or long form, lack of time, incident seemed unimportant, unit was busy, forgot to report, and not sure who is responsible for the report. Using this type of information about barriers should help to develop strategies/interventions, such as changes to processes, policies, and procedures to prevent barriers so that the staff is more engaged in the incident reporting system. Staff orientation and education should provide information so that the staff understands why and how it is done. Reporting results to staff also helps staff better understand incident reporting and why it is important. Staff members have limited time and energy to devote to "administrative" tasks, so they need to appreciate the value of these tasks. Staff must also be recognized for their contributions to CQI—emphasizing their roles and responsibilities in all aspects of the HCO's QI program—for example, for staff to effectively report incidents, such as medication errors, they must know an error has occurred, be willing to report it, know the policy and procedure for reporting, and have the time to complete the incident report procedure. Further, it is important that the staff do not fear blame and punishment and that they view this activity as part of their commitment to CQI in their daily practice.

It is not enough to rely solely on incident reporting as the major monitoring method in a CQI program. HCOs and healthcare professions have focused a lot of attention on CQI, but there is an aspect of CQI getting less attention that is also important. This issue is how staff respond when they are involved in an error. Namely, how do they cope? There is recognition now that many adverse events are system related; however, this does not mean that staff may not have negative personal reactions and responses to situations that lead to adverse events and difficulties reporting them. Staff may respond with anger if they think they are being "accused" of something.

**Table 10-4** Common Format Data Elements Present on the Complete Incident Reports (*n* = 19)

| Element Description | Number of Reports With Element |
|---|---|
| *Basic Event Information* | |
| Date the event was discovered | 19 |
| Location of the event | 19 |
| Whether the event was an adverse event, near miss, or unsafe condition | 17 |
| Narrative description of the event | 16 |
| *Patient Impact Information* | |
| Time between event and assessment of harm | 16 |
| Whether rescue steps were taken | 16 |
| Level of harm caused by event | 14 |
| Whether event prolonged patient's length of stay | 2 |
| *Contributing Factor Information* | |
| Whether and which factors contributed to event | 10 |
| Patient safety staff's summary of event and follow-up | 6 |
| Preventability of event | 6 |
| Whether event was a National Quality Forum Serious Reportable Event | 0 |
| Whether a patient handoff was associated with event | 3 |

Reproduced from U.S. Department of Health and Human Services (HHS) & Office of the Inspector General. (January 2012). Hospital incident reporting systems do not capture most patient harm. OEI-06-09-009. Retrieved from http://oig.hhs.gov /oei/reports/oei-06-09-00091.asp

Staff may experience depression with lowered self-esteem due to their view of professional status or anxiety about their work. They may become overly careful, checking and recheck-ing their work process. They may feel embar-rassed with their colleagues and supervisors. If an adverse event is not reported and patient harm occurred, staff might find that keeping this event a secret has a negative impact on them personally and professionally, such as the stress impacting their personal life. HCOs must recognize that these human responses pose a potential problem and provide support to staff as needed when errors occur—to help staff who may feel they are also victims when errors are occur.

## Global Triggers

A **global trigger** is a signal or a clue that may be used to identify a potential adverse event, not the event itself. Triggers are used for screening and alerting staff to monitor for a particular situation—for example, by review-ing the medical record or a physician order (Adler et al., 2008).

The Institute for Healthcare Improvement (IHI) provides trigger tools for measuring general adverse events and events that might occur in specific care situations, such as for intensive care, perioperative, and mental health services. Only 10% to 20% of errors are reported; however, of the errors reported, 90% to 95% do not cause any harm. This means that we need more effective methods to identify those events that have greater risk of causing harm, and triggers can help to do this (IHI, 2015a). There is danger in focusing on counting errors rather than examining errors that cause harm to patients (IHI, 2015b). The general tool monitors adverse events per 1,000 patient-days per 100 admissions and percentage of admissions with an adverse event (IHI, 2016a, 2016b). "The term alert fatigue describes how busy workers (in the case of health care, clinicians) become desensitized to safety alerts, and as a result ignore or fail to respond appropriately to such warnings. This phenomenon occurs because of the sheer number of alerts, and it is compounded by the fact that the vast majority of alerts generated by CPOE systems (and other healthcare technologies) are clinically inconsequential—meaning that, in most cases, clinicians *should* ignore them. The problem is that clinicians then ignore both the bothersome, clinically meaningless alarms *and* the critical alerts that warn of impending serious patient harm" (HHS, AHRQ, PSNet, 2019c).

# Morbidity and Mortality Monitoring

Despite many years since the publication of one of the first quality reports on patient errors (Institute of Medicine [IOM], 1999), current data indicate a modest reduction in the mortality rate associated with adverse effects of medical treatment (Sunshine et al., 2019). **Morbidity** (incidence of disease state or condition) and **mortality** (incidence of death) are important outcomes requiring monitoring. Morbidity is determined by scores based on

tested systems, such as scales rating coma level and pain and special rating scales, such as APACHE II (intensive care unit patient rating mortality risk and rate of disease) and SAPS II (acute care patient rating of mortality risk and rate of disease). The mortality rate is typically described as number of deaths per 1,000 individuals annually and includes crude death rates; perinatal, maternal, or infant rates; and rates figured by age, gender, diagnosis, and other characteristics.

Acute care HCOs typically have routine meetings in which mortality and morbidity are discussed per specific patients and events. The staff examines system factors that contribute to adverse events and adverse patient outcomes. These meetings are also used for teaching medical staff, residents, and healthcare profession students. How are morbidity and mortality measured? The discussions focus on more than just data; they include details about practice and related problems and solutions. These meetings should be interprofessional and should not emphasize blame but rather provide opportunities for staff learning, consideration of needs for changes in practice to improve outcomes, and identification of care that is effective.

## Utilization Review/ Management and Risk Management

**Utilization review/management** is used by HCOs to routinely collect data about use of services. The data describe the number of admissions, transfers, discharges, procedures, and other pertinent details and provide other types of data, such as patient diagnosis, gender, age, length of treatment, and types of treatment. This information is also used in CQI and HCO marketing to assist in understanding HCO services, finance, and other operations. In addition, HCOs need information about causes of problems, such as admission and discharge delays. These processes cause stress and also increase expenses. A tracking tool to monitor discharge in real time—and to identify reasons for delays based on predetermined categories, such as prescriptions, transportation, lack of discharge summary, and so on—can be helpful in better understanding data that indicate these are delays in discharge (Holland, Pacyna, Gillard, & Carter, 2016). It is also important to view data from a time perspective—day of week, time of day. Holland and colleagues noted that in their study using this tracking tool the most reported cause of discharge delay was lack of plans for postacute services. If an HCO identifies this type of cause, then specific strategies can be developed and then implemented to deal with the problem and thus reduce the number of delayed discharges. This is how data and analysis can assist in improving care—and in reducing stress for patients, families, and staff.

**Risk management** focuses on HCO risk for malpractice claims and thus risk for financial loss. Risk management requires that HCOs do the following (Barach & Johnson, 2013): (1) Identify risk so that the HCO knows what is going wrong, (2) analyze the risk by collecting and understanding data, and (3) control the risk by developing strategies/interventions that will help identify, manage, and prevent problems. Attorneys are involved in assisting the HCO in this monitoring. The incident reporting system is a critical source of information for CQI but also for risk management. HCO structure often combines utilization review with risk management so that staff work together or are the same staff that provide this monitoring and may also be part of the QI program. Risk managers recognize that there is always risk, and some risk can be identified and prevented or actions may be taken to reduce the risk level. Examples of methods used to collect risk management data are observation and rounds, medical record reviews, and informal feedback from staff.

Malpractice lawsuits that focus on nurses do occur. A study of closed claims reviewed 516 claims (2006–2010) and identified that the average total incurred payment per nursing claim was $204,594 (Benton, Arm, & Flynn, 2013). Out of 11 nursing specialty areas, the areas with the highest percentage of claims were adult medical/surgical (40.1%), gerontology in an aging services facility (18.0%), and obstetrics (10.3%). The study reviewed the following malpractice categories of problems noted in claims: scope of practice (1.7%); assessment (12.6%); monitoring (6.8%); treatment/care (58.6%); medication administration (14.7%); patients' rights, patient abuse, and professional conduct (5.4%); and documentation (0.2%). The licensure types included in the claims were 84.5% registered nurses and 15.5% licensed practical or vocational nurses. Acute care had the most claims (57.3%). The review of these claims indicates that some of the situations could have been prevented. Nurses need to document according to standards, clearly, and in a timely manner; follow policies and procedures; understand and follow their scope of practice; improve written and oral communication; implement effective handoff methods; and maintain clinical competence through self-assessment, staff education, and continuing education. Each nurse must feel comfortable reporting concerns to supervisors without fear of reprimand.

## STOP AND CONSIDER 10-2

Monitoring care quality is a never-ending endeavor.

# Analysis of Quality Care

Analysis of CQI data is usually done quantitatively and statistically, but multiple variables make this a complicated process for healthcare.

The HHS, HRSA (2011b) describes the key concepts of this process as follows: *"Analyzing* data is the *review* of performance data to determine if it meets the desired quality level; it is used to define a performance plan. *Interpreting* data is the process of *assigning* meaning or determining the significance, implications, and conclusions of data collected; it is used to evaluate and improve activities, identify gaps, and plan for improvement."

The drivers of CQI are people, information management, infrastructure, processes, and culture, all of which impact desired outcomes (Ettinger, 2005). People are an important component of CQI. They are needed to develop and implement CQI initiatives and then to develop and implement necessary changes. How people work together can make a difference. Even the staffing level has an impact—for example, if staffing is short and staff members are overworked, CQI efforts may be negatively impacted; namely, the HCO may see increased errors, and aspects of the QI program, such as reporting, documenting, collecting, and analyzing data, may be limited, thus harming development of improvement strategies.

Just collecting data is not enough. Analysis and interpretation of data are critical, and mistakes can be made in interpretation (Ettinger, 2005)—for example, when focusing too much on mean or average and ignoring variation, data may be misinterpreted—that is, the mean can be improved and yet the variation is still unacceptable. If the analysis focuses just on percentages and not absolute numbers, this too might not provide a clear view of a problem—for example, the HCO might identify that 95% of medication orders were administered according to procedure, but the numerical description is 5,000 errors a year or 15 per day. The latter description better indicates an unacceptable result. It is also important to recognize that much of what is done in healthcare is multifactorial, such as medication administration. When errors occur, staff need to examine many factors, including patient demographics and conditions,

unit variables such as work culture and layout of unit, staffing and competency, communication, procedures, policies, leadership, and much more (Loresto, Welton, Grim, Valdez, & Eron, 2019).

Infrastructure is the driver that focuses on physical aspects of the HCO, such as space, lighting, noise, equipment availability, function, and computer software and hardware. Processes represent another driver, are integral in all HCO functioning, and have an impact on CQI (Ettinger, 2005). HCOs use different methods to understand their processes and their impact on quality. Examples of these methods are process mapping, as well as define, measure, analyze, design, verify (DMADV) (discussed later in this chapter). Organizational culture is also a driver and has been discussed in other chapters of this text. We pay more attention to organizational culture today in healthcare. A high-performing culture has "optimistic staff and leaders, [is] open to change and innovation, [has] leaders focused on both customers (e.g., patients and others) and staff, [is] process oriented, [is] committed to excellence, and measures and shares information" (Ettinger, 2005, p. 125). Organizational culture is connected to development of a culture of safety within HCOs.

The data analysis process requires that the CQI team and staff review current performance and then, ideally, compare performance with baseline data that were collected earlier (benchmarking)—for example, data from the previous year or month. Measures/indicators guide this process to determine if there is any change and, if so, describe the change. To determine if this is acceptable, the "interpretation process provides knowledge of the changes applied to the systems, special events with a potential impact, and lessons learned from the prior month's work that forms the next steps" (HHS, HRSA, 2011b). The team may use the plan-do-study-act (PDSA) cycle, discussed elsewhere in this text and summarized in **Figure 10-4**, to guide action and make changes to improve.

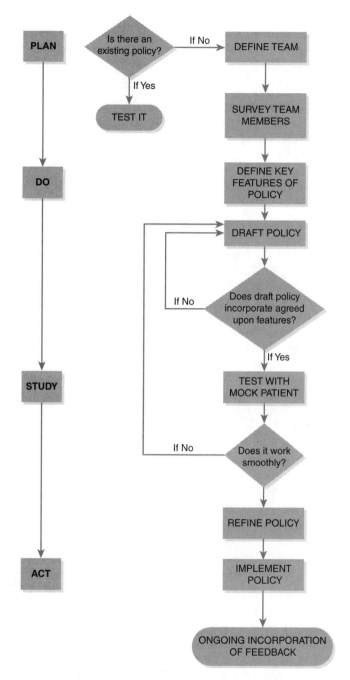

**Figure 10-4** Plan-Do-Study-Act Cycle of Policy Development

Reproduced from Bonner, L., Felker, B., Chaney, E., Vollen, K., Berry, K., Revay, B., ... Sherman, S. (February 2005). Suicide risk response: Enhancing patient safety through development of effective institutional policies. In Agency for Healthcare Research and Quality (AHRQ), Advances in patient safety (Vol. 3: Implementation issues). AHRQ publication No. 05-0021-3. Retrieved from http://www.ahrq.gov/professionals/quality-patient-safety/patient-safety-resources/resources/advances-in-patient-safety/index.html

Reproduced from National Patient Safety Foundation (NPSF). (2015). RCA2 : Improving root cause analyses and actions to prevent harm. Retrieved from http://www.ihi.org/resources/Pages/Tools/RCA2-Improving-Root-Cause-Analyses-and-Actions-to-Prevent-Harm.aspx>

If the QI team decides that progress toward improvement has not occurred, and this includes progress in all the CQI steps, it might then review any of the following (HHS, HRSA, 2011a, 2011b):

- *Ensure data systems are reliable.* Secondary sources are at risk as data are collected for reasons other than CQI and may not meet CQI requirements.
- *Reevaluate potential causes of underlying system problems.* Methods used to identify the causes, effectiveness of the methods, and analysis of results all could have led to errors in identifying causes.
- *Reevaluate changes made for improvement.* A common cause of a change failing to result in improvement is that the change was implemented inconsistently or was unexpectedly discontinued; possible reasons are communication issues, insufficient training, or resistance to change and are the typical challenges that may contribute to an unsuccessful change.
- *Increase number of changes per week/month, etc.* When a team has insufficient resources or time, it may implement changes slowly, which slows the rate of performance improvement. A recommendation for this scenario is to include other staff members to assist with incremental tasks, such as testing the changes so the CQI team can work on multiple factors simultaneously to improve systems.

It is important to focus on more than problems but also to recognize success. What does the HCO do when a CQI project is successful and helpful, meaning care has improved and there is greater understanding of positive staff engagement? HCO and team celebration is just as important as the other steps. Teams need to remember that healthcare delivery is complex, and there is no single magic answer to CQI challenges. Many problems require many changes, but celebrating success along the way is critical in engaging staff, developing a culture of safety, and improving quality care. The CQI team needs to evaluate the process overtime, make changes as needed, and recognize success when it occurs.

As Kelly and colleagues (2013) state, "Variation is the extent to which a process differs from the norm" (p. 79). Understanding variation within an HCO helps to understand connections with variation within the HCO, its processes, resources used, adverse events, and patient outcomes. HCO management must determine if the amount of variation represents acceptable performance. To better understand a process, it is necessary to include the people involved and technical concerns. Processes have requirements—which are also the criteria that are used to evaluate a process—and impact the inputs needed to design the process and also the outputs of the process. Elements that are important are inclusion of customers, such as patients and other stakeholders, and listening to their feedback—for example, What do stakeholders expect? How are services selected, designed, and improved? And how are outcomes measured?

Analysis of data requires thoughtful planning and choice of methods. Some of the common methods are described below, although root cause analysis is the most common method used in HCOs. The Connect to Current Information section at the end of this chapter provides links to sites that describe some of the following methods.

# Root Cause Analysis

**Root cause analysis (RCA)** is a method used today by many HCOs to analyze errors, supporting the recognition that most errors are caused by system issues and not necessarily individual staff issues. RCA is a system process using a structured method to analyze serious adverse events. "Initially developed to analyze industrial accidents, RCA is now widely deployed as an error analysis tool in health care. A central tenet of RCA is to identify underlying problems that increase the likelihood of errors while avoiding the trap of focusing on mistakes by individuals" (HHS, AHRQ, PSNet, 2019d).

The reasoning behind RCA may seem to imply that there is only one cause for an error. Using the Swiss cheese model of errors, discussed elsewhere in this text, however, the focus should be on multiple errors and system flaws that often intersect for a critical incident to reach the patient. Labeling one or even several of these factors as "causes" may overemphasize specific "holes in the cheese" and obscure others, decreasing understanding of the overall relationships between different layers and other aspects of system design. The RCA process includes the following steps (HHS, AHRQ, PSNet, 2019d):

1. Select the team to complete the RCA. The team should include experts related to the event—for example, if the error occurred in the intensive care unit for postcardiac surgical patients, team members should include representatives from the intensive care unit, operating room, and anesthesiology staffs, as well as other relevant healthcare professionals such as cardiac surgeons and nurses, laboratory technicians, radiologist, infusion team, pharmacy, and infection control. Management should also be represented, and staff educators may participate.
2. Create a flowchart, as described earlier in this chapter.
3. Examine the flowchart for areas of failure.
4. Use team methods to assist the team in discussing and identifying underlying causes.
5. Use CQI tools to relate data collected to possible root causes.
6. Redesign the process for improvement (if required) based on the analysis results.
7. Implement the changes first through a pilot program, and then spread to other areas as appropriate for the improvement strategy/intervention.

RCA applies in-depth analysis, follows specific steps, and should focus on the system, not individual staff. Its major purpose is to identify causes and then consider changes that might be required to reduce risk of reoccurrence.

The team analyzing the problem or error usually uses brainstorming, flowcharts, and cause–effect diagrams. The goal is to clearly describe the problem and all factors related to it. Typical contributing factors are categorized as follows:

- *Environmental factors* (e.g., work environment, staff safety, safety culture type, ethical/legal concerns)
- *Organizational factors* (e.g., staffing levels/mix, staff availability and roles, support staff, clear policies, administrative support, effective leadership, access to equipment and supplies, documentation, use of rounds and other communication methods, attitudes toward patients and families, patient-centered care)
- *Staff/team* (e.g., supervision of staff, communication, team membership, quality of teamwork, team leadership and functioning, availability of expertise)
- *Individual staff factors* (e.g., level of knowledge, competence, and experience; fatigue; stress; expectations; position description; staff safety)
- *Task factors* (e.g., clear protocols and/or guidelines, use of checklists, lab tests and other procedures, description of tasks, policies)
- *Patient factors* (e.g., stress, communication, accessible patient information, diversity factors, comorbidities, status on admission, past history, 30-day unplanned readmission, discharge plans)

Key questions that are asked during RCA include the following:

- What happened?
- Who was involved?
- When did it happen?

- Where did it happen?
- What is the severity of the actual or potential harm?
- What is the likelihood of reoccurrence?
- What are the consequences?

Many analysis methods are used during RCA, but one common method focuses on the "five whys": to better understand a problem ask why; in answer to that reason, continue to ask why to gain more depth of understanding (iSixSigma, 2019). In addition to the preceding questions, the team may ask the following questions to analyze the responses to the "why" questions (HHS, AHRQ, PSNet, 2019c).

- What proof do I have that this cause exists? (Is it concrete? Is it measurable?)
- What proof do I have that this cause could lead to the stated effect? (Am I merely asserting causation?)
- What proof do I have that this cause actually contributed to the problem I'm looking at? (Even given that the cause exists and could lead to this problem, how do I know it was not actually something else?)
- Is anything else needed, along with this cause, for the stated effect to occur? (Is it self-sufficient? Is something needed to help it along?)
- Can anything else, besides this cause, lead to the stated effect? (Are there alternative explanations that fit better? What other risks are there?)

RCA results should provide a clearer picture of the problem and options for preventing additional errors or problems, then choices can be made as to the best approach to take; however, whenever possible, evidence or best practice should also be used to support decisions. The process should include an interprofessional team of staff who are knowledgeable about the issue or problem, thereby increasing the chance that the analysis will be complete and decisions effective (HHS, AHRQ, PSNet, 2019d).

Healthcare has borrowed and adapted models and methods from a variety of industries—for example, some of the leadership theories and models that are often applied to healthcare delivery originated in other industries. RCA is one of the methods that was adopted. Despite the common use of RCA, data supporting its effectiveness are actually limited. There are problems with how RCA results are interpreted, and there is no consensus as to how an HCO should analyze data for RCA or follow-up. Another issue is that few formal mechanisms exist for analysis of multiple RCAs across institutions. Each time the RCA process is used, it might be considered to be a case study focused on a specific event in a specific HCO. In addition, there should also be an analysis of multiple RCAs from multiple HCOs to identify trends and patterns (macro and aggregate data), and then this information should be used to recommend changes in healthcare that would apply across HCOs. The Joint Commission expects its accredited HCOs to use RCA, and some states require use of RCA as part of their state HCO regulations. Outcomes may then be reported to The Joint Commission or to state regulators. So despite the need for greater supporting evidence to determine the value of using RCA, it continues to be an important analysis method.

The National Patient Safety Foundation (NPSF) issued a report in 2015 renaming RCA as RCA squared ($RCA^2$). The reason for this change is to emphasize the need for using RCA to identify adverse events, hazards, and HCOs vulnerable for future events. In doing this, the HCO must identify and take steps to prevent repetition of these events, which is the most important step in the RCA, or $RCA^2$, process. To improve RCA and establish the $RCA^2$ approach, the report makes the following recommendations (HHS, AHRQ, PSNet, 2919e):

- Leadership (e.g., CEO, board of directors) should be actively involved in the RCA and action process, supporting the process. This involvement includes approving and periodically reviewing the status of actions, understanding what a thorough RCA² report should include, and taking actions when reviews do not meet minimum requirements.

- Leadership should review the RCA² process at least annually for effectiveness.
- Blameworthy events that are not appropriate for RCA² review should be defined.
- HCOs should use a transparent, formal, and explicit risk-based prioritization system to identify adverse events, close calls, and system vulnerabilities requiring RCA² review.
- An RCA² review should be started within 72 hours of recognizing that a review is needed.
- RCA² teams should be composed of four to six people. The team should include process experts as well as other individuals drawn from all levels of the organization, and the team should consider inclusion of a patient representative unrelated to the event. Team membership should *not* include individuals who were involved in the event or close call being reviewed, but those individuals should be interviewed for information. (Some HCOs include staff members who were involved on the team.)
- Time should be provided during the normal work shift for staff to serve on an RCA² team, including attending meetings, researching, and conducting interviews.
- Common RCA² tools (e.g., interviewing techniques, flow diagramming, cause and effect diagramming, five rules of causation, action hierarchy, process/outcome measures) should be used by teams to assist in the investigation process and identification of strong and intermediate-strength corrective actions.
- Feedback should be provided to staff involved in the event as well as to patients and/or family members regarding findings of the RCA² process.

Some HCOs are now using a new rapid RCA² approach, called SWARMing (Li et al., 2015). SWARMs may be part of RCAs and are conducted without delay after a reported event. The first step is a preliminary investigation into what happened and who was involved, followed by an in-person meeting with the interprofessional team and any staff directly involved in the event. Following this, a full RCA is conducted.

# Failure Modes and Effects Analysis

**Failure modes and effects analysis (FMEA)** is one example of a prospective analysis method. This method can also be used as a retrospective method when RCA is used in combination with FMEA. When they are combined, the analysis considers the probability of failure and also consequences of failure (Wachter & Gupta, 2018). FMEA is focused on known or potential problems and errors, with the goal "to prevent errors by attempting to identify all the ways a process could fail, estimate the probability and consequences of each failure, and then take action to prevent the potential failures from occurring" (Hughes, 2008). It requires identification of all steps in the process and a description of potential problems with each step, probability, and impact. In this analysis of the problem, the team identifies the areas or steps that are at higher risk for problems (IHI, 2019a). FMEA reliability has been questioned by some experts, as there can be variation in opinions when it is used. This factor must be considered when FMEA is used.

# Fishbone Analysis

**Fishbone analysis** is a problem analysis tool. It allows the team to identify causes of a problem. It requires the team to be open and consider all possible causes and then add ideas to the fishbone graphic. Brainstorming is typically used to stimulate the review process and idea formulation. The visual can then be used to identify and discuss the possible causes.

## Define, Measure, Analyze, Design, Verify

**Define, measure, analyze, design, verify (DMADV)** is a method used by Six Sigma. Using this method, project goals and outcomes are defined; the process is analyzed; a detailed description of the process is developed; and then performance is verified. Another method used by Six Sigma is define, measure, analyze, improve, control (DMAIC), which completes the same activities described for the first two DMADV steps. In the third step, however, the process is improved by removing defects so that future performance is controlled. Six Sigma is an approach to QI that is focused on using data, reducing variation, and eliminating defects or deviations in processes. The DMADV method is typically used when a new process or product must be developed or when a process or product has been changed but more improvement is needed (iSixSigma, 2016a).

## Gap Analysis

**Gap analysis** is a method for examining current status. The analysis focuses on where the organization, department, or unit and staff want to go. The difference in current status and future vision is referred to as the "gap." The gap may then guide actions to improve. Further detailed analysis and planning are then required.

## Value Stream Mapping

**Value stream mapping** is a method used in Six Sigma. It documents, analyzes, and improves the flow of information or supplies that are needed to complete a process or produce a product (iSixSigma, 2016b). Elements include

mapping to identify the process boundaries, process steps, information flow, process data, timeline, and stakeholders; interpreting data; and planning next steps.

## Brainstorming

Brainstorming is a method used to identify the most ideas possible and can also be used during analysis to determine both prospective and retrospective views. Examples of brainstorming are I PASS the BATON, the Delphi technique, and the nominal group. These methods are discussed elsewhere in this text as methods used in the change process; however, here they may also be used in the analysis of CQI problems.

## Deep Dive

**Deep dive** is an in-depth brainstorming technique that is used ideally by an interprofessional team. All members actively participate in the process—engaging frontline staff in the change process to improve care. Deep dive focuses on ensuring that the critical participants in the workplace are involved. It is a structured approach, with a plan for implementing change, including aspects such as agenda, time spent storytelling and identifying what is disturbing staff and exploring possible resolutions, use of methods to post ideas so that they can be viewed by the team for assessment and discussion, and use of voting or selection methods. Deep dive is a critical method used in Transforming Care at the Bedside (TCAB), an important nursing initiative to improve care and engage nursing staff in the process, which is described elsewhere in this text (IHI, 2019b).

---

**STOP AND CONSIDER 10-3**

CQI analysis requires an in-depth view of a CQI problem.

# Examples of National Healthcare Measurement Programs

The number of national healthcare measurement programs has increased, particularly since the first *Quality Chasm* reports in 1999. The NQS has been very important in stimulating further development in aggregate or macro-initiatives rather than just focusing on an individual HCO's QI program (micro level). However, many measures/indicators have been developed to assist efforts to measure care. The following content provides examples of initiatives that identify multiple measures/indicators, illustrating the complexity and choices for CQI measurement (Chassin, Loeb, Schmaltz, & Wachter, 2010, pp. 1–3; HHS, CMS, 2015; NAM, 2015):

- The Medicare and Medicaid programs use the Centers for Medicare and Medicaid Services (CMS) Measures Inventory to assess their quality; it includes nearly 1,700 measures/indicators.
- The National Quality Foundation (NQF) measure database includes 620 measures. The NQF does not develop measures but rather reviews and endorses measures. Its web-based system, Quality Positioning System, provides access to the endorsed measures.
- The National Committee for Quality Assurance's Healthcare Effectiveness Data and Information Set, used by more than 90% of health insurance plans, includes 81 different measures.
- The Joint Commission requires hospitals to provide data for specified measures.

An important example of the impact of new models of care on measurement is the movement to establish accountable care methods by developing accountable care organizations (ACOs), which was a provision in the Patient Protection and Affordable Care Act of 2010 (ACA). This model focuses on replacing the fragmented and uncoordinated care system described by the *Quality Chasm* reports, recognizing the need for a system that integrates care received by a patient, with payment incentives aimed at individual and population health outcomes (Fisher, Staiger, Bynum, & Gottlieb, 2007). The CMS, the federal agency responsible for implementing the ACO model, has launched several programs to support the ACO model, including the Medicare Shared Savings Program, the Pioneer model, the Advance Payment initiative, and Medicaid ACOs. In addition, private insurers, employers, and others support ACOs, and some have established these programs. Monitoring care quality and coordination is part of the ACO model. In early 2020, 11.2 million beneficiaries are involved in this program (HHS, CMS, 2020).

**Table 10-5** describes a coordinated care model developed by the AHRQ.

Other care delivery changes such as patient-centered medical homes, clinics devoted to high-risk patients, team-based care models, and retail clinics also indicate the need for monitoring measures that meet the needs of these new models of care. Over the years there have been changes in reimbursement requirements, and reimbursement does influence QI. When people have more access to care, there is a greater chance that they will get care when needed and reach care outcomes. In addition, the increase in patients requesting care impacts the risk of complications and errors; there may be greater incidence due to the greater number of potential patients, and some of them may have complex needs. Another problem that is increasing is changes in the insurance marketplaces due to some insurers dropping out of participation. This has an impact on patients receiving care when they need care from a consistent provider.

## Centers for Medicare and Medicaid Services Quality Core Measures

The CMS bases its QI goals on four principles: (1) Eliminate racial and ethnic disparities,

**Table 10-5** Care Coordination Measures

| Type of Care Coordination | Description | Example |
|---|---|---|
| Coordination within a provider team/site | Coordination between individuals employed by or acting for a health-care organization (defined by a single administrative management) | A measure assessing adequacy and timeliness of follow-up on ordered tests in the ambulatory care setting |
| Coordination across provider teams/sites | Coordination between individuals employed by or acting for different health-care organizations that do not share institutional or administrative management systems | A measure assessing the quality of discharge documentation sent from a hospital to a long-term care facility at the time of hospital discharge |
| Coordination between providers and patient/caregiver | Coordination between healthcare workers and the patient, family members, or caregivers (often nonprofessionals) with responsibility for providing care to the patient | A measure assessing contacts between the primary care team and patients/caregivers between ambulatory visits |
| Coordination between providers and community | Coordination between healthcare workers and community-based organizations on behalf of the patient | A measure assessing communication between pediatricians and school staff for pediatric patients with developmental disorders |

Reproduced from Agency for Healthcare Research and Quality & National Quality Measures Clearinghouse. (2015, June 18). Finding care coordination measures. Retrieved from https://www.qualitymeasures.ahrq.gov/tutorial /CareCoordination.aspx https://www.ahrq.gov/gam/index.html

(2) strengthen infrastructure and data systems, (3) enable local innovations, and (4) foster learning organizations (HHS, CMS, 2019). The CMS is mandated to assess the quality of its services. This effort is also connected with the NQS, which was first described in 2011 and provides the broad aims and priorities that guide the HHS and CMS quality initiatives. The overall vision for the CMS Quality Strategy is to optimize health outcomes by improving quality and transforming the healthcare system. The CMS includes many partners to ensure a comprehensive approach. Its measure domains are as follows (HHS, CMS, 2015):

- Patient safety
- Patient and family engagement
- Care coordination
- Clinical process/effectiveness
- Population/public health
- Efficient use of healthcare resources (p. 2)

These measures are reviewed and changed when new data indicate different issues exist. **Table 10-6** describes the relationship between the NQS and the CMS Quality Strategy per measure. The CMS believes its efforts are in the best interest of all patients whether they are a CMS patient or not. Most HCOs have patients covered by CMS and thus have to follow the CMS requirements. Consequently, these requirements then impact all patient care and outcomes.

# Patient Safety Organizations

The AHRQ is mandated by Congress to support the development of patient safety organizations (PSOs), but the federal government does not fund PSOs. To be PSO certified requires that the HCO collect and analyze data in a standardized manner, such as applying the Common Formats developed by the

**Table 10-6** National Quality Strategy and CMS Quality Strategy

| National Quality Strategy Priorities | CMS Quality Strategy Goals and Objectives | Measure Domains (Abbreviated) |
|---|---|---|
| 1. Making care safer by reducing the harm caused in the delivery of care | Goal 1: Make care safer by reducing harm caused in the delivery of care. <br> ■ Improve support for a culture of safety. <br> ■ Reduce inappropriate and unnecessary care. <br> ■ Prevent or minimize harm in all settings. | Patient Safety (Safety) |
| 2. Ensuring that each person and family are engaged as partners in their care | Goal 2: Strengthen person and family engagement as partners in their care. <br> ■ Ensure all care delivery incorporates patient and caregiver preferences. <br> ■ Improve experience of care for patients, caregivers, and families. <br> ■ Promote patient self-management. | Patient and Family Engagement (Patient Engagement) |
| 3. Promoting effective communication and coordination of care | Goal 3: Promote effective communication and coordination of care. <br> ■ Reduce admissions and readmissions. <br> ■ Embed best practices to manage transitions to all practice settings. <br> ■ Enable effective healthcare system navigation. | Care Coordination (Care Coordination) |
| 4. Promoting the most effective prevention and treatment practices for the leading causes of mortality, starting with cardiovascular disease | Goal 4: Promote effective prevention and treatment of chronic disease. <br> ■ Increase appropriate use of screening and prevention services. <br> ■ Strengthen interventions to prevent heart attacks and strokes. <br> ■ Improve quality of care for patients with multiple chronic conditions. <br> ■ Improve behavioral health access and quality care. Improve perinatal outcomes. | Clinical Process/ Effectiveness (Effective Treatment) |
| 5. Working with communities to promote wide use of best practices to enable healthy living | Goal 5: Work with communities to promote best practices of healthy living. <br> ■ Partner with and support federal, state, and local public health improvement efforts. <br> ■ Improve access within communities to best practices of healthy living. <br> ■ Promote evidence-based community interventions to prevent and treat chronic disease. <br> ■ Increase use of community-based social services support. | Population/Public Health (Healthy Communities) |

*(continues)*

**Table 10-6** National Quality Strategy and CMS Quality Strategy *(continued)*

| National Quality Strategy Priorities | CMS Quality Strategy Goals and Objectives | Measure Domains (Abbreviated) |
|---|---|---|
| 6. Making quality care affordable for individuals, families, employers, and governments by developing and spreading new healthcare delivery models (affordable care) | Goal 6: Make care affordable.<br>■ Develop and implement payment systems that reward value over volume.<br>■ Use cost analysis data to inform payment policies. | Efficient Use of Healthcare Resources (Affordable Care) |

AHRQ (HHS, AHRQ, PSO, 2019a). A PSO is an entity or component of another organization that may carry out or provide services on behalf of an HCO or a healthcare provider, including the following services (HHS, AHRQ, PSO, 2019a):

1. Efforts to improve patient safety and quality of healthcare delivery
2. Collection and analysis of patient safety work product (PSWP)
3. Development and dissemination of information regarding patient safety, such as recommendations, protocols, or information regarding best practices
4. Utilization of PSWP for the purposes of encouraging a culture of safety as well as providing feedback and assistance to effectively minimize patient risk
5. Maintenance of procedures to preserve confidentiality with respect to PSWP
6. Provision of appropriate security measures with respect to PSWP
7. Utilization of qualified staff
8. Initiation of activities related to the operation of a patient safety evaluation system and provision of feedback to participants in a patient safety evaluation system

In providing these services, PSOs, acting as independent, external experts, assist HCOs in improving healthcare delivery. Since patient data are part of these services, it is important that this communication be protected. PSOs gather data from multiple HCOs and then are able to analyze aggregate data about patient safety events to better understand these events.

# Healthcare Effectiveness Data and Information Systems

Nurses primarily think about CQI in relation to healthcare providers and HCOs that provide care. However, other healthcare delivery quality issues that need to be considered other than those associated directly with clinical care, such as insurer/third-party payer quality, are also important. The Healthcare Effectiveness Data and Information Set (HEDIS®) is a tool that is supported by the National Committee for Quality Assurance. It is used by more than 90% of U.S. health plans to measure their performance, but it also provides performance measurement options for physician provider organizations (PPOs), physicians, and other HCOs. Its 81 measures cover five domains, providing data for plans to compare themselves (National Committee for Quality Assurance [NCQA], 2019). The HEDIS® report card, Quality Compass®, is an interactive web-based comparison tool that assists employers and consumers in choosing the best health insurance plan for them by comparing plans that participate in this report card or performance measurement report. The Connect to Current Information section at the end of this chapter provides a link to the HEDIS® site.

# National Healthcare Quality and Disparities Reports

*National Healthcare Quality and Disparities Reports* are discussed elsewhere in this text. In this chapter, it is important to note that these annual reports provide national data focused on specific indicators related to quality and diversity. This information is useful to HCOs as they plan their QI programs because the reports identify national elements of care delivery that are improving, and those that are not should then be considered when HCOs identify specific areas of concern for their CQI planning.

## AHRQ QI™

The AHRQ QI™ is used to "highlight potential quality concerns, identify areas that need further study and investigation, and track changes over time" (HHS, AHRQ, 2015). As an HHS agency, the AHRQ provides free software to hospitals. This software is used to collect data and submit data to the AHRQ based on indicators identified by the AHRQ. This tool allows hospitals to compare their data to national benchmarks. This is an example of a national effort used to monitor some aspects of care and provide individual hospitals with tools to collect data and guidelines for improving care. Examples of these indicators, which were identified in 2009, include the following (HHS, AHRQ, 2019):

- *Prevention quality indicators.* These indicators focus on preventing additional hospitalization or are used to indicate need for early intervention to avoid complications and change negative change in disease status. The indicators rely on use of inpatient discharge data and help communities assess needs and patient self-management needs.
- *Inpatient quality indicators.* Using hospital administrative data, these indicators focus on hospital quality care (e.g., mortality rates; utilization and volume of procedures that might be overused, underused, or misused; risk for mortality).
- *Pediatric quality indicators.* These indicators examine care in hospitals for pediatric patients.
- *Home and community-based services.* These indicators focus on Medicaid beneficiaries who are receiving home- and community-based services.
- *Patient safety indicators (PSIs).* These hospital indicators examine hospital complications and adverse events, particularly following procedures, surgery, and childbirth; includes 18 provider-level indicators established by the AHRQ to screen for adverse patient events. Use of PSI provides aggregate data per hospital applied to a number of events that are identified by the PSIs. A study, using a retrospective, multifacility, cross-sectional chart abstraction, addressed the question of whether the AHRQ PSIs could be used to improve nursing care.

## *Healthcare Cost and Utilization Project*

The Healthcare Cost and Utilization Project (HCUP) is an online resource that includes a number of databases developed and maintained by the AHRQ to provide data about hospital discharges from the majority of the states. Data from state data organizations, hospital associations, private data organizations, and the federal government are updated quarterly and annually. The HCUP, with its extensive data collection of longitudinal hospital data, is an important source for providers, policy makers, and others who need this information (HHS,

AHRQ, HCUP, 2019). Currently, the databases focus on national inpatient data, state inpatient data, state ambulatory surgery and services, pediatric services, and emergency departments. Over time, additional data and information may be added to this source.

# Multiple Roles of Nurses in Quality Improvement: Monitoring, Collecting Data, and Analyzing

As discussed in this chapter, multiple methods are used to identify and track errors or potential errors. However, no matter how much is done to identify and/or track errors, if staff do not report problems or potential problems, and then if little or nothing is done to take action to improve, CQI will not be effective. Use of these tools requires more than just applying the tools. It requires analysis and use of critical thinking. CQI has commonly been viewed as a management function. In the long run, this view removed nurses from CQI or led nurses to believe it was not their responsibility to participate, let alone lead, CQI activities. It is clear that such thinking has not been helpful. Nurses provide much of the direct care and in this role can provide quality care, intervene to prevent problems, and participate in all phases of the CQI process. Nurses should be active in monitoring, data collection, analysis, and developing strategies/interventions to prevent or respond to CQI problems. Including nurses in all levels of CQI planning increases the opportunity for the

inclusion of nursing ideas and experience in the QI program. One author concludes the following and summarizes some key points related to nursing and quality improvement: "Nurses have a social responsibility to evaluate the effect of nursing practice on patient outcomes in the areas of health promotion; injury and illness prevention; and alleviation of suffering. Quality assessment initiatives are hindered by the paucity of available data related to nursing processes and patient outcomes across these three domains of practice. Direct care nurses are integral to self-regulation for the discipline as they are the best source of information about nursing practice and patient outcomes. Evidence supports the assumption that nurses do contribute to prevention of adverse events but there is insufficient evidence to explain how nurses contribute to these and/or other patient outcomes" (Jones, 2016).

Each HCO must communicate and commit to engaging all staff, not just clinical staff, in CQI. Efforts include improving documentation, providing a cleaner and safer environment, ensuring that equipment is maintained and functioning safely, monitoring drug supplies so they are available when needed, keeping supplies current and accessible, providing nutritious and attractive meals to patients, answering telephones, and helping to keep computers working effectively.

# Summary

This chapter provides a toolbox of information about monitoring, measuring, and analyzing care quality. Methods are described to meet the CQI process elements that should be considered when an HCO develops its QI program and associated plans. There are multiple methods that an HCO may choose to use. In addition to the HCO-focused CQI initiatives, there are now more national CQI measurement initiatives that make a difference to healthcare status and influence the HCO's CQI activities. Several examples were discussed, and others are included in other sections of this text. As noted in the *Future of Nursing* report (IOM, 2010) and by other experts, the nursing profession must assume more responsibilities in

CQI activities—as individual nurses providing care, as managers and leaders, and as members of professional organizations—and nurses must participate in CQI health policy development, implementation, and evaluation. Nurses need to be familiar with the methods used and then participate in their use on a routine basis in the work environment, and they must effectively use data to inform decision making. Exemplars of quality improvement roles and responsibilities for staff nurses, nurse managers, and APRNs are found in **Exhibit 10-2**.

---

**Exhibit 10-2** **Exemplars: Quality Improvement Roles and Responsibilities**

### Staff Nurse

A sentinel event (death of a newborn) occurs in the obstetrical department. A week later a staff nurse who was with the mother during labor and a second one who was at the delivery due to change of shift are served with legal documents informing them of a lawsuit. Both nurses carry professional liability insurance. The first nurse calls her insurer and is told she must contact an attorney that they choose and to do so immediately. The second nurse says this is unnecessary because the hospital attorneys will take care of her. The latter is not necessarily correct. This nurse also should have her own attorney, and if she has insurance she should call her insurer for advice.

### Nurse Manager

The nurse manager for the eight clinics in an ambulatory care center in a large medical center recognizes the need to share QI data with staff and then engage them in the CQI process. He uses a dashboard at the monthly staff meetings to share the data and analysis and then uses this to stimulate discussion—to get ideas for improvement. The dashboard is provided by the QI progam with assistance from the nurse manager.

### Advanced Practice Registered Nurse*

Two APRNs who work in pediatrics are developing a CQI project to address parent complaints about their interactions with staff. They are discussing data collection to get data from parents, focusing on three possible methods to monitor this problem: interviews, surveys, and observation. They will conduct the interviews of parents but will need to find other staff to collect data via observation. The nurse manager agrees to pay nurses who do not work in the units to collect the data. They will need to be trained for this by the APRNs. If they do not get enough data from these two methods, they will then develop a survey, which takes more time and must be pilot tested.

---

* Advanced Practice Registered Nurse includes APRN, Clinical Nurse Specialist, Clinical Nurse Leader, and nurses with DNP.

# APPLY CQI

## Chapter Highlights

- Measurement is a complex process that is critical to the success of QI programs.
- Many methods are used to monitor care and collect data for quality improvement (QI). HCOs must choose effective methods as they plan and implement their QI program.
- Measures/indicators are an important part of an HCO's QI program. They help identify the focus of QI efforts and are used to track progress.
- HCOs use utilization review/management to better understand conditions that impact the quality of care, such as use of nursing services, diagnoses, and length of treatment. Risk management is used to identify potential risk, such as financial loss, with the goal of mitigating or eliminating the risk in a timely, effective manner.

- Many methods are used to analyze care quality; however, root cause analysis is the most common method.
- A number of national initiatives address national healthcare measurement, mostly led by the Agency for Healthcare Research and Quality (AHRQ) but also by the Centers for Medicare and Medicaid Services (CMS). Examples of initiatives, which are influenced by the National Quality Strategy (NQS), are the CMS Quality Core Measures, Healthcare Effectiveness Data and Information Systems, patient safety organizations, Healthcare Effectiveness Data and Information Systems, *National Healthcare Quality and Disparities Reports*, AHRQ QI™, and the Healthcare Cost and Utilization Project.
- Nurses need to be involved in all aspects of QI measurement.

## Critical Thinking and Clinical Reasoning and Judgment: Discussion Questions and Learning Activities

1. Develop a comparison chart of the following: dashboard, check sheet, survey, interview, observation, run chart, Pareto chart, flowchart, benchmarking, and report card.
2. What are the advantages and disadvantages of mandatory and voluntary reporting? Do you think nursing students understand this issue and the need for them to report errors as students and then as registered nurses? Why or why not?
3. Compare and contrast the methods used to analyze quality: root cause analysis,

   fishbone analysis, FMEA, DMADV, gap analysis, brainstorming, and deep dive.
4. What is the nurse's role in CQI measurement?
5. The following link provides access to state-specific healthcare quality information, providing opportunity to compare states covering over 250 healthcare quality measures. Go to your state and compare with other states. What is the highest performing state? The lowest? https://www.ahrq.gov/data/state -snapshots.html

# Connect to Current Information

- CDC: *Morbidity and Mortality Weekly Reports*
  http://www.cdc.gov/mmwr/index.html
- Examples of flowchart templates
  https://www.google.com/search?q=
  flow+charts+templates&client= safari&sa
  =X&rls=en&biw=1324&bih=1019&tb-
  m=isch&tbo=u&  source=univ&ved=
  0ahUKEwiM8Pi_253KAhXGyyYKHTXoB-
  DIQsAQINg
- Examples of run charts
  http://www.bing.com/images/search?q=r
  un+chart&qpvt=run+chart&qpvt=run
  +chart&FORM=IGRE
- Examples of fishbone charts
  http://www.bing.com/images/search?q
  =fishbone+analysis&qpvt=Fishbone
  +analysis&qpvt=Fishbone+analysis&
  FORM=IGRE
- Examples of check/tally sheets
  https://www.google.com/search?q=tal-
  ly+sheets&client=safari&rls=en&tbm
  =isch&tbo=u&source=univ&sa=X&
  ved=0ahUKEwi-6JuFp_KAhVHLSY
  KHT9uAagQsAQIHA&biw=1324&bih
  =1019
- Examples of dashboards
  *Government dashboards*

- http://dashboard.healthit.gov/dashboards
  /dashboards.php
  *Nongovernment dashboards*
  https://www.google.com/search?q
  =health+care+dashboards&client=
  safari&rls=en&tbm=isch&tbo=u&-
  source=univ&sa=X&ved=0ahUKEwi-
  YuurT-5_KAhVEPiYKHe9dDTQQsA
  QITg&biw=1324&bih=1019
- Examples of value stream mapping
  https://www.google.com/search?q=val-
  ue+stream+mapping&client=safari&
  rls=en&tbm=isch&tbo=u&source=uni-
  v&sa=X&ved=0ahUKEwitmqHZ16z
  KAhUD4CYKHcC1AM0QsAQIRA&bi-
  w=1033&bih=1012
- AHRQ QI™
  http://www.qualityindicators.ahrq.gov
- AHRQ: QI™ Toolkit
  http://www.ahrq.gov/professionals/systems
  /hospital/qitoolkit/index.html
- AHRQ: National Quality Strategy (NQS)
  http://www.ahrq.gov/workingforquality
- AHRQ: Common Formats
  http://www.pso.ahrq.gov/common
- NCQA: Healthcare Effectiveness Data and
  Information Systems (HEDIS®)
  https://www.ncqa.org

## Connect to Text Current information with the Author

Go to the update for this text to review the Blog, QI News, and Literature Review. Access this regular
update at: http://nursing.jbpub.com/Finkelman/QualityImprovement/2e.

# EBP, EBM, and Quality Improvement: Exemplar

Umberfield, E., Ghaferi, A., Krein, S., &
Manoilovich, M. (2019). Using incident reports
to assess communication failures and patient
outcomes. *Joint Commission Journal Quality
Patient Safety, 46*(6), 406–413.

## Questions to Consider

1. What is the objective(s) of this study?
2. What is the study design and sample?
   Why is this type of design effective for
   this research problem?
3. What are the results of the study?
4. Discuss the implications of this
   study to nursing practice and quality
   improvement?

# EVOLVING CASE STUDY

As the nurse manager for the operating room service, you are meeting with the medical director, with whom you have worked for 5 years. You are both overwhelmed with routine work, and now you have to prepare a plan to address CQI in your department. Administration and the QI program recommend that you use the following AHRQ website, which provides a toolkit: http://www.ahrq.gov/professionals /systems/hospital/qitoolkit/index.html

## Case Questions

*After reviewing the toolkit, you both decide to focus on the two most common quality care problems your department experiences. You are now ready to address next steps with the information you have.*

**1.** Apply the AHRQ toolkit to your department and to the two focus areas of concern that you have identified.

**2.** Describe how you will engage the staff (clinical and nonclinical) in the new initiative.

# References

Adler, L., Denham, C., McKeever, M., Purunton, R., Guilloteau, F., Moorhead, D., & Resar, R. (2008). Global trigger tool: Implementation basics. *Journal of Patient Safety, 4*(4), 245–249.

Austin, J., Jha, A., Romano, P., Singer, S., Vogus, T., Wachter, R., & Pronovost, P. (2015). National hospital ratings systems share few common scores and may generate confusion instead of clarity. *Health Affairs, 34*(3), 423–430.

Barach, P., & Johnson, K. (2013). Assessing risk and harm in clinical microsystems. In W. Sollecito & J. Johnson (Eds.), *McLaughlin and Kaluzny's continuous quality improvement in health care* (4th ed., pp. 249–274). Burlington, MA: Jones & Bartlett Learning.

Benton, J., Arm, D., & Flynn, J. (2013). Identifying and minimizing risk exposures affecting nursing practice to enhance patient safety. *Journal of Nursing Regulation, 3*(4), 5–9.

Casey, D. (2006). Fundamentals of outcomes measurement. In D. Nash & N. Goldfarb (Eds.), *The quality solution* (pp. 93–113). Sudbury, MA: Jones & Bartlett Publishers.

Chassin, M., Loeb, J., Schmaltz, S., & Wachter, R. (2010). Accountability measures—Using measurement to promote quality improvement. *New England Journal of Medicine, 363*(7), 683–688.

Donabedian, A. (1980). *Explorations in quality assessment and monitoring, Volume 1: The definitions of quality and approaches to its assessment.* Ann Arbor, MI: Health Administration Press.

Duffey, P., Oliver, J., & Newcomb, P. (2019). Evaluating the use of high-reliability principles to increase error event reporting: A retrospective review. *JONA: Journal of Nursing Administration, 49* (6), 310–314.

Ettinger, W. (2005). Basic tools for quality improvement. In D. Nash & N. Goldfarb (Eds.), *The quality solution* (pp. 115–131). Sudbury, MA: Jones & Bartlett Publishers.

Evans, S., Berry, J., Smith, B., Esterman, A., Selim, P., O'Shaughnessy, J., & DeWit, M. (2006). Attitudes and barriers to incident reporting: A collaborative hospital study. *BMJ Quality Safety in Health Care, 15*, 39–43.

Finkelman, A. (2019). *Professional nursing concepts: Competencies for quality leadership* (4th ed.). Sudbury, MA: Jones & Bartlett Publishers.

Fisher, E., Staiger, D., Bynum, J., & Gottlieb, D. (2007). Creating accountable care organizations: The extended hospital medical staff. *Health Affairs, 26*(1), 44–57.

Gottlieb, J. (2006). Analyzing quality data. In D. Nash & N. Goldfarb (Eds.), *The quality solution* (pp. 73–92). Sudbury, MA: Jones & Bartlett Publishers.

Holland, D., Pacyna, J., Gillard, K., & Carter, L. (2016). Tracking discharge delays. Critical first step toward mitigating process breakdowns and inefficiencies. *Journal of Nursing Care Quality, 31*(1), 17–23.

Hughes, R. (2008). Chapter 44: Tools and strategies for quality improvement and patient safety. In R. Hughes (Ed.), *Patient safety and quality: An evidence-based handbook for nurses.* Rockville, MD: Agency for Healthcare Research and Quality. Retrieved from http://www .ncbi.nlm.nih.gov/books/NBK2682

Institute for Healthcare Improvement (IHI). (2015a). Introduction to trigger tools for identifying adverse events. Retrieved from http://www.ihi.org/resources /Pages/Tools/IntrotoTriggerToolsforIdentifyingAEs .aspx

Institute for Healthcare Improvement (IHI). (2015b). Improvement tip: Focus on harm, not errors. Retrieved from http://www.ihi.org/resources/Pages/ImprovementStories/ImprovementTipFocusonHarmNotErrors.aspx

Institute for Healthcare Improvement (IHI). (2016a). Introduction to trigger tools for identifying adverse events. Retrieved from http://www.ihi.org/resources/pages/tools/intrototriggertoolsforidentifyingaes.aspx

Institute for Healthcare Improvement (IHI). (2016b). IHI global trigger tool for measuring adverse events. Retrieved from http://www.ihi.org/resources/Pages/Tools/IHIGlobalTriggerToolforMeasuringAEs.aspx

Institute for Health Improvement (IHI). (2019a). Failure modes and effect analysis (FMEA) tool. Retrieved from http://www.ihi.org/resources/Pages/Tools/FailureModesandEffectsAnalysisTool.aspx

Institute for Healthcare Improvement (IHI). (2019b). Transforming care at the bedside: Overview. Retrieved from http://www.ihi.org/Engage/Initiatives/Completed/TCAB/Pages/default.aspx

Institute of Medicine (IOM). (1999). *To err is human.* Washington, DC: The National Academies Press.

Institute of Medicine (IOM). (2010). *The future of nursing: Leading change, advancing health.* Washington, DC: The National Academies Press.

iSixSigma. (2016a). DMAIC versus DMADV. Retrieved from https://www.isixsigma.com/new-to-six-sigma/design-for-six-sigma-dfss/dmaic-versus-dmadv/

iSixSigma. (2016b). Value stream mapping. Retrieved from http://www.isixsigma.com/tools-templates/value-stream-mapping

iSixSigma. (2019). Determine the root cause: 5 whys. Retrieved from https://www.isixsigma.com/tools-templates/cause-effect/determine-root-cause-5-whys

Jones, T. (2016). Outcome measurement in nursing: Imperatives, ideals, history, and challenges. *Online Journal of Nursing, 21*(2). Retrieved from http://ojin.nursingworld.org/MainMenuCategories/ANAMarketplace/ANAPeriodicals/OJIN/TableofContents/Vol-21-2016/No2-May-2016/Outcome-Measurement-in-Nursing.html

Kelly, D., Johnson, S., & Sollecito, W. (2013). Measurement, variation, and CQI tools. In W. Sollecito & J. Johnson (Eds.), *McLaughlin and Kaluzny's continuous quality improvement in health care* (4th ed., pp. 77–116). Burlington, MA: Jones & Bartlett Learning.

Keroack, M., & Rhinehart, E. (2013). The investigation and analysis of clinical incidents. In B. Youngberg (Ed.), *Patient safety handbook* (2nd ed., pp. 125–142). Burlington, MA: Jones & Bartlett Learning.

Kizer, K., & Stegun, M. (2014). Serious reportable adverse events in health care. In Agency for Healthcare Research and Quality (Ed.), *Advances in patient safety* (pp. 339–352). Retrieved from http://www.ncbi.nlm.nih.gov/books/NBK20598

Levinson, D. (2012). *Hospital incident reporting systems do not capture most patient harm.* Washington, DC: U.S. Department of Health and Human Services.

Li, J., Boulanger, B., Norton, J., Yates, A., Swartz, C., Smith, A., . . . Williams, M. (2015). "SWARMing" to improve patient care: A novel approach to root cause analysis. *Joint Commission Quality Patient Safety, 41*, 494–501.

Loresto, F., Welton, J., Grim, S., Valdez, C., & Eron, K. (2019). Exploring inpatient medication patterns. A big data and multilevel approach. *JONA: Journal of Nursing Administration, 49*(6), 336–342.

Mainz, J. (2003). Defining and classifying clinical indicators for quality improvement. *International Journal for Quality in Health Care.* Retrieved from https://academic.oup.com/intqhc/article/15/6/523/1823652. doi:http://dx.doi.org/10.1093/intqhc/mzg081

National Academy of Medicine (NAM). (2015). *Vital signs: Core measures for health and health care progress.* Washington, DC: The National Academies Press.

National Committee for Quality Assurance (NCQA). (2015). Databases used for health plan measures. Retrieved from https://www.ahrq.gov/talkingquality/measures/setting/health-plan/databases.html

National Patient Safety Foundation (NPSF). (2015). RCA[2] improving root cause analyses and actions to prevent harm. Retrieved from http://www.ihi.org/resources/Pages/Tools/RCA2-Improving-Root-Cause-Analyses-and-Actions-to-Prevent-Harm.aspx

National Quality Forum (NQF). (2019). ABCs of measurement. Retrieved from http://www.qualityforum.org/Measuring_Performance/ABCs_of_Measurement.aspx

Nelson-Brantley, H., Jenkins, P., & Chipps, E. (2019). Turning health systems data into actionable information. *JONA: Journal of Nursing Administration, 49*(4), 176–178.

Press Ganey. (2019). Capture nursing-specific measures. Retrieved from https://www.pressganey.com/solutions/clinical-excellence/capture-nursing-specific-measures

Regenstein, M. (2013). Understanding the first Institute of Medicine report and its impact on patient safety. In B. Youngberg (Ed.), *Patient safety handbook* (2nd ed., pp. 1–16). Burlington, MA: Jones & Bartlett Learning.

Rosen, A. (2010, November). Are we getting better at measuring patient safety? WebM&M, Agency for Healthcare Research and Quality. Retrieved from https://psnet.ahrq.gov/perspective/are-we-getting-better-measuring-patient-safety

Sadeghi, S., Barzi, A., Mikhail, O., & Shabot, M. (2012). *Integrating quality and strategy in healthcare organizations.* Burlington, MA: Jones & Bartlett Learning.

Shojania, K. (2015). In conversation with . . . Kaveh Shojania, MD. *Perspectives on Safety.* Retrieved from https://psnet.ahrq.gov/perspective/conversation-kaveh-shojania-md

Strome, T. (2013). *Healthcare analytics for quality and performance improvement.* Hoboken, NJ: John Wiley & Sons, Inc.

Sunshine, J., Meo, N., Kassebaum, N., Collison, M., Mokdad, A., & Naghavi, M. (2019). Association of adverse effects of medical treatment with mortality in the United States. *JAMA Network Open, 2*(1):e187041. doi:10.1001/jamanetworkopen.2018.7041

The Joint Commission. (2019). Quality check and quality reports. Retrieved from https://www.jointcommission.org/en/about-us/facts-about-the-joint-commission/quality-check-and-quality-reports/

U.S. Department of Health and Human Services (HHS), Agency for Healthcare Research and Quality (AHRQ). (2014). Part IV. Selecting quality and resource use measures. https://www.ahrq.gov/sites/default/files/publications/files/perfmeas.pdf

U.S. Department of Health and Human Services (HHS), Agency for Healthcare Research and Quality (AHRQ). (2015). Chartbook on effective treatment. Retrieved from https://www.ahrq.gov/research/findings/nhqrdr/chartbooks/effectivetreatment/index.html

U.S. Department of Health and Human Services (HHS), Agency for Healthcare Research and Quality (AHRQ). (2016). Toolkit for using the Quality Indicators™ Toolkit: Fact sheet. Retrieved from http://www.ahrq.gov/research/findings/factsheets/quality/qifactsheet/index.html

U.S. Department of Health and Human Services (HHS), Agency for Healthcare Quality and Research (AHRQ). (2019). Quality improvement and monitoring at your fingertips. Retrieved from http://www.qualityindicators.ahrq.gov

U.S. Department of Health and Human Services (HHS), Agency for Healthcare Research and Quality (AHRQ), Healthcare Cost and Utilizations Project (HCUP). (2019). National HCUP databases. Retrieved from https://www.hcup-us.ahrq.gov/databases.jsp

U.S. Department of Health and Human Services (HHS), Agency for Healthcare Research and Quality (AHRQ), Patient Safety Network (PSNet). (2019a). Detection of safety hazards. Retrieved from https://psnet.ahrq.gov/primer/detection-safety-hazards

U.S. Department of Health and Human Services (HHS), Agency for Healthcare Research and Quality (AHRQ), Patient Safety Network (PSNet). (2019b). Reporting patient safety events. Retrieved from https://psnet.ahrq.gov/primer/reporting-patient-safety-events

U.S. Department of Health and Human Services (HHS), Agency for Healthcare Research and Quality (AHRQ), Patient Safety Network (PSNet). (2019c). Alert fatigue. Retrieved from https://psnet.ahrq.gov/primer/alert-fatigue

U.S. Department of Health and Human Services (HHS), Agency for Healthcare Research and Quality (AHRQ), Patient Safety Network (PSNet). (2019d). Root cause analysis. Retrieved from https://psnet.ahrq.gov/primer/root-cause-analysis

U.S. Department of Health and Human Services (HHS), Agency for Healthcare Research and Quality (AHRQ), Patient Safety Network (PSNet). (2019e). Rethinking root cause analysis. Retrieved from https://psnet.ahrq.gov/perspective/rethinking-root-cause-analysis

U.S. Department of Health and Human Services (HHS), Agency for Healthcare Research and Quality (AHRQ), Patient Safety Organization (PSO). (2019a). Frequently asked questions. Retrieved from https://pso.ahrq.gov/faq

U.S. Department of Health and Human Services (HHS), Agency for Healthcare Research and Quality (AHRQ), Patient Safety Organization (PSO). (2019b). Common Formats. Retrieved from https://pso.ahrq.gov/common

U.S. Department of Health and Human Services (HHS), Centers for Medicare and Medicaid Services (CMS), Center for Clinical Standards and Quality. (2015). 2015 national impact assessment of the Centers for Medicare & Medicaid Services (CMS) quality measures report. Retrieved from https://www.cms.gov/Medicare/Quality-Initiatives-Patient-Assessment-Instruments/QualityMeasures/Downloads/2015-National-Impact-Assessment-Report.pdf

U.S. Department of Health and Human Services (HHS), Centers for Medicare and Medicaid Services (CMS). (2019). What's the CMS quality strategy? Retrieved from https://www.cms.gov/Medicare/Quality-Initiatives-Patient-Assessment-Instruments/Value-Based-Programs/CMS-Quality-Strategy

U.S. Department of Health and Human Services (HHS), Centers for Medicare and Medicaid Services (CMS). (2020). About the program. Retrieved from https://www.cms.gov/Medicare/Medicare-Fee-for-Service-Payment/sharedsavingsprogram/about

U.S. Department of Health and Human Services (HHS), Health Resources and Services Administration (HRSA). (2010). Quality improvement. Retrieved from http://www.hrsa.gov/quality/toolbox/508pdfs/qualityimprovement.pdf

U.S. Department of Health and Human Services (HHS), Health Resources and Services Administration (HRSA). (2011a). Developing and implementing a QI plan. Retrieved from https://www.hrsa.gov/sites/default/files/quality/toolbox/508pdfs/developingqiplan.pdf

U.S. Department of Health and Human Services (HHS), Health Resources and Services Administration (HRSA). (2011b). Performance management and measurement. Retrieved from http://www.hrsa.gov/quality/toolbox/508pdfs/performancemanagementandmeasurement.pdf

U.S. Department of Health and Human Services (HHS), Office of the Inspector General (OIG). (2010). Memo to Director of the Agency for Healthcare Research and Quality: Adverse events in hospitals: Public disclosure of information about events, OEI-06-09-00360.

Retrieved from http://oig.hhs.gov/oei/reports/oei-06-09-00360.pdf

Wachter, R. (2016, January 16). How measurement fails doctors and teachers. *New York Times*. Retrieved from https://www.nytimes.com/2016/01/17/opinion/sunday/how-measurement-fails-doctors-and-teachers.html

Wachter, R., & Gupta, K. (2018). *Understanding patient safety* (3rd ed.). New York, NY: McGraw Hill.

Waldren, S. (2016, January 28). Uncertain future of meaningful use. Retrieved from https://www.aafp.org/news/opinion/20160128guestedmu.html

# Ensuring the Healthcare Environment Is Focused on Quality

| | |
|---|---|
| *Alice:* | **"Would you tell me, please, which way I ought to go from here?"** |
| *The Cheshire Cat:* | **"That depends a good deal on where you want to get to."** |
| *Alice:* | **"I don't much care where."** |
| *The Cheshire Cat:* | **"Then, it doesn't matter which way you go."** |
| *Alice:* | **"So long as I get SOMEWHERE," Alice added as an explanation.** |
| *The Cheshire Cat:* | **"Oh, you're sure to do that, if only you walk long enough."** |

Lewis Carroll, *Alice's Adventures in Wonderland (1865)*

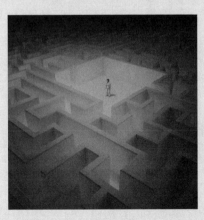

The goal of the quality improvement maze is to reach a state of quality care. As you find your way to the end of the maze, you need to care about your roles and responsibilities as a nurse in the healthcare environment that need major improvement. Just being present is not enough. You need to care and engage in continuous quality improvement and operate with direction.

## CHAPTER 11

# Creating and Sustaining Quality Care: Prevention of Quality Care Problems

## CHAPTER OBJECTIVES

At the conclusion of this chapter, the learner will be able to:

- Critique methods used to prevent or reduce quality care problems.
- Analyze the role of teamwork and the team in continuous quality improvement.
- Explain the relationship of technology and informatics in continuous quality improvement.
- Examine the multiple roles and responsibilities of nurses in preventing or reducing quality care problems.

## OUTLINE

## KEY TERMS

Bar-code medication
    administration
Call-out
Case management
Check-back
Checklist
Clinical guideline
Coaching
Comprehensive Unit-based
    Safety Program (CUSP)
Clinical decision support (CDS)
Computerized physician/
    provider order entry (CPOE)
Crew resource management
    (CRM)
Disease management

Early warning system
Electronic health record (EHR)
Electronic medical record
    (EMR)
Health informatics technology
    (HIT)
Huddle
Interoperability
Meaningful use
Medication reconciliation
Mentoring
Patient-centered rounds
Patient safety primer
Personal health record (PHR)
Policies
Procedure

Rapid response teams (RRTs)
Read-back
Safe zone
Safety walkarounds
Sensemaking
Signout
Situation-background-
    assessment-
    recommendation
Spread
Standard
Teach-back
TeamSTEPPS®
Time-out
Universal Protocol
Workflow

# Introduction

This chapter concludes the content on the measurement process used in quality improvement (QI) programs. It is easy to view continuous quality improvement (CQI) only as a process to collect data and then, through analysis, to determine the status of care quality; however, if staff stop the process here, then care is unlikely to improve. What healthcare organizations (HCOs) do with this information to make changes when needed to improve care must be planned and implemented. These approaches may be directed at preventing or reducing errors and quality problems, applied in response to situations in which errors or problems occur, and then used to prevent future similar situations. Some of the methods discussed in this chapter are also included in other chapters, as they may be used for several purposes during the measurement process. In addition to critiquing examples of methods used to accomplish this goal, this chapter examines some of the nurse's roles and responsibilities in preventing or reducing quality care problems. **Figure 11-1** describes a process map of performance management, providing a summary of content that has been described in other chapters. In this chapter, the focus is on steps 5 to 6b in the process map.

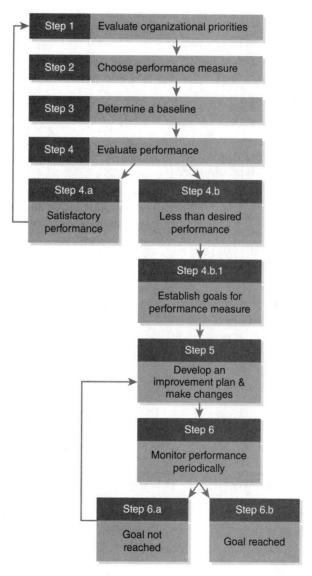

**Figure 11-1** Process Map of Performance Management Pathway

Reproduced from U.S. Department Health and Human Services & Health Resources and Services Administration. (2011, April). Performance management and measurement. Retrieved from http://www.hrsa.gov/quality/toolbox/508pdfs/ performancemanagementandmeasurement.pdf

# Examples of Methods to Prevent or Reduce Quality Care Problems

QI programs can be viewed from multiple perspectives. The most common one, and the perspective focused on throughout most of this text, is a QI program that is developed, implemented, and evaluated within an HCO. In addition, there are broader perspectives, state and national perspectives, and even a global perspective. An important aspect of CQI is sustainability, which comprises maintaining CQI by developing strategies and changes to improve care. **Figure 11-2** describes factors that influence successful CQI implementation within an HCO.

**Spread**, or actively disseminating best practice and knowledge gained from the CQI process so that individual HCOs can apply them, is an important part of application at the state and national levels (Institute for Healthcare Improvement [IHI], 2013). Steps involved in a spread plan include the following (U.S. Department of Health and Human Services [HHS], Health Resources and Services Administration [HRSA], 2011a):

- List changes to be spread.
- Evaluate new system against current system. Process mapping is helpful and identifies key differences; these are the areas that the spread team will focus on to make changes.
- Discuss potential impact or challenges that might result from adopting the redesigned system and developing a plan to manage those impacts.
- Create an action plan to make the changes and describe how you will capture information to monitor. Identify those areas you can just change and those areas where it might be better to test changes using methods such as plan-do-study-act methodology. (pp. 15–16)

Spread can lead to consideration of other changes necessary for additional improvement. The CQI team needs to consider what is needed to support spread—to hardwire or ensure that the improvement is part of the work environment and practice. Factors that may be important, although they vary with the improvement focus, are staff levels and mix, expertise, staff roles and responsibilities, staff training, supplies and equipment, health informatics, policies and procedures, organizational structure and culture, management, and so on.

After CQI problems are identified and analyzed, decisions are made about interventions or strategies to resolve or prevent

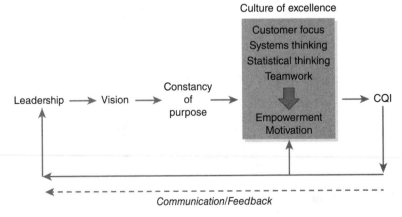

**Figure 11-2** Factors Influencing Successful CQI Implementation

problems. Development of an implementation plan is discussed in more detail in other chapters, but it is also relevant here. The focus is on best practice, which is identified by using gap analysis—what is wrong and how it can best be corrected using available evidence (evidence-based practice [EBP] and evidence-based management [EBM]). The plan includes details about actions or tasks that are needed, team member assignment to tasks, target completion date, tracking of the actual completion date, communication and/or training required with target dates and then actual dates of completion, implementation start date, and comments about completion of implementation and evaluation of outcomes (HHS, Agency for Healthcare Research and Quality [AHRQ], 2019a).

## Healthcare Organization and Professional Methods

HCOs and healthcare professions are concerned about CQI and use various strategies to engage in CQI and improve care. Some of these methods are done in collaboration with others, and some focus either on the HCO or a profession. The Connect to Current Information section at the end of this chapter provides links to sites that provide further information or examples for some of the methods described.

### Redesigning Systems and Processes

When an HCO recognizes that it has sufficient CQI problems, it may decide to undergo a redesign or transformation to improve. This situation involves the HCO and healthcare professions within the organization, as well as other staff. Some of the common factors that might indicate the need for this step include the following (Gabow, Eisert, Karkhanis, Knight, & Dickson, 2005):

- Little application of knowledge from other industries

- Enormous redundancies in care delivery processes
- Numerous patient handoffs
- Major workforce shortages
- Employee dissatisfaction
- Limited involvement of the patients and their families in hospital care
- Patient dissatisfaction (p. 3)

Redesigning the system and processes requires detailed assessment to ensure that the HCO or a specific unit in the HCO is ready to handle change, develop the description of the design or change required and structure for the redesign process, implement data collection, use effective tools to analyze the data and methods to facilitate the change, and continue to evaluate in a consistent manner. This then becomes a change cycle.

According to the AHRQ (HHS, AHRQ, 2015a): "**Workflow** is the sequence of physical and mental tasks performed by various people within and between work environments." When you think about workflow, you need to consider that workflow happens in a variety of situations, such as within a unit, clinic, department, or HCO; between HCOs, between healthcare providers and teams, and between a healthcare provider and a patient (before, during, and after an encounter); and as you think about your work, the workflow often occurs unconsciously. These instances of workflow may occur sequentially or simultaneously. Informatics has a critical role in workflow, and changes to improve workflow often involve use of informatics. Understanding the workflow process may lead to a better understanding of multiple aspects of care delivery. Often workflow is oversimplified and not considered a critical factor in CQI; however, it is important. The AHRQ website includes tools for assessing and improving workflow.

Staffing is another factor, and it has been discussed in this text. There is much literature about the need for levels of staffing that provide an effective work environment, reduce nurse fatigue and burnout, and provide nurse–patient time that reduces "rushing" and limits time with patients. Patient satisfaction and reaching patient outcomes have also been connected to staffing. Potter and colleagues (2014) discuss the complexity of meeting staffing needs: "Certainly understaffing is a threat to patient safety. However, merely increasing the number of RNs on a patient care unit may not be a panacea if the environment in which RNs work is not conducive to clinical decision-making. Better understanding is needed with respect to the conditions in an acute care environment that affect clinical decision-making" (pp. 49–50). Understanding workflow and its impact on staffing is a critical component of improving work processes. These authors anticipate greater research into staffing needs in the future: "The research team will conduct additional observations . . . so that sufficient data can be compiled to examine the association between cognitive shifts, interruptions, cognitive load, and the incidence of errors and omissions in care. Further work is also needed to explore the relationship of variables such as nurse experience, type of clinical specialty setting, and delivery of care models with clinical decision-making patterns" (p. 50).

## Position Descriptions and Performance Appraisal

HCOs use position descriptions to provide clear descriptions of position responsibilities and requirements to maintain a position, but these descriptions also must support expected care needs that staff must provide for quality care and a positive work environment. To provide greater support for staff engagement in CQI, CQI responsibilities should be included in all position descriptions for clinical and nonclinical staff. The position description is the first place where the organization demonstrates its commitment to CQI to new employees. During hiring, CQI should be discussed, such as asking about the applicant's viewpoint

of CQI and experience with CQI and at the same time providing an opportunity to discuss the relevance of CQI to the HCO and the position responsibilities. This theme is carried through to orientation, both HCO orientation and specific orientation activities per unit assigned and the new employee position.

Performance appraisal is directly related to the HCO's QI program. Using surveys, the HCO performance appraisal form, and individual interviews, performance appraisal can be an important source of CQI data. Performance appraisal includes an evaluation form to ensure that the staff are consistently evaluated using the same questions. Recording of this information from the interview may be useful in identifying needs. Self-assessment is also important as it allows staff to identify where they stand at the time of their performance evaluation, and it also helps staff improve their self-assessment skills as they provide direct care; when staff members work, they need to continually assess their own performance. Regular self-evaluation has an important impact on CQI in practice, with staff using critical thinking and clinical reasoning and judgment to prevent problems while they provide care.

First, through establishing position requirements, the expectation of staff engagement in CQI is clear. This is then discussed in performance appraisal—annual and ongoing. Staff need to consider how they have participated in CQI when they complete their self-appraisal, and then the supervisor and employee should discuss this responsibility, adding comments about appraisal of CQI participation. This assessment should not be a "blame" session but rather a constructive discussion.

The QI program also uses aggregate information from performance appraisal. For example, a nurse manager should summarize staff performance appraisal information after completing annual reviews. The results should be in aggregate form rather than containing individual identifiers. As the nurse manager assesses the unit staff involvement in CQI, the following questions might be considered: What CQI activities are staff involved in? How many staff members are involved in CQI, and how many are not? What are the barriers to participation reported by staff? What makes it easier for staff to participate in CQI? Is the staff familiar with the unit's CQI data? What does the staff think are the most critical CQI problems on the unit? What has improved in the past year? Does the staff think they are getting sufficient and clear updates about CQI? Are there methods that should be used to increase this communication, and if so, what methods? This type of aggregate information can then be combined across the HCO to provide important organization-wide CQI data, but efforts should not stop with data sharing—steps need to be taken to change and improve. During performance appraisal, the supervisor and employee should work out a specific plan for employee engagement in CQI or improvement in this area of practice.

### Clinical Ladder

Clinical ladders have been used in HCOs for some time. They are used to recognize clinical and professional competence and provide support for career advancement (Donley & Flaherty, 2008). This HCO approach recognizing staff competency and contributions to the HCO is primarily focused on direct-care or bedside nurses, addressing the concern that there is an overemphasis on management and promotion to management positions. Staff members who participate in clinical ladders need to demonstrate competencies and provide examples, often referred to as a portfolio. How does this relate to CQI? In this process nurses need to include CQI activities as one aspect of professional activities. Using a ladder assists HCOs in emphasizing CQI as a staff responsibility and pushes staff to actively participate in the development of strategies to prevent or respond to quality care concerns.

### Policies and Procedures

HCO **policies** and **procedures** serve many purposes, and most of them are connected to CQI. Policies and procedures clarify important communication and consistent processes within an HCO—to ensure care quality, consistency, and other objectives. They also help to communicate critical concerns with the expectation that staff will follow them. Changes in policies and procedures must be communicated to staff in a timely manner, and often the changes are driven by CQI needs. For example, during root cause analysis of medication errors, it was noted that the documentation procedure steps were not clear. This then led to a change in the medication administration documentation procedure, but staff must be informed about changes and then apply the changes. HCOs now use evidence to support policies and procedures whenever best evidence is available, and evidence may also drive changes in current policies and procedures.

### Evidence-Based Practice Requirements and Influence on Standardization of Care

EBP is discussed in many sections of this text. Best practice not only impacts policies and procedures but also implementation of care and, ideally, CQI activities and initiatives (e.g., assisting in identifying measures/indicators that are based on evidence). EBP and evidence-based management (EBM) improve clinical and management decision making, and they have an impact on CQI. As nurses get involved in EBP/EBM and reviewing evidence, they learn more about effective care and apply this evidence to their practice and to management in the HCO.

### Standards

As discussed in this text, standards are important to healthcare professionals, accreditors, government agencies, and HCOs. Standards are guides and should be based on best evidence. Some **standards** focus on professional issues such as competence, and others focus on patient care by identifying practice expectations. HCOs use standards that are developed by external sources such as the American Nurses Association (ANA), but they also develop their own standards, which should not conflict with critical professional or government standards. Standards then guide care, and thus they have an impact on the quality of care and should be considered during the CQI process, as they are methods for reducing quality care problems or responding to them.

## Clinical Guidelines and Protocols

*Clinical Practice Guidelines We Can Trust* (IOM, 2011) is an important report that examines the need for developing and using effective clinical guidelines. A **clinical guideline** is a written description of care for a specific patient population and should be based on best evidence whenever possible. It acts as a guide for staff; however, the guidelines should not be used automatically without careful assessment of individual patient needs, recognizing that recommendations may need to be adapted. Clinical protocols are similar to guidelines but typically are described in a chart so that the information is easy to review and use. The protocol identifies expected assessment data, actual and potential problems, interventions, timelines, outcomes, and responsibilities (Finkelman, 2019). Using clinical guidelines or protocols provides a consistent approach that has been reviewed by experts based on evidence. These tools can assist in supporting effective care. Data on the use of guidelines and adaptions can then be used in assessing quality, and they can be used to track expected outcomes to determine if they were met and also applied as a strategy to improve.

## Patient Safety Primers

**Patient safety primers** are evidence-based sources of information about patient safety available on the AHRQ website (HHS, AHRQ, PSNet, 2019a). These primers are an example of government-sponsored CQI resources that are easy to access and use. HCOs need current information for their staff as they develop, implement, and evaluate their QI programs and make changes to prevent and/or resolve CQI problems.

## Case Management

The purpose of **case management** is to get the right services to patients when needed with the goal of avoiding fragmented and unnecessary care (Finkelman, 2011). Key elements of case management are coordination and collaboration. Case managers work with individual patients, typically patients with complex needs (e.g., chronic illness). Lack of coordination and collaboration is a barrier to effective care and meeting expected outcomes, thus impacting quality care. Case management may then be a strategy used to improve care.

## Disease Management

**Disease management** services are used to better ensure patient-centered care and have an impact on quality care (Finkelman, 2019). Typically, third-party payers implement these services and then collaborate with HCOs to ensure coordinated care for patients with complex needs, such as chronic illness (e.g., diabetes, cardiac conditions, cancer, arthritis, respiratory conditions). These services focus on prevention, early detection and diagnosis, treatment, and care management, including self-management. Health literacy is an important factor for patients receiving disease management services and is discussed in other chapters.

## Patient Flow Management

Common complaints from patients relate to patient flow—for example, "I have to wait in the emergency room to go to radiology or to get a room in the hospital"; "My surgery was delayed. I do not know why but I am still waiting"; and "The paperwork for my discharge is not ready, so I cannot leave." Patient flow is how patients move through the healthcare system, which is a very complex system. Why is this problem important?

- Decreases patient satisfaction
- Impacts treatment, which may be delayed or inadequate
- Reduces effective handoffs, which increases risk of errors
- Increases staff stress
- Increases staff time
- Increases costs

The Joint Commission identifies problems with patient flow, and it has developed a standard related to patient flow that must be followed by Joint Commission–accredited hospitals, which applies to most hospitals (NEJM Catalyst, 2018). HCOs must examine causes for patient flow problems and develop strategies to resolve them (Rutherford, Provost, Kotagal, Luther, & Anderson, 2017). Common points of cause are the admission process; discharge process; emergency room (availability of treatment areas and staff and then, if required, need to transfer); and patient care services availability, such as radiology, laboratory, and patient transportation. When addressing this problem, HCOs must be recognized as systems—with emphasis on the right patient, right time, right treatment, and right setting.

## Quality Improvement Committee

HCO committee structure typically includes a QI committee that works closely with the HCO's QI program. These committees of staff and management representatives carry major responsibility for guiding the development, implementation, and evaluation of the QI program. The committee participates in all levels of CQI planning: strategic, operational, and individual CQI projects. The committee should

meet all HCO committee requirements, such as size, selection of chairperson, documentation of minutes, meeting schedule, reports, and so on. Committee membership should be representative of management; clinical staff, including a variety of healthcare professionals; medical records; admission/discharge; utilization review and risk management; health informatics; financial; staff education; and, when possible, community representatives.

HCOs use different titles for committees, and QI committees are no exception—for example, the Patient Safety Committee may go by different names, such as the Environment of Care Committee or a Quality Care Committee may include safety. The goal is to ensure a patient environment and a work environment that are safe and allow healthcare providers to function effectively. An HCO may choose to use a broader term—"quality" rather than "safety"—and many HCOs do this, as safety is a dimension of quality care.

## Utilization Review/ Management Committee

As mentioned in this text, utilization review is a rich source of data about patients and services. Some HCOs have a committee (staff and management) that assists utilization review staff in the work they do to collect data, but it is more important that the committee may assist in analyzing the data and ensuring that data and the analysis are shared and used for multiple CQI purposes. This committee is not only a source of data and analysis, but it also makes decisions that impact improvement—changes and strategies to prevent errors or resolve CQI problems related to utilization. For example, the utilization review committee might note that data indicate there are long waits for admission from the emergency department to inpatient units; however, its work should not stop there. The committee might then propose changes in the admission process to reduce this wait time—basing its recommendations on the analysis of the data and causes. In doing this, the committee demonstrates how it is part of the measurement process, and it also participates at the next level in the CQI process: intervention.

### Staff Education

This text discusses the importance of staff education. Staff competence has a direct impact on care. The ANA standards (ANA, 2010) emphasize the need for structured staff education that is based on evidence-based standards. Staff education includes orientation and all ongoing staff education. To improve care, staff education specialists need to work with HCO management staff and the QI committee to assist in identifying care needs, problems, and errors. Often staff education is the intervention chosen to improve care in response to a CQI problem; however, it is important that lack of education or competence be identified as a cause through analysis methods. It is too easy to just say, "Provide an education program to staff and the problem will be solved." Staff education specialists have a lot of contact with staff in many areas of the HCO, and their observations and interactions with staff can provide additional information about CQI. This input expands understanding of processes and CQI concerns and may be helpful in assessing outcomes for changes that are implemented to prevent errors or resolve CQI problems. In addition, staff education programs include support interventions to improve care, and staff education specialists work with staff throughout the HCO to improve care and staff engagement in CQI—for example, an education program on a new medication procedure may be provided for the nursing staff. Then staff education specialists may work with staff on the units as they apply the new procedure to support application of learning.

### Mentoring and Coaching

**Mentoring** is using a role model to assist in career development. A staff member may select a mentor for career guidance. **Coaching** is another related method used to provide career guidance and support. To be effective, it should be ongoing, and the coach should have the necessary expertise and knowledge to provide useful guidance to a nurse. A supervisor may be viewed as a coach, whereas a mentor is not a supervisor. The coach provides constructive feedback, and this then provides informal performance appraisal with self-assessment. Both of these methods include setting goals and working toward meeting them with a guide (mentor or coach). Why are mentoring and coaching related to CQI? Since both focus on improvement and advancement, they impact individual staff performance and thus impact CQI. Those who act as mentors and coaches should include discussion of CQI responsibilities and QI knowledge and competencies to assist in developing CQI competencies and engagement in CQI.

## Structured Communication Methods

As CQI needs became more important, it became clear that communication problems are a major cause of quality care concerns and errors. Understanding the need to improve communication by making it more structured and consistent led to methods and strategies to prevent errors or resolve CQI problems. Healthcare delivery systems turned to other industries, such as aviation, to adopt some methods and also developed new approaches. Typically, an HCO adopts several structured communication methods, and staff are trained in their use and then expected to apply the method(s).

### Checklists

Gawande (2010) identifies two reasons why healthcare providers may fail. The first reason is we do not know enough. Science is not clear, and so we have a partial understanding. Second, we fail due to ineptitude, or we have the knowledge but apply it incorrectly. These reasons may focus on individuals, but it is important to recognize that they have system implications. Development of knowledge is not just an individual responsibility. Not applying knowledge correctly can be due to individual staff problems, such as not keeping up with current information; not following recommendations, such as procedure requirements; and other personal reasons, such as stress and work overload, but there are also system issues. These issues might be failure of the HCO to provide sufficient information or to do so in a timely fashion, lack of staff education, inadequate staff to handle a change or the job that needs to be done, or lack of HCO knowledge of need to change. Gawande offers a simple and effective tool for reducing errors: "We need a different strategy for overcoming failure, one that builds on experience and takes advantage of the knowledge people have but somehow also makes up for our inevitable human inadequacies. And there is such a strategy—though it will seem almost ridiculous in its simplicity, maybe even crazy to those of us who have spent years carefully developing ever more advanced skills and technologies. It is a checklist" (p. 13).

A **checklist** is "an algorithmic listing of actions to be performed in a given clinical setting" (HHS, AHRQ, PSNet, 2019b). Checklists are used in a variety of ways in HCOs to reduce errors. The purpose is to make sure all steps are followed in the expected order and then to document this process. A checklist provides a consistent method of checking to make sure what needs to be done is done in a consistent, standardized way; the list helps with memory recall. As discussed in other chapters, checklists may also be used to collect data, but in this chapter we consider the checklist as a tool that helps staff focus on the required tasks to ensure greater quality care, thus reducing risk of errors.

Why does the checklist work? Research indicates that for many tasks, we operate reflexively or on "autopilot," or we use attentional behavior, which requires problem solving and planning. For some tasks, lack of concentration, distraction and disruptions, fatigue, and stress may lead us to slips or failure to complete the task. When this happens, error risk increases. So no matter how many times one has done a procedure, the checklist should be followed. The expectation is that everyone will follow the standardized checklist, all the steps in the order identified. The list should be developed by stakeholders and agreed upon for effective use. Checklists do not relieve staff of using critical thinking and clinical reasoning and judgment to ensure an effective discharge process.

The checklist is simple and requires limited, if any, training to use, but implementing checklists is not a simple process. Even though physicians may be pushed by physician leaders to use checklists (such as Atul Gawande, a surgeon), it is not easy to get staff, particularly physicians, to do this routinely. Gawande noticed that nurses used a variety of checklists, such as on rounds, and this tool kept order during rounds, or they used a checklist for a procedure to ensure that all steps were completed. Aviation uses checklists for its pilots and staff on planes, and they are also used to check the mechanical status of the plane. These practices led healthcare entities to consider use of checklists. The danger in healthcare is that some assume that the use of a checklist is equivalent to teamwork and team communication, and it is not (Shojania, 2015).

The staff need to understand the purpose of the checklist, its content, and how it may or may not affect other aspects of care. The checklist should be based on the steps in the focused procedure or action and should correspond with what is expected and realistic. Leadership must ensure that the work culture expects use of checklists and must discuss the impact on patient outcomes by providing current data for staff. When the checklist is not used, this must be addressed. Data about use and errors that might occur are valuable in understanding the CQI process and care, and they can then be used to plan and implement appropriate changes in care. A checklist is not just a tool; it is also a method to better understand processes, communication, and teamwork. This information should then be used to improve practice and outcomes.

There are two considerations for surgical checklists: (1) Do they make a difference in care quality? (2) Are they used as recommended (compliance)? A study examined compliance by using remote video auditing with real-time feedback (Overdyk, 2015). In the groups that used the auditing, there were improved rates of sign-ins, time-outs, and sign-outs. As a result of this study and other related work, the AHRQ notes that if used during surgery, this type of auditing can make a difference and should be used (Xiao, Mackenzie, & Seagull, 2015). Another problem with checklists is checklist fatigue; it becomes routine and done by rote. When thought is left out, staff may miss something important (Lyons & Popejoy, 2017). Requiring use of checklists does not ensure that they will be used or that they will reduce all errors. This is similar to long-term problems with hand-washing compliance; just requiring it does not mean it will be done or done effectively.

## Situation-Background-Assessment-Recommendation

What types of communication do nurses and physicians primarily learn and use (Narayan, 2013)? Physicians tend to use a communication style that focuses on prioritizing and lists, which appears to apply critical thinking more than does the nurse's approach of using timeline-descriptive narrative as the focus of communication. Due to these differences, there can be clashes in how communication proceeds and what is communicated or not communicated. As mentioned in this text, disruptive behavior or incivility between nurses and physicians is influenced by communication. Nurses frequently have to make decisions about when to ask for more assistance and also when to contact the physician. Given differences in how communication may be conducted, consideration

must be given to how communication can be improved to prevent problems in teamwork and QI. One recommendation is to use more structured, clear communication methods, such as **situation-background-assessment-recommendation** (SBAR or ISBAR). Use of this type of communication method typically leads to more "efficient communication that promotes effective collaboration, improves patient outcomes, and increases patient satisfaction with care" and reduces interprofessional communication problems (Narayan, 2013, p. 507). The SBAR/ISBAR elements include the following:

- **I**ntroduction (who you are)
- **S**ituation (what is going on with the patient)
- **B**ackground (information that is critical to better understand the situation)
- **A**ssessment (what you think is the problem)
- **R**ecommendation (what you would do to solve the problem)

SBAR also includes callouts and check-backs. In a **call-out**, important information is communicated to the team so that all team members hear the same information at the same time, reducing the chance of miscommunication or some team members not hearing the same information. A **check-back** occurs when the team is asked if they heard the information and understood it.

Nurses are involved in many of the situations in which SBAR could improve communication and quality of care (Haig, Sutton, & Whittington, 2006). Effective use of SBAR requires understanding, along with training of management and staff committed to its use. Care delivery is complex, and many issues arise at the same time, such as complex patient needs; need for supplies, equipment, and medications; documentation requirements; changing staffing and team composition; emergencies that might occur; and typical workday stress and possible problems with coworkers. These dynamics impact how difficult it might

---

**Exhibit 11-1** SBAR Example

---

This is an example of how SBAR might be used to focus a telephone call between a nurse and a physician. The nurse would not wait for the physician to ask these questions but rather would routinely provide the information in clear statements as indicated by SBAR.

**Situation:** *What is going on with the patient?*
   A nurse finds a patient on the floor. She calls the doctor: "I am the charge nurse on the night shift on 5 West. I am calling about Mrs. Jones. She was found on the floor and is complaining of pain in her hip."

**Background:** *What is the clinical background or context?*
   "The patient is a 75-year-old woman who was admitted for pneumonia yesterday. She did not complain of hip pain before being found on the floor."

**Assessment:** *What do I think the problem is?*
   "I think the fall may have caused an injury. Her pain is level 8 out of 10."

**Recommendation:** *What would I do to correct it or respond to it?*
   "I think she needs to be seen tonight by the orthopedic resident."

---

be to improve communication and maintain effective communication. Using an approach, such as SBAR, can help with this process.

What should you do as a nurse before you initiate SBAR in a given situation (Narayan, 2013)? You need to consider the patient situation, consider data you have or need, and use critical thinking and clinical reasoning and judgment in the process. Since part of the SBAR is sharing critical information about the patient, it is important to be clear about the information before initiating SBAR. Then you must decide if the situation is emergent (a developing situation), urgent (requiring quick response), or routine; review the patient record and compare data; and organize the information in a concise manner in the SBAR format. This information includes primary data or information about the patient's situation that is critical for the physician or other healthcare provider (e.g., nurse, advanced practice registered nurse [APRN]) to know and is directly related to the reason for the communication. Secondary data, which represent information that may not be directly related to the specific situation but are to be considered in your analysis, are also important.

SBAR communication content should be concise; it should take about 60 seconds to state it. In the first 10 seconds, it is important to get the attention of the physician or APRN to make your point. Nurses tend to use the initial contact to explain or apologize for the contact, which is typically a phone call, although it may be done in person. This approach may lead to the person who is called not listening to the rest of the message—the important parts. The SBAR step that may cause problems for the nurse calling is recommendations, something that many nurses do not feel comfortable doing or may not know how to do effectively. However, it is critical that the nurse use analysis and provide recommendations based on the nurse's work with patients and share knowledge of patients and experiences in patient care. **Exhibit 11-1** provides an SBAR example.

## CUS

When nurses are concerned that their message is not getting across, the CUS method can be used to assist in thinking through communication before trying to communicate a message. CUS is a mnemonic for the following (Leonard, Graham, & Bonacum, 2004, p. 185):

- **C**: I am *concerned* because . . .
- **U**: I am *uncomfortable* because . . .
- **S**: The *safety* of the patient is at risk because . . .

This type of method, which provides a consistent communication framework, can easily be taught to staff, but there should be discussion about the situations in which it might be used.

## Time-out

A **time-out** is a method used to stop work or care when the staff is concerned there is risk or an error has occurred. HCOs that actively use time-outs have a designated procedure to follow, and all staff should know about the procedure. Typically, any staff member may call a time-out. A common situation in which a time-out is used is in surgery—for example, when using the Universal Protocol for Preventing Wrong Site, Wrong Procedure, or Wrong Person Surgery.

## Crew Resource Management

**Crew resource management (CRM)** is a system that is used in aviation and has been applied to HCOs. CRM focuses on leadership, interprofessional communication, and effective decision making. It uses all available resources, emphasizes a no-blame culture, and focuses on clear, comprehensive standard operating procedures (HHS, AHRQ, 2015b). CRM can improve the CQI culture within an organization, but it is not an approach that solves problems quickly, nor is it a method that is used alone to improve care.

## Signout

The Joint Commission requires that its accredited HCOs use a standardized method for communication during handoffs, with individual HCOs identifying the method their staff will use. **Signout is one such method that might be used during** patient transfer handoffs. It is the transmission of information about the patient. As discussed in other chapters, checklists may also be used to collect data, but in this chapter, the checklist is considered to be a tool that helps staff focus on the required tasks to ensure greater quality care,

reducing risk of errors. HCOs should have protocols that describe how the signout should be done. Standardizing this communication better ensures more effective written and verbal signouts or more effective transfers. The environment for this communication should be one of limited interruptions and noise so that staff can focus. I-PASS is one standardized method used for signout. It includes the following (HHS, AHRQ, PSNet, 2015):

- *Illness severity.* One-word summary of the patient acuity, such as stable, unstable, observe
- *Patient summary.* Brief summary of the patient's diagnoses and treatment plan
- *Action list.* To-do items to be completed by the healthcare provider receiving the input
- *Situation awareness and contingency plans.* Directions to follow in case of changes in the patient's status, often in an "if-then" format
- *Synthesis by receiver.* An opportunity for the receiver of the message to ask questions and confirm the plan of care

## Read-Backs and Huddles

A **read-back** occurs when staff members repeat written or oral information—for example, the nurse repeats an order back to a physician to make sure the information is correct, and then the physician must confirm the information. A **huddle** is used to call a team or group of staff together to discuss a critical concern. It is a short meeting with staff focusing on a specific issue; it can be scheduled or unscheduled. HCOs should have a protocol for how and when these methods should be used. Huddles usually include a huddle sheet (checklist or worksheet). The unscheduled huddle may be used when any staff member wants to address a concern or review what needs to be done or has been done with the team. A read-back may be part of the huddle. These brief meetings should be efficient and to the point. A huddle supports CQI by identifying potential risk, near misses, or other quality problems, providing time for staff to discuss what should be done (i.e., actions), and read-back ensures that information is clearly exchanged to avoid errors and missed information.

### Change-of-Shift Reports

The nurses' work environment is complex and disorganized, involving multiple staff and other people (patients, family, visitors)—an environment that is high risk for errors. Shift reports are structured methods for exchanging information about the patients and the unit when staff are coming in and going out. It is an extremely important time for handoffs. As noted in this text, these reports may use a variety of methods or combination of methods, such as face-to-face interaction with the unit staff, the team, or individual staff in a meeting format; rounds with exchange of information in verbal and written form; and/or recorded communication. Failure to share information affects consistent care, knowledge of patient status, errors and near misses, and patient satisfaction. Shift report may also be a time to identify CQI concerns and actions that must be taken. Other information may also be shared, such as a change in a procedure or a clinical guideline that would make a difference in care provided. Improving shift reports is an important CQI strategy and not just a method to get more CQI data.

### Whiteboards

Whiteboards may seem like an unusual topic for a text on QI, but they are a simple, effective method to provide structured communication. Units use them to share critical information for staff, such as staff assignments. It is important to consider patient privacy factors when placing the whiteboards for staff access and the type of data included on the board. Information included may ensure that staff know whom to contact about individual patients and may provide other unit information. Some units have whiteboards in patient rooms to note information that the patient may need. If this is used, the information must be current, easy for the patient to read, and staff should consider patient privacy and confidentiality when adding information to the whiteboard.

### Staff Meetings

Staff meetings are held in various parts of HCOs routinely—for example, they may occur at the level of a unit, a particular department or service, or the HCO as a whole. These meetings offer many opportunities to support and engage in CQI, which should be a routine agenda item. Sharing information to update staff increases consistency and reduces staff stress due to not knowing current information; both of these factors can limit quality, interfering with effective work. These meetings are also opportunities to identify successes (improvement) and to identify problems. Staff might analyze the problem and move to solutions or set up a process for this to occur. Minutes from meetings provide documentation about issues, problems, solutions, and other details discussed, all of which might apply to CQI. Staff meetings should include time for sharing CQI results and discussing implications for the staff and the unit (e.g., department, service). Providing clear visuals, such as using some of the methods discussed in this text (e.g., dashboards) helps staff to quickly appreciate the data, move to considering implications, develop interventions/strategies, and take actions. Meetings are critical times to develop strategies to respond to quality concerns and inform staff of changes to resolve concerns.

## Other Methods

A variety of other methods, many of them clinically focused, are used to prevent CQI problems and improve care. The methods discussed in this section provide additional perspectives on CQI activities found in HCOs to prevent errors and/or resolve CQI problems.

## Rapid Response Teams

The major purpose of **rapid response teams (RRTs)** is to identify and respond when patients are experiencing deterioration in their condition. This intervention has become an important QI strategy. A systematic review examined whether RRTs could identify preventable factors (Amaral et al., 2015). The results of this review indicated that when RRTs responded, almost 20% of the patients had experienced an adverse event. Among these patients, 80% of the events were preventable. RRTs may be considered a method to assist a patient who has problems and also could be a trigger to identify potential adverse events. In another study of 15 hospitals, participants who were primarily nurse executives noted that RRTs had a positive impact on patient outcomes, including providing more timely appropriate care; reducing transfers while ensuring patients receive care in the best setting for them; and in addition to clinical outcomes, having an impact on the healthcare team through support, empowerment, reducing stress, building relationships, and staff collaboration (Smith & McSweeney, 2017). There were also comments that RRTs supported families. Staff education was also provided through the RRTs as staff learned more about clinical problems, assessment, and interventions. The HCO then benefitted with improved care and more effective CQI and cost reductions. It is important to monitor RRTs to evaluate their outcomes and process.

The AHRQ's Patient Safety Network describes their use as follows: "Patients whose condition deteriorates acutely while hospitalized often exhibit warning signs (such as abnormal vital signs) in the hours before experiencing adverse clinical outcomes. In contrast to standard cardiac arrest or 'code blue' teams, which are summoned only after cardiopulmonary arrest occurs, rapid response teams are designed to intervene during this critical period [ideally before a critical event occurs], usually for patients on general medical or surgical wards" (HHS, AHRQ, PSNet, 2019b). The AHRQ identifies three rapid response system models (HHS, AHRQ, PSNet, 2019b):

- *Medical emergency team.* Personnel include physicians (critical care or hospitalist) and nurses; responsibilities include responding to emergencies.
- *Critical care outreach.* Personnel include physicians and nurses; responsibilities include responding to emergencies, following up on patients discharged from the intensive care unit (ICU), proactively evaluating high-risk unit patients, and educating unit staff.
- *Rapid response team.* Personnel include the critical care nurse, respiratory therapist, and physician (critical care of hospitalist); responsibilities include responding to emergencies, following up on patients discharged from the ICU, proactively evaluating high-risk unit patients, and educating and acting as liaison to unit staff.

The triggers for calling any of these teams for assistance might be the same, but team members and what they do might vary. In some HCOs, when patients and families are concerned about the patient, they are encouraged to request this support. It is important for HCOs to provide guidelines to staff and to patients and families on the use of RRTs.

The **early warning system** is a "physiological scoring system typically used in general medical-surgical units before patients experience catastrophic medical events" (Duncan, McMullan, & Mills, 2012, p. 40). This system is what triggers the use of the RRT to prevent failure to rescue. The early warning system must be clear and easy to use (Wood, Chaboyer, & Carr, 2019). Some hospitals use simple charts that integrate color-coding to easily identify risk and response levels (e.g., fall risk, allergies). The rating scale is used, and depending upon the score, the decision is made to request expertise. Staff members require training to effectively use the early warning system. Use of this type of rapid assessment and decision making can lead to positive outcomes for the patient. The AHRQ recommendation is that any staff may initiate the request to call the RRT, for example, due to any of the following trigger criteria (HHS, AHRQ, PSNet, 2019b):

- Heart rate over 140/min or less than 40/min
- Respiratory rate over 28/min or less than 8/min
- Systolic blood pressure greater than 180 mm Hg or less than 99 mm Hg
- Oxygen saturation less than 90% despite supplementation
- Acute change in mental status
- Urine output less than 50 cc over 4 hours
- Staff member with significant concern about the patient's condition
- Other criteria used by some HCOs: chest pain unrelieved by nitroglycerin, threatened airway, seizure, uncontrolled pain

The HCO specific criteria for RRT use must be clear and concise and shared with staff. Any changes to the list also must be shared in a timely manner with staff. Nurse managers should ensure that all clinical staff know about the process and the criteria for calling the RRT. It is important to track data on the use of RRTs—for example, an HCO identifies an increase in critical care events that could have been prevented and then decides to implement an RRT as a strategy to help prevent these events; it is important to track outcomes from initiating an RRT option for staff.

## Safety Walkarounds

Face-to-face discussion and observations are important in the CQI process, and a critical element is direct contact with frontline staff and management. **Safety walkarounds** are a method used to communicate to staff and patients that the HCO leadership is committed to improvement—that it is engaged in the process. This direct involvement of leadership provides opportunities for observation and sharing of information that may lead to strategies (immediate or long term) to prevent harm to patients and also staff. Safety walkarounds help reduce errors because there are greater opportunities for reporting near misses and actual errors; increased information sharing and discussion; recognition of human factors, particularly those related to communication and teamwork; clarification and support of internal and external patient safety standards; and identification of environmental, equipment-related, or product-related hazards; and possible solutions are discussed (Graham et al., 2014).

Walkarounds should include critical managers (such as the nurse manager), medical director, supervisor, and frontline staff and may also include representatives from higher-level management. It is best to have a briefing before the walkaround to provide time to highlight any concerns the manager may have about the area to be visited and to identify other aspects that will be covered. Discussion during the walkaround should be open and nonjudgmental. Standardized questions may be used, which makes it easier to compare information from one unit to another. After the walkaround, a debriefing with all who participated should be held to discuss issues and identify and prioritize next steps. Follow-up is important, and when relevant, actions taken following previous walkarounds should be reviewed. It is important to have guidelines for these rounds. The guidelines should be clear about how to discuss in front of patients and families issues that may have negative implications or privacy concerns. A leader for the walkaround should be clearly designated, and some type of documentation method should be used for the pre-briefing, walkaround, and debriefing. This documentation can then be shared with staff and management who need to know about the information, and the documentation also serves as a record for CQI purposes.

## Patient-Centered Rounds

Many different types of rounds are used in HCOs, including administrative, management, safety/quality, and clinical, as well as routine rounds that staff make that are not usually structured or set for routine times. Rounds, as noted in other chapters, may be used to collect data, but they are also a strategy used to prevent or resolve quality care problems.

**Patient-centered rounds** can be configured in a number of ways for different purposes, but the critical element is that they focus on the patient and patient needs. In reality, all rounds should be patient centered. A study examined if the use of a standardized hourly rounding process (SHaRP) improved efficiency, patient satisfaction, and quality and safety metrics compared to not using a structured approach (Krepper et al., 2012). Staff were trained to use SHaRP, and the rounds were called "comfort care rounds." Patients were informed that staff would conduct the rounds hourly with a focus on ensuring a clean environment, assessing pain management needs, and assisting the patient to the toilet or in getting up. Units determined which staff would participate in the rounds. The use of this type of rounds demonstrated significant outcomes in all four areas, although the researchers recommended that more research is needed.

## Teach-Backs

**Teach-backs** occur when staff ask patients to repeat something a patient has been told—for example, in a patient education session or as care directions. This method also helps to reduce health literacy problems and thus has an impact on CQI directed at meeting expected outcomes. If the patient is not able to repeat the information, then this may mean the staff need to further assess how the information is shared and how to improve the communication.

## Safe Zones

The use of **safe zones** is an approach adopted from aviation. The goal during certain activities is to better ensure that there are no interruptions and distractions so that staff can meet their responsibilities effectively and safely. Safe zones are particularly helpful in reducing errors during medication preparation and administration. In this situation all staff are informed that the space used for the medication preparation procedure or whenever staff are involved in medication administration is a safe zone or a time period for no interruptions. In addition to these issues, frequent data flow through electronic methods can also overload staff as they provide care during these procedures, thereby impacting the safe zone.

## Universal Protocol for Preventing Wrong Site, Wrong Procedure, or Wrong Person Surgery

The Universal Protocol for Preventing Wrong Site, Wrong Procedure, or Wrong Person Surgery (often referred to simply as the **Universal Protocol**) establishes a step-by-step protocol to prevent wrong site, wrong procedure, or wrong person surgery (HHS, AHRQ, PSNet, 2006). The Joint Commission supports this protocol, as does the AHRQ. The protocol includes a time-out at the beginning of a surgical procedure, and the entire surgical team participates in the review of the protocol. Wrong site, procedure, and person events are considered to be never events or hospital-acquired complications by the Centers for Medicare and Medicaid Services (CMS), and The Joint Commission considers these events to be sentinel events for which there is zero tolerance. Since 2009, the CMS has not reimbursed for these events when their beneficiaries experience them in the hospital. This protocol is a critical strategy used by HCOs. In addition, some research focusing on the Universal Protocol has found that actions taken before or after its use must be examined, as this is when errors may still occur even though staff feel comfortable that they are using the protocol (Paull et al., 2015).

## Medication Reconciliation

With increasing use of medications and many patients taking multiple medications, there is greater risk for errors in HCOs and with patients at home. More than half of patients also have one or more unintended medication discrepancies at the time of hospital admission (Cornish et al., 2005). **Medication reconciliation** consists of formulation of a list of medications (e.g., drug name, dosage and frequency, administration method, purpose of the medication, and prescriber) and reviewing the list to ensure that there are no conflicts or errors in the medications. Healthcare providers need a clear policy and procedure for medication reconciliation, and the use of this policy and procedure should be monitored (Ketchum, Grass, & Padwojski, 2005). The Joint Commission requires its accredited HCOs to have a medication reconciliation policy and procedure in place. If this is not done, problems that can arise are omitted medication, incorrect dosage, incorrect route, incorrect timing, same medication with different formulations, allergies, and failure to discontinue contraindicated medications (Rozich, Howard, Justeson, Macken, Lindsay, & Resar, 2004). Implementing medication reconciliation is not always easy. For some patients it can take time to complete. Some patients may not know or provide accurate information. Asking patients to bring in a written list of their medications provides more accurate information, but patients should be reminded that the list should be updated and current. The AHRQ comments that medication reconciliation done by the hospital pharmacy staff offers some help in preventing this problem, but it is not sufficient. Nurses are also typically involved in medication reconciliation. Greater use of electronic records may make a difference, but more evidence is required.

Among the most common adverse events after discharge are discrepancies in medication orders, such as medication not listed or change in dose not provided (HHS, AHRQ,

PSNet, 2019c). Using medication reconciliation is also important in home care to ensure that patient medications are safe (Marrelli, 2016). Home healthcare nurses should check a patient's medication storage methods, such as medication boxes, and availability of outdated medications should be included in this process. In addition, it is important to check reasons why patients may not be following a prescribed medication routine (e.g., inability to afford medications, side effects, lack of transportation to get medications). Out-of-date medications may indicate that the patient is "stretching out" use and thus taking less medication over time, skipping doses, and so on. Medication compliance is important to patient outcomes. Access to medications should be considered, such as transportation to get medications, someone to get medications, and cost of medications—all these factors impact effective treatment and outcomes.

# Summary of Key Recommended Methods to Prevent or Reduce Quality Care Problems

Identifying high-risk situations that require responses and strategies/interventions that might be used to respond should be based on evidence and reliable sources. In 2013, the AHRQ identified the top 10 patient safety strategies/interventions (Barclay, 2013):

- Preoperative/anesthesia checklists to reduce operative and postoperative events
- Bundles, including checklists, to reduce septicemia associated with central lines
- Catheter reminders, stop orders, nurse-initiated removal protocols, other interventions to limit urinary catheter use
- Bundles to prevent ventilator-associated pneumonia, including head-of-bed elevation, sedation vacations, oral care with chlorhexidine, and subglottic suctioning endotracheal tubes
- Hand hygiene

- Do-not-use list for hazardous abbreviation
- Multicomponent interventions to help prevent pressure ulcers
- Barrier precautions to reduce health-care-associated infections
- Central line placement guided by real-time ultrasonography
- Strategies to improve venous thromboembolism prophylaxis

**STOP AND CONSIDER 11-1**

Many methods are used to prevent or reduce quality care problems, and nurses need to be actively involved in using them.

# Teams

Teams have become a major focus in healthcare delivery, particularly interprofessional teams. How do teams relate to CQI? There are many factors to consider with teams and CQI. As Robichaud and colleagues (2012) explain, "The teamwork that is required for interprofessional collaboration in healthcare is not an inherent attribute of the current system, and must be fostered. Education, training, and role modeling are important enablers" (p. 156). The term "team" does not include "I" (Weinstock, 2010). Teams are not groups of people who do their work alone and then periodically come together to collaborate but rather are groups of people (e.g. staff) who work together over time. Teams also support the critical element for effective CQI: active staff participation. Teams are an important part of today's QI programs and initiatives, and they have an impact on many of the strategies/interventions used to prevent and improve care, as many of these methods require effective staff participation.

How does interprofessional education (IPE) relate to patient and healthcare system outcomes (National Academy of Medicine [NAM], 2015)? IPE is discussed in other sections of this text, but here it is important to recognize its relevance to teams and CQI.

A critical first step in teamwork is increased effective collaboration and coordination between education and practice, which is not easy to accomplish. There is also a need for more research evidence on interprofessional collaboration. NAM notes this lack of research-based support for IPE: "Although there is a widespread and growing belief that IPE may improve interprofessional collaboration, promote team-based healthcare delivery, and enhance personal and population health, definitive evidence linking IPE to desirable intermediate and final outcomes does not yet exist" (p. 6). Linking IPE to collaborative behavior changes requires a systematic approach.

# High-Performance Teams

HCOs must assess their use of teams and teamwork. Effective teams require members (staff nurses, APRNs, nurse managers, physicians, pharmacists, HCO management, and so on) who do the following (IOM, 2003):

- Learn about other team members' expertise, background, knowledge, and values.
- Learn individual roles and processes required to work collaboratively.
- Demonstrate basic group skills, including communication, negotiation, delegation, time management, and assessment of group (team) dynamics.
- Ensure that accurate and timely information reaches those who need it at the appropriate time.
- Customize care and manage smooth transitions across settings and over time, even when the team members are in entirely different physical locations.
- Coordinate and integrate care processes to ensure excellence, continuity, and reliability of the care provided.
- Resolve conflicts with other members of the team.
- Communicate with other members of the team in a shared language, even when the members are in entirely different physical locations. (p. 56)

What outcomes are evaluated to determine team effectiveness? A systematic review of 6,934 articles included studies that used outcomes focused on length of stay, readmission, or mortality rates for general medicine patients (Pannick et al., 2015). Common outcomes such as these, however, have not been effective in assessing outcomes of interprofessional teams. They recommend that complications and preventable adverse events should be included in assessing interprofessional team outcomes.

It is common when interprofessional teams are discussed to forget that administration/management/leadership must be part of the interprofessional team concept in HCOs (Begun, White, & Mosser, 2011). High-performance teams are associated with administrators who support the need for a culture that emphasizes CQI. Administrators facilitate resources, such as budget and staffing so that care can be improved. In short, they are in the position to be a driver for success. Management must demonstrate that teamwork is integrated in all aspects of the HCO, beginning with the HCO's vision, mission, goals, and QI program. To accomplish this, administrators must understand the clinical care process and its relationship to CQI. It is also the top administrator who works with the HCO's board of directors to explain the need for CQI; the CQI process, goals, and outcomes; and the importance of a team approach. The board approves the budget, and developing, implementing, and evaluating a QI program require funding. Achieving these objectives requires collaboration and partnership between management and staff and also the board.

Interprofessional team education should include teamwork and group processes, reflection and documentation, communication, shared knowledge or a base of general common knowledge, and ethics. Effective teams must have members who meet the purpose of the team and can provide knowledge and expertise, and members should be representative of the areas of concern, such as the clinical specialty or the appropriate administrative area, such as financial, documentation, CQI, and health informatics. The typical team size is five to seven members. Too many or too few members may be a barrier to team effectiveness. Each team should strive to do the following (HHS, HRSA, 2011b):

- Gain buy-in from the leadership.
- Define roles and responsibilities.
- Recognize stages of team growth: forming, storming, norming, performing.
- Set ground rules.
- Establish an effective team meeting process.
- Set meeting agendas.
- Set meeting outcomes/actions and document. (p. 4)

The following are competencies that better ensure effective collaborative interprofessional teamwork (Interprofessional Education Collaborative [IPEC], 2016):

- Work with individuals of other professions to maintain a climate of mutual respect and shared values (values/ethics for interprofessional practice).
- Use the knowledge of one's own role and those of other professions to appropriately assess and address the healthcare needs of patients and to promote and advance the health of population (roles/responsibilities).
- Communicate with patients, families, communities, and health professionals in other fields in a responsive and responsible manner that supports a team approach to the promotion and maintenance of health and the prevention and treatment of disease (interprofessional communication).
- Apply relationship-building values and the principles of team dynamics to perform effectively in different team roles to plan, deliver, and evaluate patient/population-centered care and population health programs and policies that are safe, timely, efficient, effective, and equitable (teams and teamwork). (p. 10)

Accomplishing these competencies requires greater emphasis on IPE for all healthcare profession students so that they are prepared to work effectively on interprofessional teams.

## Teams and QI Projects

HCOs must assess not only their overall CQI process but also how their teams function and impact the process and results. Effective teamwork and communication can have a positive impact on CQI, but if not effective, this can act as a barrier and increase risk of errors due to such problems as fragmentation of care, reducing collaboration, and lack of ownership impacting taking responsibility (Rosenbaum, 2019). This assessment should include the readiness for the team to do its job (HHS, AHRQ, 2017). For example, a team working on a CQI project should consider the following questions (HHS, HRSA, 2011c):

- Has the organization identified and prioritized its desired results?
- Is there an established means to measure progress toward those results, or can it be created?
- Is there a process for tracking and measuring progress toward its desired results, which includes effective means to display data?
- Is there a communication plan that includes how individuals working to achieve the desired results can exchange and provide ongoing feedback?
- Is there an established plan to periodically review progress?
- Is there a process to intervene when needed as a means to improve progress? (p. 4)

It is easy for CQI teams to quickly get into a CQI problem without stopping to plan. This is a mistake and often leads to haphazard actions and outcomes. The HRSA recommends the use of an aim statement when undertaking an improvement process:

"An *aim statement* provides a CQI team with a focused target or a goal to achieve through its quality improvement work. An aim statement is a written declaration of what an organization wants to accomplish. An effective aim contains measurable and time-sensitive parameters for the expected results of an improvement process" (HHS, HRSA, 2011c, p. 7).

It is important to stop and consider planning, as discussed in this text. To improve CQI efforts and team results consider the following questions: (1) What will improve? (2) When will it improve? (3) How much will it improve? (4) For whom will it improve?

Unfortunately, not all dynamics of clinical teamwork can be considered positive. Collective vigilance, as described by Jeffs, Lindgard, Berta, and Baker (2012), "can potentially create risk by eroding individual professional accountability through reliance on other team members to catch and correct their errors" (p. 122). The problem of collective vigilance was observed in a study that also noted a dissimilar finding—when healthcare providers are involved in a near miss, they frequently work in isolation from other staff who might be able help identify and correct potentially harmful errors. In other words, working in a team can create overreliance on team members, but working in isolation can leave providers without a support system—for example, in home healthcare. Another factor is that "over time, adaptive processes by workers and ongoing transgressions can become accepted, routine practices that are embedded into professional interactions and can erode performance" (Amalberti, Vincent, Auroy, & de Saint Maurice, 2006; Cook & Rasmussen, 2005; Jeffs et al., p. 125). These examples do not demonstrate high-performance situations in work groups or teams and can interfere with improving care because team members do not intervene when they should. They could improve care by stepping in and noting potential or actual problems. Teams must work together and act effectively.

# The Physical Environment and Teamwork

Another aspect of teamwork, which is often forgotten, is the physical environment. Teams work and communicate in a physical space, a simple fact that impacts their work and CQI. A multisite collective case study of three rural hospitals in South Australia examined the collaborative working culture of each hospital. Gum, Prideaux, Sweet, and Greenhill (2012) describe the results as follows: "Of the cultural concepts examined, the physical design of nurses' stations and the general physical environment were a major influence on an effective collaborative practice. Factors that were important were communication barriers related to poor design, lack of space, frequent interruptions, and a lack of privacy" (p. 21). How can this type of research result be applied?

Tight space increases staff stress, and lack of space for private conversations or work meetings limits communication and planning. Lack of space for relaxation limits opportunity for team members to rest, impacts care quality and burnout, and limits opportunities for team members to have personal dialogue and get to know one another. Workspace can be problematic, increasing risk for errors—for example, limited space to move around and get supplies and equipment can be a factor as the staff prepare medications, provide direct care, or try to arrange supplies and equipment in emergencies. Decentralized nurses' stations reduce walking and provide more time for care, but they may also limit team interaction and increase risk of working in silos, providing less time to discuss care and ask questions of peers. Other spaces for staff interaction, as noted, should be provided. Space is also associated with territory and power—for example, the title "nurses' station" symbolizes the space's function for nurses, not all staff. The unit workstation has long been a place of interprofessional work, but in many HCOs, it is still referred to as the nurses' station. Staff safety is also an important factor associated with physical space, as noted in other sections of this text.

# TeamSTEPPS®

One of the most respected and common methods for team development and team function is **TeamSTEPPS®**, which was developed by the U.S. Department of Defense's Patient Safety Program in collaboration with the AHRQ. The (HHS, AHRQ, 2019b) describes TeamSTEPPS® as follows: "[TeamSTEPPS® is] an evidence-based teamwork system aimed at optimizing patient care by improving communication and teamwork skills among healthcare professionals, including frontline staff. It includes a comprehensive set of ready-to-use materials and a training curriculum to successfully integrate teamwork principles into a variety of settings." **Figure 11-3** describes this model. The goal for CQI teams should be team ownership of CQI within the HCO.

The HHS notes that if a team has tools and strategies, it can leverage to build a fundamental level of competency in each of those skills. Research has shown that the team can enhance three types of teamwork outcomes: performance, knowledge, and attitudes." This teamwork system can be described as follows (HHS, AHRQ, 2019b):"

- A powerful solution to improving patient safety within [an] organization
- An evidence-based teamwork system to improve communication and teamwork skills among healthcare professionals
- A source for ready-to-use materials and a training curriculum to successfully integrate teamwork principles into all areas of [the] healthcare system
- Scientifically rooted in more than 20 years of research and lessons from the application of teamwork principles

Applying this model provides higher-quality, safer patient care by doing the following: producing highly effective medical teams that optimize

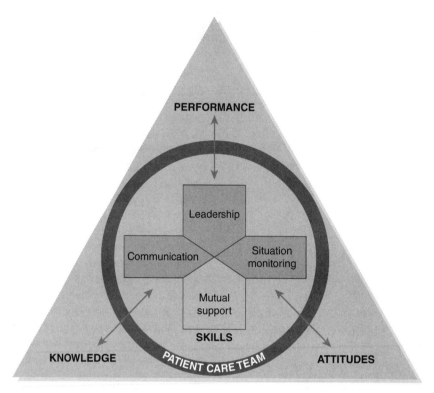

**Figure 11-3** TeamSTEPPS®

the use of information, people, and resources to achieve the best clinical outcomes for patients; increasing team awareness and clarifying team roles and responsibilities; resolving conflicts and improving information sharing; and eliminating barriers to quality and safety.

The model includes three phases. The goal of the first phase is to ensure that the HCO and its staff are ready to implement Team-STEPPS®. The training focuses on teamwork skills of leadership, communication, situation monitoring, and mutual support. The second phase focuses on structured training for trainers in the HCO and for healthcare staff. The final phase is implementation of Team-STEPPS® and sustaining it in the HCO. Training materials are evidence based and provide structured learning experience using modules, guides, videos of vignettes supporting the

model, coaching, and other methods to assist staff in understanding teamwork and implementing this teamwork model. Since this method and all its resources were developed and maintained on the Internet for easy access by the federal government, they are freely available to all HCOs and healthcare providers. **Exhibit 11-2** describes the TeamSTEPPS® model in greater detail. The Connect to Current Information section at the end of this chapter provides a link to additional information about TeamSTEPPS®.

## Examples of Types of Teams Related to CQI

With the increase in use of teams in clinical care, particularly interprofessional teams, there is greater emphasis on teams in CQI.

**Exhibit 11-2** Description of TeamSTEPPS®

---

**Three Phases of the TeamSTEPPS® Delivery System**

The three phases of TeamSTEPPS® are based on lessons learned, existing master trainer or change agent experience, the literature of quality and patient safety, and culture change. A successful TeamSTEPPS® initiative requires a thorough assessment of the organization and its processes and a carefully developed implementation and sustainment plan.

**Phase 1: Needs Assessment**

The goal is to determine the HCO's readiness for implementing TeamSTEPPS®, which requires training needs analysis. For more information about conducting a needs assessment, visit http://www.ahrq.gov/teamstepps/readiness/index.html.

**Phase 2: Planning, Training, and Implementation**

Phase 2 focuses on the planning and implementation of the TeamSTEPPS® initiative. Because TeamSTEPPS® was designed to be tailored to the organization, options in this phase include implementation of all tools and strategies in the entire organization, a phased-in approach that targets specific units or departments, or selection of individual tools introduced at specific intervals (called a "dosing strategy"). As long as the primary learning objectives are maintained, the TeamSTEPPS® materials are very adaptable.

**Phase 3: Sustainment**

The goal is to sustain and spread improvements in teamwork performance, clinical processes, and outcomes resulting from the TeamSTEPPS® initiative. The key objective is to ensure that opportunities exist to implement the tools and strategies taught, practice and receive feedback on skills, and provide continual reinforcement of the TeamSTEPPS® principles on the unit or within the department.

**Details of an HCO Site Assessment**

A site assessment includes identifying opportunities for improvement; determining the readiness of the HCO or unit/department within an HCO, such as leadership support; identifying potential barriers to implementing change; and deciding whether resources are in place to successfully support the initiative. Phase 1 assessment includes the following:

1. *Establish an organizational-level change team.* The organizational-level change team should consist of an interprofessional team that represents the healthcare professionals within the HCO. Successful change teams include organizational leaders who are committed to changing the current culture.
2. *Conduct a site assessment.* A site assessment, also called "team training needs analysis," is a process for systematically identifying teamwork deficiencies so training programs can be developed to address those deficiencies. This information is then used to identify critical training and develop training objectives and allows the program to be individualized.
3. *Define the problem, challenge, or opportunity for improvement.* The team must identify the recurring problem that threatens patient safety, determine how this problem results from existing processes and procedures, and devise a flowchart or map of the process during which the problem occurs. With information and processes properly mapped, it becomes clear what interventions are needed, what the objective of these interventions should be, and how ready the organization is to engage in these interventions.
4. *Define the goal of your intervention.* List the goals that will reduce or eliminate the risk to safe patient care. For each goal, state in one sentence what will be achieved, who will be involved (whose behavior will change), and when and where the change will occur. Ideally, a team process goal, a team outcome goal, and a clinical outcome goal will be defined.

### Details for Planning, Training, and Implementation of TeamSTEPPS®

The tools and strategies needed to address opportunities for improvement in an organization will be determined by the phase 1 assessment. The next step is to develop a customized implementation and action plan, followed by training and implementation. A brief description of the steps for planning, training, and implementation follows.

1. *Define the TeamSTEPPS® intervention.* Decide whether "whole training" (all the tools in one sitting) or "dosing" (specific tools targeted to specific interventions) is the best intervention tactic. Whole training optimizes teamwork but does not maximize learning. It can also lead to overload or uncertainty about which tools best fit improvement opportunities. Dosing is the recommended approach because it allows for direct linking of tools and strategies with specific opportunities for improvement to minimize training fatigue and overload.

2. *Develop a plan for determining the intervention's effectiveness.* A variety of ways are available to evaluate the impact of training. The plan should assess whether trainees have acquired new knowledge, skills, or attitudes at the end of training; whether individuals are taking their learning back to the workplace and using it on the job; and whether organizational objectives are being met.

3. *Develop an implementation plan.* Assess what groups will be trained, the order in which they will be trained (if not together and all at once), and what level of training they will receive. Include in the plan who will conduct training and where and when training will take place.

4. *Gain leadership commitment to the plan.* Inform leaders of all facets of the plan, including how much time will be used for training and the desired resources to support it. Leadership commitment often yields plan refinement. The key is to know what elements of the plan cannot be altered.

5. *Develop a communication plan.* Develop a plan for communicating what will be done and how the goal will be achieved. Leaders (both designated and situational) should provide information to all those in their departments or units about the initiative. It is crucial to tie together all activities that will take place with the overall goal for the initiative (i.e., improved patient safety).

6. *Prepare the HCO.* For any initiative to be fully successful, transfer of training must be achieved. Transfer is achieved by ensuring new knowledge or skills are learned and applied in the work environment. The change team must ensure the work environment is prepared to foster transfer of training so new tools and strategies are applied on the job.

7. *Implement training.* The most effective strategy for delivering the training initiative is one that involves teams of trainers that include physicians, nursing staff, and support staff. A combination of the curricula is recommended when training different sets of staff independently. The TeamSTEPPS® system includes three different medical team-training curricula and a complete suite of multimedia course materials:

   a. **Train the Trainer.** This 2.5-day training course is designed to create a cadre of teamwork instructors with the skills to train and coach other staff members.

   b. **TeamSTEPPS® Fundamentals.** This curriculum includes 4 to 6 hours of interactive workshops for direct patient care providers.

   c. **TeamSTEPPS® Essentials.** This curriculum is a 1- to 2-hour condensed version of the Fundamentals course and is specifically designed for nonclinical support staff.

### Details for Sustaining a TeamSTEPPS® Intervention

The designated change team manages sustaining interventions through coaching and observing team performance. An effective sustainment plan should account for ongoing assessment of the effectiveness of the intervention, sustainment of positive changes, and identification of opportunities for further improvements.

1. *Provide opportunities to practice.* Any TeamSTEPPS-based initiative will be much more successful if the change team accounts for opportunities to practice these behaviors. It is important to embed opportunities for practice in day-to-day functions.

2.  *Ensure leaders emphasize new skills*. Leaders play a critical role in sustainment because they are responsible for emphasizing daily the skills learned in TeamSTEPPS® training. The goal is for leaders to engage in activities that will ensure continuous involvement in teamwork.
3.  *Provide regular feedback and coaching*. Regular feedback and coaching are key to ensuring interventions are sustained. Change team members, champions from the unit, and leaders should develop and use a coaching and feedback plan that allows for sufficient observation and feedback opportunities.
4.  *Celebrate wins*. Celebrating wins bolsters further sustainment and engagement in teamwork. When using a TeamSTEPPS®-based initiative, it is critical to celebrate successes for two reasons: First, it recognizes the efforts of those who were engaged from the beginning, and second, it provides detractors or laggards a tangible example of how teamwork has improved the current operations.
5.  *Measure success*. The change team should measure success through satisfaction with training, demonstrations of learning, effective use of tools and strategies on the job, and changes in processes and outcomes. It is useful to ensure that measurement of pre-training factors is parallel with post-training factors so changes can be assessed.
6.  *Update the plan*. The final stage in any TeamSTEPPS®–based intervention is to revise the plan as the organization's needs change. The change team should determine when organizational needs have changed and ensure the sustainment plan continues to focus on the needs of the organization or unit where the intervention has been implemented.

Modified from Agency for Healthcare Research and Quality (AHRQ). (2020). TeamSTEPPS: Strategies and tools to enhance performance and patient safety. About TeamSTEPPS®. Retrieved from https://www.ahrq.gov/teamstepps/instructor/essentials/pocketguide.html

The following are some examples of specific types of teams used by HCOs to expand their CQI activities and integrate more staff in the process.

## CQI Project Teams

The HHS describes the importance of teamwork in the CQI process as follows: "For a CQI project to succeed, an organization must use the knowledge, skills, experiences, and perspectives of a wide range of people. A CQI project requires problem solving, multiple decisions, and effective solutions that involve complex systems. A comprehensive multidisciplinary [interprofessional] approach by a CQI team is preferred over individual decision makers, especially when a task is complex, creativity is necessary, the path to improvement is unclear, efficient use of resources are required, [and] cooperation is essential to implementation" (HHS, HRSA, 2011b, pp. 1–2). CQI project teams need to be flexible as they go through the process to improve care focused on a specific concern. Team members must be engaged and have a stake in the outcome. No one person has the knowledge or expertise to resolve a CQI problem; it takes a team representing multiple aspects of knowledge and expertise. Selecting members for a CQI team is critical to successful improvement. The following team member attributes should be considered:

- Respected by a broad range of staff
- Team players
- Excellent listeners
- Good communicators
- Proven problem solvers
- Frustrated with the current situation and ready for change
- Creative and able to offer solutions
- Flexible—demonstrated by their willingness to change and accept new technology
- Proficient in the areas and systems focused for improvement (p. 2)

## Crisis Management Teams

Some clinical adverse events are also referred to as sentinel events, which result in a patient(s) experiencing a permanent psychological and/or physical harm (or death) (Conway, Federico, Steward, & Campbell, 2011). Many of the strategies used to address these serious adverse events apply to all adverse events. Crisis management should be part of the response to serious events, and key leaders in the HCO should be involved as need arises. There should be policies and procedures for coping with sentinel events, including how to apply crisis management. Conway and colleagues discuss the importance of the crisis management team (CMT) in responding to a crisis event, saying the CMT's role "is to ensure that the priorities of the patients and families, staff, and organization are met, as well as to ensure enhanced communication, support, assessment, resolution, learning, and improvement following the event" (p. 11). This team should include key stakeholders and provide expertise. The purpose of the team is to determine the risk of problems occurring and of potential complications to a problem, creating a response plan, implementing the plan, and evaluating and revising the plan over time. As is true for other adverse events, risk assessment and root cause analysis should be done. The team should consider the following questions when evaluating the implementation of the plan (Conway et al., 2011):

- What worked?
- What didn't work?
- What could have been done better?
- What did you learn? (p. 13)

The team's engagement should be timely and transparent. Risk management should be involved if there are concerns about malpractice, which is not an uncommon concern with situations that require crisis management. It is often important to consider not only internal communication but also external communication, such as with the media, government agencies, and law enforcement, to effectively manage the response.

An example of a crisis for which a CMT was activated occurred in a university medical center in the fall of 2015 (CBS News, 2015; U.S. & World, 2015). A woman delivered twins; one was stillborn, and the second lived an hour. The remains of one of the infants were lost, even leading the hospital to search the city dump. This crisis required immediate examination to assist the family and prevent further events like this one. In this case, the media were involved, so managing the media was critical. HCO leadership should have a procedure for response to media, including how to communicate with the media and the police. Staff need to be informed about such a procedure as they might be the first to encounter the media—for example a telephone call might come in to the hospital or a journalist might arrive on site. Given the increase in situations in HCOs that involve guns, drugs, suicide, and violence, and to better ensure safety for patients, families, visitors, and staff, as well as ultimately to ensure quality care, all HCOs must be clear about crisis management procedures for responding to a situation's immediate and long-term demands.

## Comprehensive Unit-Based Safety Program

**The Comprehensive Unit-based Safety Program (CUSP)** was developed by the AHRQ as a framework to improve patient safety at the unit level. **Figure 11-4** illustrates this framework, which considers the implications of change.

Teams and teamwork are critical components in CUSP, which uses **sensemaking** by applying the following process (HHS, AHRQ, 2014):

- Initiate a conversation among members of an organization involved in an event/issue.
- The purpose is to reduce the ambiguity about the event/issue—literally to make sense of it.
- The conversation is the mechanism that combines that knowledge into a new, more understandable form for the members.

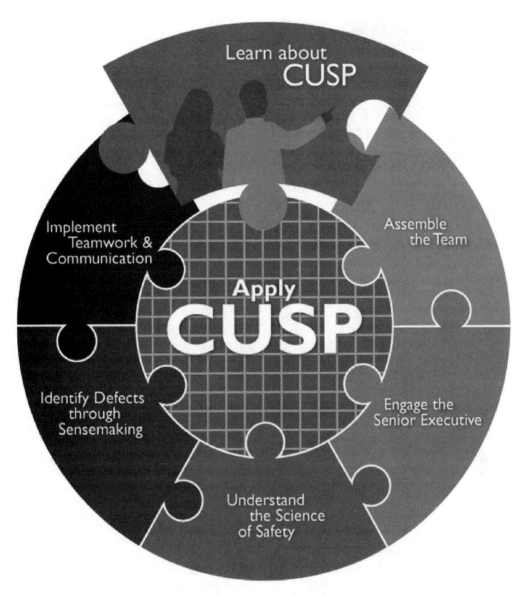

**Figure 11-4** Comprehensive Unit-Based Safety Program (CUSP)

Reproduced from Agency for Healthcare Research and Quality. (2018). Learn about CUSP. Retrieved from https://www.ahrq.gov/hai/cusp/modules/learn/index.html

- Members develop a similar representation in their minds that allows for action that can be implemented and understood by all who have participated in the conversation.

As situations are examined on a unit, staff teams gain a better understanding about what happened, why it happened, what might be done to decrease risk of reoccurrence, and how staff will know when risk is reduced. The nurse manager and unit staff work together to reduce risk and also to respond to CQI problems that occur. CUSP is commonly associated with the use of TeamSTEPPS®.

# Technology and Informatics

**Health informatics technology (HIT)** is more than technology. Today, effective solutions require consideration of technology and informatics, involving data collection methods and analysis of data; these solutions are often focused on preventing errors and resolving CQI problems (Kuziemsky & Reeves, 2012). Much of CQI depends on web-based reporting systems; anonymous, automated, integrated systems; consistent reporting methods; quality of the method, accessibility, and measurability of data; and survey and detection of adverse events. Effective HIT provides methods for secure, efficient, and effective storage and sharing of information. There are, however, problems with HIT despite its ongoing development. There still is mostly a collection of systems that are weak in supporting value-based care, and this impacts sharing information across systems to produce effective outcomes. "The pursuit of value-based care, in which we deliver better care with better outcomes at lower cost, places new demands on the healthcare system that our IT infrastructure needs to be able to support" (Adler-Milstein, Embi, Middleton, Sarkar, & Smith, 2017, p. 1036).

In 2009, the federal Health Information Technology for Economic and Clinical Health (HITECH) Act was passed. This legislation has had an impact on healthcare, with its incentives to implement new technology, such as computerized physician/provider order entry (CPOE), which is discussed later in this chapter. The law also emphasizes meaningful use. In 2016, the AHRQ issued a call for more grant proposals to gain more knowledge about HIT safety—focused on safe HIT practices related to design, implementation, usability, and safe

use of HIT by all healthcare providers (National Institutes of Health [NIH], 2016). This type of initiative demonstrates the increasing need for research and support for new initiatives to improve HIT.

With the growing recognition of the need for effective HIT, the HHS developed the Federal Health IT Strategic Plan. This plan provides direction for 2015 through 2020 focused on national healthcare delivery to ensure effective systems with all types of HCOs. The new plan for 2020–2025 was in draft form in 2020 awaiting approval (HHS, ONC, 2020). The vision and a description of the plan's goals and objectives are found in **Figure 11-5** and **Table 11-1**.

The AHRQ provides an annual HIT report that describes the work of the AHRQ Health IT Program. The current report is provided on its website. The AHRQ Health IT Program funds research to create actionable findings around "what and how health IT works best" for its key stakeholders: patients, clinicians, and health systems" (HHS, AHRQ, 2018). The report describes a broad range of research findings including safety and HIT.

Another aspect of technology and HIT is engagement of nurses in HIT, including nurse leaders at all levels. Since 2004 the Healthcare Information and Management Systems Society (HIMSS) has conducted a survey to better understand the status of nurses in HIT (HIMSS, 2017). The 2017 survey indicated that 32% of the hospitals surveyed had chief nurse informatics officers (CNIO). This is important as it indicates that these hospitals recognize the need for nursing leadership in their HIT; however, 21% did not have appropriate administrative support. The specialty of nurse informatics is increasing. "Nursing informatics (NI) is the specialty that integrates nursing science with multiple information and analytical sciences to identify, define, manage, and communicate data, information, knowledge, and wisdom in nursing practice. NI supports nurses, consumers, patients, the interprofessional healthcare team, and other stakeholders in their decision-making in all roles and settings to achieve desired outcomes. This support is accomplished through

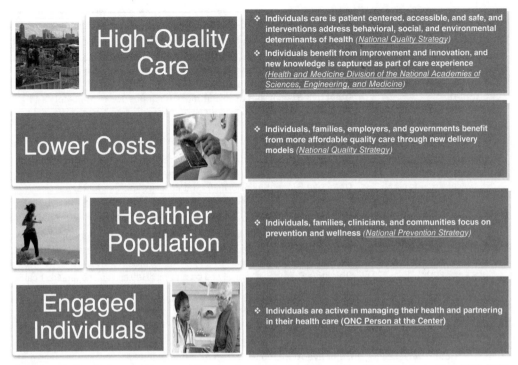

❖ Individuals care is patient centered, accessible, and safe, and interventions address behavioral, social, and environmental determinants of health *(National Quality Strategy)*

❖ Individuals benefit from improvement and innovation, and new knowledge is captured as part of care experience *(Health and Medicine Division of the National Academies of Sciences, Engineering, and Medicine)*

High-Quality Care

Lower Costs

❖ Individuals, families, employers, and governments benefit from more affordable quality care through new delivery models *(National Quality Strategy)*

Healthier Population

❖ Individuals, families, clinicians, and communities focus on prevention and wellness *(National Prevention Strategy)*

Engaged Individuals

❖ Individuals are active in managing their health and partnering in their health care *(ONC Person at the Center)*

**Figure 11-5** The Vision and Expected Results that Guide the Federal Health IT Strategic Plan 2020-2025

Reproduced from U.S. Department of Health and Human Services (HHS) & National Coordinator for Health Information Technology (ONC). (2020). Federal IT strategic plan: 2015–2020. Retrieved from https://www.healthit.gov/policy-researchers-implementers/health-it-strategic-planning

the use of information structures, information processes, and information technology" (American Nurses Association [ANA], 2015).

Healthcare delivery also uses many types of clinical technology that may or may not be directly associated with informatics and computer systems. Examples of common methods and equipment are unit-dose systems, smart administration pumps, telemetry monitoring, bar coding, telehealth equipment, and robotics in surgery. Effective use requires that healthcare professionals understand the purpose and effective use of the technology. Staff need to know how to use the equipment and participate in any maintenance or equipment checks required of clinical staff prior to use; staff need to complete required procedures for implementation and evaluation of technology use; document as required; and complete required patient assessment while using the technology. The HCO and staff need to identify and respond to CQI needs, such as data,

errors, and solutions. Equipment must be up to date, maintenance needs must be met, and records must be kept describing use and tracking problems for CQI purposes.

HIT is a rapidly changing area that is influenced by many factors. An example of an initiative to improve medication administration and management of prescriptions is a new system established by the state of New York, the first state to require that all prescriptions be created electronically (New York State Education Department [NYSED], 2017; Otterman, 2016). This change should also increase the state's ability to track use of controlled substances at a time of increased concern about the growing problem of addiction. Some difficulties with the requirement may lead to changes and adjustment in healthcare delivery—for example, when patients come to a healthcare provider, they need to know the name of the pharmacy they want to use, and if it turns out the medication is too expensive, it

**Table 11-1**  Federal Health IT Strategic Plan 2015–2020 Goals: Quick Reference Guide

|  | Goal | Objective |
|---|---|---|
| **Collect** | **Goal 1:** Expand Adoption of Health IT | **Objective A:** Increase the adoption and effective use of health IT products, systems, and services<br>**Objective B:** Increase user and market confidence in the safety and safe use of health IT products, systems, and services<br>**Objective C:** Advance a national communications infrastructure that supports health, safety, and care delivery |
| **Share** | **Goal 2:** Advance Secure and Interoperable Health Information | **Objective A:** Enable individuals, providers, and public health entities to securely send, receive, find, and use electronic health information<br>**Objective B:** Identify, prioritize, and advance technical standards to support secure and interoperable health information<br>**Objective C:** Protect the privacy and security of health information |
| **Use** | **Goal 3:** Strengthen Healthcare Delivery | **Objective A:** Improve healthcare quality, access, and experience through safe, timely, effective, efficient, equitable, and person-centered care<br>**Objective B:** Support the delivery of high-value health care<br>**Objective C:** Improve clinical and community services and population health |
|  | **Goal 4:** Advance the Health and Well-Being of Individuals and Communities | **Objective A:** Empower individual, family, and caregiver health management and engagement<br>**Objective B:** Protect and promote public health and healthy, resilient communities |
|  | **Goal 5:** Advance Research, Scientific Knowledge, and Innovation | **Objective A:** Increase access to and usability of high-quality electronic health information and services<br>**Objective B:** Accelerate the development and commercialization of innovative technologies and solutions<br>**Objective C:** Invest, disseminate, and translate research on how health IT can improve health and care delivery |

Reproduced from U.S. Department of Health and Human Services (HHS) & National Coordinator for Health Information Technology (ONC). (2015). Federal health IT strategic plan 2015-2020: Quick reference factsheet. Retrieved from https://www.healthit.gov/sites/default/files/FederalHealthIT_Strategic_Plan.pdf

will not be easy to make changes. This change in prescription procedure should reduce errors that occur due to handwriting but will require changes in the healthcare delivery system and in preparing patients. It is a system that requires an efficient electronic system for all providers. **Figure 11-6** describes the relationship of HIT to CQI, as noted by the HHS.

As HIT has expanded rapidly in healthcare, and there is now greater access to data through many types of digital records, opportunities are greater to complete effective retrospective reviews and capture more information. Real-time triggers help to catch errors in processes, providing important information to use to prevent future errors. It is also important to recognize that sometimes HIT acts

as a barrier to improvement and may actually lead to errors, just as medical equipment may help improve care but may also be associated with care problems and errors. Other examples of barriers are alarm/alert fatigue, CPOE errors, and ineffective interoperability of different electronic medical/health record systems.

Technology can assist teams by increasing communication, decision making, and sharing of information in an efficient manner (Kuziemsky & Reeves, 2012). It offers collaborative tools that can increase the team's efforts in care coordination and improve quality. However, as in our personal lives, overreliance on technology for communication reduces face-to-face interaction, which is critical to development and maintenance of team structure and function.

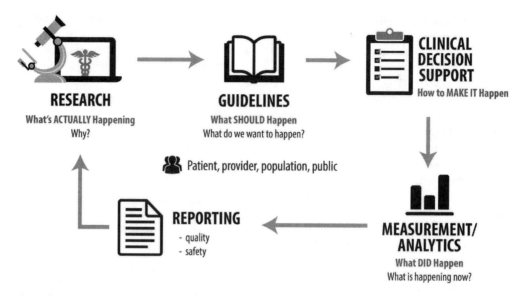

**Figure 11-6** Health IT Enabled Quality Improvement Ecosystem

Reproduced from U.S. Department of Health and Human Services & Office of the National Coordinator for Health Information Technology. (2014). Health IT enabled quality improvement: A vision to achieve better health and health care. Retrieved from https://www.healthit.gov/sites/default/files/HITEnabledQualityImprovement-111214.pdf

Care transitions and handoffs are discussed elsewhere in this text. Here, the focus is on HIT and its potential for improving transitions (Marcotte, Kirtane, Lynn, & McKethan, 2015). If HIT is integrated in plans to reduce transition problems, it then addresses the need to resolve gaps in care and quality. The discharge process requires complete and timely information. HIT can automate this information and, ideally, share it more easily among HCOs and healthcare providers. Improved information flow can fill the gap and ensure consistency and reduce errors. When medication reconciliation is part of HIT, it can prevent and reduce errors. Patient activation is required for patient-centered care. HIT can assist by increasing electronic information sharing with patients, providing patient education opportunities, and offering other resources for patients.

Nurses need to be involved in HIT to support their practice but also to better ensure their own engagement in CQI. The core healthcare professions competencies include "utilize informatics" (IOM, 2003a). Emerging technologies are important, requiring nurses to keep up to date and participate in the development, implementation, and evaluation of HIT systems. Nurses have critical roles and responsibilities related to technology; however, to make technology initiatives work effectively, nurses need to be involved in the beginning stages of HIT development within HCOs and continue their involvement through evaluation and improvement. Not only do all nurses need to know about HIT and participate in its application but nursing informatics are also a specialty that supports a nursing role in HIT (ANA, 2015). Certification and graduate programs are available for the specialty, and some HCOs have formal positions for nurses in this specialty. Nursing is also recognized by the HIMSS as important in leading and should be visible in efforts to achieve healthcare delivery transformation through technology and informatics (HIMSS, 2011).

With the growth of HIT, providers have more opportunities to improve care and reduce costs, although not all HIT meets these goals. When safety is the focus, HIT does not necessarily always demonstrate positive results. As Ehlert and Rough (2013) warn, "Technology can instill a false sense of security, leading to carelessness by healthcare professionals" (p. 470). Some AHRQ-funded researchers suggest that there is need to develop a better model or framework for HIT that focuses on safety and CQI (HHS, ONC, 2019a). The purpose of this type of model, as explained by Sitting and Singh (2015), is to "refine the science of measuring health IT-related patient safety, make health IT-related patient safety an organizational priority by securing commitment from organizational leadership, and develop an environment conducive to detecting, fixing and learning from system vulnerabilities . . . focusing on three related domains: (1) concerns unique and specific to technology; (2) concerns created by the failure to use health IT appropriately or by misuse of health IT; and (3) the use of health IT to monitor risks, health care processes, and outcomes and to identify potential safety concerns before they can harm patients."

In 2015, the HHS published a report, *Connecting Health and Care for the Nation: A Shared Nationwide Interoperability Roadmap, Draft Version 1.0*. This report provides a roadmap supporting **interoperability** or "the ability of a system to exchange electronic health information with and use electronic health information from other systems without special effort on the part of the user" (HHS, ONC, 2019b, p. 18). The key issue is access to information when needed by people, including patients. In addition, there are increased efforts to actively consider the patient and support patient-centered care in HIT. Important principles should be followed when the plan is implemented:

- Build upon the existing health IT infrastructure.
- Recognize that one size does not fit all.
- Empower individuals, giving them more access to information.
- Leverage the market, recognizing the greater need now for seamless flow of electronic clinical health information.
- Simplify.

- Maintain modularity; provide flexibility to the system, as change will be ongoing.
- Consider the current environment and support multiple levels of advancement.
- Focus on value.
- Protect privacy and security in all aspects of interoperability.
- Include scalability and universal access. (pp. 20–21)

Careful planning of use of electronic methods can reduce later planning and implementation problems, such as delays in getting information, duplication, and omissions. If there is a clear understanding and description of the process, then there is a greater chance that HIT systems will be in sync with real-world processes (Jackson, 2004). Rudman, Bailey, Hope, Garrett, and Brown (2014) describe the benefits of effective use of technology: "Technology has the potential to improve workflow and the fluid transmission of vital information on errors that surface from a system perspective, without placing blame on fallible individuals and institutions" (p. 196). It is very important to assess interfacing, particularly with pharmacy, laboratory, and radiology—ensuring that information is received in a timely manner and is correct. Errors are made, and these errors may also impact handoffs and patient flow.

Recognizing the critical need for access to CQI information and supporting evidence-based resources, in 2016 the CMS and the ONC introduced a new Internet site, eCQI Resource Center, describing it as a one-stop shop for the most current resources to support electronic clinical QI. The Connect to Current Information at the end of this chapter provides a link to this site. **Table 11-2** describes potential benefits and safety concerns of HIT components.

## Meaningful Use

A variety of communication devices are also associated with technology. There is greater use of smartphones in clinical areas and use of other devices such as tablets and laptops. These devices can have a positive impact on

**Table 11-2**  Potential Benefits and Safety Concerns of Health IT Components

### Computerized Physician/Provider Order Entry (CPOE)

An electronic system that allows providers to record, store, retrieve, and modify orders (e.g., prescriptions, diagnostic testing, treatment, and/or radiology/imaging orders).

| Potential Benefits | Safety Concerns |
|---|---|
| ■ Large increase in legible orders<br>■ Shorter order turnaround times<br>■ Lower relative risk of medication errors<br>■ Higher percentage of patients who attain their treatment goals | ■ Increases relative risk of medication errors<br>■ Increased ordering time<br>■ New opportunities for errors, such as:<br>　• Fragmented displays preventing a coherent view of patients' medications<br>　• Inflexible ordering formats generating wrong orders<br>　• Separations in functions that facilitate double dosing<br>　• Incompatible orders<br>■ Disruptions in workflow |

### Clinical Decision Support (CDS)

Monitors and alerts clinicians of patient conditions, prescriptions, and treatment to provide evidence-based clinical suggestions to health professionals at the point of care.

| Potential Benefits | Safety Concerns |
|---|---|
| ■ Reductions in:<br>　• Relative risk of medication errors<br>　• Risk of toxic drug levels<br>　• Management errors of resuscitating patients in adult trauma centers<br>　• Prescriptions of nonpreferred medications<br>■ Can effectively monitor and alert clinicians of adverse conditions<br>■ Improve long-term treatment and increase the likelihood of achieving treatment goal | ■ Wide variation in the rate of detecting drug–drug interactions among different vendors<br>■ Increases in mortality rate<br>■ High override rate of computer generate alerts (alert fatigue) |

### Bar Coding

Bar coding can be used to track medications, orders, and other healthcare products. It can also be used to verify patient identification and dosage.

| Potential Benefits | Safety Concerns |
|---|---|
| ■ Significant reductions in relative risk of medication errors associated with:<br>　• Transcription<br>　• Dispensing<br>　• Administration errors | ■ Introduction of workarounds—for example, clinicians can:<br>　• Scan medications and patient identification without visually checking to see if the medication, dosing, and patient identification are correct<br>　• Attach patient identification bar codes to another object instead of the patient<br>　• Scan orders and medications of multiple patients at once instead of doing it each time the medication is dispensed |

*(continues)*

---

**Table 11-2** Potential Benefits and Safety Concerns of Health IT Components  *(continued)*

**Patient Engagement Tools**

Tools such as patient portals, smartphone applications, email, and interactive kiosks, which enable patients to participate in their healthcare treatment.

| Potential Benefits | Safety Concerns |
|---|---|
| ■ Reduction in hospitalization rates in children<br>■ Increases in patients' knowledge of treatment and illnesses | ■ Reliability of data entered by patients, families, or unauthorized users |

*Note:* This table is not intended to be an exhaustive list of all potential benefits and safety concerns associated with health IT. It represents the most common potential benefits and safety concerns.
Reproduced with permission from Institute of Medicine. (2012). Health IT and patient safety: Building safer systems for better care. Washington, DC: National Academies Press. Courtesy of the National Academies Press, Washington, DC.

---

CQI, providing staff with more timely access to information and opportunities to search the Internet for information that was not as easily accessible in the past. For all of these devices, critical concerns are patient privacy and confidentiality. HCOs have policies and procedures that must be followed to prevent problems. These requirements should support CQI efforts to use technology and shared data, when appropriate, with appropriate persons.

Hacking, however, is a growing problem, allowing access of private information to get into the hands of people who might abuse this information. Some HCOs have even been "held hostage" by hackers who gain control of the HCO electronic systems and require that money be paid to regain access (Balakrishnan, 2016). In the future, other types of events may occur. This risk requires HCOs to be extra vigilant and to try to anticipate potential problems so that they can be prevented.

In July 2010, the ONC and the CMS issued significant new rules that have had an impact on HCOs. These rules, **meaningful use**, are criteria that hospitals and CMS-eligible providers must meet to be identified as meaningful users of HIT (HHS, 2019). If HCOs and eligible CMS providers do not meet these criteria, then the providers do not receive CMS payment for services. The criteria were developed to better ensure that services and

related HIT are meeting the recommendations from the *Quality Chasm* reports. HHS's specific meaningful use purposes are as follows:

1. Improve quality, safety, efficiency, and reduce health disparities.
2. Engage patients and their families (through electronic communication).
3. Improve care coordination.
4. Ensure adequate privacy and security protection for personal health information.
5. Improve population and public health through data collection and analysis of data.

HCOs must apply these criteria to their HIT and connect it to their CQI program. This initiative is an example of how CQI is never static and requires nurses to keep up to date with changes. Ideally, nurses should participate in health policy, providing their expertise and sharing their concerns about nursing care and the healthcare delivery system and relationship to CQI-related policy.

# Electronic Medical/Health Record

HIT includes the electronic medical/health record (EMR/EHR), patient engagement tools such as personal health records, and health information exchanges. HIT is not one product but rather multiple products and systems.

One has to consider that the use of HIT usually requires interaction with staff and this interaction can then increase risk (IOM, 2012). The work environment impacts successful use of HIT (Kutney-Lee, Sloane, Bowles, Burns, & Aiken, 2019). The EMR/EHR began to expand more than 15 years ago. "Back then, as now, we understood that EHRs carried tremendous promise for improving care. Healthcare innovators envisioned a day when a primary care clinician had a patient's latest medical history at his or her fingertips—the cardiologist's most recent consult note, the immunizations given by the local pharmacist, a link to last month's hospital discharge summary, and a real-time run-down of lab results. And, oh, by the way, notes from today's visit would be sent to patients before they leave the office. Calls for greater use of EHRs prompted a series of Federal incentive programs beginning in 2009. To date, these initiatives have provided over $37 billion in incentive payments to clinicians and hospitals to adopt health information technology, including EHRs. Since that meeting in 2005, use of EHRs in office-based practice has grown from about 24% to 86% in 2017. The growth of EHRs in hospitals is even more dramatic; in 2017, 96 percent of non-Federal acute care hospitals used an EHR. Do these trends suggest we're headed in the right direction? Definitely. At the same time, are we struggling with obstacles to further success? Indeed, we are. And thanks to new data from AHRQ's EvidenceNOW initiative, we understand more about the challenges of using EHRs among small to medium-sized primary care practices" (HHS, AHRQ, 2019c; McNellis, 2019).

The **electronic medical record (EMR)** is a digital record that includes provider medical and clinical data for a patient. The **electronic health record (EHR)** includes the same information plus more comprehensive information about the patient's history. The EMR/EHR is used to share information from one provider to another. The **personal health records (PHR)** includes the same information as the EMR and EHR, but the patient keeps the record and maintains it. These digital records help track data over time, identify when patients are due for preventive visits and screenings, monitor patient measures of certain parameters, and improve overall quality of care in practice (HealthIT.gov, 2018). Selecting, implementing, and evaluating an EMR requires a team approach. In a study reported in 2012, 71% of providers who adopted EHRs indicated they would make the same decision again. These digital systems typically also include "notification of potentially dangerous drug interactions, verify medications and dosages, and reduce the need for potentially risky tests and procedures" (HealthIT.gov). The HHS identifies the Common Clinical Data Set for electronic records, which includes the following (HHS, ONC, 2019b):

- Patient name
- Sex
- Date of birth
- Race
- Ethnicity
- Preferred language
- Smoking status
- Problems
- Medications
- Medication allergies
- Vital signs
- Care plan field(s), including goals and instructions
- Procedures
- Care team members
- Immunizations
- Unique device identifier(s) for patient's implantable device(s)
- Notes/narrative (p. 12)

EMR/EHR development and implementation began in a disorganized manner, and thus the result was great variation in hardware and software used in HCOs with limited early concern about sharing data across HCOs. There was little standardization, and now this is a problem, as there is need for more effective inter-HCO sharing and sharing with government agencies. Using a common set approach supports records with consistent content and organization within and across HCOs, improving communication, care, and ease of accessibility. The HHS ONC coordinates the department's national HIT efforts, focusing on adoption of national standards and support of interoperable exchange of health information (HHS, ONC, 2019b).

The federal government is active in developing initiatives and resources to improve electronic records. "The Office of the National Coordinator for Health Information Technology has produced the SAFER [Safety Assurance Factors for EHR Resilience] guides. These nine guides provide assessment checklists and structure for teams to assess and improve their systems in the following domains: high-priority practices, organizational responsibilities, contingency planning, system configuration, system interfaces, patient identification, CPOE with decision support, test results reporting and follow-up, and clinician communication. SAFER guides are designed for use in all types of health care settings" (HHS, AHRQ, PSNet, 2014b; HHS, AHRQ, PSNet, 2019d).

The following are examples of the potential impact digital records may have on CQI (HealthIT.gov, 2018):

- Quick access to patient information from multiple locations to assist in providing coordinated, efficient care
- Decision support, clinical alerts, reminders, medical information
- Performance-improving tools, real-time quality reporting
- Legible, complete documentation that facilitates accurate coding and billing
- Interface with labs and other sources of information
- Safer, more reliable prescribing
- Error reduction when multiple caregivers are involved in the care (i.e., care coordination)
- Improved care transitions (handoffs) between settings
- Up-to-date information for emergency care (i.e., care coordination)

Patients also benefit directly from HIT. There is reduced time needed to complete information per visit, as the provider has the information digitally. The patient can receive reminders about care needs and information, and e-prescriptions can be sent to the pharmacy. Referrals can be made electronically. In some cases, patients can access their provider electronically. Digital records also have an impact on risk management by providing timely and detailed documentation and may also help prevent liability actions, as accurate information can be provided about the care provided and use of EBP.

A recent study examined the adoption of EMR/EHRs and their impact on hospital adverse events (Furukawa, Eldridge, Wang, & Metersky, 2016; Helwig & Lomotan, 2016). This retrospective analysis of the Medicare Patient Safety Monitoring System from 2012 through 2013 included a large sample of 45,235 patients at risk for 347,298 adverse events. The focus was on fully electronic records that included physician notes, nursing assessments, problem lists, medication lists, discharge summaries, and provider orders. Fully electronic records for patients with cardiovascular conditions, surgery, and pneumonia indicated that between 17% and 30% were less likely to experience adverse events in the hospital, indicating a positive outcome when using electronic records, leading to better coordinated care with less risk of harm. Limitations in the study require further examination, such as high-alert medications in the system, safety features used, and determination of which methods had greatest influence on adverse events. Although it has long been believed that electronic records improve care, more research is needed. More nurse managers are turning to using the EMR to monitor care in their units, and more understanding of how this can be done effectively is required: how to access the data, make better use of the data, analyze the data, and then apply to improve care (Soriano, Siegel, Kim, & Catz, 2019).

As many HCOs have updated their EMR/EHRs or plan to do so, a common concern is risk of errors when using electronic documentation systems. This topic is not new, but when systems change, potential errors must be considered; moreover, the change process itself increases risk of errors. It takes about a year for an HCO and its staff to adjust to a new system, and the first year is a high-risk period for errors (Abramson et al., 2013).

Schwiran and Thede (2011) offer valuable insight into the relationship between nursing care and the EMR/EHR: "Two significant challenges have always faced nursing: (a) how to differentiate nursing's contributions to patient care from those of medicine; and (b) how to incorporate descriptions of nursing care into the health record in a manner that is commensurate with its importance to patients' welfare." In addition, greater use of EMR/EHR in measurement of causes of errors in real time offers significant data for CQI (Classen, Griffith, & Berwick, 2017). These challenges are even more important with computerized medical records. One of the underlying drivers of the latter challenge is the use (or disuse) of standardized communication among nurses. Standardized nursing terminologies (SNTs) may help in recognizing nursing interventions, improving communication among nurses and with other staff, improving patient care, providing access to data about nursing care interventions and outcomes, increasing compliance with standards of care, and providing data to help assess nursing competencies. In a study of a survey of 1,268 nurses, the respondents were asked about SNT; a large proportion of the sample had no experience or knowledge of them (Schwiran & Thede, 2011). The SNT that was the most recognizable by one-third of the respondents was that of the North American Nursing Diagnosis Association (NANDA), but these respondents had not used it since graduation. One-quarter said they had not used the Nursing Intervention Classification or the Nursing Outcome Classification since graduation. These findings raise questions about the need for SNT: Why is this type of information important? Is it integrated into electronic records? If there is conflict and lack of nursing participation in using these methods that focus on nursing terminology, what is the value of teaching them to students? Do we then confuse communication, particularly interprofessional communication? There are no clear answers to these questions, but in the future more examination of this issue is needed in order to arrive at the best approach for nursing and for healthcare delivery.

## Computerized Physician/ Provider Order Entry

**Computerized physician/provider order entry (CPOE)** is supported by the HITECH Act of 2009 and by the National Quality Forum (NQF) as a method to support quality care. When a hospitalized patient receives a medication, four steps occur: (1) ordering, (2) transcribing the order (if handwritten), (3) dispensing the medication by the pharmacists, and (4) administering medication. CPOE was developed to respond to the high rate of errors associated with the first and second steps in the medication process; more than 90% of errors occur at these two steps (HHS, AHRQ, PSNet, 2014a). Using the CPOE, a provider can enter an order directly into a computerized system, and then the pharmacist receives and reviews the information. This process eliminates some problems with treatment orders found in noncomputerized systems, such as poor handwriting, inappropriate use of abbreviations or HCO-approved abbreviations, and unclear orders. Transcribing problems may be eliminated—for example, accuracy is not dependent on a staff member's ability to transcribe orders. The order can then be clearly read by a pharmacist who has the knowledge to assess the quality of the order for the patient's needs, clinical status, and required treatment. In addition, software can often identify errors in orders and alert the provider at the time the order is entered. In addition, the extensive time nurses and other staff needed to transcribe orders is eliminated.

In 2016, the HHS reported on a review of the use of CPOE systems (HHS, AHRQ, PS-Net, 2019e). This report comments on a Food and Drug Administration (FDA) review of the safety of these systems, which noted major usability problems with all the systems tested. The following are some of the specific problems that were identified:

- Inconsistent medication naming within and across systems
- Poor medication search functions
- Difficulty interpreting displays
- Vulnerability to wrong-patient errors when multiple records were open
- A lack of standardization alerts, an abundance of irrelevant alerts, and a lack of reasons documented for alert overrides among clinical decision support functions
- Medication reconciliation modules lacking standard terms and not easily accommodating team-based reconciliation workflows

Supporting some of these comments, a study examined 10 CPOE systems and found that there was inconsistency in display medication names—for example, using generic and brand names. In these cases this increases the risk of confusion and/or errors (Quist et al., 2017).

## Clinical Decision Support

**Clinical decision support (CDS)** is used to prevent errors, may also have an impact on care omissions, and may act as a solution to improve care—for example, a CDS may alert the healthcare provider of a wrong dosage, inappropriate administration method, incorrect frequency of administration, problem with patient drug allergies, concerns about drug–drug interactions, and conflict with drug–laboratory factors when comparing laboratory results with the medication order (HHS, AHRQ, PSNet, 2019e). If there is a potential problem, this type of system would send out alerts on the computer to the healthcare provider's device. In some cases, the CDS will also send out alerts when orders should be considered for specific diagnoses—treatment that would normally be considered for the diagnosis but is not ordered.

Often CPOE is combined with a CDS; however, combining the two systems requires planning and staff training when it is implemented. One problem that has occurred and may influence how providers respond to alerts is alert fatigue. Just because the provider receives an alert on the computer that something requires attention does not mean the provider will respond or respond with correct action. Another problem is alert overrides: Does the system allow the staff member to override or cancel an alert with no action taken pertaining to the alert? This can be a problem if the alert should not be ignored—for example, one study noted that almost three-quarters of the alerts were overridden and 40% of the overrides were inappropriate (Nanji et al., 2018). CPOE and CDS systems are also expensive. HCOs also must select systems that best meet their needs, and this requires a thorough analysis of needs and equipment along with costs and staff training (Nuckols et al., 2015). Some studies recommend that there should be greater evaluation of critical drug–drug interactions on a national professional basis, as there are too many alerts given and then providers override them (Phansalkar et al., 2013). Overusing alert systems may lead to more problems. In a study that examined improvement of usability of drug–drug interaction CDS alerts, researchers identified interventions that they think should be used to improve alerts (Payne et al., 2015). Recommendations include use of consistent terminology; use of visual cues and minimal text; and consideration of formatting, content, and reporting so that usability is improved. Alerts should provide the healthcare provider with the option to reject the alert and then provide an explanation, which should be more than just "will monitor." This option is much better than just ignoring alerts, and it provides CQI data that can be tracked over time.

Wrong-patient drug orders is an example of an error that can occur when using CPOE. This is thought to be an error that is not routinely reported, particularly if voluntary reporting is the major tool used to get the data. A study that focused on automated surveillance of electronic data "hypothesized that wrong-patient orders are recognized by the healthcare provider who inputted the order shortly after entry, promptly retracted, and then reentered for the right patient" (Adelman et al., 2013, p. 305). This situation is considered to be a near miss, a type of event that happens 100 times more frequently than adverse events (IOM, 2013). The study recommends that all hospitals measure their retract-reorder events to determine if there is a problem and, if so, that they adjust their software to better ensure alerts and other methods decrease this near miss.

CDS should include the right information, shared with the right people, via the right channels, in the right formats, and at the right time. Responding to these care aspects should optimize information flow, including communication of what, who, where, when, and how. Effective use of CPOE should include the following (Ehlert & Rough, 2013):

- Relevant patient information (e.g., demographic data, laboratory and diagnostic test results) must be readily available at the time of prescribing or order entry.
- Drug–drug interaction, drug allergy, drug–laboratory, drug contraindication, and maximum–minimum dosing alerts for potentially serious mistakes must be provided. (Sensitivity of alerts can be a problem, so they need to be tracked and adjusted as needed.)
- The selection of standard order sets (medication use algorithms and guidelines for high-risk patient populations) should be automated at the point of prescribing.
- The system must be efficient and easy to use. (If too complex, physician compliance will be reduced.) (p. 475)

# Bar-Code Medication Administration

**Bar-code medication administration** uses bar codes located on the patient's identification to compare with the bar code found on orders or, in case of medications, found on the individual patient drug package. The bar code electronically confirms a patient's identity in the system and provides an alert if not the correct patient, timeline for order, or order. Many HCOs use bar-code medication administration. This technology should reduce errors and adverse events, providing an alert system at the point of care. Bar codes are now used for more than medication administration, as they are also used for many treatment actions that require patient identification. For this electronic identification method to be effective, staff must actively use it. Some systems will block the healthcare provider from moving to next steps if the bar-code procedure is not used—for example, staff may be denied access to medication storage device. **Table 11-3** provides guidelines for safe use of decentralized automated dispensing systems/devices and patient safety when using technology during medication administration.

# Medical Devices

Medical devices have had a major positive impact on CQI; however, they can also lead to errors and CQI problems. In a review of studies that examined factors related to recognition, reporting, and resolution of incidents associated with medical devices, it was noted that incidents were not commonly reported due to concern about fear of punishment, uncertainty about what should be reported and how incident reports are used, and limitations of time to complete reporting (Plisena, Gagliardi, Urbach, Clifford, & Fiander, 2015). Medical device security has also become an important topic that can impact care delivery and CQI—for example, if there are passwords/codes that must be used to access a medical

**Table 11-3** Guidelines for Safe Use of Decentralized Automated Dispensing Systems

Agree with the vendor on a documented preventive maintenance schedule that does not disrupt workflow.

Any high-risk medications stocked in devices should be accompanied by an alert system for nurses (such as a maximum-dose prompt).

Carefully select stored drugs based on the needs of the patient care unit, patient age, diagnosis, and staff expertise.

Conduct monthly expiration date checks, concomitantly verifying inventory accuracy. Configure devices to provide single-dose (or single-drug) access whenever possible, focusing such control on high-risk medications and controlled substances. Develop an ongoing competency assessment program for all personnel who use or affect the system, including direct observation and random restocking accuracy audits, as well as observation of dispensing accuracy as part of the assessment.

Develop a system to remove all recalled medications.

Develop clear, multidisciplinary system downtime procedures that are included in an ongoing competency program.

Develop strict safety criteria for selecting medications that are (and are not) appropriate for storing in devices.

Develop systems to account for narcotic waste, and routinely audit controlled substance dispenses versus patient orders and medication administration records.

Do not stock look-alike and sound-alike drugs in the same open-access drawer.

Have strict security procedures to limit unauthorized access.

Place allergy reminders for specific drugs, such as antibiotics, opiates, and NSAIDs, on appropriate drug storage pockets, or have them automatically appear on the dispensing screen.

Require all personnel to attend formal training and demonstrate competency prior to assigning them access to the system.

Require nurses to return medications to a return bin, never back to the original storage pocket or location.

Require pharmacist medication order review and approval before administration of the first dose of medication (profile dispensing), and limit medications in which profile dispensing may be overridden.

Use open-access drawers only for stocking drugs with low potential for causing patient harm if administered in error.

Whenever possible, use bar coding capabilities for restocking medications and for retrieval.

With few exceptions, maximize use of unit-dose medications in ready-to-administer form.

All actions and usage on a system must be reportable in an easily reviewed format, including identification of the user, the medication, the patient for whom the drug was dispensed, and the time of the transaction.

At medication administration, one system must be able to identify and document the medication, person administering the medication, and patient by utilizing bar code technology.

Hospital admit/discharge/transfer and medication order entry computer systems should be interfaced with automation devices to provide caregivers with warnings about allergies, interactions, duplications, and inappropriate doses at the point of dispensing and/or administration.

Information necessary to properly manage patient care must be accurate, accessible, and timely.

Pertinent patient- and medication-specific information and instructions entered into pharmacy and/ or hospital information system should be available electronically at the point of care (administration), and the system should prompt the nurse to record pertinent information before administration may be documented.

Real-time systems integration should exist from the point of prescribing (order entry) through dispensing and through documentation of medication administration.

The system must accommodate bar-coded unit-dose medications and utilize the bar code capability for drug restocking, retrieval, and administering medications.

The system should force users to confirm the intention whenever medications are accessed or administration is attempted outside of the scheduled administration time or dosage range. Such events should be signaled visibly or audibly for the user, and all such events should be electronically documented and reported daily for follow-up.

The interface with the pharmacy computer system should allow the nurse to view and access only those medications that have been ordered for the specific patient.

The nurse should be electronically reminded when a medication dose is due (and by a different mechanism when it is past due).

User access should be restricted to a unique user identification code and password or a unique bar code.

device, how does the staff member know the password/code? What happens if the password is changed? In emergencies, how does requiring a password/code impact the ability to provide care for the patient when needed? Security is important, but it has to be practical for the healthcare delivery system (HIMSS, 2016). The FDA is responsible for approval of many medical devices. In addition, as mentioned, there has been increasing concern about hacking and cybersecurity in computer systems, and these concerns may also apply to medical devices, which may have similar risks compared to typical organization computers.

An example of the impact of equipment on healthcare is found in a report to the U.S. Senate Committee on Health, Education, Labor, and Pensions, in which specific concern was identified about safety and infection risk with a medical device: the closed-channel duodenoscope.

This is, of course, a serious concern, but something else in the report is even more important. The report notes that Congress needs to "fund a national medical device evaluation system, so that the FDA can 'effectively monitor the safety of medical devices on the market rather than relying on adverse event reporting'" (Saint Louis, 2016, p. A13). The report notes that manufacturers do not always report adverse events or report them in the required time frame. The FDA provides MedWatch, an adverse event reporting program, for HCOs and staff to use. The following are examples of possible types of medical device problems that might be reported (Simone, Brumbaugh, & Ricketts, 2014):

- Electric beds (e.g., patient entrapment, electric shock)
- Negative pressure wound therapy devices (e.g., bleeding, infection)

- Patient lifts (e.g., falls)
- Infusion pumps (e.g., overdose or underdose, shock, fire)
- Peritoneal dialysis machines and components (e.g., increased intraperitoneal pressure, problems with administration sets)
- Glucose meters and strips (e.g., improper storage of strips, false high or low blood glucose values)
- Foley catheters (e.g., infection, breakage, insertion trauma)
- Gastrointestinal tubes and feeding pumps (e.g., fluid contamination, cessation of infusion) (p. 403)

The FDA expects staff to complete their own HCO incident reports in addition to reporting to the FDA. The FDA (HHS, FDA, 2016) gives the following guidelines for reporting: "Product problems should be reported to the FDA when there is a concern about the quality, authenticity, performance, or safety of any medication or device for the following reasons: suspect counterfeit product, product contamination, defective components, poor packaging or product mix-up, questionable stability, device malfunction, and labeling concerns." Even with this expectation, many problems or adverse events are not reported—for example, staff may not think a problem/event is important or may think reporting will make no difference. This failure to report then may lead to greater problems, as the FDA can do nothing to resolve these problems, such as addressing the problem with the device manufacturer. The FDA has the expertise to decide if a problem should be examined and then to determine actions that should be taken, but changes are not possible without report of problems.

## Telehealth

Telehealth is now used in a variety of settings. It is both patient centered, thereby increasing patient empowerment, and provider centered; there are benefits for both (Finley & Shea, 2019). It improves coordination, access, information sharing, and choice. This is a new area and requires nurses to get involved to ensure that nursing care is provided in the best way possible. It might be used in the home, connecting the patient to healthcare providers on a routine basis or when needed. It is also used in HCOs—for example, an intensive care unit in a rural area might use telehealth to connect to experts in larger medical centers for consultation.

A key question is this: What is the effectiveness of this expanding technology area? A systematic review of studies on this question from 233 studies that met the criteria for the review indicates that generally telehealth consultations do improve outcomes or provide services with no major difference in outcomes (Totten et al., 2019). Some systems work better than others. Virtual nursing care is expanding with greater use of electronic ICUs, use in home care, and other settings. Key questions to be considered by HCOs and nurses include the following (Boston-Fleischhuer, 2017):

1. What is the core function of the virtual acute care nurse?
2. What skills and competencies will be needed?
3. How does the virtual acute care nurse interact with the on-site care team?
4. Does the virtual acute care nurse interact with the patient and family, and if so, how?
5. With increased consumerism, how will this role and this type of care delivery be received by patients and families?
6. Will nurses derive professional fulfillment from a virtual role and therefore remain engaged?
7. How will we measure the impact of virtual nursing care? (p. 86)

In addition, to expanding telehealth, there is now movement to expand virtual clinical trials, providing access to clinical trials to more patients (NAM, 2019). Most people do not live near medical centers where clinical trials are being conducted—more than 70% of potential clinical trial participants live more than two hours from a center. Typically, trials require multiple visits, and thus getting access can be complicated for patients and their families. How might this work? Participants may be able to complete the admission and consent process remotely, attend virtual physician visits, receive drugs via shipment, monitor and report symptoms via electronic devices, and so on. This opportunity also requires careful planning and implementation of CQI for these patients.

### STOP AND CONSIDER 11-3

Health informatics may help improve care and may also act as a barrier to quality care.

# Multiple Roles of Nurses in Preventing or Reducing Quality Care Problems

Nurses are responsible for many of the aspects of daily monitoring and management of the quality of healthcare delivered to patients. The nurse's responsibilities include immediate detection and intervention when patients' clinical conditions change, although not all nurses are prepared for or effectively provide this surveillance. Expert nursing practice requires not only psychomotor and affective skills but also complex thinking processes, such as making inferences and synthesizing information to choose a course of action. Nurses constitute the surveillance system for early detection of patient complications and problems, and they are in the best position to choose a course of action. Their responsibilities include the following (Benner, Sheets, Uris, Malloch, Schwed, & Jamison, 2002; Clark & Aiken, 2003; Higuchi & Donald, 2002):

- Understand the need for and demonstrate complete participation in the medication process, including knowledge about medications.
- Assist in collecting CQI data.
- Participate in root cause analysis.
- Participate in incident reporting as required by your HCO.
- Recognize the importance of sentinel events and participate in reporting and analysis of these events.
- Use standardized, structured communication methods such as SBAR.
- Participate actively on teams; collaborate and coordinate care.
- Participate actively in the HCO accreditation process.
- Use tools provided by your HCO, such as checklists, protocols, and clinical guidelines, to improve care and participate in their selection and/or development.
- Use methods such as failure modes and effects analysis (FMEA) effectively.
- Attend and actively participate in clinical rounds and safety rounds.
- Recognize the negative impact of failure to rescue (FTR), and implement methods to reduce it.
- Consider documentation a critical component of care and take care when documenting.
- Engage with other staff and managers to develop and maintain a culture of safety.
- Recognize the need for a healthy work environment and the impact of human factors on CQI. Apply this knowledge to yourself, such as recognizing risks that increase when you are tired, work long hours, and are stressed.
- Follow all required infection control protocols.
- Ask management to share CQI data, analysis, and conduct routine discussion of outcomes with staff.
- Ensure that the workspace for clinical care and medication administration is as free as possible from disruptions and noise.

- Use EBP and EBM.
- Apply medication reconciliation as needed.
- Recognize the importance of near misses and how this type of error impacts your practice, and take action.
- Request that information and resource access be accurate and timely (e.g., receipt of lab test results, delivery of medications and supplies to the unit).
- Participate in CQI-related committees and task forces.
- Keep patient-centered care in focus at all times, and remain mindful of how it can be improved.
- Work to improve your participation in handoffs and use HCO-required methods such as checklists and standardized, structured communication methods.
- Respect all members of the staff—clinical and nonclinical.
- Participate in staff education and peer evaluation. (Potter et al., 2014, p. 39)

Healthcare professionals must participate in self-regulation and self-improvement (Benner, Malloch, & Sheets, 2010). In 2007, the National Council of State Boards of Nursing (NCSBN) began an initiative to better understand nursing practice and quality care and to develop a national database of nursing errors, referred to as the Taxonomy of Error, Root Cause Analysis, and Practice Responsibility (TERCAP®) (Benner, Malloch, & Sheets, 2010; Woods & Doan-Johnson, 2002). The TERCAP® database includes data on patient profile, patient outcome, setting, system issues, healthcare team, nurse profile, intentional misconduct or criminal behavior, safe medication administration, documentation, and practice breakdown. This database is different from the National Database of Nursing Quality Indicators (NDNQI®), which is also discussed in this text. The NDNQI® focuses on specific nursing measurement indicators, whereas the TERCAP® database is focused on nursing errors that are reported prospectively online to state boards of nursing and then analyzed and shared with the NCSBN, although not all states participate.

Why is TERCAP® important to this chapter's discussion? It recognizes the need for state and national tracking of nursing errors and, in doing so, recognizes that there must be something unique in identifying a nursing error. The work done to develop the TERCAP® database system provides information about nursing care, nursing education, errors, and quality care (Benner, Malloch, & Sheets, 2010). We need to understand more about how nursing practice impacts care and how we can learn from errors. The intent of TERCAP® is not to move backwards toward a "blame" culture within nursing education but rather forward toward a culture of safety and a better understanding of the root cause of errors from a system view, both education and practice, and from an individual view. This extensive examination of nursing practice based its framework on the five healthcare professions core competencies and the Quality and Safety Education for Nurses (QSEN) six core competencies for nurses. As noted in another chapter, these two sets of competencies do not completely agree, although they are very similar.

TERCAP® led to the identification of three major standards of nursing practice that are integral to CQI (Malloch, Benner, Sheets, Kenward, & Farrell, 2010):

- *Safe medication administration.* The nurse administers the right dose of the right medication via the right route to the right patient at the right time and for the right reason.
- *Documentation.* Nursing documentation provides relevant information about the patient and the measures implemented in response to the patient's needs.
- *Attentiveness/surveillance.* The nurse monitors what is happening with the patient and staff. The nurse observes the patient's clinical condition; if the nurse has not observed a patient, then he or she cannot identify changes and/or make knowledgeable discernments and decisions about the patient. (p. 12)

**Table 11-4** describes the TERCAP nursing practice breakdowns in greater detail.

As CQI measures are considered, one approach for HCOs to take when considering nursing practice within the HCO and CQI is to use the practice breakdowns identified in TERCAP®: medication administration, communicating patient data, attentiveness/surveillance, clinical reasoning/judgment, prevention, intervention, interpretation of orders, and professional responsibility. This type of initiative provides more opportunities for nurses to meet their CQI responsibilities as a profession and within the healthcare delivery system.

## STOP AND CONSIDER 11-4

In the course of a nurse's daily practice, the nurse has many opportunities to prevent or reduce quality care problems.

# Summary

Information in this chapter ties together the content on CQI measurement by discussing multiple methods/strategies/interventions used to prevent and reduce quality care problems and respond to them. Nurses need more knowledge not only about CQI but also about how to engage in the CQI process and change. Nurses need "opportunities to pose nursing practice questions, identify process flow, implement and monitor change, and then evaluate and chart related outcomes" (Beckel & Wolf, 2013, p. 648). Appendix A provides a list of examples of major HCOs and governmental and nongovernmental agencies that provide CQI resources for HCOs and healthcare professions. Exemplars of quality improvement roles and responsibilities for staff nurses, nurse managers, and APRNs are found in **Exhibit 11-3**.

**Table 11-4** Overview of the TERCAP Database

| Nursing Practice Breakdown | Description |
|---|---|
| Medication administration | To safely and effectively administer drugs, the nurse must assess the patient's status, actions needed, medication side effects, other medications the patient is taking, the patient's environment, and other care activities provided to the patient. If the patient is able, then the patient should be involved in the administration process. The nurse must be knowledgeable about the drug to be administered. Prevention of errors and improvement require assessment of system design and how to support effective, safe medication administration, particularly avoiding the approach of the "status quo"—doing things the way we always have. |
| Communicating patient data | Nurses have multiple ways to communicate/share patient data and assessment with others—the care team. Documentation is the primary method used, and today it has moved more to digital methods, though some HCOs still use nondigital methods. Digital methods require effective collaboration with health informatics. |
| Attentiveness/ surveillance | Nurses use surveillance to gather information and assess what is happening to the patient. This should be an active part of nursing practice. At the same time that better surveillance is needed, it can also be a burden and can increase work, and many factors can negatively impact surveillance, such as fatigue, stress, workload, lack of expertise for the situation, and so on. The Institute of Medicine particularly addresses the nurse's role in surveillance in its significant report *Keeping Patients Safe: Transforming the Work Environment* (2003b). |

*(continues)*

**Table 11-4** Overview of the TERCAP Database *(continued)*

| Nursing Practice Breakdown | Description |
|---|---|
| Clinical reasoning/ judgment | Nurses need to use clinical reasoning and judgment in their practice as they assess patients and outcomes based on data that they obtain. A nurse not selecting and using the best intervention constitutes clinical reasoning/judgment breakdown. |
| Prevention | The nurse uses interventions to prevent or reduce risks, hazards, or complications that may be related to illness or treatment. It is easier to identify lack of prevention, as one can use the outcomes of complications as the measure that prevention was not done or ineffective. Engaging the patient is a critical factor in prevention. |
| Intervention | Intervention refers to the nurse acting on behalf of the patient—an act made by the nurse. If the nurse does not execute an intervention correctly or the timing is not what it should be, then this is an intervention breakdown. Intervention does not include assessment, surveillance, and monitoring, even though these efforts do provide important information for interventions. Interventions are visible and invisible (related to surveillance). |
| Interpretation of orders | Communication of orders is an important part of care delivery, and nurses must guard against the risk of misinterpretation (e.g., incomplete orders, illegible writing, problems in transcribing orders, and digital errors). |
| Professional responsibility and patient advocacy | Nurses must speak up for their needs to provide quality care (e.g., staffing levels and mix), and they also speak for the patient to ensure patient needs are understood and met when possible. As nurses meet this practice area, they must consider professional boundaries as described by the National Council of State Boards of Nursing. |

Data from Benner, P., Malloch, K., & Sheets, V. (Eds.). (2010). *Nursing pathways for patient safety.* St. Louis, MO: National Council State Boards of Nursing and Mosby.

**Exhibit 11-3** **Exemplars: Quality Improvement Roles and Responsibilities**

**Staff Nurse**

Staff nurses applying for change in the hospital's clinical ladder process must include examples that demonstrate active participation in CQI. One of the staff nurses indicates she serves on the unit CQI Task force and describes how she used evidence-based practice with specific patients.

**Nurse Manager**

The nurse manager for intensive care notices that communication is not at the level it should be. She discusses this with the medical director of the unit. The unit includes medical residents, nursing students, pre-licensure, and two advanced practice nurses. They meet with the faculty involved with these educational experiences too. They conclude that the unit will establish clear guidelines about structured communication and train staff in these methods. They select SBAR, time-outs, improved use of change-of-shift reports, and whiteboards in the patient rooms.

**Advanced Practice Registered Nurse***

The APRNs in a hospital must be provided with the same training physicians receive to use a new computerized order system. The HCO should ask the APRNs for feedback about their use of the new system and the training.

* Advanced Practice Registered Nurse includes APRN, Clinical Nurse Specialist, Clinical Nurse Leader, and nurses with DNP.

# APPLY CQI

## Chapter Highlights

- HCOs use multiple methods/strategies/interventions to assist in preventing or reducing quality care problems—to intervene and to improve. These methods/strategies/interventions are chosen by the HCO and staff, but in some cases they are influenced by requirements from accreditors, third-party payers, and government agencies (state and federal).

- HCOs and healthcare professional organizations may develop and/or use the following methods/strategies/interventions: redesign of systems and processes, position descriptions and performance appraisal, clinical ladders, policies and procedures, evidence-based practice (EBP) requirements, standardization of care, clinical guidelines and protocols, case management, disease management, QI committees, utilization review/management committees, staff education, and mentoring and coaching.

- Documentation of CQI data, analysis, and solutions are an important part of preventing or reducing quality care problems and improving care.

- Structured communication methods are used by many HCOs to reduce problems with ineffective communication. Examples are SBAR (situation-background-assessment-recommendation), time-outs, crew resource management, signouts, read-backs, huddles, worksheets, change-of-shift reports, whiteboards, and staff meetings.

- Other methods/strategies/interventions that are more patient centered are rapid response teams; safety walkarounds; patient-centered rounds; teach-backs; safe zones; the collaborative care model; Comprehensive Unit-based Safety Program (CUSP); the Universal Protocol for Preventing Wrong Site, Wrong Procedure, or Wrong Person Surgery; and medication reconciliation.

- Teams and teamwork are critical to all aspects of CQI.

- TeamSTEPPS®, developed by the federal government, is an evidence-based approach to staff team training that is used by many HCOs.

- Technology and informatics are important in providing care. They also are used to prevent or reduce quality care problems—for example, they are used for data collection and analysis and for providing alerts to providers.

- Common health informatics technology (HIT) are electronic medical record/electronic health record (EMR/EHR), computerized physician/provider order entry (CPOE), clinical decision support (CDS), and bar-coding medication administration.

- Medical devices present safety concerns and require maintenance and correct use to prevent errors. Nurses and other staff with technology experience work together to ensure that devices are used effectively.

- Nurses need to be more actively involved in preventing or reducing quality care problems. These responsibilities require that nurses be prepared to meet them.

## Critical Thinking and Clinical Reasoning and Judgment: Discussion Questions and Learning Activities

1. Select one of the examples of methods/ strategies/interventions used to prevent or reduce quality care problems, and discuss the method and how it impacts care. Do this in a team, with each member selecting a different method/ strategy/intervention. In the team discussion, consider the pros and cons of using the method/strategy/ intervention.

2. Provide two examples of how a nurse can prevent or reduce quality care problems. Support your example with references.

3. Why are teams and teamwork important to CQI? Provide two examples to support your response. Support your examples with references.

4. What is the purpose of meaningful use? Describe how a nurse applies it?

5. Ask a staff member from a local HCO's HIT department to speak to the class about HIT. Students should prepare questions based on chapter content. Provide two examples of how nurses can prevent or reduce quality care problems using HITs. Support your examples with references.

## Connect to Current Information

- AHRQ: PocketGuide—TeamSTEPPS
  https://www.ahrq.gov/teamstepps
  /instructor/essentials/pocketguide.html
- FDA: Medical Device Safety
  http://www.fda.gov/medicaldevices/safety
  /default.htm
- HealthIT.gov
  https://www.healthit.gov
- eCQI Resource Center Sponsored by the CMS
  https://ecqi.healthit.gov

- AHRQ: CUSP Toolkit
  http://www.ahrq.gov/professionals/educa-tion/curriculum-tools/cusptoolkit/index.
  html
- The Joint Commission: Universal Protocol
  http://www.jointcommission.org/standards
  _information/up.aspx
  http://www.jointcommission.org/assets/1/18
  /up_poster1.pdf
- AHRQ, PSNet: Patient Safety Primers
  https://psnet.ahrq.gov/primers

### Connect to Text Current information with the Author

Go to the update for this text to review the Blog, QI News, and Literature Review. Access this regular update at: http://nursing.jbpub.com/Finkelman/QualityImprovement/2e.

## EBP, EBM, and Quality Improvement: Exemplar

Wittie, M., Ngo-Metzger, Q., & Lebrun-Harris, L. (2016). Enabling quality: Electronic health record adoption and meaningful use readiness in federally funded health centers. *Journal of Healthcare Quality, 38*(1), 42–51.

This large study is a major examination of the adoption and use of electronic health records.

### Questions to Consider

1. What is the design used for this study, including research question(s), sample, interventions, data collection, and analysis?

2. What are the results of the study?

3. How might you apply these results to a clinical setting to improve care?

# EVOLVING CASE STUDY

The QI program in a 250-bed hospital is examining its use of teams and how teams might impact the ability to improve care. You are an expert on teams and CQI and have been invited to speak to the group. Prior to your presentation, you are told that teams are used sporadically throughout the hospital, but they are used more effectively in medical units. Staff members have had little education about teams, and some staff see no value in them, including a variety of professions, such as nurses, physicians, and some pharmacists. The nonclinical staff often feel as though they are not part of the teams in the hospital, so they ignore the topic.

## Case Questions

1. Prepare a PowerPoint slide presentation that you will use to explain the importance of teams and teamwork to CQI. Provide three examples to demonstrate the relationship.
2. Select three of the methods/strategies/interventions to prevent or reduce quality care problems discussed in this chapter. Prepare a clear plan describing the implementation of each method/strategy/intervention along with a rationale for use with a specific quality care problem. Discuss how teams would be used.
3. What does a hospital need to do to prepare staff in the use of the methods/strategies/interventions and application to team and team process?

# References

Abramson, E., Malhotra, S., Osorio, S., Edwards, A., Cheriff, A., Cole,C., & Kaushal, R. (2013). A long-term follow-up evaluation of electronic health record prescribing safety. *Journal of American Medical Informatics Association, 20*, e52–e53.

Adelman, J., Kalkut, G., Schechter, C., Weiss, J., Berger, M., Reissman, S., . . . Southern, W. (2013). Understanding and preventing wrong patient drug electronic orders. *Journal of American Informatics Association, 20*(2), 305–310.

Adler-Milstein, J., Embi, P., Middleton, B., Sarkar, I., & Smith, J. (2017). Crossing the health IT chasm: Considerations and policy recommendations to overcome current challenges and enable value-based care. *Journal of American Medical Informatics Association, 24*(5), 1036–1043.

Amalberti, R., Vincent, C., Auroy, Y., & de Saint Maurice, G. (2006). Violations and migrations in health care: A framework for understanding and management. *Quality and Safety in Health Care, 15*(Suppl. 1), i66–i71.

Amaral, A., McDonald, A., Coburn, N., Ziong, W., Shojania, K., Fowler, R.A., . . . Adhikari, N. (2015). Expanding the scope of critical care rapid response teams: A feasible approach to identify adverse events. *BMJ Quality Safety*. Retrieved from http://qualitysafety.bmj.com/content/early/2015/06/22/bmjqs-2014-003833.abstract?sid=7588baee-666c-4b2d-98c3-026cb23fe0ba

American Nurses Association (ANA). (2010). *Nursing professional development: Scope and standards of practice*. Silver Spring, MD: Author.

American Nurses Association (ANA). (2015). *Nursing informatics: Scope and standards of practice* (2nd ed.). Silver Spring, MD: Author.

Balakrishnan, A. (2016). The hospital held hostage by hackers. Retrieved from http://www.cnbc.com/2016/02/16/the-hospital-held-hostage-by-hackers.html

Barclay, L. (2013). AHRQ identifies top 10 patient safety strategies. *Medscape Medical News*. Retrieved from http://www.medscape.com/viewarticle/780237

Beckel, J., & Wolf, G. (2013). Identification of potential barriers to nurse-sensitive outcome demonstration. *JONA: Journal of Nursing Admiinstration, 43*(12), 652.

Begun, J., White, K., & Mosser, G. (2011). Interprofessional care teams: The role of the healthcare administrator. *Journal of Interprofessional Care, 25*(2), 119–123.

Benner, P., Malloch, K., & Sheets, V. (Eds.). (2010). *Nursing pathways for patient safety*. St. Louis, MO: National Council of State Boards of Nursing and Mosby.

Benner, P., Sheets V., Uris, P., Malloch, K., Schwed, K., & Jamison, D. (2002). Individual, practice and system causes of errors in nursing: A taxonomy. *JONA: Journal of Nursing Administration, 32*(10), 509–523.

Boston-Fleischhuer, C. (2017). The explosion of virtual nursing care. *JONA, 47*(2), 85–87.

CBS News. (2015, September 29). Cincinnati hospital apologizes for lost remains of baby. Retrieved from http://www.cbsnews.com/news/university-of-cincinnati-medical-center-apologizes-for-lost-remains-of-baby

Clark, S., & Aiken, L. (2003). Failure to rescue. *American Journal of Nursing, 103*, 42–47.

Classen, D., Griffith, F., & Berwick, D. (2017). Measuring patient safety in real time: An essential method for effectively improving the safety of care. *Annals of Internal Medicine, 167*(2), 882–883.

Conway, J., Federico, F., Stewart, K., & Campbell, M. (2011). *Respectful management of serious clinical adverse events* (2nd ed.). Institute for Health Improvement Innovation Series white paper. Cambridge, MA: Institute for Health Improvement. Retrieved from http://www.ihi.org/resources/Pages/IHIWhitePapers /RespectfulManagementSeriousClinicalAEsWhite Paper.aspx

Cook, R., & Rasmussen, J. (2005). "Going solid": A model of systems dynamics and consequences of patient safety. *Quality and Safety in Health Care, 14*(2), 130–134.

Cornish, P., Knowles, S., Marchesano, R., Tam, V., Shadowitz, S., Juurlink, D., Etchells, E. (2005). Unintended medication discrepancies at the time of hospital admission. *Archives of Internal Medicine, 165*(4), 424–429.

Donley, R., & Flaherty, M. (2008). Promoting professional development: Three phases of articulation in nursing education and practice. *Online Journal of Nursing, 13*(3). Retrieved from https://ojin.nursingworld.org/MainMenu Categories/ANAMarketplace/ANAPeriodicals/OJIN /TableofContents/vol132008/No3Sept08/Phasesof Articulation.html

Duncan, K., McMullan, C., & Mills, B. (2012). Early warning. *Nursing 2012, February*, 38–44.

Ehlert, D., & Rough, S. (2013). Improving the safety of the medication use process. In B. Youngberg (Ed.), *Patient safety handbook* (2nd ed., pp. 461–493). Burlington, MA: Jones & Bartlett Learning.

Finkelman, A. (2011). *Case management*. Upper Saddle River, NJ: Pearson Education.

Finkelman, A. (2019). *Professional nursing concepts: Competencies for quality leadership* (4th ed.). Burlington, MA: Jones & Bartlett Learning.

Finkelman, A. (2020). *Leadership and management for nurses: Core competencies for quality care* (4th ed.). Upper Saddle River, NJ: Pearson Education.

Finley, B., & Shea, K. (2019). Telehealth. Disrupting time for healthcare quantity and quality. *Nursing Administration Quarterly, 43*(3), 256–262.

Furukawa, M., Eldridge, N., Wang, Y., & Metersky, M. (2016). Electronic health record adoption and rates of in-hospital adverse events. *Journal Patient Safety*, doi:10.1097/PTS.0000000000000257. Retrieved from http://journals.lww.com/journalpatientsafety/Abstract /publishahead/Electronic_Health_Record_Adoption _and_Rates_of.99605.aspx

Gabow, P., Eisert, S., Karkhanis, A., Knight, A., & Dickson, P. (2005). A toolkit for redesign in health care.

Prepared for the Agency for Healthcare Research and Quality. AHRQ Publication No. 05-0108-EF. Retrieved from http://archive.ahrq.gov/professionals /quality-patient-safety/patient-safety-resources /resources/toolkit/index.html

Gawande, A. (2010). *The checklist manifesto*. New York, NY: Metropolitan Books.

Graham et al. (2014, October). Patient safety executive walkarounds (pp. 223–235). Agency for Healthcare Research and Quality (AHRQ). *Advances in patient safety*. https://www.ncbi.nlm.nih.gov/books/NBK20582/

Gum, L., Prideaux, D., Sweet, L., & Greenhill, J. (2012). From the nurses' station to the health team hub: How can design promote interprofessional collaboration. *Journal of Interprofessional Care, 26*, 21–27.

Haig, K., Sutton, S., & Whittington, J. (2006). SBAR: A shared mental model for improving communication between clinicians. *Journal of Quality and Patient Safety, 32*(3), 167–175.

Healthcare Information and Management Systems Society (HIMSS). (2011). Position statement. *Share the vision: Transforming nursing practice through technology and informatics*. Retrieved from http://www.himss.org /library/nursing-informatics/position-statement

Healthcare Information and Management Systems Society (HIMSS). (2017). HIMSS: Medical device security, data breaches stop concern. Retrieved from https:// healthitsecurity.com/news/himss-medical-device -security-data-breaches-top-concerns81

Healthcare Information and Management Systems Society (HIMSS). (2017). 2017 nursing workforce informatics workforce survey. Retrieved from https://www .himss.org/sites/hde/files/d7/2017-nursing-informatics -workforce-full-report.pdf

HealthIT.gov. (2019). What is an electronic medical record (EMR)? Retrieved from http://www.healthit.gov /providers-professionals/electronic-medical-records-emr

Helwig, A., & Lomotan, E. (2016). Can electronic health records prevent harm to patients? Retrieved from http://www.ahrq.gov/news/blog/ahrqviews/020916 .html

Higuchi, K., & Donald, J. (2002). Thinking processes used by nurses in clinical decision making. *Journal of Nursing Education, 41*(4), 145–153.

Institute for Healthcare Improvement (IHI). (2013). How-to guide: Sustainability and spread. Retrieved from http://www.ihi.org/resources/Pages/Tools/Howto GuideSustainabilitySpread.aspx

Institute of Medicine (IOM). (2003a). *Health professions education: A bridge to quality*. Washington, DC: The National Academies Press.

Institute of Medicine (IOM). (2003b). *Keeping patients safe*. Washington, DC: The National Academies Press.

Institute of Medicine (IOM). (2011). *Clinical practice guidelines we can trust*. Washington, DC: The National Academies Press.

Institute of Medicine (IOM). (2012). *Health IT and patient safety: Building safer systems for better care.* Washington, DC: The National Academies Press.

Institute of Medicine (IOM). (2013). *Patient safety: Achieving a new standard for care.* Washington, DC: The National Academies Press.

Interprofessional Education Collaborative (IPEC) Expert Panel. (2016). *Core competencies for interprofessional collaborative practice: 2016 update.* Washington, DC. Retrieved from https://hsc.unm.edu/ipe/resources/ipec-2016-core-competencies.pdf

Jackson, K. (2004). Shedding light on medication errors. *For the Record, 16*(4), 27–29.

Jeffs, L., Lingard, L., Berta, W., & Baker, R. (2012). Catching and correcting near misses: The collective vigilance and individual accountability trade-off. *Journal of Interprofessional Care, 26,* 121–126.

Ketchum, K., Grass, C., & Padwojski, A. (2005). Medication reconciliation: Verifying medication orders and clarifying discrepancies should be standard practice. *American Journal of Nursing, 105*(11), 78–79.

Krepper, R., Vallejo, B., Smith, C., Lindy, C., Fullmer, C., Messimer, S., . . . Myers, K. (2012). Evaluation of a standardized hourly rounding process (SHaRP). *Journal for Healthcare Quality, 36*(2), 62–69.

Kutney-Lee, A., Sloane, D., Bowles, K., Burns, L., & Aiken, L. (2019). Electronic health record adoption and nurse reports of usability and quality of care: The role of work environment. *Application of Clinical Informatics, 10*(1), 129–139.

Kuziemsky, C., & Reeves, S. (2012). The intersection of informatics and interprofessional collaboration. *Journal of Interprofessional Care, 26,* 437–439.

Leonard, M., Graham, S., & Bonacum, D. (2004). The human factor: The critical importance of effective teamwork and communication in providing safe care. *Quality and Safety in Healthcare, 13*(Suppl. 1), 185–190.

Lyons, V., & Popejoy, L. (2017). Time-out and checklists. A survey of rural and urban operating room personnel. *Journal of Nursing Care Quality, 32*(1), E3–E10.

Malloch, K., Benner, P., Sheets, V., Kenward, K., & Farrell, M. (2010). Overview: NCSBN practice breakdown initiative. In P. Benner, K., Malloch, K., & V. Sheets, V. (Eds.), *Nursing pathways for patient safety* (pp. 1–29). St. Louis, MO: National Council of State Boards of Nursing and Mosby.

Marcotte, L., Kirtane, J., Lynn, J., & McKethan, A. (2015). Integrating health information technology to achieve seamless care transitions. *Journal of Patient Safety, 11*(4), 185–190.

Marrelli, T. (2016). *Home care nursing. Surviving in an ever-changing care environment.* Indianapolis, IN: Sigma Theta Tau International.

McNellis, B. (2019). The promise of electronic health records: Are we there yet? Retrieved from https://www.ahrq.gov/news/blog/ahrqviews/promise-of-electronic-health-records.html

Nanji, K., Seger, D., Slight, S., Amato, M., Beeler, P., Her, Q., . . . Bates, D. (2018). Medication-related clinical decision support alert overrides in inpatients. *Journal of American Medical Informatics Association, 25*(5), 476–481.

Narayan, M. (2013). Using SBAR communications in efforts to prevent patient rehospitalizations. *Home Healthcare Nurse, 31*(9), 504–516.

National Academy of Medicine (NAM). (2015). *Measuring the impact of interprofessional education on collaborative practice and patient outcomes.* Washington, DC: The National Academies Press.

National Academy of Medicine (NAM). (2019). *Virtual clinical trials: Challenges and opportunities.* Washington, DC: The National Academies Press.

National Institutes of Health (NIH). (2016). AHRQ announces interest in research in health IT safety. Retrieved from http://grants.nih.gov/grants/guide/notice-files/NOT-HS-16-009.html

NEJM Catalyst. (2018). What is patient flow? Retrieved from https://catalyst.nejm.org/doi/full/10.1056/CAT.18.0289

New York State Education Department (NYSED). (2017). Frequently asked questions: Electronic transmittal of prescriptions in New York State. Retrieved from http://www.op.nysed.gov/prof/pharm/pharmelectrans.htm

Nuckols, T., Asch, S., Patel, V., Keeler, E., Anderson, L., Buntin, M., & Escarc, J. (2015). Implementing computerized provider order entry in acute care hospitals in the United States could generate substantial savings to society. *Joint Commission Quality Patient Safety, 41,* 341–350.

Otterman, S. (2016, March 14). The end of prescriptions as we know them in New York. *New York Times,* pp. A22–A23.

Overdyk, F. (2015). Remote video auditing with real-time feedback in an academic surgical suite improves safety and efficiency metrics: A cluster randomized study. *BMJ Quality Safety,* doi:10.1136/bmjqs-2015-004226. Retrieved from https://qualitysafety.bmj.com/content/25/12/947

Pannick, S., Davis, R., Ashrafian, H., Byrne, B., Beveridge, I., Athanasiou, T., . . . Sevdalis, N. (2015). Effects of interdisciplinary team care interventions on general medical wards: A systematic review. *JAMA Internal Medicine, 175*(8), 1288–1298.

Paull, D., Mazzia, L., Neily J., Mills, P., Turner, J., Gunnar W., & Hemphill, R. (2015). Errors upstream and downstream to the universal protocol associated with wrong surgery events in the Veterans Health Administration. *American Journal of Surgery, 210*(1), 6–13.

Payne, T., Hines, L., Chan, R., Hartman, S., Kapusnik-Uner, J., Russ, A., . . . Malone, D. (2015). Recommendations to improve the usability of drug-drug interaction clinical decision support alerts. *Journal of the American Medical Informatics Association.* Retrieved from http://jamia.oxfordjournals.org/content/jaminfo/early/2015/03/30/jamia.ocv011.full.pdf

Phansalkar, S., van der Sijs, H., Tucker, A., Desai, A., Bell, D., Teich, J., . . . Bates, D. (2013). Drug-drug interactions that should be non-interruptive in order to reduce alert fatigue in electronic health records. *Journal of American Medical Informatics Association, 20,* 489–493.

Plisena, J., Gagliardi, A, Urbach, D., Clifford, T., & Fiander, M. (2015). Factors that influence recognition, reporting, and resolution of incidents related to medical devices and other healthcare technologies: A systematic review. *Systematic Review, 4,* 37. Retrieved from http://www.ncbi.nlm.nih.gov/pmc/articles/PMC4384231

Potter, P., Wolf, L., Boxerman, S., Grayson, D., Sledge, J., Dunagan, C., & Bradley Evanoff. (2014). An analysis of nurses' cognitive work: A new perspective for understanding medical errors (pp. 39–50). Agency for Healthcare Research and Quality (AHRQ). *Advances in patient safety*. Retrieved from https://www.ncbi.nlm.nih.gov/books/NBK20475

Quist, A., Hickman, T-T., Amato, M., Volk, L., Salazar, A., Robertson, A., . . . Schiff, G. (2017). Analysis of variations in the display of drug names in computerized prescriber-order-entry systems. *American Journal of Health System Pharmacy, 74*(7), 499–509.

Robichaud, P., Saari, M., Burnham, E., Omar, S., Wray, R., Baker, G., & Matlow, A. (2012). The value of a quality improvement project in promoting interprofessional collaboration. *Journal of Interprofessional Care, 26*(2), 158–160.

Rosenbaum, L. (2019). Teamwork—Part 1: Divided we fall; Part 2: Cursed by knowledge—Building a culture of psychological safety; and Part 3: The not-my-problem problem. *New England Journal of Medicine, 389,* 684–688; 786–790; 881–885.

Rozich, J., Howard, R., Justeson, J., Macken, P., Lindsay, M., & Resar, R. (2004). Standardization as a mechanism to improve safety in health care. *Joint Commission Journal Quality and Safety, 30*(1), 5–14.

Rudman, W., Bailey, J., Hope, C., Garrett, P., & Brown, C. (2014). The impact of web-based reporting system on the collection of medication error occurrence data (pp. 195–205). Agency for Healthcare Research and Quality (AHRQ). *Advances in patient safety*. Retrieved from http://www.ahrq.gov/professionals/quality-patient-safety/patient-safety-resources/resources/advances-in-patient-safety/index.html

Rutherford, P., Provost, L., Kotagal, U., Luther, K., & Anderson, A. (2017). *Achieving hospital-wide patient flow*. IHI White Paper. Cambridge, MA: Institute for Healthcare Improvement. Retrieved from http://www.ihi.org/resources/Pages/IHIWhitePapers/Achieving-Hospital-wide-Patient-Flow.aspx

Saint Louis, C. (2016, January 14). Medical scope is linked to infections, Senate says. *New York Times*, A13.

Schwiran, P., & Thede, L. (2011). Informatics: The standardized nursing terminologies: A national survey of nurses' experiences and attitudes. *OJIN, 16*(2). Retrieved from http://ojin.nursingworld.org/mainmenucategories/anamarketplace/anaperiodicals/ojin/columns/informatics/standardized-nursing-terminologies.html

Shojania, K. (2015, November). In conversation with . . . Kaveh Shojania, MD. *Perspectives on Safety*. Retrieved from https://psnet.ahrq.gov/perspective/conversation-kaveh-shojania-md

Simone, L., Brumbaugh, J., & Ricketts, C. (2014). Medical devices, the FDA, and the home healthcare clinician. *Home Healthcare Nurse, 32*(7), 402–408.

Sitting, D., & Singh, H. (2015). The health IT safety center roadmap: What's next? Health Affairs Blog. Retrieved from http://healthaffairs.org/blog/2015/07/21/the-health-it-safety-center-roadmap-whats-next

Smith, P., & McSweeney, J. (2017). Organizational perspectives of nurse executives in 15 hospitals on the impact and effectiveness of rapid response teams. *Joint Commission Journal on Quality and Patient Safety, 43*(6), 289–298.

Soriano, R., Siegel, E., Kim, T., & Catz, S. (2019). Nurse managers' experiences with electronic health records in quality monitoring. *Nursing Administration Quarterly, 43*(3), 222–229.

Totten, A., Hansen, R., Wagner, J., Stillman, L., Ivlev, I., Davis-O'Reilly, C., . . . McDonagh, M. (2019). Telehealth for acute and chronic care consultations. Comparative effectiveness review No. 216. AHRQ Publication No. 19-#HC012-EF. Rockville, MD: Agency for Healthcare Research and Quality.

U.S. & World Report. (2015, September 29). Ohio hospital loses newborn's remains, trash searched. Retrieved from http://www.necn.com/news/national-international/Infant-Remains-Lost-University-of-Cincinnati-Medical-Center-329958311.html

U.S. Department of Health and Human Services (HHS). (2014). More physicians and hospitals are using EHRs than before. Retrieved from http://www.hhs.gov/news/press/2014pres/08/20140807a.html

U.S. Department of Health and Human Services (HHS). (2019). Meaningful use regulations. Retrieved from https://www.healthit.gov/topic/laws-regulation-and-policy/health-it-regulation-resources

U.S. Department of Health and Human Services (HHS), Agency for Healthcare Research and Quality. (AHRQ). (2014). Identify defects through sensemaking. Retrieved from https://www.ahrq.gov/hai/cusp/modules/identify/identify.html

U.S. Department of Health and Human Services (HHS), Agency for Healthcare Research and Quality (AHRQ). (2015a). What is workflow? Retrieved from https://healthit.ahrq.gov/health-it-tools-and-resources/workflow-assessment-health-it-toolkit/workflow

U.S. Department of Health and Human Services (HHS), Agency for Healthcare Research and Quality (AHRQ).

(2015b). Plenary: TeamSTEPPS in Crisis Situations. Retrieved from https://www.ahrq.gov/teamstepps /national-meeting/2013-conference-materials/ts -crisis-situations.html

U.S. Department of Health and Human Services (HHS), Agency for Healthcare Research and Quality (AHRQ). (2017). Organizational readiness resources. Retrieved from https://www.ahrq.gov/sites/default/files/wysiyg/working forquality/nqs/toolkits/nqs-readiness-resources.pdf

U.S. Department of Health and Human Services (HHS), Agency for Healthcare Research and Quality (AHRQ). (2018). Health information technology research. 2018 year in review. Retrieved from https://healthit. ahrq.gov/2018-year-review

U.S. Department of Health and Human Services (HHS), Agency for Healthcare Research and Quality (AHRQ). (2019a). Quality and patient safety resources. Retrieved from http://www.ahrq.gov/qual/qitoolkit

U.S. Department of Health and Human Services (HHS), Agency for Healthcare Research and Quality (AHRQ). (2019b). TeamSTEPPS®: Strategies and tools to enhance performance and patient safety. Retrieved from https:// www.ahrq.gov/teamstepps/index.html

U.S. Department of Health and Human Services (HHS), Agency for Healthcare Research and Quality (AHRQ). (2019c). EvidenceNow. Retrieved from https://www .ahrq.gov/evidencenow/index.html

U.S. Department of Health and Human Services (HHS), Agency for Healthcare Research and Quality (AHRQ), Patient Safety Network (PSNet). (2006). Universal protocol for preventing wrong site, wrong procedure, wrong person surgery. Retrieved from https://psnet.ahrq.gov/issue /universal-protocol-preventing-wrong-site-wrong -procedure-wrong-person-surgery

U.S. Department of Health and Human Services (HHS), Agency for Healthcare Research and Quality (AHRQ), Patient Safety Network (PSNet). (2014a). Safety assurance factors for EHR resilience. Retrieved from https://psnet.ahrq.gov/issue /safety-assurance-factors-ehr-resilience-safer-guides

U.S. Department of Health and Human Services (HHS), Agency for Healthcare Research and Quality (AHRQ), Patient Safety Network (PSNet). (2014b). Safety assurance factors for EHR resilience: SAFER guides. Retrieved from https://psnet.ahrq.gov/issue /safety-assurance-factors-ehr-resilience-safer-guides

U.S. Department of Health and Human Services (HHS), Agency for Healthcare Research and Quality (AHRQ), Patient Safety Network (PSNet). (2014b). Computerized provider order entry. Retrieved from http://psnet .ahrq.gov/primer.aspx?primerID=6

U.S. Department of Health and Human Services (HHS), Agency for Healthcare Research and Quality (AHRQ), Patient Safety Network (PSNet). (2015). Handoffs and signouts. Retrieved from https://psnet.ahrq.gov /primers/primer/9/handoffs-and-signouts

U.S. Department of Health and Human Services (HHS), Agency for Healthcare Research and Quality (AHRQ), Patient Safety Network (PSNet). (2019a). Patient safety primers. Retrieved from https://psnet.ahrq.gov/primersx

U.S. Department of Health and Human Services (HHS), Agency for Healthcare Research and Quality (AHRQ), Patient Safety Network (PSNet). (2019b). Checklists. Retrieved from https://psnet.ahrq.gov/primer/checklists

U.S. Department of Health and Human Services (HHS), Agency for Healthcare Research and Quality (AHRQ), Patient Safety Network (PSNet). (2019c). Rapid response systems. Retrieved from https://psnet.ahrq .gov/primers/primer/4/rapid-response-systems

U.S. Department of Health and Human Services (HHS), Agency for Healthcare Research and Quality (AHRQ), Patient Safety Network (PSNet). (2019d). Medication reconciliation. Retrieved from https://psnet.ahrq.gov /primers/primer/1/medication-reconciliation

U.S. Department of Health and Human Services (HHS), Agency for Healthcare Research and Quality (AHRQ), Patient Safety Network (PSNet). (2019e). Computerized provider order entry. Retrieved from https://psnet.ahrq .gov/primer/computerized-provider-order-entry

U.S. Department of Health and Human Services (HHS). Food and Drug Administration (FDA). (2016). Product problems. Retrieved from https://www.fda.gov/safety /reporting-serious-problems-fda/product-problems

U.S. Department of Health and Human Services (HHS), Health Resources and Services Administration (HRSA). (2011a). Redesigning a system of care to promote QI. Retrieved from https://www.hrsa.gov/sites/default/files/quality /toolbox/508pdfs/redesignsystemofcaretopromoteqi.pdf

U.S. Department of Health and Human Services (HHS), Health Resources and Services Administration (HRSA). (2011b). Improvement teams. Retrieved from http://www.hrsa.gov/quality/toolbox/methodology /improvementteams/part4.html

U.S. Department of Health and Human Services (HHS), Health Resources and Services Administration (HRSA). (2011c). Readiness assessment and developing project aims. Retrieved from https://www.hrsa.gov /sites/default/files/quality/toolbox/508pdfs /readinessassessment.pdf

U.S. Department of Health and Human Services (HHS), Office of the National Coordinator for Health Information Technology (ONC). (2019a). Health IT enabled quality improvement: A vision to achieve better health and health care. Retrieved from https://www .healthit.gov/sites/default/files/HITEnabledQuality Improvement-111214.pdf

U.S. Department of Health and Human Services (HHS), Office of the National Coordinator for Health Information Technology (ONC). (2019b). Connecting health and care for the nation: A shared nationwide interoperability roadmap draft version 1.0. Retrieved from https://www.healthit.gov/sites/default

/files/hie-interoperability/nationwide-interoperability-roadmap-final-version-1.0.pdf

U.S. Department of Health and Human Services (HHS), Office of the National Coordinator for Health Information Technology (ONC). (2020). 2020–2025 Federal health IT strategic plan. Retrieved from https://www.healthit.gov/sites/default/files/page/2020-01/2020-2025FederalHealthIT%20StrategicPlan_0.pdf

Weinstock, M. (2007, March 3). There's no "I" in team. *H&HN 81*(9), 38-46.

Wood, C., Chaboyer, W., & Carr, P. (2019). How do nurses use early warning scoring systems to detect and act on patient deterioration to ensure patient safety? A scoping review. *International Journal of Nursing Studies, 94*(6), 166–178.

Woods, A. & Doahn-Johnson, S. (2002). Executive summary: Toward a taxonomy of nursing practice errors. *Nursing Management 33*(10), 45-48.

Xiao, Y., Mackenzie, C., & Seagull, J. (2015). Video to improve patient safety: Clinical and education uses. U.S. Department of Health and Human Services, Agency for Healthcare Research and Quality, Patient Safety Network. Retrieved from https://psnet.ahrq.gov/perspective/video-improve-patient-safety-clinical-and-educational-uses

## CHAPTER 12

# Nursing Leadership for Quality Improvement

## CHAPTER OBJECTIVES

At the conclusion of this chapter, the learner will be able to:

- Examine the current progress of the *Future of Nursing* report.
- Explain the importance of transformational leadership to nursing's role in continuous quality improvement (CQI).
- Critique the need for effective decision making to ensure quality care.
- Summarize the need for effective communication in leading CQI.
- Formulate a clear statement supporting the need for staff education and improving care.
- Examine the best approach to nursing leadership that supports CQI.
- Explain how the examples of nursing initiatives to improve care are important in supporting nursing leadership and nursing engagement in CQI.

## OUTLINE

## KEY TERMS

| | | |
|---|---|---|
| Accountability | Empowerment | Responsibility |
| Clinical judgment | Leadership | Shared governance |
| Clinical reasoning | Management | Supervision |
| Critical reflection | Micromanaging | Transformational leadership |
| Critical thinking | Power | |
| Delegation | Powerlessness | |

## Introduction

Throughout this text there is content about nurses and the need for more nursing leadership at all staff levels and in all settings in continuous quality improvement (CQI). This chapter focuses on highlighting some issues that nurses need to consider as they develop their own competencies in CQI and lead efforts to improve care.

The American Nurses Association (ANA) has long been active in pursuing improved care and supporting the need for a more active nursing role in CQI through education, research, publications, lobbying to improve care, collaboration with other organizations, and development of and participation in many other initiatives. The ANA website offers multiple resources on the culture of safety (ANA, 2016). Some of the topics include the culture of safety, healthy nurses, fatigue and shift work, infections, transitions of care, data and systems thinking, and other related topics—all are topics discussed in this text. It is significant that this healthcare professional organization recognizes the critical need to improve care and the nursing leadership required to support improvement.

## Progress Toward Meeting *The Future of Nursing: Leading Change, Advancing Health* Recommendations

*The Future of Nursing: Leading Change, Advancing Health* (IOM, 2010) is discussed throughout this text. The focus now is on the status of this report's evidence-based recommendations— what has been accomplished since 2010, and how does this impact nursing and its role in CQI? In 2016, a progress report was published (National Academy of Medicine [NAM], 2016), and further analysis has continued since 2016. If we support the need for improvement in healthcare delivery, then it is important to assess our own professional progress and outcomes and then develop and implement strategies/interventions to continue our efforts as a profession to improve.

After the publication of the 2010 nursing report, a major initiative was undertaken, supported by the Robert Wood Johnson Foundation, to encourage change based on *The Future of Nursing* recommendations. This initiative is The Future of Nursing: Campaign for Action (referred to here simply as the Campaign or Campaign for Action) (Campaign for Action, 2019). The American Association of Retired Persons (AARP) is also a partner with the Robert Wood Johnson Foundation (RWJF) in this campaign. Despite all the work that has been done, major problems with healthcare quality have not been eliminated—for example, one study noted that if death due to error were listed with the major causes of death in the United States, it would rank third (Makary, 2016). Results like this emphasize the challenges we face in healthcare delivery to improve care and health of patients and how nurses must step up to guide and engage in the efforts.

As discussed in many chapters in this text, since 1999 and the first *Quality Chasm* reports, there has been greater concern in our view of the healthcare delivery system related to quality, diversity and disparities, teams and interprofessional teamwork, cost, collaboration, care coordination, patient-centered care, and integration of the Triple Aim (better care, healthy people/healthy communities, affordable care). The 2016 progress report recommendations are related to all of these issues, and even more so than in 2010, as there is now greater understanding of the CQI problem. For the focus of this text and chapter, the following list identifies *The Future of Nursing* report's recommendations and provides a summary of some of the progress and relevance to CQI (Campaign for Action, 2020: IOM, 2010):

1. *Remove scope of practice barriers.* In 2010, 13 states met the criteria for full practice authority, and since then, more states have been added. Some states have made some changes but still do not fully meet the criteria. The Centers for Medicare and Medicaid Services (CMS) has expanded the scope of practice for CMS payment;

however, medical staff membership and hospital privileges for advanced practice registered nurses (APRNs) continue to be based on state laws and business preferences rather than federal law—and many states have expanded APRN scope of practice as has the U.S. Department of Veterans Affairs.

*Relevance to CQI:* This outcome is not fully met, but there has been steady improvement. How does scope of practice impact CQI? It impacts nursing practice—what nurses do. In the case of this report, the focus was on APRNs. What APRNs and also registered nurses (RNs) can do in their practice is directed by state nurse practice acts, and as noted, this is improving. Healthcare organizations (HCOs) must ensure that clinicians of all professions follow the requirements to meet the standards.

2. *Expand opportunities for nurses to lead and diffuse collaborative improvement efforts.* The National Academy of Medicine explains the need to expand nursing care models to meet the changing demands of health care (NAM, 2016). Some of these new models are accountable care organizations, nurse-managed health centers/ clinics (NMHCs), and others. These new models support and assist in meeting this recommendation. Data reported in early 2020 indicate that 30 million people in the United States receive care from an ACO (Dartmouth College, 2020). The CMS has invested in developing ACOs for its beneficiaries. NMHCs have also expanded across the United States.

*Relevance to CQI:* Collaboration is a critical component of care today, and it is important for effective interprofessional teamwork, one of the healthcare professions core competencies identified in the *Quality Chasm* reports (IOM, 2003). Effective CQI requires care coordination and collaboration from many stakeholders (clinical and nonclinical), including many professional organizations, professional education programs, accrediting organizations, government agencies, and third-party payers. The new models provide new opportunities for nurses to lead and collaborate, and in the future, it is hoped other models will be developed—and nursing roles and responsibilities will expand. Schools of nursing are offering more required clinical courses and/or activities that include both registered nurse students and graduate students of other health professions.

3. *Implement nurse residency programs.* At the time of the publication of *The Future of Nursing* report, staff turnover and retention were of concern, and these continue to be concerns. Nurses participating in residency programs is one method that may reduce this problem, and the report focused on these programs for new graduates. The progress report notes that these programs should also be available for nurses transitioning to new settings and for APRNs. In 2011, the National Council of State Boards of Nursing (NCSBN) engaged in research about transition-to-practice programs (NCSBN, 2019). Residency programs vary, but the progress report notes that they do have value in helping nurses develop competencies important in improving practice and self-confidence in practice. Similar programs for nurses are also needed in outpatient settings. Most states now have some hospitals offering nurse residency programs.

*Relevance to CQI:* This result indicates there has been progress, although more programs are needed. These programs are costly to develop and implement. The American Association of Colleges of Nursing (AACN) provides a model and standards for nurse residency programs focused on graduates with a baccalaureate degree in nursing (BSN), although not all existing residency programs are accredited (AACN, 2019). The programs can be particularly helpful in encouraging nurses to participate in CQI by including nurse residency content and experiences related to evidence-based practice (EBP), CQI, and evidence-based management (EBM).

4. *Increase the proportion of nurses with a baccalaureate degree to 80% by 2020.* In 2018, 57% of practicing nurses had achieved a BSN, indicating steady improvement in this recommendation. There are other important improvements, such as the number of four-year nursing (BSN) programs increased and more employers are requiring BSN degrees. However, the progress report indicates a need to continue to focus on improving nursing education programs; also, funding for degrees must be monitored and improved, which is a barrier to increasing enrollment.

*Relevance to CQI:* Leaders are needed in all types of healthcare settings to improve care. Education is needed to prepare competent nurses who can assume roles that include CQI activities, meeting the healthcare core competency related to quality improvement (IOM, 2003). Nurses with BSN degrees typically have a positive impact on the quality of care. There are now more opportunities for nurses who do not have BSN degrees to obtain the degree, and many more HCOs are requiring BSNs and supporting nurses to expand their education. This trend will likely continue.

5. *Double the number of nurses with a doctorate by 2020.* The recommendation does not specify details as to type of doctorate (e.g., doctorate in nursing practice [DNP], PhD in nursing, PhD in another field) or

number of degrees per type. Enrollment in total has increased. Major barriers are funding and number of faculty and their experience. The number of nurses with doctoral degrees has increased and met the recommendation for this degree. Since the publication of *The Future of Nursing*, the terminal degree for advanced practice registered nursing has changed to DNP; consequently, these programs are transitioning to this degree.

Relevance to CQI: It is expected that nurses with the highest degree would serve in leadership positions in HCOs, on faculty, and in other positions, such as policymaking and leadership in the government at local, state, and federal levels. All need to guide nursing engagement in CQI.

6. *Ensure that nurses engage in lifelong learning.* The progress report (NAM, 2016) states the following: "Continuing education and competence have not kept pace with the needs of the increasingly complex, team-based healthcare system. Nurses and other providers will increasingly need to update skills for providing care in both hospital and community-based settings" (p. 7). We need more data about continuing education, particularly about its impact on patient outcomes. As noted in other chapters, there have been greater efforts to understand and support interprofessional continuing education (IOM, 2009). In addition, we need to better understand the implications of the relationship between nurse certification, credentialing, and lifelong learning and the impact of these efforts on practice and patient outcomes as well as on collaboration and leadership.

Relevance to CQI: Education, including lifelong learning, is discussed in other chapters, and it is critical in maintaining and developing knowledge and competencies. Lifelong learning should include content and

experiences related to CQI. This is a rapidly changing area, and one in which nurses must actively participate. If we expect staff to engage in interprofessional teams within the context of CQI and practice, interprofessional initiatives are particularly important.

7. *Prepare and enable nurses to lead change to advance health.* There has been progress with the campaign and the development of the Interprofessional Education Collaborative (IPE, 2016) supported by the Josiah Macy Jr. Foundation. These competencies are important and should be included in academic and staff education. They are discussed in other chapters in this text. *The Future of Nursing* report recommended that there be 10,000 nurses on boards by 2020. As of January 2020, 7,100 were identified as serving on boards, and thus they were serving in a critical position for healthcare decision making.

Relevance to CQI: There are many types of leadership, and nurses are involved or need to be more involved in leadership. Hospital boards direct the vision and goals of the hospitals, including CQI, and thus are important. Nurses need to actively participate in all types of leadership activities. Communicating the need for nursing leadership and what nurses can offer has progressed, but this effort has primarily focused on nurses. More needs to be done to inform other healthcare professionals, patients, families, and other relevant parties about the roles of nurses, and not just during the annual National Nurses Week.

8. *Build an infrastructure for the collection and analysis of interprofessional healthcare workforce data.* This text discusses measurement—how it works and barriers to success. The progress report notes similar concerns in assessing *The Future of Nursing* recommendations. Data must be

collected and analyzed to drive decisions. The Affordable Care Act of 2010 included a provision to establish the National Healthcare Workforce Commission, focused on all healthcare professions, including nursing. This commission should be considered an important resource for gathering workforce data and analysis; however, there have been funding problems for the commission. The goal was for this commission to be a source of information and provide guidance to healthcare professions to ensure a sufficient number of competent healthcare providers entering the healthcare delivery system, a problem noted in the *Quality Chasm* reports (IOM, 2003). States have increased their efforts to collect data on nurse education programs, supply of nurses, and demand for nurses.

One workforce problem that *The Future of Nursing* report noted was nursing workforce diversity, and it continues to be a problem identified in the 2016 progress report. Data about diversity in nursing is collected. Important focus points are recruitment, retention, and success in nursing education programs monitored long term. Diversity must be a workforce priority. The campaign's 2020 data indicate that in 2018 prelicensure RN program graduates were 85.9% female and 14.0% male, which is an increase in men in nursing, with some 30% of students in all nursing degree programs representing minority populations. Other data collected indicate the following findings from the National Sample Survey of Registered Nurses (NSSRN), administered by the Health Resources and Services Administration (U.S. Department of Health and Human Services [HHS], HRSA, 2020):

- An estimated 3,957,661 licensed registered nurses live in the United States. In 2017, roughly 83% (3,272,872 RNs) held a nursing-related job.

- The average age of an RN was 50 years; however, most nurses (53%) were less than 50 years old.
- Nurses are more diverse today than shown in the 2008 NSSRN study. Both minority groups and men have seen a slight increase within the RN population.
- Most of the RN workforce is college educated (63.9%). Of them, nurses with a master's or doctorate degree accounted for 19.3%.
- Advanced practice RNs account for approximately 11.5% of the nursing workforce.
- Telehealth capabilities were reported in 32.9% of nurses' workplaces. Among them, 50.3% of nurses used telehealth in their practice.
- Median earnings for full-time RNs were $73,929, while part-time RNs earned a median amount of $39,985.

The 2016 progress report identifies barriers to data collection that must be addressed: lack of consistent national indicators to provide consistent state-to-state data, lag time in data collection and reporting, lack of standardized databases, and need to use proxy measures to assess progress toward *The Future of Nursing* recommendations. The lack of effective national infrastructure (the commission) to meet this recommendation continues to be a major problem.

*Relevance to CQI:* Workforce data are important to CQI. This information provides greater understanding of the current status of problems related to staffing levels and mix and competent staff (for all healthcare professions, not just nursing). This information can then be used to develop strategies to address workforce problems and also address problems with recruitment and retention as a component of ensuring quality care and reducing errors. The information can also be used to support requests for health professions education funding and to identify improvements that might be needed in health professions education programs.

The Campaign for Action now tracks results that flow from the original *The Future of Nursing* report. Its vision is "Everyone in America can live a healthier life, supported by nurses as essential partners in providing care and promoting equity and well-being" (Campaign for Action, 2020). The Future of Nursing 2020-2030 now extends the work of the original report and will examine the following (NAM, 2019):

- The role of nurses in improving the health of individuals, families, and communities by addressing social determinants of health and providing effective, efficient, equitable, and accessible care for all across the care continuum, as well as identifying the system facilitators and barriers to achieving this goal
- The current and future deployment of all levels of nurses across the care continuum, including in collaborative practice models, to address the challenges of building a culture of health
- System facilitators and barriers to achieving a workforce that is diverse, including gender, race, and ethnicity, across all levels of nursing education
- The role of the nursing profession in ensuring that the voices of individuals, families, and communities are incorporated into design and operations of clinical and community health systems
- The training and competency-development needed to prepare nurses, including advanced practice nurses, to work outside of acute care settings and to lead efforts to build a culture of health and health equity, and the

extent to which current curriculum meets these needs
- The ability of nurses to serve as change agents in creating systems that bridge the delivery of health care and social needs care in the community
- The research needed to identify or develop effective nursing practices for eliminating gaps and disparities in health care
- The importance of nurse well-being and resilience in ensuring the delivery of high-quality care and improving community health

---

**STOP AND CONSIDER 12-1**

Some years after the publication of *The Future of Nursing* report, we still have much work to do to meet its recommendations.

---

# Transformational Leadership

Leadership is required in all healthcare settings, such as hospitals, clinics, home care, long-term care, and community or public health services. Today, managers must make more complex decisions and carry more accountability. Ideally, all managers should be leaders, but this is not always the case. This chapter focuses on the nature of leadership and how it can improve care for patients and also improve the HCO work environment. Some staff members are in formal management positions, and others are not, but all, including staff nurses, need to understand leadership to work effectively in the healthcare environment. **Transformational leadership** has been identified in various reports and by professional organizations as an important leadership approach for healthcare delivery and nursing leadership and management (Finkelman, 2019, 2020). The *Quality Chasm* reports, particularly *Leadership by Example* (IOM,

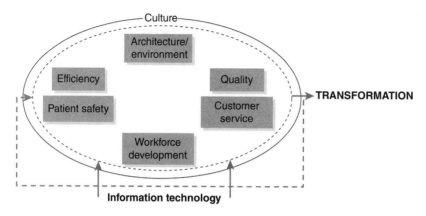

**Figure 12-1** Perspectives for Transformation

Reproduced from Agency for Healthcare Research and Quality (AHRQ). (2004). A toolkit for redesign in health care: final report. AHRQ Publication No. 05-0108-EF. Retrieved from https://www.ahrq.gov/patient-safety/resources/resdesign-tool/kit4.html

2002), *Keeping Patients Safe* (IOM, 2004), and *The Future of Nursing* (IOM, 2010), support use of transformational leadership.

As is true for CQI and change models, leadership theories and models have changed and adapted, and new ones have been added. Moving from autocratic, bureaucratic, and laissez-faire approaches, the more current emphasis is on transformational leadership. There are other types of models, and many of them incorporate elements of transformational leadership. Transformational leaders are better able to transform the system. As we recognize the need to consider redesigning and improving the status of care quality in the United States, this approach is important to nursing and to the discussion about CQI. **Figure 12-1** describes one perspective of transformation.

## Description

**Leadership** is a term that is formally defined, but it is also a term that requires individuals to apply their personal views of leadership— what it means to them and how they view it in others. Concepts that relate to leadership include the following:

- *Advocacy.* The act of speaking for another and providing support
- *Authority.* The power to act

- *Autonomy.* The capacity to determine one's own action
- *Motivate.* To get another person to do something that may require extra effort

Leadership is the ability to influence, inspire, and guide others. It may be confused with **management**, which ensures that the structure and resources exist to accomplish the job. Management focuses on four functions:

1. *Planning.* Identify the short- and long-term objectives and related actions with a timeline.
2. *Organizing.* Arrange resources needed to accomplish the work that needs to be done. Examples of resources are competent and sufficient staff, supplies, equipment, space, and budget.
3. *Leading.* Guide the process of work, which may require directing, delegating, coordinating, influencing, ensuring a positive work environment, and applying other methods to ensure that work is done effectively.
4. *Controlling.* Ensure that outcomes are met, evaluating and adapting as need.

Managers hold specific positions in an organization, such as nurse manager, director of health informatics, director of quality improvement, pharmacy supervisor, or laboratory manager. Position descriptions for a manager position integrate the four functions.

## Leadership Characteristics, Knowledge, and Competencies

Leaders are found in all types of HCOs. Some are in formal management positions, and some are not. There are myths about leadership, such as the following, that are commonly mentioned when leadership is discussed (Goffee & Jones, 2000):

- *Everyone can be a leader.* People may have leadership potential, but not everyone can be an effective leader.
- *Leaders deliver business results.* Leaders do not always deliver expected outcomes.
- *People who get to the top are leaders.* Many people in high positions in HCOs do not function as leaders, although they may have been more effective leaders when in lower positions.
- *Leaders are great coaches.* Not all leaders are great coaches. Some leaders are better at inspiring and influencing, and some are less able to share important competencies for development of staff.

Why is it important to identify myths? We sometimes make assumptions that then lead to poor leadership working relationships, and often management and staff mention these myths. Leaders can be developed with additional education and mentoring, but leaders are not perfect and may function at different levels of effectiveness. Leaders make mistakes, and some leaders may be better at different aspects of leadership than others. We all have encountered managers whose behavior made us wonder how they reached their position. They are promoted to the point where they are not effective. With clinical staff, the assumption often is made that if you are a competent nurse, then you would be an effective manager. This is not always the case. Different characteristics and competencies are required for a management position compared to a clinical staff position. A question commonly asked is this: Is a manager a leader? The manager holds a formal leadership position and should be a leader, demonstrating leadership competencies; however, many managers are not leaders or are not viewed by others as leaders.

Successful leaders and managers also should be able to assess staff mood, morale, and the work environment to effectively guide staff and ensure a positive work environment. Staff often recognizes managers who are also leaders, although they may not mention leadership to describe the manager. They might say the manager is interested in more than just "getting the job done" or that the manager seems to care, understands the work processes and impact on staff and outcomes, and engages staff in the process of improving. Staff would not say this manager abstains from decision making or is not available and leaves them on their own but, rather, that the manager is there in the workplace with them. The effective manager uses knowledge management by bringing together staff with a variety of knowledge levels and expertise and making the whole greater than any individual staff member—focusing on teamwork. We are told frequently that teamwork is critical to effective healthcare. We know that this is complex. Those who have worked in teams, whether they are teams of nursing staff or interprofessional teams, know there is much to do to develop and maintain effective teams—and even times when we think it would be easier to just do everything by ourselves.

Whenever possible, a proactive approach prevents problems, improves communication and problem solving, and demonstrates more concern for staff and outcomes. Facilitating staff engagement is a critical method for reaching outcomes. The manager also considers what staff are doing and whether the work can be done more effectively, improving performance. They determine resources that are needed and identify changes in processes to reach better productivity. To accomplish this, the manager requires staff feedback and staff participation in the change process.

Leaders exhibit a number of important characteristics. They need to have self-understanding, or self-awareness. This trait enables them to understand and assess and influence others. Trusting oneself is a critical characteristic. Rigidity does not help a leader; rather, the ability to be flexible at appropriate times results in more effective leadership. Leaders often challenge the status quo. Leaders care about people. Honesty is an important characteristic. Staff members usually recognize leaders who are not honest with them. Leaders use advocacy effectively. Just as is true with managers, there are ranges of effective leaders; some are more effective than others. Leaders also focus on staff strengths, not staff weaknesses. This approach develops staff self-confidence.

The term *transformational* in transformational leadership emphasizes change, and this is a critical aspect of this leadership style. Change and improvement are considered critical aspects of successful organizations. HCOs require leaders and managers who appreciate that change is needed and also know how to engage in change and bring staff into the process. Effective leadership does not mean the staff are always told what they must do and that there is no flexibility (as in autocratic and bureaucratic styles of leadership). Nor does it mean that the leader or manager turns all decision making and planning over to the staff (as in a laissez-faire style of leadership). The transformational leader is very involved in the process of work and change, but this leader knows how to assess staff and their needs, how to guide them, reward them, provide constructive criticism, and create and maintain a positive work environment. Transformational leaders guide staff in developing a vision that provides a perspective of the organization in the future: *This is where we want to be.* The mission statement then connects to the vision and establishes goals and purpose—how we will get to the vision. Issues and factors that drive the need to change the view of HCO leadership include the following:

- Greater need for teams and effective teamwork, including team leaders and members (followers)
- Greater recognition that the specific characteristics of a situation impact leaders and managers
- Increased use of collaboration and coordination
- Need to improve communication
- Increased recognition of need to engage all staff
- Emphasis on change and how to use it as opportunity
- Recognition that factors such as feelings, self-esteem, and listening and responding impact leadership, staff, and work outcomes
- Need for understanding and development of the knowledge worker
- Need for effective use of EBP and EBM

Related to all of these issues and factors is CQI, which cannot be effectively managed without considering how nurses will respond to them. Establishing and maintaining a culture of safety now constitute an important part of HCO leadership.

To better understand leadership and its relationship to CQI, it is important to identify the areas in which managers must be knowledgeable to be effective and meet their responsibilities:

- Clinical practice
- Communication and relationship building
- Collaboration
- Coordination
- Change process
- Planning and decision making (strategic, operational, project)
- Teams and teamwork
- Guiding and teaching staff
- Delegation
- Budgeting and healthcare financing
- Problem solving and use of critical thinking
- Crisis management

- Performance appraisal
- CQI planning, measurement, and process
- Evidence-based practice and evidence-based management
- Accreditation
- Staffing, including recruitment and retention
- Risk management and utilization management
- Health informatics
- Ethics and legal concerns
- Conflict resolution and negotiation
- Diversity and disparities
- Regulatory compliance
- Policy and procedures, including development and implementation

The competencies required of a leader are the same as those of a manager, although the degree of emphasis placed on each competency may vary depending on the leader's position. The following competencies are required for effective leadership:

- Analyze information and the environment to understand current status, respond to current status and problems, and project future problems.
- Use collaboration and coordination.
- Plan effectively (strategic, operational, project).
- Communicate clearly and in a timely manner.
- Influence and motivate others.
- Create and innovate.
- Ask staff for feedback routinely and apply as appropriate.
- Share information with staff so they can understand decisions and recognize progress.
- Apply the CQI process, including effective measurement.
- Engage staff in CQI.
- Empower others.
- Work effectively on leadership teams and leading teams.
- Recognize success in others.
- Advocate for patients and their families and for staff.

- Work toward consistent transparency and ethical decision making.

Effective leadership requires that the leader step back and see the "big picture," and this must be an ongoing process. This is a critical element of transformational leadership.

Leaders and managers gain their leadership knowledge and competencies from a variety of sources. Many have completed formal academic work and may have graduate degrees. Some managers had management content integrated in their professional degree programs, such as leadership and management content in prelicensure programs. The third source is staff education and continuing education. This education should include leadership development, methods to improve management, such as time management, priority setting, using the change process effectively, planning methods, budgeting, quality improvement and measurement, and current trends and issues related to health policy and standards.

Staffing, which includes selecting, orienting, and retaining staff, is a key management function. A manager who is a leader will ensure that at the beginning of the process every potential job candidate knows about the leadership style of the manager and how this impacts staff. It is not easy to retain staff. Staff turnover is disruptive and costly, and it often negatively impacts quality care. The more that staff are involved in work processes and decision making, the more committed they will be to the organization and the work unit. Involving staff requires a culture that allows for open staff communication. The effective leader knows this, strives to establish and maintain such a culture, and supports a culture of safety. Engaging potential staff in CQI, even during the selection and hiring process, can be very beneficial to the potential employee and the HCO.

## Power and Empowerment

Power and empowerment are critical aspects of effective leadership and also are important to CQI. **Power** is about "influencing decisions, controlling resources, and affecting behavior. Power can be used constructively or destructively" (Finkelman, 2020, p. 327). To empower is to enable to act. **Empowerment**, however, means that some may gain power and some may lose power and prestige. In organizations that truly practice shared participation in decision making, middle management tends to lose the most, turning over power and authority to teams. Not only does power mean you can influence others and decisions, but you can often get things done more effectively. When the HCO or its leaders/managers empower staff to work in teams, the teams have authority to make and implement decisions. Management provides guidance and resources but does not dictate. Empowerment does not mean the staff make all decisions and that there are no guidelines and boundaries, but these are limited.

**Powerlessness** also occurs in organizations when staff feel like they have no influence and cannot influence decisions. This situation is very negative and impacts staff morale and productivity. Some managers prefer that staff do not have power, but this situation is not effective leadership and management. It represents destructive use of power.

There are various types of power, and each is based on the source of the power (Finkelman, 2019, 2020). Most power is legitimate, originating from a formal position, such as a manager position. Some staff gain power due to their experience and/or knowledge, special qualities, or ability to influence others, or as a reward. Another type of power originates when one is in a position to punish someone, which is a negative type of power. A manager may have all or some of these types of power. Staff do not, however, have to be in a formal management position to have some of these types of power. Within a work unit, staff will have different types of power—for example, nurses on a unit may go to one particular nurse, whom they consider an expert, to ask questions or to get information (expert and information power). Other staff may go to a staff member for advice because that staff member seems to care about the team members and responds quickly (referent power). Nurse managers in a hospital may pick one nurse manager to represent them with upper management because this nurse manager seems to be able to influence or persuade others. There is variation in leadership and how it is viewed and applied—all healthcare organizations and providers need to recognize this.

## Staff Engagement

Transformational leaders encourage staff to be active in work processes and decision making. This type of leadership supports "moving a profession, an institution, or some aspect of health care down a new path with different expectations, structures, and ways of conceptualizing how the mission can be achieved in light of changing conditions" (McBride, 2011, p. 179). This leader collaborates with staff to develop the vision by considering this question: Where do we want to be? The staff must be brought into the process of asking the following: (1) How do we get there? (2) How do we know we have reached our outcomes? Change is a critical and ever-present situation in transformational leadership. The leader knows this and needs to communicate to staff the value of the change process. Staff need to view the work team and their own team membership as critical to success. What can the leader do to engage staff and establish a positive work environment that supports CQI (Finkelman, 2019, 2020; IOM, 2002, 2010; McBride, 2011)?

- Recognize the value of knowledge; provide staff with opportunities to expand knowledge through staff education and other methods, such as access to academic programs.
- Ensure that staff have the information and resources they need to do their work.
- Encourage staff to share information and knowledge with the team and through other methods, such as presentations at

professional meetings, publishing articles, and so on.

- Avoid micromanaging; include staff in the decision-making process.
- Listen and respond to staff.
- Recognize staff, team, and individual successes.
- Provide mentoring and coaching opportunities for staff.
- Engage staff in decision making at all levels.
- Apply standards, policies and procedures, EBP, and EBM.
- Engage staff in evaluation of outcomes at all levels and in CQI.
- Use performance appraisal as a time to recognize accomplishments and provide constructive feedback. Support staff self-assessment.
- Support effective teamwork and expand team competencies.
- Reinforce positive feedback throughout work processes; do not just wait to do this at the annual performance appraisal.
- Ask staff for feedback about leaders' abilities and outcomes; use this information to improve leadership.
- Recognize that disagreement and conflict may occur; negotiate to meet outcomes.
- Be flexible whenever possible.
- Recognize differences/diversity as opportunities.

## STOP AND CONSIDER 12-2

Transformational leadership requires engagement of both the leader and the staff.

# Decision Making

Decision making is part of daily practice for every nurse in all settings and positions. Effective decision making, however, is a problem for many nurses. CQI requires effective decisions. Sometimes these decisions must be made quickly, and sometimes they are made after data collection and data analysis. This text discusses CQI measurement. For nurses to participate in CQI decisions, they need to understand measurement and participate in the process. In this way, nurses can be more active and more effective in making decisions about strategies/interventions to improve care and in working toward their implementation.

**Shared governance** is used more often today in HCOs because it supports transformational leadership and greater use of shared decision making—thereby engaging the staff. It may be applied to the entire organization, or it could be used primarily in one department, such as nursing or patient services. Shared governance means that the staff are encouraged to provide input in decision making and a structure is in place to facilitate this process (Di Fiore et al., 2018). To reach this goal, the staff require timely access to information. Accountability and responsibility are important at all levels in shared governance, although staff may have different accountability and responsibilities in their daily work to change or improve work processes and outcomes. In this type of organization, there is more collaboration among all levels of staff. There are councils and committees where much of the planning and decision making occur. The structured top-down chain of command is then reduced. Communication is critical in this type of organization. It must be clear, timely, and shared with appropriate staff members. This system might be called decentralized decision making because decisions are made at levels of the organization other than the top. Most decisions are made at the lower levels, where work is done. This structure does not mean that organization-wide decisions are not made or that high-level leaders do not make decisions. It does mean there is more two-way communication and decision-making flow.

Leaders need to have self-confidence, which impacts their decision making. They often work in situations that are high stress, which may negatively impact self-confidence. The leader needs to reassure others that he or she is able to lead and will be there when needed. This requires self-confidence. How can self-confidence be developed and maintained? Leaders must be able to convince themselves that their ability to lead is effective. When times get tough—and they will—leaders need to be able to maintain a feeling of self-confidence. Using a mentor may help during these times. Participation in activities outside work that provide release of stress is important. Working 24/7 is not helpful. The staff do not want to work with an exhausted, stressed leader. Being a leader can be lonely, particularly if one is in a high position or in an organization in which there are few managers—for example, a clinic that may have one or just a few managers compared to an acute care or long-term care facility with several layers of managers.

## Process: Critical Thinking and Clinical Reasoning and Judgment

Nursing has traditionally emphasized critical thinking; however, more must be done to focus on clinical reasoning and judgment (Benner, Hughes, & Sutphen, 2008; Benner, Sutphen, Leonard, & Day, 2010). **Critical thinking** is concerned with questioning, recognizing the importance of knowledge, intuition, and application of knowledge. Practice and CQI, however, also require use of clinical reasoning and judgment, creative thinking, evaluation of evidence, and application of standards of practice. **Critical reflection** is also an important component of critical thinking and "requires that the thinker [the nurse] examine the underlying assumptions and radically question or doubt the validity of arguments, assertions, and even facts of the case" (Benner, Hughes, & Sutphen, 2008, p. 3). This type of thinking is important when one examines practices that may require improvement. **Clinical judgment**—staff making decisions about clinical concerns and treatment—requires use of **clinical reasoning**. Benner

and colleagues (2008) describe clinical reasoning as follows: "Clinical reasoning stands out as a situated, practice-based form of reasoning that requires a background of scientific and technological research-based knowledge about general cases, more so than any particular instance. It also requires practical ability to discern the relevance of the evidence behind general scientific and technical knowledge and how it applies to a particular patient" (p. 4).

Not only are critical thinking and clinical reasoning and judgment important to effective practice, thus helping ensure quality care, but also they are necessary in implementing an effective CQI process. We tend to focus on collecting data, but analysis is what makes the final difference and provides direction for decisions and development of strategies to improve. Nurses need to use these methods of thinking and their expertise in the analysis phase of the CQI process.

## Leadership: Risk and Success

Sometimes effective leaders have to take risks; however, risks must be considered very carefully. Leaders are able to evaluate pros and cons or costs and benefits and then arrive at a decision. They are not naïve about risks, recognizing that some decisions will fail. When they do, leaders use these experiences to learn more about how they lead and make decisions to improve care and their leadership and management. Collecting the best data possible, using effective analysis, and including others in the process may reduce risk in decision making when guiding CQI activities.

Rath and Conchie (2008) offer the following insights: "Effective leaders surround themselves with the right people and build on each person's strengths. Yet in most cases, leadership teams are a product of circumstances more than design. . . . Executive team members are selected or promoted primarily on knowledge or competence. . . . Rarely are people recruited to an executive team because their strengths are the best complement for those of the existing team members. . . . What's worse, when leaders do recruit for strength, they all too often pick people who act, think, or behave like themselves, albeit unintentionally in most cases" (p. 21). Ineffective selection of team members can lead to work team problems and ineffective outcomes; however, sometimes teams must learn to work together effectively regardless of member characteristics or competencies. This type of situation requires even more effective team leadership.

There is no perfect world. Although much can be said about the importance of effective leadership, finding one person who has all the needed knowledge and competencies can prove impossible. In addition, people and situations change. A person could be a very effective leader in situations that require long-term planning and in-depth analysis, but the same leader may not be so effective in a crisis situation. In the first situation, the leader may have the ability to work with staff and influence them over a long period, building confidence and motivating staff. In the second situation, leadership is needed quickly to understand the problem, engage staff, meet outcomes and take actions, and handle stress. The leader may not be able to do this effectively.

There are times when a manager or leader makes the wrong decision. How these instances are handled with staff says a lot about the manager or leader and can have an impact on the leader's self-confidence and ability to function effectively. The best approach is to admit to staff that an error was made and to not focus on excuses. Be clear about the reason(s) for the mistake, and explain the steps that will be taken to resolve the issue and prevent future similar mistakes. This is not easy to do, but the staff has greater respect for this type of response. The leader will gain credibility and support through honesty. Staff members want to believe in their managers—that they can lead and manage, they can guide staff and the organization, and they will be there when needed. The process of decision making

is a key time when the staff observes and experiences leader competencies, and it may be a time of high stress, particularly if the staff do not trust the leader's decision-making ability.

Leaders encounter times that do not go as they planned or as they explained to staff. Often, these situations are beyond the control of the leaders, but in some situations managers higher up in the HCO may be in control, depending on factors in the HCO or the healthcare environment, such as laws and standards that must be followed. Despite this loss of control, the leader must still implement the CQI activities as planned by the quality improvement (QI) program. The best approach with staff is to be honest and transparent, and then collaborate with staff to make the situation as positive as it can be (O'Neil & Chow, 2011). The quality of responses to unexpected change may or may not support trust and open communication. In many situations, it is easier to blame others or even deny that the situation is not going as expected, but these approaches do not provide effective leadership. Self-awareness helps all leaders identify their own strengths and weaknesses. Each leader has a unique combination of strengths and weaknesses; knowing what these are helps a leader be even more effective. However, this is an ongoing challenge as the leaders develop over time and encounter difficult, complex situations.

## Delegation and Quality Improvement

It may seem unusual to discuss delegation in content about QI, but delegation and QI are related. What is delegated, by whom, to whom, and when all impact patient and HCO outcomes. Delegation applies to all staff, even nonclinical staff. Work is delegated in all parts of an HCO, including clinical, laboratory, radiology, dietary, physical therapy, clinics, medical records, healthcare informatics, human resources, staff education, admissions, administration, housekeeping, maintenance, security, and other areas. **Delegation** involves transferring a specific task to be performed by another person, or empowering another to act. This process gives someone the responsibility and authority to complete a task. The person to whom a task is transferred should be competent, demonstrating required knowledge, skills, and experience to complete a task. Accountability is also part of the delegation process. When delegating responsibility, the person delegating (the delegator) must answer for the subsequent actions taken or decisions made. **Accountability** occurs when a person assumes ownership for his or her work. In doing so, outcomes become more important to the person, and it is clearer to others who are the person(s) answerable for the work. **Responsibility** is the acceptance of or obligation to do something. It is a two-way process—one person allocates responsibility and another person accepts it. Responsibility cannot be totally delegated, as the delegator has ultimate responsibility for the task. Effective responsibility includes reliability, dependability, and obligation (Marthaler & Kelly, 2008). **Supervision** is an integral part of ensuring CQI and involves directing, guiding, and evaluating performance.

The decision to delegate is the critical issue. It requires the delegator to follow the steps in the delegation process (ANA, 2013). The Connect to Current Information section at the end of the chapter provides a link to a site with delegation information. This process integrates the five rights of delegation (ANA; Finkelman, 2019, 2020):

- *Right task.* The task required for a specific patient or situation
- *Right circumstances.* Appropriate setting, available resources, and other factors relevant to the task's completion
- *Right person.* Right person delegating the right task to the right person, who then performs the task
- *Right directions/communication.* Clear, concise description of the task, including the objective(s), limits, and expectations

- *Right supervision.* Appropriate monitoring, evaluation, intervention (as needed), and feedback

CQI requires use of effective delegation as staff make clinical and management decisions to meet patient and HCO outcomes. Delegation should not be a barrier to effective work practice but, rather, another strategy used to improve care and outcomes.

> **STOP AND CONSIDER 12-3**
>
> Effective decision making requires ongoing improvement.

# Communication: Impact on Leadership in Quality Care

Information is a critical part of leadership and CQI. Interpretation of information may lead to clear understanding, but it also may lead to confusion, poor decision making, an increase in staff frustration, and poor CQI outcomes. Effective leaders are interested in people, and communicating with people is critical to the work environment. This is not to say that all leaders are overly social but, rather, that they are focused on people, like to work with people, and can assess where people stand on issues. They know which people should be involved in the change process and in decision making, including who should not be left out and why. They are effective communicators with a variety of types of people and in a variety of situations, even difficult or negative situations. Communication in HCOs is a critical element in stressful situations, requiring understanding of stress and the need to manage stress for effective communication. It is accepted that communication problems are a common cause of errors, so anything that can be done to improve communication is important to CQI. Other chapters in this text discuss structured communication methods now used in many HCOs, such as

SBAR (situation-background-assessment-recommendation). Nurse leaders/managers need to ensure that staff understand these methods and apply them when required.

# Leadership: Ensuring that Staff Are Up to Date and Engaged in Continuous Quality Care Status

As noted in other chapters, prelicensure, graduate, and lifelong education (e.g., continuing education) are important to the nursing profession as well as to all HCOs. Nursing leaders in education, whether this is in nursing academic programs or in staff education programs, need to ensure that CQI is part of the content and learning experiences. There is no doubt that we need more of this content in all educational experiences for nurses and for nursing students at all levels, from prelicensure to advanced nursing practice and the doctoral level. It should be integrated throughout the curriculum and also include focused content on CQI so that students recognize its importance. It is also clear, as discussed in this text, that to develop effective interprofessional teams, there is need for more effective and routine interprofessional education (IPEC, 2016; NAM, 2015). Quality care is not easy to define; nor is there a definition that most agree on; however, understanding its meaning is an important element in developing effective CQI programs. In one study in a medical center, a number of themes or trends of interest were identified by nurses in their perceptions of quality care: leadership, staffing, resources, timeliness, effective communication/collaboration, professionalism, relationship-based care, environment/culture,

simplicity, outcomes, and patient experience (Ryan et al., 2017). These themes correspond to common views of quality care.

Engaging staff in CQI should be approached from a variety of levels. One approach is the unit design and processes, all of which impact quality care and also staff satisfaction and the work environment. When unit design is assessed and then changed, staff should be involved in these decisions. Incorporating nurse input and also best practice and management evidence has a greater chance of improving care (Tafelmeyer, Wicks, Brant, & Smith, 2017). The nurse manager must ensure that this occurs and recognize that staff feedback is important.

# Nursing Leadership and CQI

The American Organization for Nursing Leadership (AONL), formerly the American Organization of Nurse Executives (AONE), has long supported CQI and nurses' roles in the process to improve care. Its guiding principles include principles that are directly related to CQI. In addition, the AONL integrates in its resources the need to develop leadership and also CQI competencies for clinical nurses and nurse managers. **Exhibit 12-1** describes principles for collaborative relationships between clinical nurses and nurse managers. Effective collaboration is critical to improving care. When clinical nurses and nurse managers work together, communicate, respect one another, and turn to one another for assistance, patient-centered care will be more effective and quality of care will be a top priority. Goals are established to meet outcomes for patients and clinical nurses, and nurse managers work toward these goals with all staff working with each other and not against one another. In addition, the AONL

**Exhibit 12-1** ANA/AONL Principles for Collaborative Relationships Between Clinical Nurses and Nurse Managers

**Effective Communication Principles**
- Engage in active listening to fully understand and contemplate what is being relayed.
- Know the intent of a message, and the purpose and expectations of that message.
- Foster an open, safe environment.
- Whether giving or receiving information, be sure it is accurate.
- Have people speak to the person they need to speak to, so the right person gets the right information.

**Authentic Relationships Principles**
- Be yourself. Be sure actions match words, and those around you are confident that what they see is what they get.
- Empower others to have ideas, to share those ideas, and to participate in projects that leverage or enact those ideas.
- Recognize and leverage each others' strengths.
- Be honest 100% of the time—with yourself and with others.
- Respect others' personalities, needs, and wants.
- Ask for what you want, but stay open to negotiating the difference.
- Assume good intent from others' words and actions, and assume they are doing their best.

**Learning Environment and Culture Principles**
- Inspire innovation and creative thinking.
- Commit to a cycle of evaluating, improving, and celebrating, and value what is going well.
- Create a culture of safety, both physically and psychologically.
- Share knowledge, and learn from mistakes.
- Question the status quo. Ask "what if" rather than saying "no way."

Data from American Nurses Association (ANA) & American Organization for Nursing Leadership (AONL). (2012, May). ANA/AONL principles for collaborative relationships between clinical nurses and nurse managers. Retrieved from https://www.nursingworld.org/~4af4f2/globalassets/docs/ana/ethics/principles-of-collaborative-relationships.pdf

describes the role of the nurse executive in patient safety, noting that the nurse executive needs to lead cultural change, provide shared leadership so that staff at all levels are engaged and assume responsibility, build external partnerships for collaboration, and develop leadership competencies around patient safety that focus on safety technology, leadership, culture of safety, and a practice environment of safety (AONL, 2019a).

It is important to understand the connection between the microsystem (unit level) and patient quality. **Table 12-1** describes the key characteristics that clinical nurses and nurse managers need to consider when they

evaluate the unit's culture and care improvement. **Table 12-2** provides a list of critical questions nurses and managers should ask as they work to improve.

Effective nurse leadership leads to positive outcomes for HCOs. Staff retention is higher, and through word of mouth people often apply for positions that allow them to work with a known effective leader. Leadership impacts work outcomes such as productivity, budget goals met, and higher-quality care. When staff morale is higher, all aspects of the work environment, productivity, and quality are positively affected. Leadership and innovation are now often discussed together.

**Table 12-1** Linkage of Microsystem Characteristics to Patient Safety

| Microsystem Characteristics | What This Means for Patient Safety |
|---|---|
| 1. Leadership | ■ Define the safety vision of the organization<br>■ Identify the existing constraints within the organization<br>■ Allocate resources for plan development, implementation, and ongoing monitoring and evaluation<br>■ Build in microsystems participation and input to plan development<br>■ Align organizational quality and safety goals<br>■ Engage the board of trustees in ongoing conversations about the organizational progress toward achieving safety goals<br>■ Recognition for prompt truth-telling about errors or hazards<br>■ Certification of helpful changes to improve safety |
| 2. Organizational support | ■ Work with clinical microsystems to identify patient safety issues and make relevant local changes<br>■ Put the necessary resources and tools in the hands of individuals |
| 3. Staff focus | ■ Assess current safety culture<br>■ Identify the gap between current culture and safety vision<br>■ Plan cultural interventions<br>■ Conduct periodic assessments of culture<br>■ Celebrate examples of desired behavior, for example, acknowledgment of an error |
| 4. Education and training | ■ Develop patient safety curriculum<br>■ Provide training and education of key clinical and management leadership<br>■ Develop a core of people with patient safety skills who can work across microsystems as a resource |
| 5. Interdependence of the care team | ■ Build PDSA* cycles into debriefings<br>■ Use daily huddles to debrief and to celebrate identifying errors |
| 6. Patient focus | ■ Establish patient and family partnerships<br>■ Support disclosure and truth around medical error |
| 7. Community and market focus | ■ Analyze safety issues in community, and partner with external groups to reduce risk to population |
| 8. Performance results | ■ Develop key safety measures<br>■ Create feedback mechanisms to share results with microsystems |
| 9. Process improvement | ■ Identify patient safety priorities based on assessment of key safety measures<br>■ Address the work that will be required at the microsystem level |
| 10. Information and information technology | ■ Enhance error-reporting systems<br>■ Build safety concepts into information flow (e.g., checklists, reminder systems) |

* PDSA: Plan-Do-Study-Act

Reproduced from Barach, P., & Johnson, J. (2013). Assessing risk and harm in the clinical microsystem. In W. Sollecito & J. Johnson (Eds.), *McLaughlin & Kaluzny's continuous quality improvement in health care* (4th ed., pp. 249–274). Burlington, MA: Jones & Bartlett Learning.

**Table 12–2** Questions Senior Leaders Could Ask About Patient Safety

What information do we have about errors and patient harm?

What is the patient safety plan?

How will the plan be implemented at the organizational level and at the microsystem level?

What type of infrastructure is needed to support implementation?

What is the best way to communicate the plan to the individual microsystems?

How can we foster reporting—telling the truth—about errors?

How will we empower microsystem staff to make suggestions for improving safety?

What training will staff need?

Who are the key stakeholders?

How can we build linkages to the key stakeholders?

What stories can we tell that relate the importance of patient safety?

How will we recognize and celebrate progress?

Reproduced from Barach, P., & Johnson, J. (2013). Assessing risk and harm in the clinical microsystem. In W. Sollecito & J. Johnson (Eds.), *McLaughlin & Kaluzny's continuous quality improvement in health care* (4th ed., pp. 249–274). Burlington, MA: Jones & Bartlett Learning.

How does this apply to nurse leaders who are actively engaged in CQI? "The healthcare systems operate between past models and the need to evolve. Innovation leadership skills are about adaptive problem solving, building a culture of improvement, facilitating a growth mindset, supporting proactive thinking not reaction, and preparing organizations to stay relevant in the face of changing market factors. Innovation occurs on a continuum from subtle to disruptive but not in any defined order" (Edmonson & Weberg, 2019). This requires teamwork and support for teams, emphasizing information sharing and making sure it can be effectively accessed, developed, and applied to a shared vision—not one developed only by leadership. A constant struggle for healthcare leaders is the balance between system optimization/standardization and creating/adopting innovation. "High-performing organizations have integrated the role of performance improvement and innovation. Organizations that focus solely on performance improvement will only optimize what's currently known and won't adapt to new challenges. And organizations that focus solely on innovation will create many novel solutions but fail to optimize them for organizational efficiency. Only organizations that combine both can become efficient at adaptation and systemness" (Edmonson & Weberg).

**Micromanaging**, or being overly involved in the details of others' everyday work functions, limits a person's views and understanding of processes and outcomes. For effective strategic thinking, it is important to consider the entire HCO and its components (departments, units, and so on) and also the external environment—connecting aspects of all to arrive at an understanding of the organization, its structure and function, vision and mission, and expected outcomes. HCO strengths and weaknesses should also be part of this understanding. Maintaining a broad perspective is very important when involved in CQI; data and details are important, but

Nursing Leadership and CQI

ignoring the "big picture" and system are critical weaknesses of relying too much on micromanaging. Sometimes leaders have to use intuition or their gut reaction to step outside the box and broaden their perspective even when engaged in the CQI measurement process. In many cases, if this is not done, then strategic planning may not be as effective. Strategic planning requires understanding of multiple systems and how they interact.

Leadership walkarounds are an important method for nurse leaders at all levels offering opportunity to engage with staff, patient care, and CQI and assess the culture of safety. Some HCOs and their nurse leaders are using electronic methods to document data from these rounds (Schoster & Gormley, 2018). The goal is application of what is learned during walkarounds—to improve and initiate effective change and communication.

A critical leadership role is the role of advocate, a role that all staff should demonstrate. Advocacy includes supporting rights of patients and focusing on patient-centered care but also making sure rights are actually protected. Advocacy is implemented by sharing information with patients, ensuring that informed consent is complete, providing privacy during care, and ensuring that ethical principles are followed. When staff advocate for the patient, they are demonstrating leadership. A staff member who demonstrates leadership works with others collaboratively, works to motivate others as the staff member would want to be motivated, understands the organization and need to meet outcomes, and strives to improve practice and functions of the organization. When staff members engage in CQI, they are advocating for the patient in daily practice (clinical or management) and participating in CQI activities within the HCO.

Healthy, positive work environments are the responsibility of the HCO, leadership and management, and staff. This type of work environment has a positive impact on quality care, productivity, staff satisfaction and retention, and organization outcomes. It promotes staff engagement and innovation in problem solving. As discussed in other chapters, staff problems such as incivility/bullying or even the extreme of violence impact CQI. Nurse leaders need to address the problems, but staff also need to assume responsibility and participate in resolving problems. Nurses at all levels in HCOs should be involved and guide others to improve the work environment. As Davis (2011) states, "Leaders set the tone for the organization. . . . This translates into ensuring that the clinical environment enables staff to practice in a setting whereby their mutual interactions are one of respect and support" (p. 26). The following list identifies some strategies that the leader or manager may use to address or prevent incivility and support a healthy work environment; however, for these strategies to be effective, staff must also commit to resolving the problem(s) (Pearson & Porath, 2005).

- *Set zero-tolerance expectations.* These expectations must come from top leadership and [be] communicated throughout the organization, and then implemented. Management needs to provide a method for reporting problems in applying these expectations.
- *Take an honest look in the mirror.* Leaders/managers must be role models. If there is incivility in the management team, then zero tolerance is not practiced and staff will follow the lead of managers, increasing staff incivility.
- *Weed out trouble before it enters the organization.* It is best to hire civil employees, although employers may not always know whether an applicant is or is not civil when hiring. Employers should check references and find out as much as possible.
- *Teach civility.* Common competencies needed for effective civility are effective communication, conflict resolution, negotiation, ability to deal with difficult people, stress management, listening, and coaching.

- *Put your ear to the ground and listen carefully; pay attention to warning signals.* Leadership must avoid limiting staff input and must prevent feelings of staff hopelessness and fear of repercussion. This requires listening to staff and sharing with staff.
- *When incivility occurs, hammer it.* Leadership should not wait for incivility to get worse. It needs to be dealt with as soon as it is recognized.
- *Heed warning signals.* Common signals are situations in which the staff is not allowed to provide input, feelings of hopelessness among staff that problems will be resolved, and fearfulness among staff that if they report an instance of incivility, they will suffer repercussions.
- *Don't make excuses for powerful instigators.* Do not overlook those who stimulate incivility. Managers need to be held accountable for dealing with incivility.
- *Invest in post-departure interviews.* Most staff members that leave positions because of incivility do not report it prior to leaving. Routine post-departure interview may get to this information, which is very valuable for the manager. (pp. 9, 12–14)

---

**STOP AND CONSIDER 12-6**

Nurse leaders, both formal and informal, impact CQI, but lack of leadership is a barrier to effective care.

# Examples of Nursing Initiatives to Improve Care

Nurses and nursing organizations have a long history of involvement in various QI initiatives. Several of the current important initiatives are described in this section, and additional examples are discussed in other chapters.

# Magnet Recognition Program®

The Magnet Recognition Program® is the only recognition program focused on the nursing service within healthcare organizations (American Nurses Credentialing Center [ANCC], 2019). It provides standards of excellence that many HCOs follow today. When these HCOs meet the Magnet standards, the HCO may be given this recognition. The Magnet standards expect the use of effective leadership and staff engagement in these activities. Structural and process factors, such as adequate staffing, nurse education, collaboration and interprofessional relationships and teams, and nurse autonomy and responsibility, are also considered important. As has been discussed in this text, patient-centered care is critical to effective outcomes. The Magnet Recognition Program® is an example of a program that strongly emphasizes engagement of nurses in CQI (Beard & Sharkey, 2013). The expectation is that Magnet hospitals will excel in CQI and EBP.

The National Database of Nursing Indicators® (NDNQI) is the only nursing database that tracks specific nursing-sensitive indicators related to nursing structure, processes, and patient outcomes, emphasizing the key concepts noted in QI models (Press Ganey®, 2019). The original database was developed with ANA support and administered through several academic nursing programs, but now it is administered through Press Ganey. HCOs voluntarily participate in the database, and thus not all HCOs are involved; currently an estimated 2,000 U.S. hospitals and 98% of Magnet-recognized HCOs participate in the NDNQI (Press Ganey, 2019). The database provides a monitor for relationships between its specific indicators and outcomes, including hospital-acquired conditions (HACs). When the NDNQI is used, it should be integrated into the HCO's CQI plan.

Transforming Care at the Bedside (TCAB) is another example of a nursing initiative focused on CQI. In 2003, the Institute for

Healthcare Improvement (IHI) in collaboration with the Robert Wood Johnson Foundation developed TCAB (IHI, 2019). TCAB is discussed in other chapters; however, it is important to recognize it as an example of nursing participation at the CQI direct-care level. It also provides opportunities to expand nursing engagement at all levels in an HCO's CQI activities. Publications that describe TCAB projects support the need for EBP and EBM to improve care.

In summary, the AONL's guiding principles provide guidelines about quality and safety for the nurse in future care delivery (AONL, 2019b). Given the need to develop competencies related to CQI, it is critical that all nurses are currently and in the future included in improving their own practice, whether that practice is in the clinical area or management. **Exhibit 12-2** describes the AONL principles focused on future needs. Nurses should understand and participate in the application of the National Quality Strategy (NQS), which is discussed in many chapters of this text (HHS, AHRQ, 2017).

If nurse leaders want to develop and maintain a culture of excellence, they need to consider the following important elements (Sollecito & Johnson, 2013):

- *Customer focus.* Emphasizing the importance of both internal and external customers
- *Systems thinking.* Maintaining a goal of optimizing the systems as a whole and thereby creating synergy
- *Statistical thinking.* Understanding causes of variation and the importance of learning from measurement; having the ability to use data to make decisions
- *Teamwork.* Teams of peers working together to ensure empowerment, thereby creating the highest levels of motivation to ensure alignment of the organization, the team, and the individual around the CQI vision
- *Communication and feedback.* Maintaining open channels of communication and feedback to make adjustments as needed, including modifying the vision to achieve higher levels of quality in a manner

---

**Exhibit 12-2** Exemplars: Quality Improvement Roles and Responsibilities

**Staff Nurse**

A staff nurse is delegating care to nurse assistants on his team. He recognizes he must do this carefully as delegation has an impact on daily practice. He decides to not delegate personal care to one nursing assistant who is new but rather to work directly with the assistant providing opportunity to orient and supervise to better ensure the patient gets the care needed. After this experience the nurse decides he can delegate this type of care to the new assistant who is competent to provide for most patients.

**Nurse Manager**

A hospital has decided to apply for Magnet status. The nurse manager group is meeting to discuss this initiative. All of the managers recognize that it is their responsibility to lead this effort and to engage their staff.

**Advanced Practice Registered Nurse***

The APRN who works on a surgical unit is assigned overall routine review of CQI on the unit. The nurse manager also expects the APRN to report on results at the staff meetings and periodically to provide staff education based on CQI needs.

* Advanced Practice Registered Nurse includes APRN, Clinical Nurse Specialist, Clinical Nurse Leader, and nurses with DNP.

consistent with a learning organization, including feedback that is fact based and given with true concern for individuals' organizational success (p. 64)

Sharing these elements with all staff establishes expectations that all staff need to be committed to effectively meeting these elements and leads to improve care.

## National Alliance for Quality Care

The ANA manages the NAQC (NAQC, 2019). This is a partnership of the leading U.S. nursing organizations, consumers, and other key stakeholders. Its mission is "To Advance the highest quality, safety, and value of consumer-centered health care for all individuals-patients, their families, and their communities." To achieve this aim, the NAQC will work to ensure the following:

- Patients receive the right care at the right time by the right professional.
- Nurses actively advocate and are accountable for consumer-centered, high-quality health care.
- Policymakers recognize the contributions of nurses in advancing consumer-centered, high quality health care.

The NAQC provides resources on its website for nurses to use in their practice and provides opportunities for nurses to discuss, collaborate, and lead in quality improvement.

### STOP AND CONSIDER 12-7

Nursing initiatives may impact CQI and require ongoing innovation.

## Summary

Nursing leadership should not just focus on nurses in formal management positions, such as nurse executives, supervisors, and nurse managers. Nursing leadership must be part of every nurse's practice, whether this is clinical, management, education, or research. For nurses to become active and positive leaders in CQI, each nurse must be knowledgeable about CQI, engage in the CQI process, and commit to quality care for all patients in all types of settings and healthcare situations. This requires that the profession commit to this goal and collaborate within the profession and externally.

In 2008, an article on the role of nurses in hospital CQI noted the importance of this role and related challenges such as "scarcity of nursing resources, difficulty engaging nurses at all levels—from bedside to management, growing demands to participate in more, often duplicative, QI activities; the burdensome nature of data collection and reporting; and shortcomings of traditional nursing education in preparing nurses for their evolving role in today's contemporary hospital setting" (Draper, Felland, Liebhaber, & Melichar, 2008, p. 1). We continue to face these challenges, although there is now more recognition that we must resolve them.

There is no doubt that nurses are involved in CQI, and this involvement has increased. There is, however, great need for more involvement. Quality care is not just about medical care. With nurses providing 24/7 care in hospitals, they have major responsibilities in hospitals and in other types of HCOs, and nurses should have greater influence over CQI. They are directly involved in ensuring that care meets the aims of safety, timeliness, effectiveness, efficiency, equity, and patient-centeredness (STEEEP®) (Sandford, 2011). Nurse leaders need to work toward more effective linkage of nursing, quality, and finance.

The ANA social policy statement supports the need for nurse accountability (ANA, 2010). Competence is a critical element of professional practice, and competence is directly related to quality care. The standards of professional practice provide a clear guideline for practice expectations (ANA, 2015a). The profession's code of ethics emphasizes that nurses have a social contract with the public, and this relates to nursing's relationships and communication with patients (ANA, 2015b). The nursing process includes steps that focus on quality and CQI, particularly outcome identification and evaluation. EBP is also a critical component of nursing practice, supporting best practice to achieve outcomes, as is the use of EBM to respond effectively to management and CQI issues.

In addition, the major nursing reports that have examined nursing and its role in the healthcare delivery system have had an impact. *Keeping Patients Safe* even focuses on quality in its title, and in this report, as noted earlier, nurses are not only recognized for what they do to ensure quality care but also for what they could do if they were better prepared in CQI (IOM, 2004). *The Future of Nursing* report focuses mostly on degrees and expansion of scope of practice, but it also discusses the need for nursing leadership in quality improvement (IOM, 2010). The roles of nurses and nursing leaders are threaded throughout this text.

Kennedy, Murphy, and Roberts (2013) discuss the NQS and its implications for nursing, noting particularly that nurses need to be more involved in supporting and applying the NQS (HHS, AHRQ, 2017). The ANA and other professional nursing organizations, such as specialty nursing organizations, have long been engaged in healthcare policy development by providing expert testimony to state and federal legislative bodies, serving on committees, lobbying, and working with regulatory bodies such as the NCSBN and individual state boards of nursing. Further, they have assisted in the accreditation of HCOs and nursing academic programs. These efforts require ongoing work, work that is really never completed—for example, how can NQS be integrated into nursing? Other chapters also expand on this critical question. Kennedy and colleagues (2013) advocate for the role of effective leadership: "Leadership makes a difference. If nurses do not engage in discussions about quality in healthcare, their ideas and opinions will not be heard. Nurses can take on leadership roles to influence healthcare delivery, improving quality, safety, and efficiency, and bring evidence for decision-making to the point of care to empower patients as partners. Collectively, nurses must respond to the challenges and opportunities." Exemplars of quality improvement roles and responsibilities for staff nurses, nurse managers, and APRNs are found in Exhibit 12-2.

# APPLY CQI

## Chapter Highlights

- *The Future of Nursing* report is a significant report that discusses critical aspects of nursing practice, including leadership and CQI.
- The progress report, *The Future of Nursing*, indicated that after five years more work must be done to achieve the recommendations.
- Transformational leadership is the recommended model for leadership today in HCOs. Nurses need to develop their leadership knowledge and competencies to support this model of leadership. This duty applies to all nurses, not just nurses in management positions.
- Decision making has a direct impact on CQI—from the perspective of making the best clinical decisions to better ensure quality care and from the perspective of the CQI process when decisions are made to address QI problems.

- Ineffective communication is one of the major causes of quality care problems and errors. Effective communication must be part of all CQI efforts and leadership. Ongoing efforts must be made to maintain effective communication through the care and management process.
- Staff need to be prepared to assume roles in CQI. This should begin in academic programs (prelicensure and graduate) and continue in staff education and continuing education. Nurse leaders and managers need to ensure that this preparation occurs. Each nurse must assume responsibility for his or her own lifelong learning, including content and experience related to CQI.

- Nursing leadership can make a difference in effective CQI, but it requires leadership knowledge and competencies.
- Accountability and responsibility are critical elements of CQI and leadership, impacting decision making, power and empowerment, teams, delegation, and effectiveness of nurses in their practice and in their CQI activities.
- Examples of nursing initiatives that assist in improving care are the Magnet Recognition Program®, National Database of Nursing Quality Indicators® (NDNQI®), Transforming Care at the Bedside (TCAB), and work done by the American Nurses Association (ANA), and other organizations, such as specialty nursing organizations and the American Organization for Nursing Leadership (AONL).

# Critical Thinking and Clinical Reasoning and Judgment: Discussion Questions and Learning Activities

1. Review the Campaign for Action: https://campaignforaction.org Discuss the following questions with your team:
   a. What is the importance of this initiative?
   b. Which of the recommendations do you think is particularly important, and why?
   c. There is a lot to explore on this website. Take time to discuss it with your student team.
   (You might want to review the original report, *The Future of Nursing: Leading Change, Advancing Health* [IOM, 2010].)

2. Describe in your own words the meaning of *transformational leadership*. Include your view of its relationship to nursing. Provide three examples of when you have observed this type of leadership in the practice setting. How do the examples relate to CQI?

3. Ask three nurse managers to come to a class session. Each manager should present a short commentary on his or her personal view of leadership and its relationship to CQI. Students should prepare questions for the question-and-answer session.

4. Review the document found at https://www.ncsbn.org/Delegation_joint_statement_NCSBN-ANA.pdf You can download this document as a PDF. This document describes a delegation decision tree. Consider the following in your review by identifying a task you want to delegate. Then apply this task to the decision tree as you answer the questions in the decision tree and consider the key points. You will see in the decision tree that if you answer "no" to a question, the tree takes you in a different direction.

Consider your own experiences when you have been the delegator or the delegatee. Write down your answers to the following questions:

  a.  What was the situation?

  b.  How did the process relate to what you are learning about in this chapter?

  c.  Was it effective or not? Why?

  d.  What would you have done differently?

  e.  Which do you prefer to be, the delegator or a delegatee, and why?

Review your answers. Develop a list of steps you will take to improve when you are either the delegator or a delegatee. Periodically use this process to improve.

5.  Describe in writing the relationship of decision making to CQI and incorporate the relationship of accountability, responsibility, and communication. Provide two examples to support your description.

6.  Consider how you will demonstrate leadership as a staff nurse. Write a two-page description and then share it in a discussion group in class or online.

## Connect to Current Information

- American Organization of Nurse Leaders (AONL): Quality Safety Resources
  https://www.aonl.org/resources/quality-safety-resources
- Nursing Alliance for Quality Care (NAQC)
  http://www.naqc.org
- Campaign for Action
  http://campaignforaction.org
- National Council of State Boards of Nursing (NCSBN): Delegation
  https://www.ncsbn.org/1625.htm
- ANA Principles for Delegation
  https://www.nursingworld.org/~4af4f2/globalassets/docs/ana/ethics/principlesofdelegation.pdf
- National Database of Nursing Quality Indicators® (NDNQI®)
  https://www.pressganey.com/about

- NCSBN: Transition to Practice (TTP)
  https://www.ncsbn.org/transition-to-practice.htm
- NCSBN: Taxonomy of Error, Root Cause Analysis, Practice-responsibility® (TERCAP®)
  https://mn.gov/boards/assets/TERCAP.pdf_tcm21-37541.pdf
- Institute for Healthcare Improvement: Transforming Care at the Bedside (TCAB)
  http://www.ihi.org/engage/initiatives/completed/TCAB/Pages/default.aspx
- American Nurses Credentialing Center: Magnet Recognition Program®
  https://www.nursingworld.org/organizational-programs/magnet

### Connect to Text Current information with the Author

Go to the update for this text to review the Blog, QI News, and Literature Review. Access this regular update at: http://nursing.jbpub.com/Finkelman/QualityImprovement/2e.

## EBP, EBM, and Quality Improvement: Exemplar

Armstrong, G., Dietrich, M., Barnsteiner, J., & Mion, L. (2017). Nurses' perceived skills and attitudes about updated safety concepts. *Journal of Nursing Care Quality, 32*(3), 226–233.

### Questions to Consider

1. What is the objective(s) of this study?
2. What is the study design and sample? Why is this type of design effective for this research problem?
3. What are the results of the study?
4. Discuss the implications of this study to nursing practice and quality improvement?

# EVOLVING CASE STUDY

The HCO administration has concluded an extensive staff survey about CQI. The results indicate that the staff, particularly nursing staff, are not engaged in CQI. Many do not see it as their responsibility. In describing their view of CQI activities, nurses say it is their job to provide "good" care and someone else takes care of the "administrative stuff." There is also a notable decrease in the number of incident report submissions. The chief nurse executive called a special meeting of her administrative staff and all nurse managers.

## Case Questions A

*You are asked to present background information as found in this chapter at the special meeting.*

1. What would you present? (Prepare PowerPoint slides.)
2. Based on the content of your presentation, what are three questions you would ask the staff group to consider?

## Case Questions B

*To give the staff group time to consider the presentation and discussion, a second meeting is scheduled for a week later. At this meeting you need to address the following questions:*

1. What do you think should be done to improve leadership for all nursing staff? Be specific.
2. What specific strategies might be used to engage nurses in CQI?
3. How would you assess outcomes for these two efforts? Be specific.

# References

American Association of Colleges of Nursing (AACN). (2019). Vizient/AACN nurse residency program. Retrieved from https://www.aacnnursing.org/Nurse-Residency-Program

American Nurses Association (ANA). (2010). *Social policy statement: The essence of the profession.* Silver Spring, MD: Author.

American Nurses Association (ANA). (2013). *Principles for delegation.* Silver Spring, MD: Author. Retrieved from https://www.nursingworld.org/~4af4f2/globalassets/docs/ana/ethics/principlesofdelegation.pdf

American Nurses Association (ANA). (2015a). *Scope and standards of practice.* Silver Spring, MD: Author.

American Nurses Association (ANA). (2015b). *Guide to the code of ethics with interpretive statements.* Silver Spring, MD: Author.

American Nurses Association (ANA). (2016). 2016 culture of safety. Retrieved from http://www.nursingworld.org/MainMenuCategories/ThePracticeofProfessionalNursing/2016-Culture-of-Safety

American Nurses Credentialing Center (ANCC). (2019). ANCC Magnet Recognition Program® overview. Retrieved from https://www.nursingworld.org/organizational-programs/magnet

American Organization of Nursing Leadership (AONL). (2019a). AONE guiding principles for the role of the nurse executive in patient safety. Retrieved from https://www.aonl.org/sites/default/files/aone/role-nurse-executive-patient-safety.pdf

American Organization of Nursing Leadership (AONL). (2019b). Guiding principles for future patient care delivery. Retrieved from https://www.aonl.org/guiding-principles-future-patient-care-delivery

Beard, E., & Sharkey, K. (2013). Innovation amidst radical cost containment in health care. *Nursing Administration Quarterly, 37*(2), 116–121.

Benner, P., Hughes, R., & Sutphen, M. (2008). Clinical reasoning, decision-making, and action: Thinking critically and clinically. In R. Hughes (Ed.), *Patient safety and quality: An evidence-based handbook for nurses* (Chapter 6). Washington, DC: Agency for Healthcare Research and Quality. Retrieved from http://archive.ahrq.gov/professionals/clinicians-providers/resources/nursing /resources/nurseshdbk/index.html

Benner, P., Sutphen, M., Leonard, V., & Day, L. (2010). *Educating nurses: A call for radical transformation.* San Francisco, CA: Jossey-Bass.

Campaign for Action (2019). Campaign for action. Retrieved from https://campaignforaction.org

Campaign for Action (2020). Campaign for action dashboard. Retrieved from https://campaignforaction.org/wp-content/uploads/2020/01/r2_CCNA-0029_2019-Dashboard-Indicator-Updates_1-28-20.pdf

Dartmouth College (2020). National Survey of Accountable Care Organizations (NSACO). Retrieved from https://tdi.dartmouth.edu/research/our-research/accountable-care-organizations/national-survey-acos

Davis, C. (2011). Creating a safe work environment, a plan for success. *Nurse Leader, 9*(8), 25–27.

Di Fiore, T., Zito, A., Berardinelli, A., Bena, J., Morrison, S., Keck, D., . . . Albert, N. (2018). Staff perceptions of decision-making in a shared governance culture. *JONA: Journal of Nursing Administration, 48*(11), 561–566.

Draper, D., Felland, L., Liebhaber, A., & Melichar, L. (2008). The role of nurses in hospital quality improvement. Retrieved from http://www.hschange.org/CONTENT/972/?words=Draper

Edmonson, C., & Weberg, D. (2019). Leadership styles that promote innovation. Retrieved from https://www.americannursetoday.com/leadership-styles-that-promote-innovationFinkelman, A. (2019). *Professional nursing concepts: Competencies for quality leadership* (4th ed.). Burlington, MA: Jones & Bartlett Learning.

Finkelman, A. (2020). *Leadership and management for nurses: Core competencies for quality care* (4th ed.). Upper Saddle River, NJ: Pearson Education, Inc.

Goffee, R., & Jones, G. (2000, Sept.–Oct.). Why should anyone be led by you? *Harvard Business Review,* 63–71.

Institute for Healthcare Improvement (IHI). (2019). Transforming Care at the Bedside. Retrieved from http://www.ihi.org/engage/initiatives/completed/TCAB/Pages/default.aspx

Institute of Medicine (IOM). (2002). *Leadership by example: Coordinating government roles in improving healthcare quality.* Washington, DC: The National Academies Press.

Institute of Medicine (IOM). (2003). *Health professions education: A bridge to quality.* Washington, DC: The National Academies Press.

Institute of Medicine (IOM). (2004). *Keeping patients safe: Transforming the work environment of nurses.* Washington, DC: The National Academies Press.

Institute of Medicine (IOM). (2009). *Redesigning continuing education in the health professions.* Washington, DC: The National Academies Press.

Institute of Medicine (IOM). (2010). *The future of nursing: Leading change, advancing health.* Washington, DC: The National Academies Press.

Interprofessional Education Collaborative (IPEC). (2016). *Core competencies for interprofessional collaborative practice.* Retrieved from https://aamc-meded.global.ssl.fastly.net/production/media/filer_public/70/9f/709fedd7-3c53-492c-b9f0-b13715d11cb6/core_competencies_for_collaborative_practice.pdf

Kennedy, R., Murphy, J., & Roberts, D. (2013). An overview of the National Quality Strategy: Where do nurses fit? *OJIN: The Online Journal of Issues in Nursing, 18*(3). Retrieved from http://ojin.nursingworld.org/National-Quality-Strategy.html

Makary, M. (2016, May 3). Medical error—The third leading cause of death in the U.S. *BMJ.* Retrieved from http://www.bmj.com/content/353/bmj.i2139/rr-40

Marthaler, M., & Kelly, P. (2008). Delegation of patient care. In P. Kelly (Ed.), *Nursing leadership and management* (2nd ed., pp. 340–367). Clifton Park, NY: Delmar.

McBride, A. (2011). *The growth and development of nurse leaders.* New York, NY: Springer Publishing Company.

National Academy of Medicine (NAM). (2015). *Measuring the impact of interprofessional education on collaborative practice and patient outcomes.* Washington, DC: The National Academies Press.

National Academy of Medicine (NAM). (2016). *Assessing progress on the Institute of Medicine report* The Future of Nursing. Washington, DC: The National Academies Press.

National Academy of Medicine (NAM). (2019). *The future of nursing 2020-2030. A consensus study from the National Academy of Medicine.* Washington, DC: The National Academies Press. Retrieved from https://nam.edu/publications/the-future-of-nursing-2020-2030

National Council of State Boards of Nursing (NCSBN). (2019). Transition to practice. Retrieved from https://www.ncsbn.org/transition-to-practice.htm

Nursing Alliance for Quality Care (NAQC). (2019). Welcome to the Nursing Alliance for Quality Care. Retrieved from https://www.nursingworld.org/naqc

O'Neil, E., & Chow, M. (2011). Leadership action for a new American health system. *Nurse Leader, 9*(12), 34–36.

Pearson, C., & Porath, C. (2005). On the nature, consequences and remedies of workplace incivility: Not time for "nice"? Think again. *Academy of Management Executive, 30*(2), 7–18.

Press Ganey®. (2019). Clinical excellence. Retrieved from https://www.pressganey.com/solutions/clinical-excellence

Rath, T., & Conchie, B. (2008). *Strengths based leadership: Great leaders, teams, and why people follow.* New York, NY: Gallup Press.

Ryan, C., Powlesland, J., Phillips, C., Raszewski, R., Johnson, A., Banks-Enorense, K., . . . Welsh, J. (2017). Nurses' perceptions of quality care. *JONA: Journal of Nursing Care Quality, 32*(2), 180–185.

Sandford, K. (2011). Making the business case for quality and nursing. *Nurse Leader, 9*(1), 28–31.

Schoster, S., & Gormley, D. (2018). CNO rounding using an electronic tracking tool. *JONA: Journal of Nursing Administration, 48*(7/8), E1–E4.

Sollecito, K., & Johnson, J. (2013). Factors influencing the application and diffusion of CQI in health care. In W. Sollecito & J. Johnson (Eds.), *McLaughlin and Kaluzny's continuous quality improvement in health care* (4th ed., pp. 49–74). Burlington, MA: Jones & Bartlett Learning.

Tafelmeyer, J., Wicks, R., Brant, J., & Smith, L. (2017). Incorporating nurse input and evidence into newly designed unit to improve patient and nursing outcomes. *JONA: Journal of Nursing Administration, 47*(12), 603–609.

U.S. Department of Health and Human Services (HHS), Agency for Healthcare Research and Quality (AHRQ). (2017). About the National Quality Strategy (NQS). Retrieved from https://www.ahrq.gov/workingforquality/about/index.html

U.S. Department of Health and Human Services (HHS), Health Resources and Services Administration (HRSA). (2020). 2018 National Sample Survey of Registered Nurses. Brief summary report. Retrieved from https://bhw.hrsa.gov/health-workforce-analysis/data/national-sample-survey-registered-nurses

# Appendix A

# Examples of Major Healthcare Organizations and Agencies, Governmental and Nongovernmental, Related to Quality Improvement

Agency for Healthcare Research and Quality (AHRQ)

AHRQ QI

AHRQ Safety Primers

Alliance for Home Health Quality and Innovation (AHHQI)

Alliance for Pediatric Quality

Ambulatory Quality Alliance (AQA)

American Association of Colleges of Nursing (AACN)

American Health Informatics Community (AHIC)

American Nurses Association (ANA)

American Nurses Association National Center for Nursing Quality

American Organization for Nurse Leadership (AONL)

Association for Prevention Teaching and Research (APTR)

Baldridge Performance Excellence Program

Center for Studying Health System Change (HSC)

Consumers Advancing Patient Safety (CAPS)

Future of Nursing: Campaign for Action

Healing Environment

Healthcare Cost and Utilization Project (HCUP)

Healthcare Effectiveness Data and Information Set (HEDIS)

Healthcare Information and Management Systems Society (HIMSS)

Health Research and Educational Trust (HRET) (Disparities Toolkit)

Health Resources and Services Agency (HRSA)

Hospital Compare (Medicare)

Hospital Consumer Assessment of Healthcare Providers and Systems (HCAHPS)

Improvement Science Research Network (ISRN)

Initiative on The Future of Nursing: Campaign for Action

Institute for Healthcare Improvement (IHI)

Institute for Safe Medication Practices (ISMP)

Interdisciplinary Nursing Quality Research Institute (INQRI)

Joint Commission International

Kaiser Family Foundation (KFF)

Leapfrog Group

Magnet Recognition Program

National Center for Nursing Quality (NCNQ)

National Committee for Quality Assurance (NCQA)

National Council of State Boards of Nursing (NCSBN)

National Database of Nursing Quality Indicators (NDNQI)

National Guideline Clearinghouse

National Healthcare Quality Report and Disparities Reports (QDR)

National Institute of Nursing Research (NINR)

National Institute for Occupational Safety and Health (NIOSH)

National Institutes of Health (NIH)

National League for Nursing (NLN)

National Patient Safety Foundation (NPSF)

National Patient Safety Goals (The Joint Commission)

National Priorities Partnership (part of NQF)

National Quality Forum (NQF)

National Quality Measures Clearinghouse

National Quality Strategy (NQS)

Nursing Alliance for Quality Care (NAQC)

Occupational Safety and Health Administration (OSHA)

Partnership for Patients

Patient-Centered Outcomes Research Institute (PCORI)

Patient Safety Indicators (PSIs)

Patient Safety Network (PSNet)

Quality Interagency Coordination Task Force (QuIC)

Quality and Safety Education for Nurses (QSEN)

Six Sigma

Taxonomy of Error Root Cause Analysis and Practice Responsibility (TERCAP)

The Joint Commission

The PROTECT Initiative: Advancing Children's Medication Safety

Transforming Care at the Bedside (TCAB)

Transition into Practice (TIP)

U.S. Department of Health and Human Services (HHS)

U.S. Department of Health and Human Services (HHS), Centers for Disease Control and Prevention (CDC)

U.S. Department of Health and Human Services (HHS), Centers for Medicare and Medicaid Services (CMS)

U.S. Department of Health and Human Services (HHS), Food and Drug Administration (FDA)

VA National Center for Patient Safety

VA Nursing Outcomes Database (VANOD)

World Health Organization (WHO)

World Health Organization (WHO), Interprofessional Teams

World Health Organization (WHO), Taxonomy for Patient Safety

World Health Organization (WHO), World Health Alliance for Patient Safety

# Glossary

**30-day unplanned readmission** Unplanned readmission of a patient to an acute care setting within 30 days of discharge.

**accountability** A person's responsibility for his or her actions and the outcomes of those actions.

**accreditation** A method used to assess organizations and determine if they meet minimum established standards.

**active error** An error that results from non-compliance with a procedure that involves a frontline worker (i.e., direct care worker).

**adverse event** An injury resulting from a medical intervention, not from the patient's underlying condition.

**advocacy** Support of a cause or action on another's behalf.

**alarm/alert fatigue** Failure of the staff to quickly respond to or a tendency to ignore alarms that occur too frequently or that are often false.

**autonomy** The ethical principle that patients have the right to determine their own rights.

**bar code medication administration** Use of bar codes located on the patient's identification to compare with the bar code found on orders or, in the case of medications, found on the individual patient drug package.

**baseline data** Data collected prior to a change has occurred to compare conditions after the change.

**benchmarking** The act of comparing a situation before a change is implemented to the situation after a change is implemented.

**beneficence** The ethical principle that nurses should not inflict harm and should safeguard the patient.

**blame culture** A professional environment in which errors are examined with a focus on assigning blame to individuals.

**brainstorming** A method used to identify as many ideas as possible so that the ideas can then be assessed to determine if they can be used or should be eliminated.

**bullying** Harmful, deliberate actions intended to embarrass, offend, or distress another person.

**call-out** A communication approach in which the person communicates important information to the team so that everyone hears the same information at the same time, reducing the chance of miscommunication or some team members not hearing the same information.

**case management** A patient care effort designed to get the right services to patients when needed with the goal of avoiding fragmented and unnecessary care.

**certification** Authorization to provide care in a given capacity. Through standardized examination, nurses can demonstrate expertise in a specialty area and validate knowledge for certification as determined by the American Nurses Credentialing Center.

**change** A difference in some aspect of the care dynamic, involving the patient, system, healthcare services, and so on.

**change agent** An individual or team who focuses on a problem or change issue and possible approaches to take.

**check sheet** A simple form used to collect and document data that allows staff to quickly indicate whether an expected action or observation occurred.

**check-back** A communication approach in which the person asks the team if they heard the information and understood it.

**checklist** A list designed to indicate the order in which steps are to be followed and to document this process.

**clinical decision support (CDT)** A method used to prevent errors and omissions by monitoring situations and alerting clinicians of patient conditions, prescriptions, and treatment to provide evidence-based clinical suggestions to health professionals at the point of care.

**clinical guideline** A written description of care for a specific patient population based on evidence.

**clinical judgment** The process of making decisions about clinical concerns and treatment.

**clinical reasoning** The application of experience and research in reasoning through clinical scenarios.

**coaching** A method used to provide career guidance and support.

**code of ethics** A set of ethical standards that guide a care provider's behavior.

**code of silence** A professional environment in which staff do not feel safe in speaking up, even when they know something is wrong, and thus do not help effect change or help other team members.

**collaboration** The act of partnering with another qualified provider to bring about optimal patient care.

**collaborative care model** An initiative to increase patient engagement by focusing on managing the health of a population rather than on treating a specific diagnosis.

**common format** A set of definitions and reporting formats developed by the Agency for Healthcare Research and Quality that offer healthcare organizations consistency across data sources when reporting data external to the healthcare organization.

**comparative effectiveness research** The review of evidence-based practice to provide healthcare providers with state-of-the-science information to make the best quality and cost decisions for patients.

**compassion fatigue** A type of cumulative stress experienced by nurses through repeated exposure to emotionally difficult situations.

**competency** A level of performance that is expected within the nursing profession.

**comprehensive unit-based safety program (CUSP)** A program developed by the Agency for Healthcare to better ensure quality care. Teams and teamwork are critical components in CUSP.

**computerized physician/provider order entry (CPOE)** A computerized method to support quality care in which four steps occur when a hospitalized patient receives a medication: (1) ordering, (2) transcribing the order (if handwritten), (3) dispensing the medication by the pharmacists, and (4) administering medication.

**consonant culture** An organizational culture that encourages development of a collaborative team environment.

**continuing education** Formal transmission of a predetermined body of knowledge. Related activities are frequently provided with designated accreditation and generate "credits" for practitioners, necessary for most state licensure and other credentialing processes.

**continuous quality improvement (CQI)** Measures taken by a healthcare organization to ensure that the best possible care is provided during each patient encounter, that the potential for errors is minimized, and that patient encounters are properly documented to enable later review and improvement.

**coordination** Organization of care across all elements of the healthcare system.

**core measure set** Standards relevant to a given field used to objectively assess the efficacy of change efforts.

**crew resource management (CRM)** A method to support quality care that focuses on leadership, interprofessional communication, and effective decision-making, using all available resources, emphasizing a no-blame culture, and focusing on clear, comprehensive standard operating procedures.

**critical reflection** The act of questioning clinical practices and assumptions in an effort to improve patient care.

**critical thinking** Examination of knowledge, intuition, and application of knowledge.

**cultural competence** A set of congruent behaviors, attitudes, and policies that come together in a system or agency or among professionals, enabling effective work in cross-cultural situations.

**culture** The prevailing attitudes and beliefs of an organization.

**culture of safety** An organizational culture in which all members share a sense of accountability in creating a safe, effective care environment.

**dashboard** A clear visual depiction of data in one view.

**data** Objective, informative details that are presented without interpretation.

**database** A method used to organize data so information is easy to store, manage, and access.

**decision tree** A method of identifying solutions to a problem by treating each potential solution as a "trunk" from which the potential positive and negative outcomes "branch."

**deep dive** An in-depth brainstorming technique that is used ideally by an interprofessional team.

**define and measure-analyze-design-verify (DMADV)** A means of assessing care quality by which project goals and outcomes are defined, the process is analyzed, a detailed description of the process is developed, and then performance is verified.

**delegation** The act of transferring a specific task to another person, or empowering another to act.

**delphi technique** A problem-solving technique in which staff respond to a questionnaire that focuses on a particular problem, and responses are discussed through multiple rounds until the problem is understood at its most refined level.

**diagnostic error** Failure to make the appropriate diagnosis given the available evidence.

**disclosure** The act of informing a patient that an error occurred, assuming the patient does not already know.

**discrimination** A cause of unequal patient treatment that occurs when healthcare providers view, and consequently treat, patients differently based on their race, ethnicity, sex, or other characteristics not relevant to the health condition at hand.

**disease management** Use of services to better ensure patient-centered care and improve the quality of care.

**disease-specific measure/indicator** A quality indicator used by healthcare organizations that focuses on a disease and applies to patients with that disease.

**disparity** See *healthcare disparity*.

**dissonant culture** An organizational culture that blocks the development of a collaborative team environment.

**diversity** Variation in the characteristics of a population, based on gender, religion, ethnicity, and so on.

**early warning system** A method of measuring patients' physiological status to anticipate and thus prevent catastrophic medical events.

**electronic health record (EHR)** A digital record that includes the same information as the EMR plus more comprehensive information about the patient's history.

**electronic medical record (EMR)** A digital record that includes provider medical and clinical data for a patient.

**empowerment** The act of giving power to someone to act.

**enterprise data warehouse** A data resource that provides a collection of databases that can be accessed and analyzed.

**error** An unintended and undesired outcome.

**error of execution** Failure to execute a planned action.

**error of planning** Failure to anticipate the patient's needs or prepare the correct course of action.

**ethical dilemma** A situation in which a choice must be made but none of the options are ideal.

**ethics** An understanding of proper practice behaviors learned through an organized system, such as standardized ethics code developed by a professional group.

**evidence-based management (EBM)** The use of current research to improve the performance of healthcare organizations.

**evidence-based practice (EBP)** The use of current research to make clinical decisions.

**failure mode and effects analysis (FMEA)** An analysis method focused on known or potential problems and errors, with the goal of preventing errors by understanding and addressing all the ways a system could fail.

**failure to rescue (FTR)** A missed opportunity to provide care that would have prevented complications.

**fishbone analysis** A problem analysis tool that uses a fishbone graphic to allow a team to identify and address all possible causes of a problem.

**flowchart** A format used to describe data that enables reviewing or updating of information and that helps keep it current.

**fraud** Intentional deception for one's own gain; it is a criminal act.

**frontline safety** Direct care practices in which staff consider patient safety and quality in their daily work.

**frontline staff** The staff members responsible for providing direct care staff. These staff members often get lost in the big picture but make the biggest difference in quality improvement, regardless of the type or size of the healthcare organization.

**GANTT chart** A type of chart used to display progress in a project over time.

**gap analysis** A method for examining current status by focusing on where the organization, department, or unit and the staff want to go. The difference in current status and future vision is referred to as the "gap."

**generic measure/indicator** A quality indicator used by healthcare organizations to assess factors that are relevant to most patients.

**global trigger** A signal or a clue that may be used to identify a potential adverse event, not the event itself.

**groupthink** The tendency of a group member to go along with the group's proposed idea even though the member does not agree with the idea.

**handoff** The transitioning of a patient from one form of care to another, such as from one clinical site or healthcare provider to another.

**harm** Impaired functioning, whether physical, emotional, or psychological, that causes pain, injury, or distress.

**health informatics technology (HIT)** The use of technology to study healthcare information and communication systems to improve decision-making and other tasks.

**health literacy** A person's understanding of his or her own health status and of the variables that lead to good health.

**healthcare delivery measure** A measure of care delivered to individuals and populations defined by its relationship to clinicians, clinical delivery teams, delivery organizations, or health insurance plans.

**healthcare disparity** A difference in the quality of health care received by one party versus that received by another party for the same condition. Health disparities in the United States are often based on racial and ethnic differences.

**healthcare equity** Attainment of the highest level of health for all people.

**healthcare inequality** The difference in health status or in the distribution of health determinants between different population groups.

**high-reliability organization (HRO)** A healthcare organization that uses a three-step approach to achieve a high level of reliability: Prevent failure, identify and mitigate failure, and redesign processes.

**high-risk** A situation in which there is greater chance of near misses and errors occurring.

**hospital-acquired condition (HAC)** A condition that develops after admission to the hospital that could have been prevented through appropriate care measures.

**huddle** A short meeting with staff focusing on a specific issue; it can be scheduled or unscheduled.

**human error** Failure to achieve a desired outcome that can be attributed to skill-, rule-, or knowledge-based performance.

**human factors and ergonomics** Physical, cognitive, and organizational factors that can have an impact on errors.

**human failure** A source of error attributed to an individual provider.

**incidence** An estimate of how frequently new events, cases, etc., develop.

**incident report** A standardized form created by an organization that addresses specific incidents to ensure that staff provide all relevant details relating to the incident.

**incivility** Unprofessional conduct such as rude and discourteous behavior, gossiping and spreading rumors, or refusing to help others in the work situation.

**indicator** An aggregate measure for a specific operation.

**interoperability** The ability of health systems to easily share electronic health information with one another.

**interprofessional education** Education for individuals from different professions offered together to promote collaborative working in their professional practice.

**just culture** An organizational culture in which individuals are not blamed for errors that may be considered organizational shortcomings but are held accountable for negligent or otherwise inappropriate care delivery.

**justice** The principle that patients should be treated fairly.

**lapse** Failure to check something that is part of the procedure.

**latent conditions** Factors that are not readily apparent within an organization that contribute to errors.

**latent error An error due to latent conditions.** See *latent conditions*.

**lateral violence** Acts of violence occurring between coworkers (e.g., nurse to nurse).

**leadership** The act of guiding others toward a desired outcome.

**lean approach** An approach to quality improvement that focuses on value to the customer (i.e., the patient), with efforts made to reduce waste in time, effort, and cost—doing more with less.

**learning healthcare system** A healthcare system that values and builds upon clinical research and that strives to use population-based data to improve patient interventions and outcomes.

**lifelong learning** Voluntary and self-motivated pursuit of knowledge for either personal or professional reasons.

**linguistic competence** The capacity of an organization and its personnel to communicate effectively and convey information in a manner easily understood by diverse audiences, including persons of limited English proficiency, those who have low literacy skills or are not literate, and those with disabilities.

**macrosystem** The broadest level of the healthcare system, such as the healthcare organization under which several distinct hospitals operate.

**macroview** The perspective of healthcare quality focused on the broader issues, from a local, state, federal, or even global perspective.

**malpractice** Failure to provide a level of care appropriate to the provider's professionally licensed capacity.

**management** The act of ensuring that the structure and resources exist to accomplish a job.

**meaningful use** Criteria defined by the Centers for Medicare and Medicaid Services that hospitals and providers must meet to be identified as meaningful users of health informatics technology.

**measure** A standard used as a reference point to compare outcomes.

**medication error** A preventable event in which medication, while still under the control of the provider, is used in a manner that causes patient harm.

**medication reconciliation** The act of formulating a list of medications for a patient (e.g., drug name, dosage and frequency, administration method, and purpose of the medication) and reviewing the list to ensure that there are no conflicts in the medications.

**mental fatigue** Reduced mental performance owing to an overload of mental task demands.

**mentoring** Use of a role model to assist in career development.

**mesosystem** A level of the healthcare system beneath the macrosystem in which the departments, clinical centers, or services operate.

**metric** A means of comparing an aspect of care to a specified criterion.

**micromanagement** Overinvolvement in the details of subordinates' everyday work functions, thus limiting their views and understanding about processes and outcomes.

**microsystem** A level of the healthcare system beneath the mesosystem in which the clinical units, the smallest unit of the system, operate; it is here that the patient has the most influence.

**microview** The perspective of healthcare quality focused on the healthcare provider, which can be a healthcare organization or an individual healthcare provider such as a physician, nurse, or pharmacist.

**missed care** Nursing care that is delayed, partially completed, or not completed.

**mistake** A wrong decision, often related to inexperience, inadequate training, or even negligence.

**misuse** An avoidable event that prevents patients from receiving the full potential benefit of a service.

**morbidity** Incidence of disease state or condition.

**mortality** Incidence of death.

**near miss** An instance in which an error almost happened, but staff caught the problem before it became an error.

**negligence** Failure to provide a level of care that would be expected of a reasonably prudent person.

**nominal group** A brainstorming method in which each group member records his or her ideas related to an issue, and the ideas are then shared anonymously and voted on by the group to determine the most important ideas.

**nursing regulation** Professional oversight intended to ensure nursing services provide for the public's health, safety, and welfare.

**omission** Failure to provide assessment, planning, or interventions, possibly leading to problems for the patient and affecting expected outcomes.

**operational plan** A plan relating to the quality improvement program that describes the steps needed to ensure outcomes are met, describes roles and responsibilities, identifies timelines, plans evaluation, and describes the revision process.

**organizational culture** The values, beliefs, traditions, and communication processes that bring a group of people together and characterize the organization.

**organizational failure** A source of error attributed to staff orientation and training, policies, procedures, and use of clinical pathways or protocols.

**organizational readiness** The likelihood that staff and the organization are prepared to handle change.

**outcome** The result of a patient intervention or treatment, whether acute or long-term.

**outcome measure/indicator** A means by which an organization evaluates the efficacy of its interventions and practices.

**overuse** An instance in which the potential for harm from the provision of a service exceeds the possible benefit.

**Pareto chart** A vertical bar graph with bars ordered from longest to shortest to prioritize the frequency of causes related to one another.

**pass the problem** A problem-solving method in which participants are divided into two groups and, through a back-and-forth process, develop a list of strategies to address given problems, ending in a group presentation and discussion of all the identified strategies.

**patient-centered care** Care that respects differences among patients, that seeks to provide optimal patient care that minimizes suffering and ensures continuity of care, and that values the patient's involvement in his or her own care.

**patient-centered rounds** Clinical rounds that can be configured in a number of ways for different purposes, but the critical element is they focus on the patient and patient needs.

**patient safety primer** Evidence-based sources of information about patient safety available on the Agency for Healthcare Research and Quality's website.

**pay for performance** A payment model by which providers and healthcare organizations are financially incentivized to provide care that meets defined care standards.

**performance management** A forward-looking process used to set goals and regularly check progress toward achieving those goals.

**performance measure** A measure of the quality of care provided by a healthcare system in which specific measurable elements are used as a quality meter.

**performance measurement** A forward-looking process used to set goals and regularly check progress toward achieving those goals.

**personal health record (PHR)** A digital record that includes the same information as the EMR and EHR, but the patient keeps the record and maintains it.

**PERT chart** A visual or graphic representation describing a project or a process using boxes and arrows to illustrate the sequence of tasks. PERT stands for program evaluation review technique.

**physical fatigue** Physical discomfort and decreased ability to perform physically due to an overload of physical task demands.

**plan-do-study-act** Often called the PDSA or Deming cycle, a rapid cycle change method used by healthcare organizations to assist in responding to change and planning.

**point of care** Direct care experiences when the healthcare provider and patient intersect for care, such as for assessment and intervention.

**point-of-care learning** A subset of workplace learning that occurs at the time and place (whether virtual such as simulation or actual) of a health professional-patient encounter.

**policy** A description intended to clarify important communication and consistent processes within a healthcare organization to ensure care quality, consistency, and other objectives that staff are expected to follow.

**population health measure** A measure that addresses health issues of individuals or populations defined by residence in a geographic area or a relationship to organizations that are not primarily organized to deliver or pay for healthcare services (such as schools or prisons).

**power** The ability to influence decisions, control situations and resources, and affect others' behavior.

**powerlessness** The inability to influence decisions or control situations.

**presenteeism** A potential source of errors in which staff are at work but are not functioning at their fullest, often due to a medical problem, whether physical or psychological.

**prevalence** The rate of the number of cases at a given time divided by the number in the at-risk population.

**primary CQI data** Information collected in original sources for the purpose of continuous quality improvement (CQI).

**proactive change** Change that is planned based on assessment of need.

**procedure** A step-by-step description of a task or clinical activity that staff are expected to follow.

**process** The manner in which the parts of the healthcare system function independently and interact.

**process measure/indicator** A means by which an organization evaluates the processes that it has in place to address specific scenarios.

**project plan** A plan relating to the quality improvement program that focuses on specific needs, such as a change in the medication administration procedure for the emergency department.

**qualitative data** Data that provide information about descriptive characteristics, used to make inferences based on observable data, not measurable data.

**quality care** The competent provision of services with effective communication, involvement of the patient in decision-making, and cultural sensitivity.

**quality gap** A deficiency in healthcare delivery resulting from a system that is fragmented and poorly organized, confusing, and complex, leading to treatment overuse, underuse, and misuse.

**quality improvement plan** A detailed, organizational work plan for a healthcare organization's continuous quality improvement activities.

**quantitative data** Data that focus on numbers and frequencies so that measurable data can be obtained and statistics used to analyze the data.

**rapid cycle model** An approach to quality improvement that is used to test small changes recommended by frontline staff and actively engage staff in the continuous quality improvement process, recognizing that small changes can impact the healthcare organization with positive outcomes.

**rapid response team (RRT)** A team formed to identify and quickly respond when patients are experiencing deterioration in their condition.

**reactive change** Change that occurs in response to a development that requires that an improvement be made.

**read-back** The act of repeating written or oral information to ensure the message was properly received.

**reasonably prudent nurse** A nurse who acts in the same manner as would any other nurse who has similar education and experience and average intelligence, judgment, foresight, and skill, given the same care scenario.

**red rules** Rules that must be followed to ensure continuous quality improvement.

**reliability** (1) The extent to which repeated measurements yield similar results. (2) The state of being failure-free that develops in an environment over time; *over time* is a critical aspect, as it is not a onetime viewpoint of quality, but rather consistent, effective performance.

**report card** A summary report of the status of a healthcare organization's quality of care.

**responsibility** The acceptance of an obligation to do something.

**risk management** An assessment of a healthcare organization's risk for malpractice claims and thus risk for financial loss.

**root cause analysis (RCA)** A method used by many healthcare organizations to analyze errors, supporting the recognition that most errors are caused by system issues and not necessarily individual staff issues.

**run chart** A display of data that illustrates or plots change and patterns over time.

**safe zone** An atmosphere created to ensure that during certain activities there are no interruptions and distractions so that staff can meet their responsibilities effectively and safely.

**safety** The assurance patients will not be harmed through the care they receive.

**safety walkaround** A communication method in which the healthcare organization's leadership directly interacts with direct care staff and patients to receive and provide feedback, thus demonstrating the organization's commitment to continuous quality improvement and helping to reduce adverse events.

**science of improvement** An approach to quality improvement that emphasizes the use of research, innovative methods, and the rapid cycle method, with focus on three questions: (1) What are we trying to accomplish? (2) How will we know that a change is an improvement? (3) What changes can we make that will result in improvement?

**scope of practice** The performance expectations relating to tasks common to all registered nurses.

**secondary CQI data** Information collected from secondhand sources, such as those primarily used in care delivery (e.g., a preoperative checklist), for the purpose of continuous quality improvement (CQI).

**self-determination** A nurse's assessment of his or her own ability to meet the demands of a given care scenario, taking into account such factors as scope of practice, skills and competencies, and factors relating to the patient and clinical setting.

**self-management** The patient's ability to meet his or her own health needs, promoted by healthcare providers through patient-centered care.

**self-regulation** Efforts made by nurses to maintain their competence, often through

required continuing education for licensure and/or certification.

**sentinel event** An unexpected event that happens to patients resulting in major negative outcomes, such as an unexpected death or a critical physical or psychological complication that can lead to major alteration in the patient's health.

**sentinel measure** A quality indicator used by healthcare organizations to identify outcomes that are intrinsically undesirable and that must always be addressed (sentinel event).

**shared governance** An approach to decision-making in which staff have substantial input and there is a structure to facilitate this process.

**signout** The transmission of information about the patient during a patient transfer (i.e., handoff).

**situation, background, assessment, recommendation (SBAR)** A structured communication approach designed to ensure consistent, clear communication.

**six hat method** A brainstorming method used by teams to better understand proposals for change. During the process, team members assume one of the roles (hats) and discuss the proposal from that perspective.

**Six Sigma** An approach to quality improvement that includes three key elements: (1) measure work output, (2) apply the process throughout all departments in an organization, until it eventually becomes part of the organization's culture, and (3) maintain a goal of no more than 3.4 errors per 1,000,000 operations.

**slip** An error that occurs due to failure to be clear, such as during documentation.

**social determinants of health** The everyday factors in a person's life that contribute to his or her overall health. Assessing these factors should take into consideration the equity with which money, power, and resources are distributed within a society.

**solution analysis** A problem-solving method that considers each of the possible solutions and then ranks them according to how effective the solution might be in meeting the objective, cost, time, and feasibility.

**spread** Active dissemination of best practice and knowledge gained from the continuous quality improvement process so that individual healthcare organizations can apply them.

**stakeholder** Any party that has a strong enough interest in an issue to want to give input and engage in actions relating to the issue.

**standard** A measure, determined by a professional body, of practice, service, or education.

**standardization** Efforts to make work consistent by regulating procedures, equipment, supplies, and so on.

**STEEEP** A quality improvement framework that is based on the six aims identified in the *Quality Chasm* series (safety, timeliness, effectiveness, efficiency, equity, and patient-centeredness).

**strategic plan** A plan relating to the quality improvement program that considers long-term goals and outcomes, noting the gaps or what needs to be improved over time.

**stress** An adverse human experience that occurs when demands exceed the person's resources.

**structure** The manner in which the parts of the healthcare system's elements are put together and come together to impact quality.

**structure measure/indicator** A means by which an organization evaluates its resources and how well those resources function as a system.

**supervision** The act of directing, guiding, and evaluating performance.

**surveillance** Oversight of patient care intended to prevent adverse outcomes.

**Swiss cheese model** A model for understanding errors that focuses on system failure and recognizes that there is potential for an error in any process.

**system thinking** Seeing the whole, how its parts interrelate, and how these parts all impact workflow.

**systematic review** A summary of evidence focused on a specific clinical question that provides critical appraisal of the evidence to determine if bias exists.

**tally sheet** See *check sheet.*

**teach-back** The act of asking patients to repeat something they have been told to ensure the message was properly received.

**teamSTEPPS** A method designed to optimize patient care by using training approaches and relevant materials to improve communication and teamwork skills among healthcare professionals, including frontline staff.

**technical failure** A source of error attributed to unavailable or malfunctioning physical equipment.

**time-out** A method used to stop work or care when staff are concerned there is risk or an error has occurred.

**transformational leadership** An approach to leadership focused on improving care for patients and also improving the organization's work environment. This approach emphasizes that all staff, whether in formal management positions or not (including staff nurses), need to understand leadership to work effectively in the healthcare environment.

**triple aim** A quality improvement framework that is designed to (1) improve the patient experience of care, (2) improve the health of populations, and (3) reduce the per capita cost of health care.

**underuse** Failure to provide a service that would have produced a favorable outcome for the patient.

**universal protocol** A step-by-step protocol to prevent wrong site, wrong procedure, or wrong person surgery.

**utilization review/management** An assessment routinely performed by a healthcare organization to collect data about use of services.

**validity** The degree to which an evaluation method measures the intended variable.

**value stream mapping** A means of assessing care quality that documents, analyzes, and improves the flow of information or supplies that are needed to complete a process or produce a product.

**veracity** The ethical principle that patients should be told the truth.

**workaround** The act of avoiding a work-related problem instead of addressing and resolving it.

**workflow** The sequencing of tasks involved in a work process.

**workplace learning** An educational approach that allows individuals or groups to acquire, interpret, reorganize, change, or assimilate a related cluster of information, skills, and feelings, and a means by which individuals construct meaning in their personal and shared organizational lives.

**workplace violence** A work-related event that is physically and/or psychologically distressing to an employee.

# Index

Note: Locators followed by *b, f,* and *t* indicates boxes, figures, and tables respectively.